FOURTH EDITION

Concepts of Chemical Dependency

Harold E. Doweiko

Brooks/Cole Publishing Company

I(T)P® An International Thomson Publishing Company

Pacific Grove • Albany • Belmont • Bonn • Boston • Cincinnati • Detroit • Johannesburg • London
Madrid • Melbourne • Mexico City • New York • Paris • Singapore • Tokyo • Toronto • Washington

Sponsoring Editor: *Eileen Murphy*
Marketing Team: *Lauren Harp, Jean Thompson*
Editorial Associate: *Julie Martinez*
Production Editor: *Kirk Bomont*
Manuscript Editor: *Charlotte Saikia*
Interior Design: *Publications Development
   Company of Texas*

Interior Illustration: *Publications Development Company of Texas*
Cover Design: *Sharon Kinghan*
Cover Photo: *Kathleen Olson*
Art Editor: *Lisa Torri*
Project Management and Typesetting: *Publications Development
   Company of Texas*
Printing and Binding: *Malloy Lithographing, Inc.*

For more information, contact:

BROOKS/COLE PUBLISHING COMPANY
511 Forest Lodge Road
Pacific Grove, CA 93950
USA

International Thomson Publishing Europe
Berkshire House 168-173
High Holborn
London WC1V 7AA
England

Thomas Nelson Australia
102 Dodds Street
South Melbourne, 3205
Victoria, Australia

Nelson Canada
1120 Birchmount Road
Scarborough, Ontario
Canada M1K 5G4

International Thomson Editores
Campos Eliseos 385, Piso 7
Col. Polanco
11560 México D. F. México

International Thomson Publishing GmbH
Königswinterer Strasse 418
53227 Bonn
Germany

International Thomson Publishing Asia
60 Albert Street
#15-01 Albert Complex
Singapore 189969

International Thomson Publishing Japan
Hirakawacho Kyowa Building, 3F
2-2-1 Hirakawacho
Chiyoda-ku, Tokyo 102
Japan

Printed in the United States of America

10 9 8 7 6 5 4 3 2 1

Library of Congress Cataloging-in-Publication Data
Doweiko, Harold E., [date]
   Concepts of chemical dependency / Harold E. Doweiko — 4th ed.
      p.   cm.
   Includes bibliographical references and index.
   ISBN 0-534-35755-5 (pbk.)
   1. Substance abuse.   I. Title.
RC564.D68   1999
362.29—dc21   97-51593
                                                   CIP

*In loving memory
of my wife, Jan*

Contents

11   Opiate   135

12   Over-the-Counter Analgesics   155

13   Hallucinogens   173

14   Inhalants and Aerosols   187

Preface

There have been a number of major advances in our understanding of the addictive disorders since the third edition of *Concepts of Chemical Dependency* was published in 1996. To keep this text as current as possible, hundreds of changes have been made. Numerous references have been deleted because ongoing research has made them obsolete. New discoveries in the fields of neurology, neuropsychology, and neuropsychopharmacology have provided new awareness of the effects of recreational chemicals within the brain and how abused drugs disrupt the normal functions of the central nervous system.

As a result of the discoveries made in the last decade, as well as the changing face of alcohol/drug use disorders, it has been necessary to review and revise this text so that it might remain current. The understanding, identification, and treatment of the addictive disorders is undergoing a revolution. New discoveries have reshaped traditional beliefs about, and treatment methods for, substance abusers. There are few generally accepted answers, a multitude of unanswered questions, and few interdisciplinary boundaries to limit one's exploration of, or contribution to, the field of substance abuse rehabilitation.

This new edition of *Concepts of Chemical Dependency* includes significant changes. Each chapter has been revised to include the latest research.

The chapter on basic pharmacology helps the reader understand *why* the drugs of abuse work the way they do. The chapter on cocaine use and abuse has been revised to include the latest information on cocaine's effects on the body, and the chapter on narcotic analgesics has also been updated. The chapter on adolescent drug use includes the latest information on chemical use by adolescents as revealed by the ongoing National Institute on Drug Abuse surveys. Also in this edition of *Concepts of Chemical Dependency* is more information on new self-help groups, such as Rational Recovery, that are emerging as alternatives to the traditional Alcoholics Anonymous. The ongoing debate over whether drugs should be legalized has made an extensive revision of the chapter on Drugs and Crime necessary.

Several reviewers have inquired why this text does not address caffeine addiction. There are several reasons for the decision not to include caffeine in the current edition of *Concepts*. First, the current evidence seems to suggest that, as addictions go, the addiction to caffeine is relatively benign. Second, the chemical structure of caffeine is so different from the other drugs of abuse that it falls into a class of its own. Third, the pattern of use of caffeine is somewhat different than those of the other drugs of abuse. Finally, for sociological and political reasons, the use of caffeine is not viewed as a serious problem in the United States at this time. Rather than cross this boundary in terms of social perception, a discussion on caffeine addiction was not included in this edition.

Although every effort has been made to include the latest information, there is always a lag between when discoveries are announced in the press or professional journals and when the research can be incorporated into a new edition of *Concepts*. This is one reason the field of addictive medicine is so exciting: it is constantly changing. There are few generally accepted answers, a multitude of unanswered questions, and, as compared to the other branches of science, few interdisciplinary boundaries to limit one's exploration of the field.

Disclaimer

This text was written in an attempt to share the knowledge and experience of the author with others interested in the field of substance abuse. While every effort has been made to insure that the information reviewed in this text is accurate, this book is *not* designed for, nor should it be used as, a guide to patient care. Further, this text provides a great deal of information about the current drugs of abuse, their dosage levels, and their effects. This information is provided not to advocate or encourage the use/abuse of chemicals. Rather, this information is reviewed in order to inform the reader of current trends in the field of drug abuse/addiction. This text is not intended as a guide to self-medication, and neither the author, or publisher, assumes any responsibility for individuals who attempt to use this text as a guide for the administration of drugs to themselves, others, or as a guide to treatment.

Acknowledgments

It would not be possible to mention each and every person who has helped to make this book a reality. However, I would like to thank Jim Plantikow, for his continued feedback and support. His knowledge and his experience as a "front line" therapist working in a dual disorders program have made him a valuable source of feedback. I have found him to be a worthy resource in my struggle to understand the person abusing or addicted to chemicals.

Most certainly, I must mention the library staff at Lutheran Hospital-La Crosse for their assistance in tracking down many obscure references. These individuals have provided uncomplaining service as part of their everyday routine, and deserve my warmest thanks.

I would also like to thank the reviewers who read the manuscript, offering valuable suggestions and insights: Bettie Dibrell, Central Piedmont Community College; Iris Heckman, Washburn University; Leonard Hamilton, Rutgers University; and Ron Jackson, University of Washington.

Finally, I would like to thank my wife, Jan, for all of her support. Until her untimely death, she happily read each chapter of each edition. When I was asked to begin work on the fourth edition, she again volunteered to help review material for the edition now in your hands. She corrected my spelling (many, many times over) and encouraged me when I was up against the brick wall of writer's block. Her feedback was received with the same openness that any author receives "constructive criticism." She persisted with her feedback about each edition and more often than not she was right. She was both my best friend and my editor-in-chief. I will miss her.

Harold E. Doweiko

CHAPTER ONE

Why Worry about Recreational Chemical Use in the United States?

It is almost impossible to open a newspaper or listen to the news without learning that yet another celebrity has been stopped by the police and found in possession of marijuana, cocaine, or some other controlled substance. Such news stories certainly generate a great deal of interest among the public, but these reports only hint at the extent of the problem of drug and alcohol abuse in the United States. Recreational chemical abuse/addiction is intertwined with virtually every other problem that human service professionals deal with. Consider, for example, how recreational chemical use impacts just the health care crisis in the United States:

- At any given time, up to one-half of those patients seen in the typical hospital emergency room are there either directly or indirectly due to chemical abuse (Evans & Sullivan, 1990).

    The medical treatment of alcoholism and drug addiction, in combination with the psychiatric consequences of these disorders, accounts for up to 60% of hospital usage in the United States (Ciraulo, Shader, Ciraulo, Greenblatt, & von Moltke, 1994a).
- Either directly or indirectly, substance abuse is the most common "disease" encountered by the modern physician (American Medical Association, 1993a).

Recreational drug use is not simply a drain on the general medical resources of the United States. The use of chemicals for personal pleasure also puts a strain on the mental health support system of this country:

- Either directly or indirectly, chemical abuse plays a role in a third to a half of those individuals seen for psychiatric emergencies (Evans & Sullivan, 1990).
- The most common cause of psychotic conditions in young adults is alcohol/drug abuse (Cohen, 1995).
- The abuse of illicit drugs is a major cause of ischemic stroke in adults, increasing the user's risk of such an event 1100% (Martin, Enevoldson, & Humphrey, 1997).
- The economic cost of chemical abuse in the United States is more than $300 billion a year (American Psychiatric Association, 1995).
- Alcohol use is a known risk factor in suicide attempts. Fully 25% of those people who successfully commit suicide are addicted to alcohol (Hyman & Cassem, 1995).

Alcohol and drug abuse are often an unspoken component of family or marital violence situations, being involved in approximately 56% of domestic abuse cases (Gentillelo, Donovan, Dunn, & Rivara, 1995). In addition, an estimated 675,000 or more children in the United States are mistreated by an alcohol- or drug-abusing caretaker each year (Bays,

1990). Finally, alcohol/drug use is a part of the wave of crime that has been flooding the United States:

- Alcohol is implicated in half of all homicides committed in the United States (National Foundation for Brain Research, 1992).
- Researchers have suggested that between 40% (Liu et al., 1997) and 60% (Hingson, 1996) of the people in the United States will be involved in an alcohol-related motor vehicle accident at some point in their lives.

Researchers have long been aware of the relationship between substance abuse and victimization:

- The team of Liebschutz, Mulvey, and Samet (1997) found that 42% of a sample of 2322 women who were seeking treatment for substance use problems had a history of having been physically or sexually abused at some point in their lives. A quarter of these women said that they were in danger of being victimized again, in the near future.
- Of a sample of 802 inpatients being treated for alcoholism, 49% of the women and 12% of the men reported that they had been the victim of some form of sexual abuse (Windle, Windle, Scheidt, & Miller, 1995).

The list goes on and on. Indeed, as one examines the full scope of recreational chemical use and abuse in the United States, it becomes increasingly evident that ours is a drug-centered society and that recreational substance abuse extracts a terrible toll from everyone living in this country. Collectively, we are either using one or more recreational chemicals, are worried about the effects of recreational drug use on one or more members of our families, are suffering from the pain caused by another person's substance abuse, or are being exposed to endless reports in the mass media about the latest public figure to enter a rehabilitation program because of addiction to recreational chemicals. No matter where we turn, we are faced with the problem of recreational substance abuse.

Who "Treats" Those Who Are Addicted to Chemicals?

Recreational chemical use is an ongoing problem for society. Indeed, the media speaks knowingly of the "disease" of addiction. Although the addictive disorders are classified as diseases, health care professionals generally are not trained to intervene and treat those who are addicted to chemicals. As hard as it may be to believe, *less than 1% of the typical medical school curriculum addresses alcohol or drug abuse* (Selwyn, 1993).

The study of the addictive disorders is required in only 8 of 126 American medical schools sampled (Dube & Lewis, 1994), and overall, "physician training about substance abuse is deficient" (Committee on Substance Abuse, 1995, p. 439). In the typical medical school, "Medical students and house staff learn to view alcoholics as patients to avoid" (Delbanco, 1996, p. 803). Given this attitude, it should not be surprising that "primary care physicians are prone to miss the diagnosis of alcoholism in 50% to 70% of adult patients" (Alexander & Gwyther, 1995, p. 220). Wing (1995) went even further, stating that only one in every ten patients who is dependent on alcohol is ever properly diagnosed.

The team of Bernstein, Tracey, Bernstein, and Williams (1996) examined the ability of Emergency Department physicians to detect alcohol-related problems in more than 210 patients. The patients completed an evaluation process that included three different tests: the Ever A Problem (EAP) quiz, the CAGE (discussed in Chapter 26), and the QED Saliva Alcohol Test (SAT). Forty percent of the patients were positive for an alcohol use problem on at least one of the three measures utilized. The authors found that less than a quarter of the patients identified as having a possible alcohol use problem by these evaluation tools were referred for further evaluation or treatment. The authors concluded that a major reason physicians did not refer alcohol-abusing patients for treatment was their professional belief about the hopelessness of intervening successfully with such problems.

Despite the known relationship between alcohol use and traumatic injury, almost three quarters of the trauma treatment centers studied do not screen for alcohol abuse/addiction when treating patients (Gentillelo et al., 1995). Further, although the benefits of professional treatment of alcoholism have been demonstrated time and again, many physicians continue to consider it "untreatable" (Rains, 1990, p. 40). At best, physicians are "often pessimistic about the efficacy of treatment" for substance abuse or addiction (Group for the Advancement of Psychiatry, 1990, p. 1295). For example, only 40% of general practice physicians are motivated to work with the alcoholic patient (Alexander & Gwyther, 1995).

This diagnostic blindness is not limited to physicians. As mentioned earlier in this chapter, alcohol use/abuse is a known risk factor for family violence, yet marital/family therapists only rarely ask the proper questions to identify alcohol or drug abuse and dependence. When a substance use problem within a marriage or family is not uncovered, therapy proceeds in a haphazard fashion. Vital clues to a very real illness within the family are missed, and the attempt at therapy is ineffective unless the addictive disorder is identified and addressed.

Despite the obvious relationship between substance abuse and psychopathology, Youngstrom (1991) reported that of the approximately 68,000 psychologists who are members of the American Psychological Association (APA), "only 504 identified substance abuse as their primary specialty, and 789 list it as their secondary specialty" (p. 14). Since this represents less than 2% of the psychologists who belong to APA, the professional response to the problem of substance abuse has obviously been far short of the need. No matter whether substance abuse/addiction is a true disease, the health care and mental health professions have not trained practitioners to recognize its symptoms or provide effective treatment.

These findings are important because they show that the mental health and health care professions have responded to the problem of substance abuse/addiction with a marked lack of attention, and minimal professional training. But is this, perhaps, because drug use/abuse in the United States is such a minor problem that it is unnecessary for large numbers of professionals to be trained to deal with it? In the next section, we examine the scope of the problem of substance use/abuse, and you can decide whether it really is as serious as it appears.

The Scope of the Problem of Chemical Abuse and Addiction

Although recreational chemical use, abuse, and addiction are widespread in the United States, several factors make it difficult to identify the full scope of the problem. First, the very nature of drug/alcohol use problems means that people will tend to hide evidence that they abuse recreational chemicals. Second, different researchers may define substance abuse in different ways and reach different conclusions based on their research data. Third, the process of psychosocial research based on demographic data makes it difficult for the average layperson to understand how different scientists might reach opposite conclusions based on their respective research samples.

A fourth factor that makes it difficult for the average citizen to understand the true scope of recreational drug/alcohol abuse is the coverage of the mass media, which focuses on "breaking" news, not long-term problems. If a dam were to burst, sending a flood of water downstream to destroy an unsuspecting village, a thousand reporters would converge on the scene of the disaster. But, how many reporters would have taken the time to document the slow deterioration of the dam in the months and years before the final moments in which the dam failed? The same process is at work when the media investigates substance abuse: attention centers on the dramatic new developments, not the slowly evolving trends so characteristic of the problem.

Finally, the public has become increasingly skeptical about passing fads that evolve from media-generated issues. The media hype (with its rapidly shifting focus from one drug of abuse to another), the conflicting conclusions of researchers, and the uneven emphasis placed on the problem of drug/alcohol abuse by different political leaders have combined to make the average person wonder whether substance abuse still is a problem and, if so, how serious a problem it might be. The research studies presented in this section illustrate the confusion that seems to surround the issue of chemical use/abuse in the United States.

A Word about Demographic Research

Students who review research based on demographic data frequently ask how it is possible for different researchers to reach disparate conclusions, often on research based on the same data. The answer to this problem is simple: because the population is so large, researchers must limit themselves to information drawn from small samples.

In one variation of an old fable, four blind men in India encounter an elephant for the first time. One of the men, holding the elephant's trunk, concludes that this animal is very much like a snake. Another, feeling the elephant's leg, disagrees, stating that the elephant is like a tree. The third man, feeling the flank, argues with the first two, insisting that the elephant is like a wall. The last man, holding on to the tail, says the others are mistaken—an elephant is like a rope. These men all were feeling the same animal, and yet each arrived at a widely different conclusion based on his "sample" (what he could feel). However, if 50 blind men were to touch the same elephant, the summary of their samples would give a much more accurate approximation of what the animal looked like.

Thus, this text reviews a large number of studies. This approach (despite what some students might think!) is not intended to frighten or punish the reader. Rather, these summaries of many research studies, each of which draws on a small sample of subjects, may suggest the overall pattern of the alcohol/drug use trends in the United States.

The Scope of the Problem

One of the most dramatic, and frightening, estimates of the scope of substance use problems in the past century was offered a decade ago (Franklin, 1987). At the height of the drug-use "crisis" of the 1980s, the author suggested that when drug rehabilitation professionals examined the statistics on alcohol and illegal drug abuse, combined with the abuse of prescription drugs, they would find "perhaps one in every five Americans (is) hopelessly addicted to

something—and another one or two (are) steady users" (p. 59).

If Franklin's (1987) estimate of 20% of the population of this country as being addicted is accepted, then this means that approximately 53 million of the estimated 265 million people in the United States are addicted to chemicals, while another 53 to 106 million Americans are steady users. Although these figures are indeed alarming, other estimates have never suggested a problem of this magnitude.

Nevertheless, a small number of research studies came relatively close to the estimate offered by Franklin (1987). The first of these studies, by Kessler et al. (1994), and a subsequent study using the same data (Kessler et al., 1997) reached some interesting conclusions about the extent of alcohol abuse/addiction in the United States. The data from each study incorporated the responses of a sample of 8098 individuals who took part in the National Comorbidity Survey. The sample was selected to approximate the characteristics of the population of the United States as a whole, in order to estimate the percentage of the population that would meet diagnostic criteria for one of 14 psychiatric conditions, both in the preceding 12 months and during their lifetime.

Kessler et al. (1994) concluded:

1. More than 14% of their respondents had a lifetime history of alcohol dependence.
2. More than 7% of their sample were dependent on alcohol in the past 12 months.
3. More than 4% of their sample had used a drug for recreational purposes at some point in their lives, but were not dependent on chemicals.
4. More than 7% of their sample would meet the criteria for a diagnosis of drug dependence at some point in their lives.

However, Kessler et al. (1997) observed that their interpretation of the data obtained from the National Comorbidity Survey was based on a rather liberal definition of alcohol/drug abuse and addiction, and that other researchers might reach different conclusions from this data if they used different criteria to define the problem behaviors being studied.

In a similar study, Warner, Kessler, Hughes, Anthony, and Nelson (1995) examined the response pattern of 8098 individuals, again selected to be representative of the entire U.S. population. The authors found that fully 51% of their sample admitted to having used an illicit chemical at least once, although only 15% had done so in the 12 months preceding their participation in the study. Because homeless people tended to be underrepresented in their research sample, and there is a known relationship between homelessness and chemical abuse, the authors suggested that the percentage of American adults who had ever used an illicit substance might be higher than the 51% figure found in their research sample.

The results obtained by Werner et al. (1995) and Kessler et al. (1994) were significantly different from those suggested by the *Harvard Mental Health Letter* ("Treatment of Drug Abuse," 1995). This publication suggested that from 5% to 10% of the adults in the United States had a "serious alcohol problem" (p. 1). According to this journal, another 1% to 2% of the adults in this country "have a serious illicit drug problem."

Approximately a decade ago, the team of Regier et al. (1990) attempted to examine the lifetime prevalence rates of various forms of mental illness, including alcohol and substance use disorders, in the United States. Their findings suggested that, at any given point in time, only 2.8% of the population would meet the criteria for a diagnosis of either alcohol abuse or dependence. Another 1.3% of the population would meet the diagnostic criteria for a drug abuse or dependence problem at any given point in time, according to Regier et al.

The authors also concluded that, over the course of their lives, 13.5% of the population would meet the criteria for either alcohol abuse or dependence. Another 6.1% of the population would meet the criteria for a diagnosis of substance abuse or dependence, according to Regier et al. (1990). If we assume that the population of the United States is approximately 265 million persons and apply the figures suggested by Regier et al. and Kessler et al. (1994), we can reach some interesting conclusions. On the basis of the study by Regier et al., it would appear that at any given time about 7.4 million Americans would meet the diagnostic criteria for alcohol abuse or dependence. Another 3.4 million Americans would qualify for a diagnosis of drug abuse or dependence.

In contrast to these estimates, the conclusions of Kessler et al. (1994) suggest that (given a population estimate of 265 million people) 18.2 million people in the United States were physically dependent on alcohol at some point in the preceding 12 months and 10.4 million Americans had used a recreational chemical other than alcohol in the same 12-month period. This latter estimate was slightly below the *Playboy* ("The Drug Index," 1995) estimate of 11.8 million Americans who were thought to have used an illicit drug in the past 30 days. Kessler et al. also suggested 35.8 million Americans would become physically dependent on alcohol at some point in their lives and 16.2 million would become dependent on a recreational drug.

Galanter and Frances (1992) offered a slightly higher estimate that 15% of the population meet the diagnostic criteria for alcohol abuse at some point in their lives. The authors offered a lifetime prevalence rate of 6% for drug abuse in this country. Again, by applying these prevalence figures to a population of approximately 265 million persons, it would appear that 40 million people in the United States will meet the criteria for a formal diagnosis of alcohol abuse at some point in their lives. Another 16 million Americans will, sooner or later, meet the diagnostic criteria for drug abuse, according to the authors.

Now compare the previous estimates with what researchers have found out about the drug abuse problem in the United States. R. White (1993) suggested that only 12 million Americans might be classified as "frequent users" (p. 26A) of illicit chemicals. This estimate did not attempt to separate those who are addicted to one or more drugs from those who are not physically addicted to chemicals. Kotz and Covington (1995) estimated that 8% of the population of the United States was addicted to alcohol.

The intravenous drug addict is often seen as a stereotype of the addicted person. Yet, there are only between 1.1 million and 1.8 million intravenous drug users in this country (Selwyn, 1993). This estimate includes both those who are addicted and those who are abusing intravenous drugs but are not addicted to them. This number works out to less than 1% of the estimated population of the United States. These estimates, and the predictions reviewed earlier, are significantly lower than the estimated 20%

of the population (or an estimated 52 million Americans) who were presumed to be addicted to chemicals, and the additional estimated 20% of the population who were abusing chemicals, suggested by Franklin (1987). The reader might consider Franklin's figures as a "worst case" estimate that has not been supported by the research data.

However, the wide differences between the estimates of the scope of substance abuse/addiction in this country underscore a serious shortcoming in the field of substance abuse rehabilitation: the lack of clear data. Depending on the research study being cited, substance abuse is/is not a serious problem, is/is not getting worse (or, better), will/will not be resolved in the next decade, and is something that parents should/should not worry about.

The underlying truth is that large numbers of people use one or more recreational chemicals, but only a small percentage of people who use them ultimately become addicted to the chemical(s) being abused (Peele, Brodsky, & Arnold, 1991). For example, only one in every four drug abusers was classified as a "hard-core" user by the Office of National Drug Control Policy (1996).

Estimates of Substance Abuse

Alcohol Use, Abuse, and Addiction

Surprisingly, the use of alcohol in the United States has been declining since around 1980; it actually has dropped about 15% since then (Musto, 1996). But alcohol remains a popular recreational chemical in the United States, and it is estimated that 90% of the adults in the United States will consume alcohol at least once in their lives (Schuckit, 1995). Half of the adults in the United States consume alcohol on a regular basis (Lieber, 1995).

Although alcohol is a popular recreational substance, it is also potentially addictive. Approximately 10% of those who drink alcohol will become addicted to it (Kotz & Covington, 1995). However, researchers disagree as to the exact scope of the problem of alcohol addiction. Various estimates have been offered, suggesting that 6 million (Ellis, McInerney, DiGiuseppe, & Yeager, 1988), to 10 million (Bays, 1990) to 12 million (L. Siegel, 1989) to perhaps as many as 20 million (Kotz & Covington, 1995; Lieber, 1995) adults in the

United States are addicted to alcohol. This number does not include another estimated 1 million (Ellis et al., 1988) to 3 million children and adolescents (Turbo, 1989) who are also thought to be addicted to alcohol.

Researchers agree that, to a large degree, alcohol abuse/addiction might be said to be a "male disease." The majority of those who abuse, or who are addicted to, alcohol are male. But this does not mean that it is exclusively a male problem. The ratio of male to female alcohol abusers/addicts is thought to fall between 2:1 and 3:1 (Blume, 1994; Cyr & Moulton, 1993; Hill, 1995). These figures suggest that significant numbers of women are also abusing, or are addicted to, alcohol.

Because alcohol can be legally purchased by adults over the age of 21, many people tend to forget that it is also a drug. The grim reality is that this legal chemical makes up the greatest part of the drug abuse/addiction problem in this country. Franklin (1987) stated, for example, that alcoholism alone accounts for 85% of drug addiction in the United States. This is not surprising, as alcohol is the most commonly abused chemical in the world (Lieber, 1995).

Narcotics Abuse and Addiction

When many people hear the term "drugs of abuse," narcotics are the drugs they think of, especially heroin. Although narcotic analgesics have the reputation of being addictive, only about half of those who abuse these drugs become addicted (Jenike, 1991). The Office of National Drug Control Policy (1996) estimated that 500,000 people in the United States use heroin at least once a week, while an additional 229,000 use this chemical less than once a week. This total is close to the estimate of 1 million Americans who use heroin at least once a week offered by Kaufman and McNaul (1992). Another estimate of 800,000 people in the United States as being addicted to heroin was offered by Abt Associates, Inc. (1995a). About half of the individuals addicted to heroin in the United States are thought to live in New York City (Kaplan, Sadock, & Grebb, 1994; Witkin & Griffin, 1994).

A significant percentage of those addicted to heroin are women. Kaplan and Sadock (1990) gave a ratio of three male heroin addicts for every female.

Given the estimate of 800,000 heroin addicts, this would mean that approximately 200,000 women are addicted to heroin in the United States. Estimates of the scope of narcotics addiction are, for the most part, based on data drawn from public treatment programs and social service agency reports (Eisenhandler & Drucker, 1993). Individuals who utilize these services are, to a large degree, indigent and dependent on public services. As discussed in Chapter 11, there is a hidden population of opiate users in the United States: those individuals who have regular jobs and thus have private health care insurance despite their addiction to opiates. Few of these users are included in the estimate of 800,000 active heroin addicts in the United States.

The truth is that there are many hidden cases of opiate abuse/addiction in the United States. Health care professionals know very little about these people. For example, it is known that some pharmaceutical narcotic analgesics are diverted to the illicit drug market. However, virtually no information is available on the person who abuses or is addicted to pharmaceutical narcotics, but who never uses heroin. Thus, the estimated 400,000–800,000 intravenous heroin addicts must be accepted only as a minimal estimate of narcotics addiction in this country.

Cocaine Abuse and Addiction

Although there is evidence to suggest that cocaine abuse peaked in the mid-1980s, it still remains a popular drug of abuse. Angell and Kassirer (1994) estimated that 1.6 million Americans use cocaine on a regular basis. However, the authors did not differentiate between those who were addicted to the drug, and, those who used cocaine infrequently. In a report issued by the RAND Corporation on the subject of drug policy in this country, it was estimated that there are currently 7 million cocaine users in the United States ("Study: Cocaine Treatment," 1994). Of this number, 1.7 million were thought to consume cocaine at least once a week, using 8 times as much cocaine as the other 5.3 million combined.

Cornish, McNicholas, and O'Brien (1995) offered a different estimate of the number of people in the United States who are using cocaine. The authors suggested that there are 3 million cocaine users in this country, of whom approximately 855,000 use the drug at least once a week. The Washington-based research group Abt Associates, Inc. (1995a) suggested that there were 2.1 million hard-core cocaine users (those who used cocaine more than 2 times a week), and 4 million occasional users (defined by the authors as those who used cocaine less than 2 times a week).

Surprisingly, despite its reputation for causing addiction, only a fraction of those who use cocaine every actually become addicted to it. Musto (1991) estimated that between 3 and 20% of those who had used cocaine would go on to become addicted to this substance. In support of this estimate, consider that of the 3 million Americans who use cocaine, only 855,000 do so once a week or more (Cornish et al., 1995). Other researchers have suggested that only one cocaine user in six (Peele et al., 1991), to one in twelve (Peluso & Peluso, 1988) is actually addicted to the drug. The rest are cocaine abusers, but do not seem to be addicted.

Marijuana Abuse/Addiction

Researchers have only recently concluded that it is possible to become addicted to marijuana in the traditional sense of the word. The possibility of an individual going through withdrawal symptoms as a result of chronic marijuana use will be discussed in more detail in Chapter 10.

Marijuana is the most commonly abused *illegal* drug in the United States (Kaufman & McNaul, 1992) as well as Canada (Russell, Newman, & Bland, 1994). It is estimated that 68 million (Kaufman & McNaul, 1992) people in the United States have used marijuana at some point in their lives. This number means that approximately 25% of the entire population of the United States has used marijuana at least once. It is estimated that there are 9 million regular users of marijuana in this country (Angell & Kassirer, 1994, p. 537). However, the authors did not identify what they meant by "regular" users of this substance. The Department of Health and Human Services estimated that 3.3 million people in the United States (a small fraction of those who have tried marijuana) use the drug on a daily basis.

Hallucinogenic Abuse

As with marijuana, investigators have questioned whether one may become addicted to hallucinogenics. For this reason, this text speaks of the "hallucinogenic abuse." Perhaps as many as one-fifth of Americans below the age of 25 have used hallucinogenics at one time or another (Kaplan & Sadock, 1990). According to the authors, however, hallucinogenic use is actually quite rare, and of those young adults who have used hallucinogenic drugs, no more than 2% will have done so in the past 30 days. These figures suggest that the problem of *addiction* to hallucinogenics is exceedingly rare.

Tobacco Addiction

Tobacco is a special drug. Like alcohol, it is legally sold to adults. Tobacco products are also readily obtained by adolescents, who make up a significant proportion of users. Researchers estimate that approximately 46 million Americans smoke cigarettes (Brownlee et al., 1994). Of this number, an estimated 24 million smokers are male, and 22.3 million are female.

The Cost of Chemical Abuse and Addiction in the United States

Although the total number of people in this country who abuse, or are addicted to, recreational chemicals is limited, recreational substance use still extracts a terrible toll from society. It is difficult to estimate the total financial cost of drug abuse and addiction, if only because substance abuse includes so many hidden faces. McGinnis and Foege (1993) noted that, in the year 1990, 9000 deaths were directly attributed to chemical abuse. However, when one stops to consider the impact of drug-related infant deaths, overdose, suicide, homicide, motor vehicle deaths, and drug-abuse-related disease (e.g., hepatitis, HIV infection, pneumonia, endocarditis), the true cost of drug abuse/addiction is closer to 25,000 (Office of National Drug Control Policy, 1996) to 30,000 (Samet, Rollnick, & Barnes, 1996) premature deaths a year. These figures do not reflect the estimated 100,000 (Lieber, 1995) to 200,000 (Hyman & Cassem, 1995; Kaplan et al., 1994) people who die each year from alcohol use/abuse, or the 450,000 to 500,000 people who die each year from tobacco-related illness.

The use of recreational chemicals accounts for between one-fourth and one-third of all deaths in the United States each year (Hurt et al., 1996). In addition to deaths discussed in the preceding paragraph, the combination of alcohol and drugs is thought to cause another 7600 deaths each year in the United States, while heroin/morphine abuse results in some 6500 deaths. Cocaine is estimated to cause some 8100 deaths in the United States each year (Hilts, 1996). As these figures suggest, chemical use, or abuse, is a significant factor in premature death, illness, loss of productivity, and medical expenses. However, because chemical abuse/addiction has so many hidden faces, behavioral scientists have only a rough estimate of the annual impact of alcohol/drug use problems in the United States.

The Cost of Alcohol Abuse

Kaplan et al. (1994) placed the cost of alcohol use/abuse alone at $600 for every man, woman, and child in the United States. However, the authors did not specify what factors they considered in reaching this estimate. In attempting to calculate the annual financial cost of alcohol abuse and addiction in this country, it is necessary to include direct and indirect costs, such as the cost of alcohol-related criminal activity, motor vehicle accidents, destruction of property, the cost of social welfare programs, private and public hospitalization costs for alcohol-related illness, and the cost of public and private treatment programs.

Researchers disagree as to the economic impact of alcohol abuse/addiction in the United States. Rice (1993) suggested that the cost of alcohol use/abuse in the United States was $98.6 billion a year, while the estimate of $100 billion per year was offered by both Lieber (1995) and the team of McCrady and Langenbucher (1996). An even higher estimate of the annual impact of alcohol abuse/addiction of $100 billion to $130 billion each year was offered by Angell and Kassirer (1994). Cornish et al. (1995) disagreed with this figure and concluded that the annual economic impact of alcohol use disorders was $136 billion per year. Finally, Bernstein et al. (1996) suggested that the annual yearly cost of alcohol use/abuse in the United States was "more than $150 billion" (p. 69).

In recent years, politicians have spoken at length about the need to control the rising cost of health care in the United States. Alcohol use disorders are significant factors in the growing health care financial crisis. Although only 5% to 10% of the general population has an alcohol use problem, 10% to 20% of ambulatory patients and 20% to 40% of those patients in hospitals suffer from some complication of alcohol use/abuse (Blondell, Frierson, & Lippmann, 1996). Further, between 15 and 30% of the nursing home beds in this country are occupied by individuals whose alcohol use has contributed to their need for placement (Schuckit, 1995). Many of these beds are supported, at least in part, by public funds, making chronic alcohol abuse a major factor in the growing cost of nursing home care for the elderly.

Alcohol use was a factor in 41% of motor vehicle accident deaths in 1995 (Hingson, 1996). Whether accident victims ultimately survive their injuries or succumb, they require emergency medical treatment. Further, alcohol use/abuse is thought to be a factor in 40% of all cases of traumatic injury (McCrady & Langenbucher, 1996). Individuals who have been injured require medical treatment that ultimately is paid for by the public in the form of higher insurance costs and higher taxes. Alcohol use disorders are thought to account for 15% of the money spent for health care in the United States each year (McCrady & Langenbucher, 1996). Yet despite the pain and suffering that alcohol causes each year, only 5% (Samet et al., 1996) to 10% of alcohol-dependent individuals are ever identified and referred to a treatment program (Wing, 1995).

Kales, Barone, Bixler, Miljkovic, and Kales (1995) examined the problems of mental illness and substance use in a rural sample of homeless people. The authors found that almost 60% of their sample of 100 individuals have had either an alcohol or recreational drug use problem at some time in their lives. While their sample was drawn from a rural setting rather than a large city, the findings were consistent with earlier studies based on urban samples of homeless people. Thus, it would seem that substance use problems often coexist with homelessness. Some estimates of the yearly cost of providing social service support (housing, medical treatment, food, etc.) to this population might be as high as $23,000 per client (Whitman, Friedman, & Thomas, 1990). When one considers the number of homeless in this country, these figures amount to a massive investment of social support dollars that must also be included in the annual cost of recreational chemical use in the United States.

The Cost of Tobacco Use

Although tobacco is legally produced and can be consumed by adults without legal problems, its use extracts a terrible cost. Tresch and Aronow (1996) estimated that the annual cost of direct health care for cigarette smokers, combined with lost productivity as a result of smoking-related illness, is an estimated $65 billion per year in the United States.

The Cost of Substance Abuse

Various estimates of the financial cost of drug abuse and dependence in this country have been advanced. Researchers believe that between $50 billion (Bugliosi, 1996) and $150 billion (Collier, 1989) are spent each year in the United States just to buy illicit recreational chemicals. But this is not the total cost of illicit substance abuse. When one factors in the estimated financial impact of premature death or illness caused by substance abuse, lost wages from those who lose their jobs as a result of substance abuse, the financial losses incurred by victims of drug-related crimes, and the expected costs of drug-related law-enforcement activities, the indirect economic loss caused by illicit drug use in the United States might range from $76 billion to $150 billion (Angell & Kassirer, 1994) or $160 billion per year (Hyman, 1996).

White (1993), on the other hand, suggested that the cost of substance abuse, when measured in terms of law enforcement, treatment, medical care, insurance costs, and the financial impact of drug-related crime, was closer to $300 billion each year in the United States. No matter which of these estimates you believe, it is clear that drug abuse is an expensive luxury.

Drug Use as an American Way of Life

In the preceding paragraph, drug abuse was identified as a "luxury." To illustrate how we have, as a nation, come to value recreational chemical use, consider that money spent on illicit recreational chemicals is not used to buy medical care, food, shelter, or clothing for people in the United States; it is spent simply to obtain illegal chemicals for personal pleasure. The annual expenditure for illicit recreational chemicals in the United States is greater than the *total combined income* of the 80 poorest Third World countries (Corwin, 1994).

There is no possible way to fully estimate the personal, economic, or social impact of chemical addiction in the United States. When one considers the possible medical costs incurred, lost productivity, and other indirect costs from hidden drug abuse and addiction, one can begin to appreciate the impact that chemical abuse and addiction has on society.

Why Is It So Difficult to Understand the Drug Abuse Problem in the United States?

For the past two generations, politicians have spoken about society's "war" on drug use/abuse. One of the basic strategies of this ongoing war has been the exaggeration of the dangers associated with chemical use (Musto, 1991; Peele, 1994). This technique is known as *disinformation*, and it seems to have been almost an unofficial policy of the government's antidrug efforts to distort and exaggerate the scope of the problem, and the dangers associated with recreational drug use.

An excellent example of this policy is the statement by U.S. Representative Vic Fazio, who in calling for legislation to control access to certain chemicals that might be used to manufacture illicit methamphetamine, spoke of "a generation of meth-addicted crank babies . . . rapidly filling our nation's hospitals" ("Politicians Discover," 1996, p. 70). This statement came as a surprise to health care professionals: there was no epidemic of methamphetamine-addicted babies. But, this did not prevent this false statement from being offered as a fact in the United States House of Representatives.

Although for more than two generations, the media has presented drugs in such a negative light that "anyone reading or hearing of them would not be tempted to experiment with the substances" (Musto, 1991, p. 46), such scare tactics have not been found to work. In the mid-1980s, the media presented report after report of the dangers of chemical abuse. Yet at this same point in time, Holloway (1991) found that 5.5 million Americans (about 2% of the population of approximately 260 million) were addicted to illegal drugs. Admittedly, this estimate did not include those addicted to alcohol. Gazzaniga (1988) arrived at a different estimate,

stating that perhaps 10% of the population "falls into addictive patterns with drugs" (p. 143). This would be about 26 million Americans, based on a population estimate of 260 million. Obviously, the reports in the media did not prevent these people from becoming addicted to chemicals.

It is not the goal of this text to advocate substance use. But, there are wide discrepancies between the scope of recreational drug use as reported in the mass media, and, scientific research. For example, Franklin (1987) stated that 20% of the population was addicted to chemicals, with another 20% being on the cusp of addiction. Yet scientific research reveals that only a small percentage of the population of the United States has a history of using illicit chemicals. Given these wide discrepancies, it is difficult to reach any conclusion but that much of what has been said about the drug abuse crisis in the United States has been tainted by misinformation, or disinformation. To understand the problem of recreational chemical use/abuse, it is necessary to look beyond the "sound bytes" or the "factoids" of the mass media and the politicians.

Summary

It has been estimated that between 2 and 10% of American adults either abuse or are addicted to alcohol/drugs. While this percentage would suggest that large numbers of people are using illicit chemicals in this society, it also implies that the drugs of abuse are not universally addictive. The various forms of dependency reflect different manifestations of a unitary disorder: chemical abuse/addiction. Finally, although drug addiction is classified as a disease, most physicians are ill prepared to treat substance-abusing patients.

In this chapter, we have examined the problem of recreational drug use and its impact on society. Later chapters in this book provide detailed information on specific drugs of abuse, their effects on the user, the consequences of their use, and, information on the rehabilitation process for those who are abusing or addicted to chemicals. This information is intended to help you better understand the problem of recreational substance use in this country.

CHAPTER TWO

What Do We Mean When We Say Substance Abuse and Addiction?

Chapter 1 examined how substance abuse/addiction is an underrecognized social problem. Like many problem areas, the world of substance abuse and drug rehabilitation has its own language. In this chapter, some of the more common concepts and terms used in the field of substance abuse and chemical dependency treatment are discussed.

The Continuum of Chemical Use

A common misperception about recreational chemicals is that the *use* of alcohol or drugs means that the person is *addicted* to them. The truth, however, is that only a percentage of those who begin to use alcohol/drugs will become addicted. Recreational alcohol/drug use, like most forms of human behavior, falls on a continuum—complete abstinence is one extreme, while physical addiction to a chemical is the opposite end point (McCrady & Epstein, 1995). In between these extremes are various patterns of chemical use that differ in the intensity with which the person engages in substance use and the consequences of this behavior for the individual.

In their discussion of illegal substance use, Cattarello, Clayton, and Leukefeld (1995) suggested:

> People differ in their illicit drug use. Some people never experiment; some experiment and never use again. Others use drugs irregularly or become regular users, whereas others develop pathological and addictive patterns of use. (p. 152)

In this statement, the authors identified five patterns of recreational chemical use: (a) total abstinence; (b) a brief period of experimentation, followed by a return to abstinence; (c) irregular, or occasional, use of illicit chemicals; (d) regular use of chemicals; and (e) the pathological or addictive pattern of use that is the hallmark of the physical dependence on chemicals.

Yet even the last point on the continuum, the addictive use of drugs, might be further subdivided. Peele et al. (1991) pointed out that an individual's specific pattern of drug use might range from "moderate excess to severe compulsion" (p. 133). In other words, even the end point of the chemical use continuum, the compulsive use of drugs, might itself be viewed as a continuum.

This is because there are no firm boundaries between the points on a substance use continuum (Sellers et al., 1993)—the points along the continuum are arbitrary. Only the end points, total abstinence and active physical addiction to chemicals, remain relatively fixed. The main advantage of a drug-use continuum such as the one suggested by Cattarello et al. (1995) is that it allows for the classification of chemical use of various intensities and patterns. Drug use/abuse/addiction thus becomes a behavior, not a "condition" that either is or is not present. A continuum allows for the classification of intermediate steps between the two extreme points of total abstinence and physical addiction.

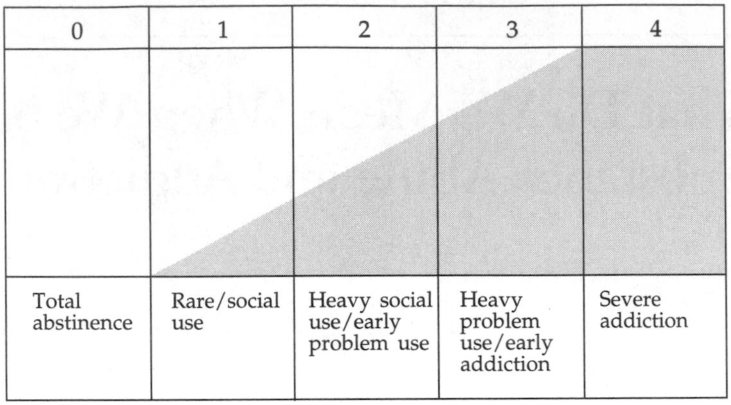

0	1	2	3	4
Total abstinence	Rare/social use	Heavy social use/early problem use	Heavy problem use/early addiction	Severe addiction

FIGURE 2.1   The continuum of chemical use.

Figure 2.1 illustrates the continuum used to view the phenomenon of recreational alcohol/drug use in this text.[1]

Level 0. Total Abstinence

This is the first point in the continuum presented in Figure 2.1. Individuals in this category would abstain from any and all recreational alcohol or chemical use.

Level 1. Rare/Social Use

This level would include experimental use and the first part of the level of irregular use, on the continuum suggested by Cattarello et al. (1995). The individual in this category would only rarely use alcohol or chemicals for recreational purposes. This person would not experience any social, financial, interpersonal, medical, or legal problems that are the hallmark of the pathological use of chemicals. Further, the person whose substance use falls at this level would not demonstrate the loss of control over chemical use found at higher levels of the continuum. The chemical use would not result in any form of danger to the person's life.

Level 2. Heavy Social Use/Early Problem Use of Drugs

A person whose chemical use falls at this point in the continuum (a) would use chemicals in a way that is clearly above the norm for his/her social group, or (b) begin to experience legal, social, financial, occupational, and personal problems associated with chemical use. This level would overlap between the end of the stage of irregular use, and the stage of regular chemical use, on the continuum suggested by Cattarello et al. (1995).

At this level, the individual might try to hide, or deny, the problems that rise as a result of the chemical use. Many persons who reach this point in the continuum will learn from their experience, and alter their behavior so that they are unlikely to encounter future problems. Further, these individuals have not lost control over their chemical use. It is *loss of control* that is the essential component of an addictive disorder (S. A. Brown, 1995; Gordis, 1995). Thus, at this level, the user is not addicted to chemicals.

Level 3. Heavy Problem Use/Early Addiction

This person's alcohol or chemical use has reached the point where there is a serious problem. Indeed, this person may be addicted to chemicals, although he/she may argue this point. For some of the drugs of abuse, one begins to see medical complications associated with addiction. Also at this phase,

---

[1] The team of Carey, Cocco, and Simons (1996) utilized a similar continuum in their work with dual-diagnosis clients (discussed in Chapter 22). But they suggested that the assessor evaluate the client's alcohol and other drug use separately.

the individual will demonstrate classic withdrawal symptoms when unable to continue the use of drugs/alcohol.

This person is often preoccupied with substance use and cannot predict how much he/she will use. Thus, the individual has slipped into a pattern of chemical use marked by loss of control, a characteristic sign of addiction. Further, by this point, the individual has started to experience legal, financial, social, occupational, and personal problems either directly or indirectly caused by chemical use.

Level 4. Severe Addiction to Drugs

At this point on the continuum, the person demonstrates the classic addiction syndrome, in combination with multiple social, legal, financial, occupational, and personal problems found in chemical addiction. The person also will demonstrate medical complications associated with chemical abuse, and may be near death as a result of chronic addiction. This individual is addicted beyond any shadow of a doubt in the assessor's mind.

Notice that the preceding sentence read that the person was "addicted beyond any shadow of a doubt in the assessor's mind." Even at this level of substance use, the addicted individual may try to rationalize away or deny problems associated with alcohol or drug use. More than one elderly alcoholic has tried to explain away abnormal liver function as being the aftermath of a childhood illness. To an impartial outside observer, however, the person at this level is clearly addicted to alcohol or drugs.

This classification system, like all others, is imperfect. The criteria used to determine the level at which an individual might fall are arbitrary and subject to discussion. As Vaillant (1983) observed in his text on alcoholism, it is often "the variety of alcohol related problems, not any unique criterion, that captures what clinicians really mean when they label a person alcoholic" (p. 42). It is a constellation of various symptoms, rather than the existence of any single symptom, that identifies alcoholism, or any other drug dependency.

As discussed in later chapters, however, some individuals use these drugs, perhaps even on a regular basis, but do not become addicted to narcotics. The long continuum of drug use styles ranges from total abstinence through occasional substance use, to the extreme of physical addiction.

Definitions of Terms Used in This Book

To understand the phenomenon of substance abuse, it is necessary to develop a common language, so that individuals who study this problem can understand each other when they discuss their work. The world of substance abuse seems to have a language all its own. This makes drug abuse terminology rather confusing to the newcomer to the field.

- *Substance abuse.* Use of a drug by an individual when there is no legitimate medical need to do so. In the case of alcohol, the person is drinking in excess of accepted social standards (Schuckit, 1995). Thus, current social standards or accepted medical practice are used to classify the individual's chemical use as either being appropriate or abusive.

- *Social use.* The use of a substance as defined by traditional social standards. When we speak of "social use," it usually means the rare or infrequent use of that drug, in a social setting. Alcohol is the chemical most frequently used within a social context, often during religious or family functions. In some circles, marijuana is also used within a social context, although its use is less acceptable than that of alcohol.

- *Drug of choice.* The preferred recreational drug used by a person. At one point, clinicians spoke about the individual's drug of choice as an important component of the addictive process. The theory was that a person's preferred drug provided an important clue to the nature of his/her addiction. However, clinicians no longer put much weight on the individual's drug of choice because the nature of addiction itself is changing (Walters, 1994). In this era of polypharmacology[2], it is rare for an addicted person to use just

[2]A term that denotes a person who is using more than one substance at once. In the "old days," the person was more likely to be using just one chemical, such as alcohol or heroin. Especially since the mid-1970s, however, individuals who use chemicals have not been limiting themselves simply to one substance.

one chemical. For example, many stimulant users drink alcohol or use benzodiazepines to control the side effects of cocaine or amphetamines. Thus, clinicians no longer emphasize the concept of the patient's drug-of-choice.

- *Addiction.* Morse and Flavin (1992) offered an updated definition of alcoholism that might be viewed as a model for all forms of drug addiction. In their opinion, alcoholism is:

> . . . a primary, chronic, disease with genetic, psychosocial and environmental factors influencing its development and manifestations. The disease is often progressive and fatal. It is characterized by impaired control over drinking, preoccupation with the drug alcohol, use of alcohol despite adverse consequences, and distortions in thinking. (p. 1013)

In this definition, one finds all of the core concepts used to define drug addiction. Each form of drug addiction: (a) is viewed as a primary disease; (b) has multiple manifestations in the person's social, psychological, spiritual, and economic life; (c) is often progressive; (d) is potentially fatal; (e) is marked by an inability to control the use of the drug; (f) shows preoccupation with chemical use; and (g) causes the individual to develop a distorted way of looking at the world that supports continued use of the chemical, despite the many consequences inherent in the chemical's use.

In addition to the preceding features, addiction to a chemical is marked by (a) the development of *tolerance* to the effects of that chemical and (b) a *withdrawal syndrome* when the drug is discontinued (Schuckit, 1995).

Tolerance develops over time, as the individual's body struggles to maintain normal function despite the presence of one or more foreign chemicals. Technically, there are several subforms of tolerance. In this text, discussion is limited to two subforms: (a) metabolic tolerance and (b) pharmacodynamic tolerance.

Metabolic tolerance develops when the body becomes more effective in biotransforming a chemical into a form that can be easily eliminated from the body. (The process of biotransformation is discussed in Chapter 3.) The liver is the main organ in which the process of biotransformation is carried out. In some cases, the constant exposure to a chemical causes the liver to become more efficient at breaking down the drug, making a given dose less effective over time.

Pharmacodynamic tolerance is a term applied to the increasing insensitivity of the central nervous system to the drug's effects. When the cells of the central nervous system are continuously exposed to a chemical, they will often try to maintain normal function by making minute changes in their cell structure to compensate for the drug's effects. The cells of the central nervous system then become less sensitive to the effects of that chemical, and the person must use more of the drug to achieve the initial effect.

- *Withdrawal syndromes.* In brief, the major recreational chemicals will, if used for a long enough time, bring about a withdrawal syndrome. The exact characteristics of the withdrawal syndrome will vary depending on the class of drugs being used, the length of time that the person used the chemical(s), and other factors such as the individual's state of health. But, each group of drugs will produce certain physical symptoms when the person stops taking the drug. A rule of thumb is that the withdrawal syndrome will include the opposite symptoms of those induced by a given chemical.

In clinical practice, a withdrawal syndrome is evidence that pharmacodynamic tolerance has developed, because the syndrome is triggered by the absence of the chemical that the central nervous system had previously adapted to. When the drug is discontinued, the central nervous system must go through a period of readaptation, as it learns to function normally without the drug molecules being present. During this period, the individual experiences the physical signs of withdrawal.

Alcohol, which is a central nervous system depressant, functions as a chemical "brake" on the cells of the central nervous system, much like the brakes on your car. If you were to try driving with the brakes engaged, you might eventually force the car to go fast enough to meet the posted speed limits. But, if you were then to suddenly release the pressure on the brakes, the car would suddenly leap forward because the brakes were no longer fighting the forward motion of the car. You would have to ease up on the gas pedal and slow down the engine enough to keep you within the posted speed limit.

During that period of readjustment, the car would, in a sense, be going through a withdrawal phase. Much the same thing happens in the body when the individual stops using drugs. The body must adjust to the absence of a chemical that, previously, it had learned would always be there. This withdrawal syndrome, like the presence of tolerance to the drug's effects, provides strong evidence that the individual is addicted to one or more chemicals.

The Growth of New "Addictions"

In addition to the tendency for the popular press to exaggerate the dangers associated with chemical abuse, there is a disturbing trend to speak of larger and larger numbers of people as being "addicts." Now, many substance abuse professionals speak of addiction to food, sex, gambling, men, women, play, television, shopping, credit cards, making money, carbohydrates, shoplifting, unhappy relationships, the Internet, and a multitude of other nondrug behaviors or substances (Peele, 1989; Peele et al., 1991). The expansion of the definition of the term *addiction* does not appear to have an end in sight.

In this text, we limit the term *addiction* to the physical dependence on the traditional drugs of abuse. Since substance abuse often blends into an addiction to that same chemical, this text often uses the terms *substance use, chemical dependency, substance abuse*, and *addiction* interchangeably. But these terms are applied only to drug abuse and addiction.

What Do We Really Know about the Addictive Disorders?

If you were to watch the television talk shows or read a small sample of the self-help books on the market, you would be left with the impression that researchers fully understand the causes and treatment of drug abuse. *Nothing could be further from the truth.* Much of what we think we know about

addiction is based on mistaken assumptions, clinical theory, or, at best, incomplete data.

An excellent example of how incomplete data can influence the evolution of treatment theory is that much of the research on substance abuse is based on a distorted sample of people: those who are in treatment for substance abuse problems (Gazzaniga, 1988). Virtually nothing is known about those people who use chemicals on a social basis but never become addicted, or those individuals who are addicted to chemicals but never enter treatment programs. Are the people in treatment representative of all drug or alcohol addicts, or just those people who are in treatment for one reason or another?

The term *chippers* refers to a subpopulation of drug users about which virtually nothing is known. They seem to be able to use a chemical (even one that is supposedly quite addictive) only when they want to, and then can discontinue using the drug whenever they choose to do so. Researchers cannot even make an educated guess as to their number. It is thought that chippers use chemicals in response to social pressure and then discontinue the drugs when the social need for them to do so has passed. But this is only a theory, and it might not account for the phenomenon of chipping.

A second reason for flawed research on substance abuse is the assumption that all chemical abuse is the same. There is a difference between *abusers* of a chemical, and those who are *addicted* to that substance (Peele, 1985). Much of the clinical research conducted in the first half of this century failed to differentiate between those who were abusing alcohol and/or drugs, and those who were addicted to them.

A third reason much of the research in the field of substance abuse rehabilitation is flawed is that a significant proportion of this research is carried out either in Veterans Administration (VA) hospitals or public facilities such as state hospitals. Patients in these facilities, however, are not automatically representative of the typical alcohol/drug dependent person. To be admitted to a VA hospital, the individual must have successfully completed a tour of duty in the military. The simple fact of having completed a term of military service means that the person is different from those people who either never enlisted in the military or who enlisted but were unable to complete a tour of duty. The alcohol/drug addict who is employed and able to afford treatment in a private treatment center might be far different from the indigent alcohol/drug dependent person who must be treated in a publicly funded treatment program.

It is also important to keep in mind that those who seek treatment for their substance abuse problem are not representative of all substance abusers. Addicts who seek treatment are different from those addicts who do not (Carroll & Rounsaville, 1992). As a group, those addicts who do not seek treatment seem to be better able to control their substance use, and have shorter drug use histories, than people who seek treatment.

This may be why the majority of those who abuse chemicals either stop, or significantly reduce, their chemical use without professional intervention (Carroll & Rounsaville, 1992; Humphreys, Moos, & Finney, 1995; *Mayo Clinic Health Letter*, 1989; Peele, 1985, 1989; Tucker & Sobell, 1992). The *Mayo Clinic Health Letter* concluded, "Despite the widespread availability of drugs and their addictive qualities, millions of Americans who once used them regularly appear now to have given them up" (p. 2). It may be that only a minority of those who begin to use recreational chemicals lose control over their substance use and require professional intervention.

Further, only a small proportion of the available literature on the subject of drug addiction addresses forms of addiction other than alcoholism. An even smaller proportion addresses the impact of recreational chemical use on women (Griffin, Weiss, Mirin, & Lange, 1989). Much of the research conducted to date has assumed that alcohol/drug use is the same for men and women, overlooking possible differences in how men and women come to use chemicals, the effects that recreational chemicals might have on men and women, and the differing impact that addiction might have on men and women.

Further, although it has long been known that children and adolescents abuse chemicals, there still is virtually no research on the subject of drug abuse/addiction for this group. Yet, as discussed in Chapter 23, child and adolescent drug and alcohol abuse is a serious problem. Youngsters who abuse chemicals are not simply small adults. It is thus not possible to automatically generalize from research done on adults to the effects of substance abuse on children or adolescents.

Much of what we think we know about addiction is based on research that is limited at best, seriously flawed in many cases, and, all too often, simply nonexistent. Yet this is the foundation on which an entire "industry" of treatment has evolved. It is not the purpose of this text to deny that large numbers of people abuse drugs, or that such drug abuse carries with it a terrible cost in personal suffering. Nor is its purpose to deny that many people are harmed by drug abuse. Admittedly, people become addicted to chemicals. The purpose of this section is to make the reader aware of the shortcomings of the current body of research on substance abuse.

The State of the Art: Unanswered Questions, Uncertain Answers

There is much confusion in the professional community over the problems of substance abuse/addiction. Even in the case of alcoholism, which is perhaps the most common of the drug addictions, there is an element of uncertainty about its essential features. For example, 30% to 45% of all adults will have at least one transient alcohol-related problem such as blackouts or legal difficulties (Kaplan et al., 1994). Yet this does not mean that 30% to 45% of the adult population is alcoholic. Rather, this fact underscores the need for researchers to more clearly identify the features that might identify the potential alcoholic.

What Constitutes a Valid Diagnosis of Chemical Dependency?

A basic unanswered question is where to draw the line between casual use of a given chemical, problem use of that same chemical, and addiction to one or more drugs. No clear lines separate problematic and nonproblematic use of a recreational substance. Rather, as Vaillant (1983) suggested, "It is not who is drinking but *who is watching*" (p. 22, italics added for emphasis) that defines whether or not alcoholism is present. Peele (1985) agreed with this statement, noting that what we define as alcoholism is actually "a social convention" (p. 35).

Are there valid diagnostic signs of drug addiction that are not simply matters of social convention? The diagnosis of chemical dependency, especially in its earlier states, is difficult (Lewis, Dana, & Blevins, 1988). In the final analysis, a diagnosis of drug addiction may be called a value judgment. This professional opinion may be made easier by lists of suggested criteria such as the ones found in the American Psychiatric Association's *Diagnostic and Statistical Manual of Mental Disorders, Fourth Edition (DSM-IV*, 1994), but even in advanced cases of drug dependency, evaluating whether the individual is addicted is not always a clear-cut process.

The *Harvard Mental Health Letter* ("Treatment of Drug Abuse," 1995) identified three elements necessary to the diagnosis of alcoholism or drug addiction:

1. *Compulsion/Loss of Control.* The person will use more of the chemical in question than he/she intended, or is unable to cut back on the amount used or unable to stop using the chemical in question.
2. *Tolerance.* The person has built up tolerance to the effects of the chemical(s) and develops withdrawal symptoms when the chemical is stopped.
3. *Impairment.* A medical disease is involved, which is to say the chemical use has caused one of many possible medical, social, psychological, legal, or vocational complications. Included in this criterion is the concept of preoccupation with further use of the chemical and the centering of one's recreational activities around the chemical.

Nevertheless, the diagnosis of chemical dependency remains an opinion made by one person, about another individual's chemical use. The fact that this opinion is offered by a trained professional and called a "diagnosis" does not alter the fact that it is simply an opinion. The point being made here is that there is still much to be learned, and many questions that must be answered, about how to objectively evaluate a given individual's chemical use pattern to provide an accurate diagnosis.

What Is the Relationship between Alcohol/Drug Use and Violence within the Family?

In Chapter 1, it was noted that there is a relationship between alcohol/drug use and violence within the family. It is wrong to automatically assume, however, that the substance use *caused* the violence. Indeed, there is evidence that suggests that, at least in some families, the violence might have taken place even if one or more members of that family did not use these chemicals (Steinglass, Bennett, Wolin, & Reiss, 1987). In such families, the alcohol/drug use and the violence may reflect the presence of yet another form of familial dysfunction that has yet to be identified. The point to keep in mind, however, is that the relationship between alcohol/drug use and violence within the family is not automatically a simple one of cause and effect. Behavioral science has a great deal more to learn about this complex relationship.

What Is the Role of News Media in the Development of New Chemical Use Trends?

One of the most serious unanswered questions facing mental health or substance abuse professionals is whether mass media has been a positive or a negative influence on those who have not started to experiment with alcohol or drugs. There is a prohibition against chemical use, coupled with legal sanctions against the importation or use of many drugs. Because of this prohibition, the sale or use of drugs or alcohol (for those who are under the legal drinking age) is newsworthy.

The charge has been made that media reports have served not to discourage chemical use, but to make these drugs appear more attractive to many who otherwise might not have been motivated to try them. For example, it is likely that the media reports of the dangers inherent in the use of inhalants actually contributed to the aura surrounding their abuse (Brecher, 1972). The same claim has been made for the abuse of the amphetamine known as "ice" (Cotton, 1990). Media reports often include information on how to use the drug in question, highlight the profits earned by those who sell the drug, and describe the potent effects of using that chemical.

Overstated media coverage of drug arrests and of the risks associated with the use of recreational chemicals, not to mention the profits associated with the sale of controlled substances, has contributed to a certain public fascination with drug abuse. The Dutch experiment in dealing with the drug problem (discussed in Chapter 34) supports the theory that, when legal sanctions are removed, recreational drugs become less attractive to the average individual, and casual use declines.

For many years in Holland, substance abuse was seen not as a legal problem, but as a public health issue. It was only after large numbers of foreign chemical users moved to Holland to take advantage of this permissiveness that Dutch authorities began utilizing law enforcement to control substance use. The point to remember is that a great deal of evidence suggests the media has actually contributed to substance abuse in this country by glamorizing and exaggerating the mystery that surrounds the street drug world. Thus, the question must be asked: Whose side is the media on?

Summary

In this chapter, the concept of a continuum of drug use was introduced. Research studies were reviewed outlining the extent of the problem of drug abuse and of addiction to different chemicals. The actual and hidden costs of chemical use/abuse were explored. Often, this is reflected solely in financial or economic terms. However, it is important that society not lose sight of the hidden impact that substance abuse has on the individual's spouse, family members, and the entire community. Unanswered questions about chemical abuse were raised, and the media's role in the evolution of the substance abuse problem was discussed.

CHAPTER THREE

An Introduction to Pharmacology[1]

It is virtually impossible to discuss the effects of drugs of abuse without touching on pharmacological concepts. In this chapter, the basic principles of pharmacology are reviewed to help you better understand the impact of different drugs of abuse on the user's body.[2]

A good starting point is to clear up two common misconceptions about recreational chemicals. First, recreational chemicals are not unique: they work in the same way as other pharmaceuticals by changing (strengthening or weakening) a potential that already exists within the cells of the body (Ciancio & Bourgault, 1989; Williams & Baer, 1994). The drugs of abuse, all of which exert their desired effects in the brain, modify the normal function of the neurons of the brain.

The second misconception about the drugs of abuse is that they are somehow different from legitimate pharmaceuticals. This is not true. Many drugs of abuse are—or were once—legitimate pharmaceuticals used by physicians to treat disease and control human suffering. Thus, the drugs of abuse obey the same laws of pharmacology that apply to the other medications in use today.

The Prime Effect and Side Effects of Chemicals

One rule of pharmacology is that introducing a chemical into the body always involves an element of risk (Laurence & Bennett, 1992). *Every* chemical agent presents the potential to harm the individual, although the degree of risk depends on factors such as the specific chemical being used and the individual's state of health. For example, an athlete's foot infection, which is caused by a fungus, presents a localized site of action on the surface of the body. The patient is unlikely to need more than a topical medication that can be applied directly to the infected region, making it easy to limit the chemical's impact on the organism as a whole.

For the drugs of abuse, however, the site of action for each of the recreational chemicals lies deep within the central nervous system (CNS). As discussed in Chapter 2, there is increasing evidence that the various drugs of abuse ultimately affect the limbic system of the brain. However, these drugs act much like a blast of shotgun pellets spewing from a scattergun: they reach not only the brain, but also many other organ systems in the body.

For example, as discussed in Chapter 9, cocaine causes the user to experience a sense of well-being and euphoria. These are the *primary effects* of the cocaine abuse. But the chemical has a number of side effects, including causing the user's coronary arteries to constrict. Coronary artery constriction is

---

[1] This chapter is designed to provide the reader with an overview of the fundamental principles of pharmacology. It is not intended to serve as, nor should it be used for, a guide to patient care.

[2] Individuals interested in reading more on pharmacology can find a wide range of texts in any medical or nursing school bookstore.

hardly a desired effect and may be the cause of heart attacks in cocaine users.[3] Such unwanted effects of a chemical are often called *secondary effects*, or *side effects*. The side effects of a chemical may range from minor discomfort to a life-threatening event for the user.

A second example is aspirin, which inhibits the production of chemicals known as prostaglandins at the site of an injury. This helps to reduce the individual's pain from an injury. But, the body also produces prostaglandins within the kidneys and stomach, where the chemical helps to modify the function of these organs. As an unwanted side effect, aspirin tends to nonselectively block prostaglandin production *throughout* the body, including the stomach and kidneys. This effect of aspirin may put the user's life at risk, as the aspirin interferes with the normal function of these organs.

The therapeutic effect/side effect phenomenon often occurs when a person with a bacterial infection of the middle ear (a condition known as *otitis media*) takes an antibiotic such as penicillin. The desired outcome is for the antibiotic to destroy the bacteria causing the infection in the middle ear. However, a common side effect is drug-induced diarrhea, as the antibiotic interferes with normal bacteria growth patterns in the intestinal tract.

Thus, all pharmaceuticals—and the drugs of abuse—have both desired effects and numerous, possibly undesirable, side effects.

Drug Forms and How Drugs Are Administered

A drug is, essentially, a foreign chemical that is introduced into the individual's body to bring about a specific, desired response. Antihypertensive medications are used to control excessively high blood pressure, while antibiotics are used to eliminate unwanted bacterial infections. The recreational drugs are introduced into the body, as a general rule, to bring about feelings of euphoria, relaxation, and relief from stress. The specific form in which a drug is administered will have a major effect on the speed with which that chemical is able to work and the way that the chemical is distributed throughout the body. In general, the drugs of abuse are administered by either the *enteral* or *parenteral* route.

Enteral Forms of Drug Administration

Medications are administered by the enteral route *orally, sublingually, or rectally* (Ciancio & Bourgault, 1989; Williams & Baer, 1994). The most common form of oral administration is the *tablet*. Shannon et al. (1995) define tablet as "a compounded form in which the drug is mixed with a binding agent to hold the tablet together before administration. . . . Most tablets are designed to be swallowed whole" (p. 8).

Many drugs of abuse are administered as tablets, including aspirin, the hallucinogens LSD and MDMA, and some forms of amphetamine. Amphetamine tablets are frequently made in illicit laboratories and are known on the street by names such as "white cross" or "cartwheels."

A second common form for oral medication is the *capsule*. This is a modified tablet, with the medication being inside a gelatin container. The capsule is designed to be swallowed whole, and once it reaches the stomach the gelatin breaks down, allowing the medication to be released into the gastrointestinal tract (Shannon et al., 1995).

Medication is available in many other forms, according to the authors. For example, some medications are administered orally as liquids. Antibiotics and some over-the-counter analgesics often are prescribed in liquid forms, especially for young children. Dosage of a liquid drug can be easily tailored to the patient's weight, and is an ideal form for patients who have trouble swallowing pills or capsules. Of the drugs of abuse, alcohol is the most prominent example of a chemical that people use in liquid form.

Some medications, and a small number of the drugs of abuse, can be absorbed through the blood-rich tissues under the tongue. A chemical that enters the body by this method is said to be administered *sublingually*. The sublingual method

---

[3] Shannon, Wilson, and Stang (1995) refer to a chemical's *primary effects* as the drug's *therapeutic effects* (p. 21). However, their text is devoted to medication and its uses, not to the drugs of abuse. To keep the differentiation between the use of a medication in the treatment of disease, and the abuse of chemicals for recreational purposes, this text will use the term primary effects.

of drug administration is considered a variation on the oral form of drug administration. Certain drugs, like nitroglycerin and fentanyl (discussed in Chapter 11) are well absorbed by the sublingual method of drug administration. For the most part, however, the drugs of abuse are not administered through sublingual means.

Parenteral Forms of Drug Administration

Parenteral drug administration involves injecting the medication directly into the body. There are several forms of parenteral administration that are commonly used in the worlds of both medicine and drug abuse. First, there is the *subcutaneous* method of drug administration. In this process, a chemical is injected just under the skin. This allows for the drug to avoid the dangers of passing through the stomach and gastrointestinal tracts. However, drugs that are administered in a subcutaneous injection are absorbed more slowly than are chemicals injected either into muscle tissue or into a vein. As described in Chapter 11, heroin addicts often use subcutaneous injections, a process that they call "skin popping."

A second method of parenteral administration involves the *intramuscular* injection of a medication. Muscle tissues have a good supply of blood, and medications injected into muscle tissue will be absorbed into the general circulation more rapidly than when injected just under the skin. As discussed in Chapter 15, it is quite common for individuals abusing anabolic steroids to inject the chemical(s) being used into the muscle tissue.

The third method of parenteral administration is the *intravenous* (or IV) *injection*. A chemical injected into a vein is deposited directly into the general circulation (Schwertz, 1991). Of the drugs of abuse, heroin, cocaine, and some forms of amphetamine are examples of chemicals administered by intravenous injection.

Because of the speed with which the chemical reaches the general circulation when administered this way, there is a distinct potential for undesirable reactions. Intravenously administered drugs allow the body little time to adapt to the arrival of the foreign chemical (Ciancio & Bourgault, 1989). This is one reason users of intravenously administered chemicals such as heroin frequently experience a

wide range of adverse effects in addition to the desired euphoria.

It cannot be assumed that using a parenteral method of drug administration means the chemical in question will have an instantaneous effect. The speed at which all forms of drugs administered by parenteral administration begin to work is influenced by a number of factors discussed later in this chapter.

Other Forms of Drug Administration

There are several additional methods of drug administration that at least need to be briefly identified. Some chemicals can be absorbed through the skin, a process that involves a *transdermal* method of drug administration. Eventually, chemicals absorbed transdermally reach the general circulation and are then distributed throughout the body. Physicians take advantage of the potential offered by transdermal drug administration to provide the patient with a low, steady blood level of a chemical. Although a drawback of this method is that it is a slow way to introduce a drug into the body, it is a useful method for certain agents. An example is the skin patch used to administer nicotine to patients who are attempting to quit smoking. Some antihistamines are administered transdermally, especially for motion sickness. There also is a transdermal patch available for the narcotic analgesic fentanyl, although its success in providing analgesia has been quite limited.

Occasionally, a chemical may be administered *intranasally* by "snorting" the material. This deposits the chemical on the blood-rich tissues of the sinuses, where it is absorbed into the general circulation. Both cocaine and heroin powders can be — and frequently are — snorted.

The process of snorting is similar to the process of *inhalation*, which is used by both physicians and illicit drug users. Inhalation of a compound takes advantage of the fact that the blood is separated from exposure to the air by a layer of tissue that is less than 1/100,000 of an inch (or, 0.64 micron) thick (Garrett, 1994). Many chemical molecules are small enough to pass through the lungs into the general circulation, as is the case with surgical anesthetics. Some of the drugs of abuse, such as heroin and cocaine, may also be abused by inhalation when they are smoked.

In another form of inhalation, the particles being inhaled are suspended in the smoke. These particles are small enough to reach the deep tissues of the lungs, where they are then deposited. In a brief period, the particles are broken down into smaller units until they are small enough to pass through the walls of the lungs and reach the general circulation. This is the process that takes place when tobacco products are smoked.

Each subform of inhalation takes advantage of the fact that the lungs offer a blood-rich, extremely large surface area through which chemical agents can be absorbed (Benet, Kroetz, & Sheiner, 1995). Further, depending on how quickly the chemical being inhaled can cross over into the general circulation, it is possible to introduce chemicals into the body relatively quickly. Researchers have found, however, that the actual amount of a chemical absorbed through inhalation tends to be variable. There are at least two reasons for this variance. First, the individual must inhale at just the right time to allow the chemical to reach the desired region of the lungs. Second, some chemicals pass through the tissues of the lung only very poorly and thus are not well absorbed by inhalation.

For example, as discussed in Chapter 10, the individual who smokes marijuana must use a different technique than the person who smokes tobacco, to get the maximum effect from the chemical inhaled. The variability in the amount of chemical absorbed through the lungs limits the utility of inhalation as a means of administering medications. However, for some of the drugs of abuse, inhalation is the preferred method. There are a number of other methods for introducing pharmaceuticals into the body (e.g., rectally, or through enteral tubes). However, the drugs of abuse are generally introduced into the body by injection, orally, intranasally, or through smoking.

Bioavailability

In order to work, the drug(s) being abused must enter the body in sufficient strength to achieve the desired effect. Pharmacists refer to this as the *bioavailability* of the chemical. Bioavailability is the *concentration of the unchanged chemical at the site of action* (Loebl,

Spratto, & Woods, 1994; Sands, Knapp, & Ciraulo, 1993). The bioavailability of a chemical in the body is influenced, in turn, by the following factors (Benet et al., 1995; Sands et al., 1993):

1. Absorption.
2. Distribution.
3. Metabolism (or "biotransformation").
4. Elimination.

Absorption

Except for topical agents, which are deposited directly on the site of action, chemicals must be absorbed into the body. The concentration of a chemical in the serum, and at the site of action, is influenced by the process of absorption (Loebl et al., 1994). The process of absorption involves the movement of drug molecules from the site of entry, through cell boundaries, to the site of action.

The human body is composed of layers of specialized cells that are organized into specific patterns to carry out certain functions. For example, the cells of the bladder are organized to form a muscular reservoir for the storage and excretion of waste products. The cells of the circulatory system are organized to form tubes (blood vessels) that contain the cells and fluids of the circulatory system.

As a general rule, each layer of cells the drug must pass through to reach the general circulation will slow the absorption down that much more. For example, just one layer of cells separates the air in our lungs from the general circulation. Drugs that are able to pass across this boundary may reach the circulation in just a few seconds. In contrast to this, a drug that is ingested orally must pass through several layers of cells before being able to reach the general circulation from the gastrointestinal tract. Thus, the oral method of drug administration is generally recognized as being one of the slowest methods by which a drug might be admitted into the body (see Figure 3.1).

There are several specialized *cellular transport mechanisms* that drug molecules can take advantage of, to pass through the walls of the cells at the point of entry. These cellular transport mechanisms are complex and function at the molecular level. Some drug molecules simply diffuse through

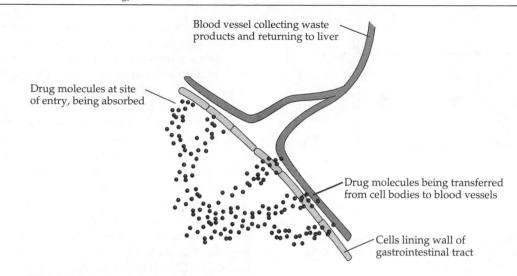

Blood vessel collecting waste products and returning to liver

Drug molecules at site of entry, being absorbed

Drug molecules being transferred from cell bodies to blood vessels

Cells lining wall of gastrointestinal tract

FIGURE 3.1   The process of drug absorption.

the cell membrane, a process known as *passive diffusion*, or *passive transport* across the cell boundary. This is the most common method of drug transport into the body's cells, and operates on the principle that chemicals tend to diffuse from areas of high concentration to areas of lower concentration. Other drug molecules take advantage of one of several molecular transport mechanisms that move essential molecules into (and out of) cells. Collectively, these molecular transport mechanisms provide a system of *active transport* across cell boundaries and into the interior of the body.

Specialized absorption-modification variables influence the speed at which a drug is absorbed from the site of entry. These include the *rate of blood flow* at the site of entry, and the *molecular characteristics of the drug molecule* being admitted to the body. However, for the purposes of this text, it is important simply to remember that the process of absorption refers to the movement of drug molecules from the site of entry to the site of action.

Distribution

The process of *distribution* refers to how the chemical molecules are moved about in the body. This includes both the process of drug transport and the pattern of drug accumulation within the body. For example, as discussed in Chapter 13, PCP tends to

accumulate both within the brain and within adipose (fat) tissues in the body.

Drug Transport

Once a chemical has reached the general circulation, that substance can then be transported to the site of action even though the main purpose of the circulatory system is not to provide a distribution system for drugs! In the circulatory system, a drug molecule is a foreign substance that takes advantage of the body's own chemical distribution system to move from the point of entry to the site of action. There are several ways a chemical can use the circulatory system to reach the site of action. Chemicals that are classified as *water-soluble* drugs mix freely with the blood plasma. Because water is such a large part of the human body, the drug molecules from water-soluble chemicals are rapidly and easily distributed throughout the fluid in the body. Alcohol is an excellent example of a water-soluble chemical. Shortly after being ingested, alcohol is rapidly distributed throughout the body to all blood-rich organs including the brain.

Other drugs utilize a different approach. Their chemical structure allows them to "bind" to fat molecules within the blood known as *lipids*. Because of this, these chemicals are often called *lipid-soluble*. Because fat molecules are used to build cell walls

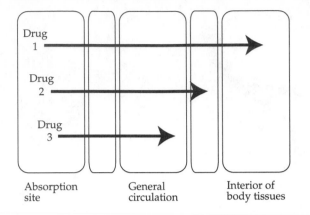

Absorption   General   Interior of
site   circulation   body tissues

Drug 1 is lipid-soluble, and because lipids penetrate the
    cell wall, it is able to penetrate into the interior of
    virtually all body tissues.

Drug 2 is not lipid-soluble. The drug is able to penetrate
    as far as the body fluids that surround each cell,
    but it cannot penetrate into the interior of the
    body tissues.

Drug 3 is protein-bound. It can penetrate only as far as the
    general circulation until it becomes "unbound," at
    which time it will move into category 1 or 2.

FIGURE 3.2 Example of drug penetration into body
compartments based on absorption characteristics.

within the body, lipids have the ability to rapidly
move out of the circulatory system into the body tissues
(Figure 3.2). Indeed, one characteristic of
blood lipids is that they are constantly passing out of
the circulatory system and into the body tissues.

Thus, lipid-soluble chemicals are distributed
throughout the body, especially to organs with a high
concentration of lipids. Compared with the other
organ systems in the body, which are made up of between
6 and 20% lipid molecules, fully 50% of the
weight of the brain consists of lipids (Cooper,
Bloom, & Roth, 1986). Thus, chemicals that are
highly lipid-soluble tend to rapidly concentrate
within the tissues of the brain. The ultrashort and
short-acting barbiturates are good examples of drugs
that are lipid-soluble. Although all the barbiturates
are lipid-soluble, there is a considerable range in the
speed with which various barbiturates can bind to
lipids. The speed at which a given barbiturate will
begin to have an effect will depend, in part, on its
ability to form bonds with lipid molecules. For the

ultrashort-acting barbiturates, which are extremely
lipid-soluble, the effects may be felt within seconds
after they are injected into a vein. This is one reason
the ultrashort duration barbiturates are so useful
as surgical anesthetics.

Remember that drug molecules are foreign substances
in the body. Their presence may be tolerated,
but only until the body's natural defenses
against chemical intruders can eliminate the foreign
substance. The body will thus be working to detoxify
(biotransform) and eliminate the foreign chemical
molecules in the body almost from the moment
that they arrive. One way that drugs avoid the danger
of biotransformation or elimination before they
have an effect is to join with protein molecules in
the blood. The chemical structures of many drugs
allow the individual molecules to bind with protein
molecules in the general circulation, especially the
one known as *albumin.* For this reason such chemicals
are said to become "protein-bound" (or, if they
bind to albumin, "albumin-bound").[4]

The advantage of protein binding is that while a
drug molecule is protein-bound, it is difficult for the
body to either metabolize or excrete it. The strength
of the chemical bond that forms between the chemical
and the protein molecules will vary. Some drugs
form stronger chemical bonds with protein molecules
than do others. The strength of this chemical
bond then determines how long the drug will remain
in the body before elimination.

The dilemma is that, while they are protein-bound,
drug molecules are also unable to have any
biological effect. Thus, to have an effect, the molecule
must be free of chemical bonds ("unbound").
Fortunately, although a chemical might be strongly
protein-bound, a certain percentage of the drug
molecules will always be unbound. For example, if
75% of a given drug's molecules are protein-bound,
then 25% of that drug's molecules are said to be unbound,
or free. It is this unbound fraction of drug
molecules that is able to have an effect on the bodily
function because it is biologically active. The protein-bound
molecules are unable to have any effect

---

[4] In general, acidic drugs tend to bind to albumin, while basic drugs
tend to bind to alpha$_1$-acid glycoprotein (Ciancio & Bourgault,
1989).

at the site of action and are biologically inactive (Rasymas, 1992; Shannon et al., 1995). Thus, for chemicals that are largely protein-bound, the unbound drug molecules must be extremely potent.

For example, the antidepressant amitriptyline is 95% protein-bound. This means that only 5% of a given dose of this drug is actually biologically active at any time (Ciraulo, Shader, Greenblatt, & Barnhill, 1995). Another drug that is strongly protein-bound is diazepam. Over 99% of the diazepam molecules that reach the general circulation will become protein-bound. Thus, the sedative effects of diazepam (see Chapter 7) are actually caused by the small fraction (approximately 1%) of the diazepam molecules that remain unbound.

As noted, unbound drug molecules may easily be metabolized and excreted (the process of metabolism and excretion of chemicals is discussed later in this chapter). Thus, an advantage of protein binding is that the protein-bound drug molecules form a reservoir of unmetabolized drug molecules. These unmetabolized molecules are gradually released back into the general circulation as the chemical bond between the drug and the protein molecules weakens. The newly released molecules then replace those that have been metabolized or excreted.

It is the *proportion* of unbound to bound molecules that remains approximately the same. Thus, if 75% of the drug were protein-bound and 25% was unbound when the drug was at its greatest concentration in the blood, then after some of that drug had been eliminated from the body, the proportion of bound to unbound drug would continue to be approximately 75:25. Although, at first glance, the last sentence might seem to be in error, remember that as some drug molecules are being removed from the general circulation, some protein-bound molecules are also breaking the chemical bonds to the protein molecules, to once again become unbound. Thus, while the amount of chemical in the general circulation will gradually diminish as the body biotransforms or eliminates the unbound drug molecules, the proportion of bound:unbound drug molecules will remain essentially unchanged.

The characteristic of protein binding actually is related to another trait of a drug: the biological half-life of that chemical. This topic is discussed in detail later in this chapter. However, protein binding allows the drug in question to have a longer duration of effect. The gradual release of the protein-bound molecules back into the general circulation over an extended period lengthens the total time during which that drug is present in sufficient quantities to remain biologically active.

Metabolism and Biotransformation

Because drugs are foreign substances, the natural defenses of the body try to eliminate the drug almost immediately. In some cases, the body is able to eliminate the drug without the need to modify its chemical structure. Penicillin is an example of a drug that is excreted unchanged from the body.

As a general rule, however, the chemical structure of drugs must be modified before they can be eliminated from the body. This process was once referred to as *detoxification*, but as researchers have learned how the body prepares a drug molecule for elimination, the term detoxification has been replaced with the term drug *metabolism* or, more accurately, *biotransformation*. The process of drug biotransformation takes place mainly in the liver, usually through enzymes produced by the region of the liver known as the *microsomal endoplasmic reticulum*. Technically, the new compound that emerges from each step of the process of drug biotransformation is known as a *metabolite* of the chemical that was admitted to the body. The original chemical is occasionally called the *parent compound* of the metabolite.

In general, metabolites are less biologically active than the parent compound. However, there are exceptions to this rule. Depending on the substance being biotransformed, the metabolite might actually have a psychoactive effect of its own. On rare occasions, a drug might actually have a metabolite that is actually more biologically active than the parent compound. This is why pharmacologists prefer to use the term biotransformation instead of detoxification.

While the liver is the organ in which drug metabolism is carried out, some biotransformation might also be carried out by other organs within the user's body. For example, as discussed in Chapter 4, at least some alcohol is biotransformed in the stomach, even before it is absorbed into the circulation.

Although we speak of drug biotransformation as if it were a single process, in reality there are four different subforms of metabolism (Ciraulo et al., 1995):

1. Oxidation.
2. Reduction.
3. Hydrolysis.
4. Conjugation.

The specifics of each form of drug metabolism are complex and best reserved for pharmacology texts. It is enough for the reader to remember that there are four different processes that are collectively called drug metabolism, or biotransformation. Many chemicals must go through more than one step in the biotransformation process, in preparation for the next step: *elimination*.

A major goal of the process of metabolism is to transform the foreign chemical into a form that can be rapidly eliminated from the body (Clark, Bratler, & Johnson, 1991). But this process does not take place instantly. Rather, the process of biotransformation is accomplished through chemical reactions facilitated by enzymes produced in the body. This process is carried out over a period of time, and depending on the drug involved, there are often a number of intermediate steps before that chemical is ready for elimination from the body.

In general, the goal of biotransformation is to change the chemical structure of the foreign substance to make it less lipid-soluble, and thus more easily eliminated from the body. There are two major subtypes of drug metabolism. In the first subtype, a constant fraction of the drug is biotransformed per hour. This is called a *first order biotransformation* process. Certain antibiotics are metabolized in this manner, with a set percentage of the medication in the body being biotransformed each hour. Other chemicals are eliminated from the body by what is known as a *zero order biotransformation* process. Drugs that are biotransformed through a zero order biotransformation process are metabolized at a set rate, no matter how high the concentration of that chemical in the blood. Alcohol is an example of a chemical that is biotransformed through a zero order biotransformation process.

As discussed in Chapter 4, alcohol is biotransformed at the rate of about what a person ingests when drinking one regular mixed drink,[5] or one 12-ounce can of beer, per hour. Whether the person ingests just one can of beer or one mixed drink, or 20 cans of beer or 20 mixed drinks in an hour, his or her body can biotransform only the equivalent of one can of beer/mixed drink per hour, for alcohol is biotransformed through a zero order biotransformation process.

Most of the chemicals that are administered orally must pass through the stomach, to the small intestine, before they can be absorbed. However, the human circulatory system is designed in such a way that chemicals absorbed through the gastrointestinal system are carried first to the liver. This makes sense, in that the liver is given the task of protecting the body from toxins. By taking chemicals absorbed from the gastrointestinal tract to the liver, the body is able to begin to break down any toxins in the substance that was introduced into the body, before those toxins can damage other organ systems.

One effect of this process is that the liver often biotransforms many orally administered medications before they have had a chance to reach the site of action. This is called *first pass metabolism*. First pass metabolism is one reason it is so hard to control pain through the use of orally administered narcotic analgesic medications. When taken by mouth, a significant part of the dose of an orally administered narcotic analgesic such as morphine will be metabolized by the liver into inactive forms *before* reaching the site of action.

Elimination

In the human body, biotransformation and elimination are closely intertwined. Indeed, some authorities on the subject of pharmacology consider these to be a single process, since one goal of the process of drug metabolism is to change the foreign chemical into a water-soluble metabolite that can then be easily removed from the circulation (Clark et al., 1991).

The most common method of drug elimination is through the kidneys (Benet et al., 1995). However, the biliary tract, lungs, and sweat glands may also

---

[5] A "regular" drink is 1 ounce of distilled spirits, 1 can 3.2 beer, or 4 ounces of wine.

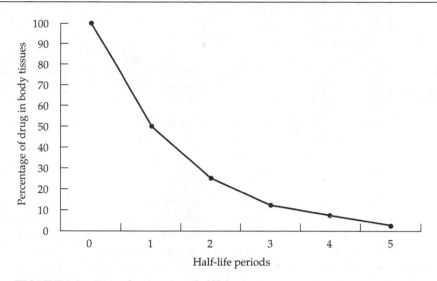

FIGURE 3.3 Drug elimination in half-life stages.

play a role in drug elimination (Shannon et al., 1995). For example, a small percentage of the alcohol that a person has ingested will be excreted when that person exhales. A small percentage of the alcohol in the system is also eliminated through the sweat glands. These characteristics of alcohol contribute to the characteristic smell of the intoxicated individual.

As discussed earlier in this chapter, some drugs are eliminated from the body virtually unchanged. These chemicals are introduced into the body in a form that may easily be removed from the general circulation without biotransformation. For example, penicillin is rapidly removed from the blood by the kidneys and is excreted in the urine in its active form. As discussed in Chapter 14, many of the inhalants, as well as many of the surgical anesthetics, are also eliminated from the body without being metabolized to any significant degree.

The Drug Half-Life

The speed at which the body is able to metabolize/eliminate a drug(s) illustrates a helpful concept that physicians use to estimate the period of time during which a chemical remains biologically active. This is the *biological half-life* of that chemical (sometimes abbreviated by the symbol $t_{1/2}$). The half-life of a chemical is the time needed for the individual's body to reduce the amount of active drug in the circulation by one-half (Benet et al., 1995). The concept of $t_{1/2}$ is based on the assumption that the individual ingested only one dose of the drug. While the $t_{1/2}$ concept is often a source of confusion even among health professionals, it allows health care workers to roughly estimate how long a drug's effects will last when that chemical is used at normal dosage levels.

A popular misconception is that it only takes two half-lives for the body to totally eliminate a drug. In reality, 25% of the original dose remains at the end of the second half-life period, and 12% of the original dose still is in the body at the end of three half-life periods. As a general rule, it takes five half-life periods for the body to eliminate virtually all of a single dose of a chemical (Williams & Baer, 1994). Figure 3.3 illustrates this process.

Generally, drugs with long half-life periods tend to remain biologically active for a longer time. The reverse is also true: chemicals with a short biological half-life tend to be active for shorter periods. This is where the process of protein binding comes into play: drugs with longer half-lives tend to become protein-bound. As stated earlier, protein binding allows a reservoir of an unmetabolized drug to gradually be released back into the general circulation, as the drug molecules become unbound. This allows a chemical to remain in the circulation at a sufficient concentration to have an effect for an extended period of time.

The Effective Dose

The concept of the *effective dose* (ED) is based on dose-response calculations, in which pharmacologists calculate the percentage of a population that will respond to a given dose of a chemical. Scientists usually estimate the percentage of the population that is expected to experience an effect by a chemical at different dosage levels. For example, the ED_{10} is that dosage level where 10% of the population will achieve the desired effects from the chemical being ingested, whereas the ED_{50} is the dosage level where 50% of the population would be expected to respond to the drug's effects. For medications, the goal is to find a dosage level that achieves response in the largest percentage of the population. However, you cannot simply keep increasing the dose of a medication; sooner or later you will raise the dosage level to the point where people start to become toxic, and quite possibly die, from the effects of the chemical.

The Lethal Dose Index

Drugs are, by their very nature, foreign to the body. By definition, drugs that are introduced into the body will disrupt its function in one way or another. Indeed, a characteristic of both legitimate pharmaceuticals and the drugs of abuse is that the person who administered that chemical hopes to alter the body's function to bring about a desired effect. But, chemicals introduced into the body hold the potential to disrupt the function of one or more organ systems to the point where it is no longer possible for those systems to function normally. Chemicals may even disrupt the body's activities to the point where the very life of the individual is in danger.

Scientists express this continuum as a form of modified dose-response curve. Instead of calculating the percentage of the population that would be expected to benefit from a certain exposure to a chemical, scientists calculate the percentage of the general population that would, in theory, die if exposed to a certain dose of a chemical or toxin (see Figure 3.4).

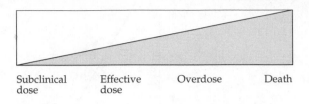

| Subclinical dose | Effective dose | Overdose | Death |

FIGURE 3.4   Theoretical range of a drug's effects on the user.

This figure is then expressed in terms of a *lethal dose* (or LD) ratio. The percentage of the population that would die as a result of exposure to that chemical/toxin source is identified as a subscript to the LD heading. Thus, if a certain level of exposure to a chemical or toxin resulted in a 25% death rate, this would be abbreviated as the LD_{25} for that chemical or toxin. A level of exposure to a toxin or chemical that resulted in a 50% death rate would be abbreviated the LD_{50} for that substance.

For example, as discussed in Chapter 4, a person with a blood alcohol level of .350 mg/mL would stand a 1% chance of death, without medical intervention. Thus, a blood alcohol level of .350 mg/mL is the LD_{01} for alcohol. It is possible to calculate the potential lethal exposure level for virtually every chemical. These figures provide scientists with a way to calculate the relative safety of different levels of exposure to chemicals or radiation and a way to determine when medical intervention is necessary.

The Therapeutic Index

In addition to their potential to benefit the user, drugs also have negative effects. Since they are foreign substances being introduced into the body, there is a danger that, if used in too large an amount, the drug might actually harm, rather than help, the person.

Scientists have devised what is known as the Therapeutic Index (TI) as a way to measure the relative safety of a chemical. The TI is the ratio between the ED_{50}, and the LD_{50}, that is, between the effectiveness of a chemical and the potential for harm inherent in using it. A smaller TI means that there is only a small margin between the dosage level needed to achieve the therapeutic effects, and the

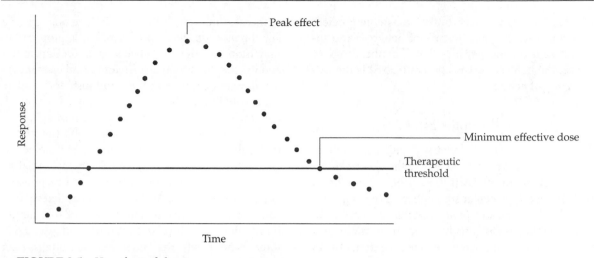

FIGURE 3.5   Hypothetical dose-response curve.

dosage level at which the drug becomes toxic to the individual. A large TI suggests that there is considerable latitude between the normal therapeutic dosage range, and the dosage level at which that chemical might become toxic to the user.

As noted in the following chapters, many drugs of abuse have a small TI. These chemicals are potentially toxic to the user. For example, the ratio between the normal dosage range and the toxic dosage range for the barbiturates is only about 3:1. In contrast, the ratio between the normal dosage range and the toxic dosage level for the benzodiazepines is estimated to be about 200:1. Thus, relatively speaking, the benzodiazepines are much safer than the barbiturates.

Peak Effects

The effects of a chemical within the body develop over a period of time, until the drug reaches what is known as the *therapeutic threshold*. The therapeutic threshold is the point at which the concentration of a specific chemical in the body allows it to begin to have the desired effect on the user. The chemical's effects become stronger and stronger until, finally, the strongest possible effects from a dose of that drug are reached. This is the period of *peak effects*. Then, gradually, the impact of the drug becomes less and less pronounced as the chemical is eliminated or biotransformed over a period of time. Eventually, the concentration of the chemical in the body falls

below the therapeutic level. As shown in Figure 3.5, scientists have learned to calculate dose-response curves, to estimate the potential for a chemical to have an effect at any given point in time after it was administered.

The period of peak effects following a single dose of a drug varies from one chemical to another. For example, the peak effects of an ultrashort-acting barbiturate might be achieved in a matter of seconds following a single dose, while the long-term barbiturate phenobarbital might take hours to achieve its strongest effects. Thus, clinicians must remember that the period of peak effects following a single dose of a chemical will vary for each chemical.

The Site of Action

To illustrate the concept of the *site of action*, consider the case of a person with an athlete's foot infection. This condition is caused by a fungus that attacks the skin. The individual with this infection wants to get rid of it and goes to the pharmacy, where several excellent over-the-counter antifungal compounds are available. The person selects one, and then applies it to the infected area on his body, to cure the condition.

Although it is not the purpose of this chapter to sell antifungal compounds, this example illustrates the use of a drug at the *site of action*. To put it simply, the site of action is where the drug being used will have its prime effect. In the case of the medication for athlete's foot, the site of action is the infected skin on the person's foot. For the drugs of abuse, the central nervous system (CNS) is the primary site of action.

Receptor Sites

The *receptor site* is the exact spot either in the cell wall, or within the cell itself, where the chemical carries out its main effects (Olson, 1992). Most drugs bind to specific receptor sites either on the cell wall, or with one of various proteins within the cell itself. The receptor site is usually a pattern of molecules that, by coincidence, allow a single drug molecule to attach itself to the target portion of the cell at that point. For example, bacteria that are susceptible to the antibiotic penicillin have a characteristic receptor site, the enzyme transpeptidase, that allows the antibiotic to work against that specific germ. This enzyme carries out an essential role in bacterial reproduction. By blocking the action of transpeptidase, penicillin prevents the multiplication of the bacteria. Eventually, as the individual bacteria cells continue to grow without being able to multiply, they destroy themselves.

The drugs of abuse achieve their main effects by altering the function of the individual nerve cells *(neurons)* within specific regions of the CNS. Drugs accomplish this by either simulating, or influencing, the action of chemical messengers *(neurotransmitters)* that pass between neurons. These neurotransmitters are the means by which neurons communicate with each other. By altering the action of certain neurotransmitters in specific regions of the brain, it is possible to alter the individual's subjective perception of the world around him/her.

Although the adult human brain is perhaps the most complex, and most certainly the most compact, organ in the body, the individual neurons actually do not touch each other. Rather, microscopic examination of the brain reveals that the neurons are separated by small spaces, known as the *synapse.* To pass information across this gap, one neuron will release a small amount of a chemical from the end of its axon. Some of these molecules will drift across the synapse to receptor sites located on the cell wall

of the next neuron in the circuit. The analogy of a key slipping into the slot of a lock is appropriate to understanding the fit between a neurotransmitter and its receptor site. If a sufficient number of receptor sites are occupied at the same instant, the electrical potential of the receiving neuron is changed, and it will pass the message on to the next cell.

Following the release of the neurotransmitter molecules, the first neuron will activate molecular "pumps" that absorb as many of the free-floating neurotransmitter molecules that were just released as possible, for reuse. At the same time, that neuron will also work to manufacture more of that neurotransmitter for future use, storing both the reabsorbed and newly manufactured neurotransmitter molecules in special sacks within the nerve cell until needed. Figure 3.6 is a diagram of the neurotransmitter process.

All the known chemicals that function as neurotransmitters within the CNS fall into two groups: those that stimulate the neuron to release a chemical message to the next cell, and, those that inhibit the release of neurotransmitters. By altering the flow of these two classes of neurotransmitters, the drugs of abuse alter the way that the CNS functions.

Upregulation and Downregulation

The individual neurons of the CNS are not passive participants in the process of information transfer. Each neuron is constantly adapting itself to the level of activity demanded of it by either increasing, or decreasing, the possible number of neurotransmitter receptor sites on the cell wall. If a neuron is subjected to high levels of a given neurotransmitter, or a similar chemical, that nerve cell will respond by increasing the number of possible receptor sites in the cell wall. This will give the neurotransmitter molecules a larger number of possible "targets" (receptor sites), reducing the frequency with which that neuron will be required to "fire." Scientists call this process *upregulation* and it is one reason a person becomes tolerant to a drug's effects.

In many cases, if there is a significant drop in the number of neurotransmitter molecules being released by one neuron, the next neuron in line will decrease the total number of possible receptor sites by absorbing/inactivating some of the receptor sites

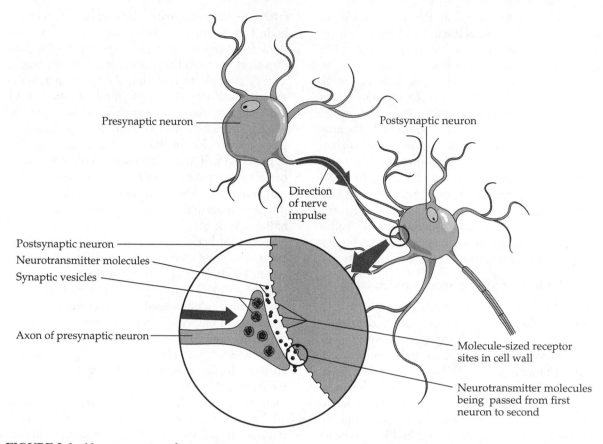

Presynaptic neuron

Postsynaptic neuron

Direction
of nerve
impulse

Postsynaptic neuron

Neurotransmitter molecules

Synaptic vesicles

Axon of presynaptic neuron

Molecule-sized receptor
sites in cell wall

Neurotransmitter molecules
being passed from first
neuron to second

FIGURE 3.6 Neurotransmitter diagram.

in the cell wall. This is the process of *downregulation,* by which a neuron decreases the total number of receptor sites necessary to cause it to fire. To better understand the process of upregulation/downregulation, remember that for a given neuron to fire, a *certain percentage* of the receptor sites must be occupied at the same instant. If there is a surplus of neurotransmitter molecules arriving at the receptor sites, the neuron will be forced to fire frequently, possibly causing false signals. To reduce this occurrence, the neuron increases the total number of possible receptor sites, but the *critical percentage required to activate that neuron remains the same.*

For example, assume that 70% of the receptor sites must be occupied in the same instant, before a given neuron can fire. Rather than firing each time 70% of 200 receptor sites are occupied by a neurotransmitter molecule, the process of upregulation

allows a neuron to increase the number of receptor sites to perhaps 400. It would require a large number of neurotransmitter molecules to reach the critical figure of 70% of these 400 receptor sites, allowing that neuron to reduce its firing rate. During periods of neurotransmitter surplus, neurons in many regions of the brain will upregulate the number of receptor sites. During times of neurotransmitter deficit, these same neurons will tend to downregulate the number of receptor sites to try and maintain a relatively constant firing rate.

Tolerance and Cross-Tolerance

The concept of drug tolerance was introduced in Chapter 2. In brief, tolerance is a reflection of the body's ongoing struggle to maintain normal function. Because a drug is a foreign substance, the body will attempt to continue its normal function, despite the presence of the chemical. Part of the process of adaptation in the CNS is the upregulation/downregulation of receptor sites, as the neurons attempt to maintain a normal level of firing.

As the body adapts to the effects of the chemical, the individual will find that he/she no longer achieves the same effect from the original dose and must use larger and larger doses to maintain the original effect. When a chemical is used as a neuropharmaceutical (i.e., intentionally introduced into the body by a physician to alter the function of the CNS in a desired manner), tolerance is often referred to as *neuroadaptation.* If the drug being used is a recreational substance, the same process is usually called "tolerance." However, neuroadaptation and tolerance are essentially the same biological adaptation.

The Concepts of Drug Agonist and Antagonist

To understand how the drugs of abuse work, it is necessary to introduce the twin concepts of drug *agonist* and *antagonist.* A drug agonist mimics the effect(s) of a chemical that is naturally found in the body (Shannon et al., 1995). The agonist either tricks the body into reacting as if the endogenous chemical were present, or it enhances the effect(s) of the naturally occurring chemical. For example, as discussed in Chapter 11, morphinelike chemicals found in the human brain help to control the level of pain that the individual experiences. Heroin, morphine, and the other narcotic analgesics mimic the actions of these chemicals and, for this reason, can be classified as agonists of the naturally occurring painkilling chemicals.

The antagonist blocks the effects of a chemical already working within the body. In a sense, aspirin might be classified as the prostaglandin antagonist, because aspirin blocks the normal actions of the prostaglandins. Antagonists may also block the effects of certain chemicals introduced into the body for one reason or another. The drug Narcan blocks the receptor sites in the CNS that opiates normally bind to in order to have their effect. Narcan thus is an antagonist for opiates and is of value in reversing the effects of an opiate overdose.

Because the drugs of abuse either simulate the effects of actual neurotransmitters or alter the action of existing neurotransmitters, they either enhance or

retard the frequency with which the neurons of the brain fire (Ciancio & Bourgault, 1989). The constant use of any of the drugs of abuse forces the neurons to go through the process of neuroadaptation, as they struggle to maintain normal function despite the artificial stimulation/inhibition caused by the drugs of abuse. Depending on whether the drug(s) of abuse cause a surplus/deficit of neurotransmitter molecules, the neurons in many regions of the brain will upregulate/downregulate the number of receptor sites, in an attempt to maintain normal function. This will affect the individual's responsiveness to that drug over time, which is part of the process of tolerance.

When the body begins to adapt to the presence of one chemical, it often also becomes tolerant to the effects of other drug(s) that use the same mechanism of action. This is the process of *cross-tolerance.* For example, a chronic alcohol user often requires higher doses of CNS depressants than a nondrinker to achieve a given level of sedation. Physicians have often noticed this effect in the surgical theater: chronic alcohol users require larger doses of anesthetics to achieve a given level of unconsciousness than nondrinkers. Because anesthetics and alcohol are both classified as CNS depressants, the individual's development of cross-tolerance requires the administration of a larger dose of many anesthetics, before surgery can proceed.

The Blood-Brain Barrier

The blood-brain barrier (BBB) is a unique structure in the human body. Its role is to function as a gateway to the brain by permitting only certain necessary molecules to pass through to the brain. For example, oxygen and glucose, both essential to life, will pass easily through the BBB (Angier, 1990). The BBB exists to protect the brain from toxins or infectious organisms. To this end, endothelial cells that form the lining of the BBB have established tight seals, with overlapping cells.

Initially, students of neuroanatomy may be confused by the term blood-brain barrier, for when we speak of a "barrier," we are usually describing a single structure. But the BBB actually is the result of a unique feature of the cells that form the capillaries through which cerebral blood flows. Unlike capillary walls throughout the rest of the body, those of the cerebral circulatory system are securely joined together. Each endothelial cell is tightly joined to its neighbors, forming a tight tubelike structure that protects the brain from direct contact with the general circulation. Thus, many chemicals in the general circulation are blocked from entering the CNS. However, the individual cells of the brain require nutritional support, and some of the very substances needed by the brain are those blocked by the endothelial cell boundary. Thus, water-soluble substances like glucose or iron, needed by the neurons of the brain for proper function, are blocked by the lining of the endothelial cells.

To overcome this problem specialized "transport systems" have evolved in the endothelial cells in the cerebral circulatory system. These transport systems selectively allow needed nutrients to pass through the BBB and reach the brain (Angier, 1990). Each of these transport systems selectively allows one specific type of water-soluble molecule, such as glucose, to pass through the lining of the endothelial cell, to reach the brain.

But lipids also pass through the lining of the endothelial cells and are able to reach the central nervous system beyond. Lipids are molecules of fat and are essential elements of cell walls, which are made up of lipids, carbohydrates, and protein molecules,

arranged in a specific order. As the lipid molecule reaches the endothelial cell wall, it gradually merges with the molecules of the cell wall, and passes through into the interior of the endothelial cell. Later, it will also pass through the lining of the far side of the endothelial cell, to reach the neurons beyond the lining of the blood-brain barrier.

Summary

In this chapter, we have examined some of the basic components of pharmacology. It is not necessary for students in the field of substance abuse to have the same depth of knowledge possessed by pharmacists to understand how the recreational chemicals achieve their effects. However, it is important for the reader to learn the basic concepts of pharmacology, in order to recognize how the drugs of abuse achieve their primary and secondary effects. Drug forms, methods of drug administration, and biotransformation/elimination were discussed in this chapter.

Other concepts discussed include those of a drug's bioavailability, the therapeutic half-life of a chemical, the effective dose and lethal dose ratios, the therapeutic dose ratio, and the role of receptor sites in processing a drug through the body. The student should understand these concepts before starting to review the drugs of abuse discussed in the following chapters.

CHAPTER FOUR

An Introduction to Alcohol

A *Brief Summary of the Acute Effects of the First Recreational Chemical*

Historians believe that, thousands of years ago, early humans learned about intoxication by watching animals eat fermented fruits from the forest floor. Observing this behavior, our ancestors must have wondered why the animals seemed to go out of their way to ingest the fermented fruits. So, one or two brave souls tried some of the fermented fruit, become intoxicated themselves, and promptly spread the word to their friends (R. L. Siegel, 1986). Over time, prehistoric humans went about trying to reproduce the effect and eventually discovered how to produce alcoholic beverages.

The regular use of alcohol thus probably became commonplace well before the advent of written history. It is not unrealistic to say that "alcohol and the privilege of drinking have always been important to human beings" (S. A. Brown, 1995, p. 4). Indeed, alcohol could be viewed as a yardstick for measuring cultural development. As Beasley (1987) suggested:

> Virtually all cultures in time and place—whether hunter-gatherers or farmers; whether technologically advanced or primitive—share two universals: the development of a noodle and the discovery and use of the natural fermentation process. (p. 17)

Some anthropologists now believe that early civilization came about in response to the need for a stable home base from which to brew *mead*, a form of beer made from fermented honey (Stone, 1991). If this theory is correct, then it would seem that

human civilization owes much to alcohol, which is also known as ethanol, or *ethyl alcohol.*[1]

A Brief History of Alcohol

The earliest written records of beer making date back only 4,000 years, to approximately 1800 B.C. (Stone, 1991). However, historical evidence suggests that a form of beer was in common use around the year 8000 B.C. (Ray & Ksir, 1993).[2] This beer was quite unlike modern brews. The thick liquid was quite nutritious and provided necessary vitamins and amino acids to the diet of the drinker. When compared with the beer of our prehistoric ancestors, modern beer is very thin and almost anemic.

The earliest written record of wine making is found in an Egyptian tomb from around the year 3000 B.C. (*Los Angeles Times*, 1996a). At about this same time, the ancient Egyptians worshiped Osiris both as the god of wine and as the ruler of the dead (Bohn, 1993). But the production of wine would seem to date back much further than 3000 B.C. By using special equipment to examine the residue of

---

[1] Other forms of alcohol also exist, but these are not normally used for human consumption and will not be discussed further here. It is enough to understand that ethyl alcohol has been with us for a long, long time.

[2] Remember that the year 2000 is approaching. Thus, 8000 B.C. was 10,000 years ago.

clay pots found in Iran, archaeologists have recently discovered evidence that suggests that ancient Sumerians might have used wine made from fermented grapes in the year 5400 B.C. (*Los Angeles Times,* 1996a). Beer and wine are also mentioned several times in Homer's *Iliad* and *Odyssey,* legends that date back thousands of years. Thus, a significant body of evidence indicates that humans have known how to produce alcoholic beverages, and have recognized something of their effects on the user, for thousands of years.

How Alcohol Is Produced

By whatever means, somehow humans discovered that if you crush certain fruits and allow the juice or pulp to stand for a period of time in a container, alcohol is produced. We now know that unseen microorganisms called yeast, which float in the air, settle on the crushed fruit and multiply, and begin to digest the sugars in the fruit through a chemical process called *fermentation.* The yeast breaks down the carbon, hydrogen, and oxygen atoms it finds in the sugar for food, and in the process produces molecules of ethyl alcohol and carbon dioxide as waste.

Thus, alcohol is actually a waste product of certain yeast as these microorganisms grow. Like other waste products, it is a poison, a toxin. When the concentration of alcohol in a certain area reaches about 15%, it becomes toxic to the yeast. The microscopic yeast begin to die, and fermentation stops. Thus, since before the time of Babylon, humans have been able to produce alcoholic beverages with a concentration of alcohol as high as about 15%.

Several thousand years elapsed before humans learned to obtain alcohol concentrations above the 15% limit imposed by the nature of yeast. This is accomplished by the process of *distillation,* which appeared just over 1100 years ago, around the year A.D. 800. At some point, an unknown experimenter discovered that alcohol boils at a much lower temperature than does water. Because this is true, the steam that forms when wine is boiled contains more alcohol than water vapor. By heating wine, then collecting the vapor and letting it cool down into a liquid again, it is possible to obtain a liquid with an alcohol

content far higher than the 15% limit found in wine. This process is called distillation.

In the process of distillation, wine is heated, causing some of the alcohol content to boil off as a vapor, or steam. The steam is then collected in a special cooling coil, which allows the vapor to cool down, forming a liquid again. This liquid contains a higher concentration of alcohol, and a lower concentration of water, than did the original mixture. The liquid, with its higher alcohol content, then drips from the end of the coil into a container of some kind. This device is the famous "still" of lore and legend.

For thousands of years, wine or beer was considered a necessary part of any meal. For example, Homer's *Iliad* and *Odyssey* describe people drinking wine with meals.[3] Even today, in some parts of the world, people drink wine with meals on a regular basis. Further, wine may supply valuable vitamins and minerals to the individual's diet. In the process of distillation, however, many vitamins and minerals in the original wine are lost. Further, when the body breaks down alcohol, it finds empty calories. As discussed later in this chapter, when alcohol is metabolized by the body, it is eventually transformed into a form of carbohydrate and carbon dioxide. While the body obtains carbohydrate from the metabolism of alcohol, it does so without the protein, vitamins, and minerals that it needs. Over time, this may contribute to a state of vitamin depletion called *avitaminosis* (see Chapter 5).

Within two centuries of its discovery, the process of distillation had spread from Arabia, where it was developed, to Europe. It is reported that by the year A.D. 1000, Italian winegrowers were distilling wine to produce drinks with higher concentrations of alcohol, mixing the obtained distilled "spirits" with various herbs and spices to produce different flavors. This mixture was then used for medicinal purposes. Distilled spirits were viewed as the ultimate medicines in Europe, where they were called the *aqua vitae,* or the water of life (Ray & Ksir, 1993). Since at least the Renaissance, there have been attempts to control or regulate alcohol use in Europe and the

---

[3] When the Puritans arrived in Massachusetts in 1620, they carried with them 14 tons of water, and 42 tons of beer (Freeborn, 1996).

New World. These attempts at regulation have been almost uniformly unsuccessful.

Alcohol Today

Over the past 900 years since the development of the distillation process, fermented wines using various ingredients, different kinds of beer, and distilled spirits combined with flavorings have emerged. With the march of civilization, some degree of standardization has resulted in uniform definitions of classes of alcohol, although some regional variation still exists.

Today, most American beer has an alcohol content of between 3.5% and 5% (R. Herman, 1993). As a class, wine continues to be made by allowing fermentation to take place in vats containing grapes, or other fruits. Occasionally, the fermentation involves other products than grapes, such as the famous rice wine from Japan called *sake*. In this country, wine tends to have an alcohol content ranging from 8% to 17% (R. Herman, 1993), and there are only minor variations in how different wines are made.

In addition to wine, there are the "fortified" wines. These are produced by adding distilled wine to fermented wine, to raise the total alcohol content to about 20%. This class contains the varieties of sherry and port (R. Herman, 1993). Finally, there are the "hard liquors," the distilled spirits, whose alcohol content may range from 20% to 95% (in the case of "Everclear" and similar distilled spirits). These beverages are often mixed with fruits and seasonings, to give them characteristic flavors.

Scope of the Problem of Alcohol Use

Alcoholic beverages are moderately popular drinks. Approximately 90% of the adults in the United States have consumed alcohol at some point in their lives (Schuckit, 1995a). Given its popularity, many people are surprised to learn that alcohol consumption in the United States peaked almost two centuries ago, around the year 1830. At that time, the annual per capita consumption of alcohol was an estimated 7.1 gallons of pure alcohol (Heerema, 1990; Musto, 1996). Within the last generation, alcohol use in the United States peaked at about 2.76 gallons of pure alcohol per person, in the year 1980. By 1996 this

figure had fallen 15%, to about 2.35 gallons of pure alcohol per person per year in the United States (Musto, 1996).

When one stops to consider that the majority of those who consume alcohol do so less than once a week, it becomes apparent that a minority of those who use alcohol consume a disproportionate amount of this beverage. In reality, 10% of those who drink consume 50% of the alcohol used in this country (Kaplan et al., 1994). These are the individuals whose alcohol use will interfere with their physical health, and, their social well-being. The impact of excess alcohol use is discussed in detail in Chapter 5. In this chapter, we focus on the casual drinker.

The Pharmacology of Alcohol

Ethyl alcohol, or simply "alcohol," is usually consumed orally in a liquid form. Actually, alcohol may also be introduced into the body intravenously, or even as a vapor. However these methods are very dangerous and are used by physicians only in extremely rare cases. This section covers orally administered alcohol in great detail since in the majority of cases people drink the alcohol that enters their body.

The alcohol molecule is quite small and is soluble in both water and lipids. Because of this characteristic, alcohol molecules are rapidly distributed to all blood-rich tissues throughout the body, including the brain. Because alcohol is so easily soluble in lipids, high concentrations of alcohol in the brain are rapidly achieved. The alcohol that a person consumes is distributed not only to the brain but throughout the body. Since alcohol also diffuses into muscle and fat tissues, an obese or muscular person would normally have a slightly lower blood alcohol level than would a lean person after a given dose.

When a person drinks on an empty stomach, the first alcohol molecules will appear in the bloodstream in as little as one minute (Rose, 1988). Ultimately, between 10% (Kaplan et al., 1994) to 20% (Julien, 1992) of the alcohol will be immediately absorbed into the circulation through the stomach lining. The remainder of the alcohol is absorbed through the small intestine, after the stomach empties its contents into the intestinal tract. If the person has consumed alcohol as part of a meal, the food will slow the absorption of the alcohol until the stomach empties its contents into the small intestine, with the result being that less of the alcohol is absorbed through the stomach lining.

It was once thought that the speed at which the alcohol entered the bloodstream, and thus was biotransformed by the liver, was determined by how quickly the stomach empties into the small intestine. This is to say that it was once thought that, sooner or later, all of the alcohol that was ingested would be absorbed (Julien, 1992).

However, research (Frezza et al., 1990) suggests that for some drinkers the process of alcohol biotransformation actually begins in the gastrointestinal tract. At least for some drinkers, the body begins to break down the alcohol even before it reaches the general circulation. The authors found that people produce an enzyme in the gastrointestinal tract known as *gastric alcohol dehydrogenase*. This enzyme begins to break down alcohol in the stomach, even before it reaches the bloodstream. The authors found that gastric alcohol dehydrogenase levels are highest in rare social drinkers, and are significantly lower in those individuals who ingest alcohol on a regular basis. Further, men produced more of this enzyme than did women, a discovery that the authors concluded might explain why women often have higher blood alcohol levels than men after drinking a similar amount of alcohol.

A popular folk remedy for the hangover is for the individual to ingest aspirin before drinking, so that the aspirin is already in the system for the morning after. Surprisingly, research has suggested that the use of aspirin an hour prior to drinking alcohol will decrease the effectiveness of gastric alcohol dehydrogenase. This will result in a higher blood alcohol level for the rare social drinker than had been intended (Roine, Gentry, Hernandez-Munoz, Baraona, & Lieber, 1990).

Within the brain, alcohol has a number of effects on the cellular and regional levels. On the cellular level, researchers have suggested several different theories to explain the effects of alcohol on the brain. It was once thought that alcohol's effects were caused by its ability to disrupt the structure and the function of the lipids in the walls of the neurons. Along with protein molecules, lipid molecules help to form the cell walls of the neurons in the brain. This theory dates back to the turn of the century (Tabakoff & Hoffman, 1992) and is known as the *membrane fluidization theory* or the *membrane hypothesis.*

In the late 1970s, researchers developed the techniques needed to measure actual alcohol-induced changes in the membranes of neurons. They discovered that alcohol is able to disrupt the structure of lipids, making it more difficult for the neurons to maintain normal function. However, researchers are still not sure which lipids are affected by alcohol or which components within the neuron are most sensitive to alcohol's effects. There are strong reasons to question whether the membrane hypothesis can account for alcohol's observed effects.

Another theory suggests that on the cellular level alcohol disrupts the normal function of neurons in the brain by interacting with protein molecules within the walls of brain cells (Tabakoff & Hoffman, 1992; Tsai, Gastfriend, & Coyle, 1995). These protein molecules help to form the ion channels and neurotransmitter receptor sites in the walls of neurons. Other protein molecules help to form some of the enzymes found in the brain (Tabakoff & Hoffman). It is thought that through the interaction with protein molecules in a neurotransmitter receptor site or sites, alcohol is able to interfere with the normal function of individual neurons and cause the characteristic feeling of intoxication for the drinker.

The neurons of the brain are actually microscopic chemical-electrical generators that produce a small electrical "message" by actively moving sodium and calcium ions into the cell and back out again. The sodium and calcium ions pass through the cell wall through special channels formed by protein molecules. Researchers think that at least some of alcohol's effects might be caused by the ability of this chemical to interact with the protein molecules that form the sodium/calcium ion channels.

Any chemical that interacts with the protein molecules that form sodium/calcium ion channels in the cell wall of the body's tissues will affect how those cells function. Neuropsychopharmacologists have discovered that alcohol inhibits the action of the amino acid *N-methyl-D-aspartate* (NMDA), which functions as an excitatory amino acid within the brain (Hobbs, Rall, & Verdoorn, 1995; Tsai et al., 1995). Alcohol does this by blocking the influx of calcium atoms through the ion channels normally activated when NMDA binds at those sites. In a very real sense, alcohol might be said to be an NMDA antagonist (Tsai et al.).

At the same time, alcohol enhances the influx of chloride atoms through an ion channel at the receptor site utilized by gamma-aminobutyric acid (GABA) (Marshall, 1994). GABA is the main inhibitory neurotransmitter in the brain (Tabakoff & Hoffman, 1992). Neurons that utilize GABA are found in the cortex, cerebellum (which is a region of the brain involved in motor coordination, among other things), the hippocampus (a region of the brain involved in memory formation) the superior and inferior colliculi regions of the brain, the amygdala, and the nucleus accumbens.

By blocking the effects of the excitatory amino acid NMDA while facilitating the inhibitory neurotransmitter GABA in these regions of the brain, alcohol depresses the action of the central nervous system. Evidence suggests that the euphoria that some drinkers experience from alcohol is brought on by the ability of this chemical to activate the endorphin reward system within the brain (Nutt, 1996; Volpicelli, Clay, Watson, & Volpicelli, 1994). However, other researchers believe that alcohol's euphoric effects are brought on by its ability to stimulate the release of the neurotransmitter dopamine, especially in the nucleus accumbens region of the brain, which is thought to be the brain's "pleasure center." By stimulating the release of dopamine in this part of the brain, alcohol causes the user to experience a sense of pleasure, or euphoria.

Alcohol also stimulates the release of the neurotransmitter serotonin in many regions of the brain. Researchers have discovered that when alcohol is used in low to moderate concentrations, it seems to potentiate the effects of serotonin at one of the subtypes of receptor sites used by this neurotransmitter (Hobbs et al., 1995). This receptor site is located on certain neurons that inhibit behavioral impulses, and it is this action that seems to account at least in part for alcohol's disinhibitory effects.

Scientists still do not completely understand, or agree, how alcohol affects the function of either individual neurons or different regions of the human brain. But they generally agree that alcohol is a potent drug of abuse affecting the normal function of virtually every neuron in the central nervous system.

The Biotransformation of Alcohol

About 95% of the alcohol that reaches the blood is metabolized by the liver before it is excreted (Brennan, Betzelos, Reed, & Falk, 1995). The other 5% of the alcohol found in the bloodstream is excreted unchanged through the lungs, skin, and the urine (Ashton, 1992; Brennan et al., 1995). Alcohol is biotransformed at about the rate of one-third of an ounce of pure alcohol per hour in the normal, healthy individual. This is accomplished in two steps. First, the liver produces an enzyme known as *alcohol dehydrogenase* (ADH), which breaks the alcohol down into acetaldehyde. Unlike many of the enzymes produced in the body, which play multiple roles in different organs, ADH has no known function other than to metabolize alcohol (Goodwin, 1989). The exact reason for this specialization is not known.

Acetaldehyde is toxic and, if left in the body, will cause significant harm. Fortunately, many different parts of the body produce a second enzyme, *aldehyde dehydrogenase*, which breaks acetaldehyde down into acetic acid.[4] Ultimately, alcohol is biotransformed into carbon dioxide, water, and fatty acids (carbohydrates). These latter are the source of the empty calories obtained by the body when the individual ingests alcohol (Goodwin, 1989). As discussed in Chapter 5, chronic alcohol abusers can obtain a significant portion of his/her daily energy requirements from the empty calories obtained from alcohol.

The Speed of Alcohol Biotransformation

A rule of thumb for estimating the rate at which the body can metabolize alcohol is that the liver can biotransform about one mixed drink of 80 proof alcohol, or one can of beer, per hour (Maguire, 1990). As

---

[4]The medication Antabuse (disulfiram) works by blocking the enzyme aldehyde dehydrogenase. This allows acetaldehyde to build up in the blood, causing the individual to become ill from its toxic effects.

discussed in Chapter 3, however, alcohol is biotransformed through a zero order biotransformation process. The rate at which alcohol is metabolized by the liver is "independent of the concentration of alcohol in the blood" (Julien, 1992, p. 72). If a person drinks at about the rate of one ounce of whiskey (or one 5-ounce glass of wine, or a 12-ounce can of beer) per hour, the individual's body can metabolize the alcohol at a rate fairly close to the speed at which that person is consuming alcohol. If, as is often the case, the person consumes more than one ounce of whiskey, or one can of beer, per hour, the amount of alcohol in the bloodstream increases, possibly to the point where the drinker becomes intoxicated.

The Alcohol-Flush Reaction

After drinking even a small amount of alcohol, a small group of people in this country, and perhaps 50% of the population of Asia, experience what is known as the *alcohol-flush reaction*. The alcohol-flush reaction is caused by a genetic mutation found predominantly in persons of Asian descent. Because of this genetic mutation, the liver is unable to manufacture sufficient aldehyde dehydrogenase for it to rapidly metabolize the acetaldehyde manufactured in the first stage of alcohol biotransformation.

Persons with the alcohol-flush syndrome will experience symptoms such as facial flushing, heart palpitations, dizziness, and nausea as the blood levels of acetaldehyde climb to 20 times the level typically seen in individuals consuming the same amount of alcohol. As discussed earlier, acetaldehyde is a toxin, and the person with a significant amount of this chemical in his/her blood will become quite ill. This phenomenon is thought to be one reason heavy drinking is so rare in persons of Asian descent.

The Blood Alcohol Level

Because it is not possible to measure the alcohol level in the brain of a living person, physicians have developed an indirect measure of the amount of alcohol in a person's body. This is accomplished through a measurement known as the blood alcohol level (BAL). The BAL is a measure of the level of alcohol actually in a given person's bloodstream. It is reported in terms of milligrams of alcohol per 100

milliliters of blood (mg/mL). A BAL of 0.10 is thus one-tenth of a milligram of alcohol per 100 milliliters of blood.

Surprisingly, researchers have discovered that there is only a mild relationship between the BAL and the individual's *subjective* level of intoxication. For reasons that are still not clear, the individual's subjective level of intoxication is highest when the BAL is still rising, a phenomenon known as the *Mellanby effect* (Lehman, Pilich, & Andrews, 1994). Further, as discussed in Chapter 5, individuals who drink on a chronic basis become somewhat tolerant to the intoxicating effects of alcohol. Thus, a person who is tolerant to the effects of alcohol may have a rather high BAL, while appearing relatively normal.

Although the BAL provides a *crude* estimate of the individual's level of intoxication, it is far from perfect. Further, several factors can affect the BAL achieved by two people who consume a similar amount of alcohol. For example, the body size (volume) of the drinker influences the BAL. Remember that once it is in the body, the alcohol molecule rapidly diffuses into *all* body tissues. Because larger individuals have a greater body mass, the alcohol has a greater body volume to diffuse into.

To illustrate this confusing characteristic of alcohol, consider the hypothetical example of a person who weighs 100 pounds, who consumed two regular drinks in one hour's time. Blood tests would reveal that this individual had a BAL of 0.09 mg/mL (slightly below legal intoxication in most states) (Maguire, 1990). But, an individual who weighs 200 pounds would, after consuming the same amount of alcohol, have a measured BAL of only 0.04 mg/mL. Each person would have consumed the same amount of alcohol, but it would be more concentrated in the smaller individual, resulting in a higher BAL.

Other factors influence the speed with which alcohol enters the blood and raises the individual's blood alcohol level, but Figure 4.1[5] provides a rough estimate of the blood alcohol levels that might be

[5] This chart is provided only as an illustration and is not sufficiently accurate to be used as legal evidence or as a guide to "safe" drinking. Individual blood alcohol levels from the same dose of alcohol vary widely, and these figures provide an average blood alcohol level for an individual of a given body weight.

Weight (pounds)

		100	120	140	160	180	200	220
	2	.07	.06	.05	.05*	.04	.04*	.03
	3	.10	.09	.07	.07*	.06	.05	.05*
	4	.14	.11	.10	.08	.08*	.07	.06
	5	.18	.14	.12	.11	.10	.08	.08*
	6	.20	.18	.14	.12	.12*	.10	.09
	7	.25	.20	.18	.16	.12	.12*	.11
	8	.30	.25	.20	.18	.16	.14	.12

Number of drinks in one hour

*Rounded off   Level of legal intoxication
                                          (0.10 blood alcohol level)

FIGURE 4.1   Approximate blood alcohol levels.

achieved through the consumption of different amounts of alcohol. This chart is based on the assumption that one "drink" is either one 12-ounce can of standard beer or one mixed drink (one ounce of 80 proof liquor).

Subjective Effects of Alcohol in the Average Drinker

At Normal Doses

Both as a toxin, and as a psychoactive agent, alcohol is quite weak. To achieve a significant degree of intoxication, the user must ingest an amount of alcohol that is millions of times higher than the dosage level at which the other drugs of abuse have an effect (Hyman & Cassem, 1995). However, when consumed in sufficient quantities, alcohol does have an effect on the user. Indeed, it is for its psychoactive effects that most people consume alcohol.

At low to moderate dosage levels, the individual's expectations play a role in interpreting the effects of alcohol (S. A. Brown, 1990; Smith, Goldman, Greenbaum, & Christiansen, 1995). It is now apparent that ". . . expectancies are closely linked to actual

drinking practices of both adolescents and adults" (p. 17). The individual's expectations for alcohol not only influence how he/she interprets the effects of alcohol when drinking, but also play a role in shaping the individual's drinking behavior.

The team of Smith et al. (1995) examined the expectations for alcohol held by a sample of 461 adolescents, and compared the individual's expectations with his/her drinking pattern over a 2-year period. The authors found a positive relationship between the individual's expectations for alcohol and his/her drinking pattern. Those individuals who had more positive expectations for alcohol were found to be more likely to initiate drinking or increase their alcohol intake than those adolescents who did not hold such expectancies.

There is evidence to suggest that some people begin to form expectations for alcohol in childhood, perhaps as early as 8 years of age (Gordis, 1995). Brown, Creamer, and Stetson (1987) explored the expectations for alcohol by adolescents who did and did not abuse it. It was found that adolescents who abused alcohol were more likely to anticipate a positive experience when they drank than their nondrinking counterparts. This finding was attributed to the home environment of the individual. Homes where parents reported positive experiences with alcohol were more likely to have adolescents who abused alcohol than homes with adolescents who did not drink.

Thus, at low to moderate dosage levels, one factor that influences the effect that alcohol has on the individual is his/her expectancies for alcohol. These expectations and subjective interpretation of alcohol's effects may be at least as important as the pharmacological effects of the alcohol consumed in shaping the individual's subjective interpretation of the drinking experience (S. A. Brown, 1990).

After one or two drinks, the individual experiences a second effect of alcohol, the *disinhibition effect*. As stated earlier, researchers now believe that the disinhibition effect is caused when alcohol interferes with the normal function of inhibitory neurons in the cortex. This is the part of the brain most responsible for higher functions, such as abstract thinking and speech. The cortex is also the part of the brain where much of our voluntary behavior is planned. As the alcohol interferes with cortical nerve function, one tends to temporarily forget social inhibitions (Elliott, 1992; Julien, 1992). During periods of alcohol-induced disinhibition, the individual may engage in behavior that, under normal conditions, he/she would never carry out. It is this disinhibition effect that may contribute to the relationship between alcohol use and aggressive behavior. For example, researchers have long been aware that between 40% and 50% of those who commit homicide used alcohol prior to the commission of the murder (Parker, 1993).

Individuals with either developmental or acquired brain damage are especially at risk for the disinhibition effects of alcohol (Elliott, 1992). This is not to say, however, that the disinhibition effect is seen *only* in individuals with some form of neurological trauma. Individuals without any known form of brain damage may also experience alcohol-induced disinhibition.

Intoxicating Doses

For a 160-pound person, two drinks in an hour's time would result in a BAL of 0.05mg/mL. At this level of intoxication, the individual's reaction time

and depth perception become impaired (Hartman, 1995). Four drinks in an hour's time will cause a 160-pound person to have a BAL of 0.10 mg/mL or higher (Maguire, 1990). At this level of intoxication, the individual's reaction time is even more impaired than before; he/she will have problems coordinating muscle actions (a condition called *ataxia*). One consequence of the alcohol-induced increase in reaction time is that individuals with a BAL between 0.10 and 0.14 mg/mL are 48 times as likely as the nondrinker to be involved in a fatal car accident (*Alcohol Alert*, 1996).

A person with a BAL of 0.15 mg/mL would be above the level of legal intoxication in every state and would definitely be experiencing some alcohol-induced physical problems. The individual with a BAL of 0.15 mg/mL would experience a signficant increase in reaction time, to the point where he/she would have serious difficulty reacting in time to avoid an accident while driving (Lingeman, 1974). Individuals with a BAL of 0.15 mg/mL are between 25 times (Hobbs et al., 1995) and 380 times (*Alcohol Alert*, 1996) as likely as a nondrinker to be involved in a fatal car accident.

The person who has a BAL of 0.20 mg/mL will experience marked ataxia (Matuschka, 1985). The person with a BAL of 0.25 mg/mL would stagger around and have difficulty making sense out of sensory data (Kaminski, 1992; Ray & Ksir, 1993). The person with a BAL of 0.30 mg/mL would be stuporous and, although conscious, would be unlikely to remember what happened during this state of intoxication. With a BAL of 0.35 mg/mL, the stage of surgical anesthesia is achieved (Matuschka, 1985). At high dosage levels, alcohol's effects are analogous to those seen with the anesthetic ether (Maguire, 1990).

The amount of alcohol in the blood necessary to bring about a state of unconsciousness is only a little less than the level necessary to bring about a fatal overdose. This is because alcohol has a Therapeutic Index (TI) of between 1:4 and 1:10 (Grinspoon & Bakalar, 1993): The minimal effective dose of alcohol (i.e., the dose at which the user becomes intoxicated) is a significant fraction of the lethal dose. Thus, when a person drinks to the point of losing consciousness, he/she is dangerously close to the point of overdosing on alcohol. Because of alcohol's low TI, it is very easy to die from an alcohol overdose, something that occasionally happens. Even experienced drinkers have been known to die from an overdose of alcohol. About 1% of drinkers who achieve a BAL of 0.35 mg/mL will die without medical treatment (Ray & Ksir, 1993).[6]

At or above a BAL of 0.35 mg/mL, alcohol is thought to interfere with the activity of the nerves that control respiration (Lehman et al., 1994). Since a BAL of 0.35 mg/mL or above may result in death, *all cases of known or suspected alcohol overdose should be immediately treated by a physician.* A BAL of 0.40 mg/mL will result in about a 50% death rate from alcohol overdose without medical intervention (Bohn, 1993). The LD_{50} is thus around 0.40 mg/mL.

Segal and Sisson (1985) reported that the approximate lethal BAL in human beings is 0.50 mg/mL, while Lingeman (1974) notes that the fatal concentration of alcohol in the blood lies somewhere between 0.50 and 0.80 mg/mL. In theory, the LD_{100} is reached when the nontolerant drinker has a BAL between 0.50 and 0.80 mg/mL. However, there are cases on record where an alcohol-tolerant person was still conscious and able to talk with a BAL as high as 0.78 mg/mL (Bohn, 1993; Schuckit, 1995a).

The effects of alcohol on the rare drinker are summarized in Table 4-1.

Remember that alcohol is a toxin, or poison. When the person has consumed a great deal of alcohol, the body will call on several defense mechanisms in an attempt to limit its exposure to this chemical. When the level of alcohol in the stomach rises to extremely high levels, the stomach will begin to excrete higher levels of mucus and will also close the pyloric valve between the stomach and the small intestine (Kaplan et al., 1994). These actions slow down the absorption of the alcohol that is still in the stomach, giving the body more time to metabolize the alcohol in the blood.

These actions will also contribute to feelings of nausea and possibly cause the drinker to vomit. Vomiting allows the body to rid itself of the alcohol the drinker has ingested, but sometimes this may

happen when the individual is unconscious. At such times, the individual may aspirate some of the material being regurgitated, which will then contribute to the development of a condition known as aspirative pneumonia. This is a very real, if rarely discussed, danger of drinking.

Medical Complications of Alcohol Use in the Average Drinker

The Hangover

The exact mechanism by which alcohol causes one to suffer from a "hangover" is not well understood (Ray & Ksir, 1993). It is known that both the stomach and the brain react to alcohol's toxic effects. The drinker who has ingested enough alcohol will experience a hangover the next day. Some symptoms of a hangover are malaise, headache, tremor, and nausea (Kaminski, 1992). While the alcoholic hangover may, at least in severe cases, make the victim wish for death (O'Donnell, 1986), in general it is self-limiting.

The hangover is seldom seen as a medical emergency. Usually, the victim treats his/her suffering with such remedies as antacids, bed rest, solid foods, fruit juice, and aspirin (Kaminski, 1992).

TABLE 4-1   Effects of Alcohol on the Rare Drinker

Blood alcohol level (BAL)	Behavioral and physical effects of alcohol on rare drinker
0.02	Feeling of warmth, relaxation
0.06	Skin becomes flushed. Person is talkative, coordination slightly impaired.
0.05–0.09	Euphoria, ataxia, loss of many inhibitions
0.10–0.19	Slurred speech, severe ataxia, mood instability, drowsiness, nausea
0.20–0.29	Lethargy, combativeness, stupor, incoherent speech, vomiting
0.30–0.39	Coma, respiratory depression
Above 0.40	Death

Sources: Based on material provided by Lehman, L. B., Pilich, A., & Andrews, N. (1994). "Neurological Disorders Resulting from Alcoholism." *Alcohol Health & Research World,* 17, 306–309; Morrison, S. F., Rogers, P. D., & Thomas, M. H. (1995). "Alcohol and Adolescents." *Pediatric Clinics of North America,* 42, 371–389.

---

[6]Thus, the LD_{01} dosage level for alcohol is about 0.35 mg/mL.

Some experts believe that the hangover is a symptom of an early alcohol withdrawal syndrome (Ray & Ksir, 1993). Thus, the individual suffering from a hangover, be it after a single night or a more protracted period of drinking, might be viewed as going through a mild withdrawal process.

The Effects of Alcohol on Sleep

Alcohol, while a CNS depressant, interferes with the normal sleep cycle. Although alcohol, like the other depressants, may bring about sleep, it does not allow for a normal dream cycle. This effect is not noted for the person who drinks only on a social basis. However, in the chronic alcoholic, the cumulative effects may be quite disruptive; this impact on the normal sleep cycle is discussed in the following chapter.

Even the occasional drinker should be aware, however, of the impact of alcohol on the ability to breathe during sleep. Even moderate amounts of alcohol within two hours of going to sleep can contribute to sleep apnea (*Science Digest*, 1989). Sleep apnea is a disorder in which the individual's ability to breathe is disrupted during sleep. Other complications caused by sleep apnea include high blood pressure, a disruption of the normal heart rate, and, possibly, death. Individuals who consumed even moderate amounts of alcohol prior to sleep were found to experience twice as many apnea episodes as when they abstained from alcohol. Thus, persons with a respiratory disorder, especially sleep apnea, should not drink, especially during the hours prior to going to sleep.

Drug Interactions Involving Alcohol[7]

In addition to the potentiation effect from combining alcohol with CNS depressants, alcohol interacts with many other medications. For example, individuals who take nitroglycerin, a medication often used in the treatment of heart conditions, frequently develop significantly reduced blood pressure levels, possibly to the point of dizziness and loss of consciousness, if they drink while using this medication (*Alcohol Alert*, 1995; Pappas, 1990). Patients taking the antihypertensive medication Inderal (propranolol) should not drink, as the alcohol will decrease the effectiveness of the blood pressure medication (*Alcohol Alert*, 1995). Further, patients taking the anticoagulant medication warfarin should not drink, as moderate to heavy alcohol use can cause the user's body to biotransform the warfarin more quickly than normal (*Alcohol Alert*, 1995; Graedon & Graedon, 1995).

There is some evidence that the antidepressant amitriptyline might enhance alcohol-induced euphoria (Ciraulo, Creelman, Shader, & O'Sullivan, 1995). Using a mixture of alcohol and certain antidepressant medications such as amitriptyline, desimipramine, or doxepin might cause a person to experience problems concentrating since alcohol will potentiate the sedation caused by these medications (Ciraulo, Creelman, et al., 1995; Sands, Knapp, & Ciraulo, 1993).

Surprisingly, there is some animal research that suggests individuals who take beta carotene, and who drink to excess on a chronic basis, may experience a greater degree of liver damage than heavy drinkers who do not take this vitamin supplement (Graedon & Graedon, 1995). When combined with aspirin, alcohol may contribute to bleeding in the stomach because both alcohol and aspirin are irritants to the stomach lining; using them together increases the chances of damage to the stomach lining (Sands et al., 1993). While acetaminophen does not irritate the stomach lining, the chronic use of alcohol causes the liver to release enzymes that transform the acetaminophen into a poison, even when the drug is used at recommended dosage levels. Thus, active alcoholics are advised not to use acetaminophen for the relief of pain.

Patients taking oral medications for diabetes should not drink, as the antidiabetic medication may negate the body's ability to metabolize alcohol. This may possibly result in acute alcohol poisoning from even moderate amounts of alcohol for the individual who combines alcohol and oral antidiabetic medications. Further, because the antidiabetic medication prevents the body from biotransforming alcohol, the individual will remain intoxicated far longer than he/she would normally. In such a case,

---

[7]The list of potential alcohol-drug interactions is extensive. Patients who are taking either a prescription or over-the-counter medication should not consume alcohol without first checking with a physician or pharmacist to determine whether there is a danger for an interaction between the two substances.

the individual might underestimate the time before which it would be safe to drive a motor vehicle.

Patients who are on the antidepressant medications known as monoamine oxidase inhibitors (MAOIs) should not consume alcohol. The fermentation process produces an amino acid, tyramine, along with the alcohol. Ordinarily, this is not a problem. Indeed, tyramine is found in certain foods, and it is a necessary nutrient. But, tyramine interacts with the MAOIs, causing dangerously high, and possibly fatal, blood pressure levels. Patients who take MAOIs are provided a list of foods that they should avoid while they are taking their medication, and these lists also caution the individual against drinking while taking these drugs.

The effects of alcohol are similar to other drugs that have a depressant effect on the central nervous system. The CNS depressants make up a class of drugs that includes narcotic analgesics, the barbiturates and barbituratelike drugs, the benzodiazepines, antihistamines, and a number of other chemicals. So similar are the effects of the CNS depressants to alcohol that one class of drug *potentiates* the effects of the other. Potentiation is a process where one drug will enhance or exaggerate the action of another, similar, drug. The potentiation effect of alcohol and the CNS depressants may be fatal, as the chemicals combine to produce a greater degree of CNS depression than either one could achieve individually (*Alcohol Alert*, 1995).

Researchers have found that the calcium channel blocker Verapamil inhibits the process of alcohol biotransformation, increasing the period of time in which alcohol might cause the user to be intoxicated. At one point, it was thought that patients who are using the medications Zantac (ranitidine)[8] and Tagamet (cimetidine) should not drink while taking these drugs. Sicherman (1992) warned that patients who drink alcohol while taking prescribed doses of these antiulcer medications experience a faster rise in blood alcohol levels than persons who are not taking these medications. Patients who drank while on Tagamet (cimetidine) experienced a 92% increase

in measured blood alcohol levels compared with nonmedicated drinkers. The author warned that patients might exceed the legal limit for intoxication after only two or three drinks, if they drank while taking these medications.

It should be noted that although both cimetidine and ranitidine were once available only by prescription, they are now available as over-the-counter medications, without a physician's prescription. However, Wormsley (1993) challenged the conclusion of Sicherman (1992), noting the earlier study of the effects of alcohol and ranitidine was flawed. Wormsley noted that Sicherman's (1992) research study used fasting subjects or the use of atypical dosing schedules that did not reflect how this medication would be used in real life by patients. When these variables were controlled for, Wormsley concluded that there was no evidence to suggest that ranitidine use resulted in higher blood alcohol levels.

But, when one considers the damage that alcohol can cause to the user's gastrointestinal tract (discussed in detail in Chapter 5), it would appear wise for patients to avoid alcohol if they are taking ranitidine to help their ulcers heal, even if there is no irrefutable evidence of a significant clinical interaction between alcohol and ranitidine.

Patients who are taking the antibiotic medications chloramphenicol, furazolidone, metronidazole, or the antimalarial medication quinacrine should not drink alcohol. The combination of these antibiotics with alcohol may produce a painful reaction similar to that seen when patients on Antabuse (disulfiram) consume alcohol (Meyers, 1992). Patients who are taking the antitubercular drug Isoniazid (INH) should also avoid the use of alcohol. The combination of these two chemicals will reduce the effectiveness of Isoniazid and, may increase the individual's chances of developing hepatitis.

Because of the potentiation effect between narcotic analgesics and alcohol, both of which are CNS depressants, patients who are using narcotic analgesics should not drink. Also, alcohol combines with the analgesic Darvon (propoxyphene), and can cause potentially dangerous levels of CNS depression or even death (Sands et al., 1994).

Alcohol is a potent pharmacological agent, and it is not possible to list all the potential interactions

[8]The most common brand name is given first, with the generic name in parentheses.

between alcohol and the medications currently in use. Thus, before mixing alcohol with any medication, a physician should be consulted, to avoid potentially dangerous interactions between pharmaceutical agents and alcohol.

Alcohol Use and Accidental Injury or Death

Alcohol is a popular recreational beverage. Advertisements in the media proclaim the benefits of recreational alcohol use at parties, social encounters, or as a way to celebrate good news. What these advertisements often fail to mention is that recreational alcohol is associated with an increased risk of accidental injury, or even premature death, for the drinker, or those about him/her.

There is a known relationship between alcohol use and motor vehicle accidents. Despite a protracted campaign to reduce "drunk driving" in this country, alcohol-related motor vehicle accidents are the leading cause of death for individuals between the ages of 15 and 24 in the United States (Committee on Substance Abuse, 1995). It is difficult to determine whether the campaign against drunk drivers is having any effect and, if so, how strong an effect it is exerting on driving patterns in the United States. The percentage of people killed in alcohol-related motor vehicle accidents declined from 43% of all traffic fatalities in 1986 to 37.4% in 1992 (Gordis, 1996b). But, by 1995, the percentage of alcohol-related motor vehicle accident fatalities had gone back up to 41% of all fatal accidents (Hingson, 1996). In 1995, a total of 17,274 people died in alcohol-related motor vehicle accidents in the United States.[9]

Some forms of motor vehicle transportation are more dangerous than others. It has been estimated that 60% of all boating fatalities are alcohol-related (*Alcohol Alert*, 1994), and an estimated 70% of motorcycle drivers who are killed in an accident are thought to have been drinking prior to the accident (Colburn, Meyer, Wrigley, & Bradley, 1993). These figures indicate that alcohol-related motor vehicle accidents remain a significant cause of premature death in this country.

Alcohol use is a factor in 41% of all fatal injuries due to falling, and 42% of all deaths associated with fires (Rice, 1993). Further, approximately 30,000 individuals lose their lives each year because of other alcohol-related accidental injuries[10] (e.g., drownings, injuries at home) (McGinnis & Foege, 1993). Researchers have found that 42% of those individuals treated at one major trauma center had alcohol in their blood at the time of admission (Milzman & Soderstrom, 1994). No matter how you look at it, even casual alcohol use carries with it a significantly increased risk of accidental injury or death.

Summary

This chapter provides a brief history of alcohol—the first recreational chemical. The process of beer making was discussed, as was the manner in which wine is obtained from fermented fruit. The use of distillation to achieve concentrations of alcohol above 15% was reviewed, and questions surrounding the use of alcohol were discussed. Alcohol's effects on the rare social drinker were considered, as well as some of the more significant interactions between alcohol and pharmaceutical agents. The history of alcohol consumption and the pattern of alcohol use in the United States also were mentioned.

---

[9] To further illustrate the scope of the problem of people driving motor vehicles while under the influence of chemicals, Brookoff, Cook, Williams, and Mann (1994) found that when special urine toxicology testing was conducted, 59% of those reckless drivers who were not under the influence of alcohol at the time they were involved in a motor vehicle accident were found to be under the influence of marijuana or cocaine at the time of the accident.

[10] This number is part of the 200,000 alcohol-related deaths discussed in Chapter 5.

Chronic Alcohol Abuse and Addiction

The focus of Chapter 4 was the acute effects of alcohol on the "average," or rare social drinker. Alcohol has a strong potential to be abused and to cause the user to become physically addicted. Simple alcohol abuse—and most certainly the chronic use of alcohol—contribute to a wide range of physical, social, and emotional problems for the drinker. Given its potential for harm, one could argue that if alcohol were only to be discovered today, its use might never be legalized (Miller & Hester, 1995).

Scope of the Problem

Chronic alcohol intoxication was first recognized as a disease by Domitius Ulpinus in A.D. 276 (J. W. Campbell, 1992). Despite its long history as a drug of abuse, alcohol remains the most popular recreational chemical in the United States, accounting for an astounding 85% of the drug addiction problem in this country (Franklin, 1987). This fact illustrates the complex nature of alcohol use: it is a recreational substance that, if used often enough and in sufficient quantities, becomes a drug of abuse. If alcohol is abused for an extended period, the user can become physically addicted. This is the state known as *alcoholism*, or alcohol dependence.

The hallmark of alcohol abuse/addiction is a pattern of alcohol-related problems in the individual's social life, interpersonal relationships, and educational or vocational activities, or legal predicaments that might be attributed to the use of alcohol. Not all those people who experience a *single* alcohol-related problem are *dependent* on it. The American Psychiatric Association (1994) estimated that fully 60% of the men and 30% of the women who consume alcohol have at least one transient alcohol-related problem (e.g., blackouts, discussed later in this chapter). Kaplan et. al. (1994) reported that 30% to 45% of those who drink alcohol experience a transient sign of alcohol abuse. The vast majority of these individuals do not go on to become physically dependent on alcohol.

However, studies of the health of the nation's population suggest that about 13.5% of the population either abuse alcohol or become physically dependent on it at some point in their lives (Regier et al., 1990). Thus, a significant minority of those who experience one symptom of alcohol use problems go on to demonstrate additional symptoms. These people can be said to have an alcohol abuse problem. It is only when the individual is physically dependent on alcohol that he/she is said to have developed the disease of alcohol addiction (alcoholism).

Estimates of the scope of the problem of alcohol dependence vary. Bays (1990) suggested that there are about 10 million alcohol-dependent adults in the United States. Beasley (1987) presented a higher figure, reporting that between 10 and 15 million Americans are dependent on alcohol, with an additional 10 million being "on the cusp of alcoholism" (p. 21). Nor is the problem of alcohol abuse/addiction limited to adults. It is estimated that between 1 million

(Ellis et al., 1988) and 3 million (Turbo, 1989) children and adolescents are also addicted to alcohol.

Alcoholism is predominately a male disease in the sense that male alcoholics outnumber female alcoholics by a ratio of about 2:1 (Blume, 1994). However, if it is assumed that the alcohol use of about 10 to 15 million individuals in this country is beyond the range of just social drinking, then between 6 and 10 million men and 3 to 5 million women either abuse alcohol, or are addicted to it.

Clinicians who specialize in substance abuse often hear a client deny being an alcoholic; instead, the person claims to be "only a problem drinker." Schuckit, Zisook, and Mortola (1985) explored whether there are significant differences between individuals who are physically addicted to alcohol and those who might be said to be "problem drinkers." The authors found that a group of men identified as only being abusers of alcohol was virtually identical to another group diagnosed as being alcohol dependent. The two major differences between these groups were that the alcohol-dependent group took more drinks when they did drink and were likely to have had more alcohol-related medical problems.

On the basis of their research, the authors concluded that it was "not clear whether the distinction between alcohol abuse and alcohol dependence carries any important prognostic or treatment implications" (p. 1403). When the individual's use of alcohol has reached the point where the user is experiencing physical, legal, social, and financial problems, the distinction between "problem drinking" and "alcoholism" is so vague as to become meaningless.

What the research suggests is that, at least for some individuals, their alcohol use will progress from social use through abuse, to the point of physical dependence. The progression to alcohol dependence usually takes between 10 (Meyer, 1994) and 20 years (Alexander & Gwyther, 1995) of heavy drinking. However, the physical dependence on alcohol has lifelong implications for the individual. Once a person becomes dependent on alcohol, even if that person stops drinking for a period of time, he/she will again become dependent on alcohol "in a matter of days to weeks" if he/she resumes drinking (Meyer, 1994, p. 165). Thus, the individual

who becomes dependent is unlikely to be able to return to nonabusive drinking.

The "Typical" Alcohol-Dependent Person

Individuals with an alcohol use problem are "masters of denial" (Knapp, 1996, p. 19). They often have a thousand and one rationalizations to explain why they cannot possibly have an alcohol use problem: they always go to work; they never go to the bar to drink; they know ten people who drink as much, if not more, than they do. One of the most common rationalizations offered by the person with an alcohol use problem is that he/she has nothing in common with the stereotypical skid row derelict. In reality, only about 5% of those people who are dependent on alcohol fit the image of the skid row alcoholic (Knapp). The majority of those with alcohol use problems might best be described as "high functioning" (Knapp, p. 12) alcoholics, who have jobs, responsibilities, families, and images to protect. Often, the alcohol-dependent person expends a great deal of effort to keep his/her alcohol problem hidden and protect his/her public image. In many cases, high-functioning alcoholics keep their growing dependence on alcohol hidden from virtually every person in their lives. But, in secret moments of dread, they know that their use of alcohol is somehow different from that of the nonalcoholic drinker.

Alcohol Tolerance, Dependence, and Craving: Signposts of Alcoholism

There are specific signs that suggest the drinker has moved past simple social drinking and may have an alcohol use problem or even be physically dependent on alcohol and its effects. These signs are *tolerance*, *dependence*, and *craving*.

Tolerance

As the individual repeatedly consumes alcohol, his/her body will begin to make certain adaptations to try to maintain normal function in the continual presence of the foreign chemical. First, the individual's liver will begin to become more efficient at biotransforming alcohol, at least in the earlier stages of the person's drinking career. This is known as *metabolic tolerance* to alcohol. During clinical interviews, it is not uncommon for alcohol-dependent individuals to admit that they need to drink far more alcohol to become intoxicated than they did five or ten years ago. A drinker might admit, for example, that he could become intoxicated on "just" a six-pack of beer when he was 21. But, this same person might admit that, now, it takes 12 to 18 cans of beer before he can reach that same level of intoxication. This is a reflection of his growing tolerance to alcohol's effects. Compare the effects of alcohol for the chronic drinker in Table 5-1 with those shown in Table 4-1 (in Chapter 4).

Behavioral tolerance is another expression of tolerance to alcohol's effects. Where a novice drinker might appear quite intoxicated after five or six beers, the chronic drinker might appear sober despite being legally intoxicated. If judged only on the basis of physical appearance, a chronic alcoholic often appears relatively sober, at least to the untrained observer, although a blood test would reveal that the individual's blood alcohol level is far in excess of the legal limit.

Another form of tolerance is *pharmacodynamic tolerance*. In pharmacodynamic tolerance, the cells of the central nervous system attempt to carry out their normal function despite the continual presence of alcohol. The cells of the brain become less and less sensitive to the intoxicating effects of the chemical, and the individual must use more of the drug to achieve the same effect.

TABLE 5-1   Effects of Alcohol on the Chronic Drinker

Blood alcohol level (BAL)	Behavioral and physical effects of alcohol on chronic drinker
0.05–0.09	No to minimal effect
0.10–0.19	Mild ataxia, euphoria
0.20–0.29	Mild emotional changes, ataxia
0.30–0.39	Drowsiness, lethargy, stupor
Above 0.40	Coma

Source: Based on material provided by Lehman, L. B., Pilich, A., & Andrews, N. (1994). "Neurological Disorders Resulting from Alcoholism." *Alcohol Health & Research World, 17,* 306–309.

In general, clinicians do not identify each subform of tolerance that a specific patient has developed in his/her drinking career. Rather, if any of these subtypes are present, the patient simply is said to be "tolerant" to the effects of alcohol. But even if the patient has become tolerant, the lethal dose of alcohol does not change (Matuschka, 1985). Chronic alcohol users may overdose on alcohol in the same manner as the novice drinker. Thus, *any suspected alcohol overdose should immediately be evaluated and treated by a physician.*

Also, the physical adaptations that the drinker's body goes through to maintain normal function are not permanent. Over time, the drinker actually may become *less* tolerant to alcohol's effects. Thus, it is not uncommon for late-stage alcoholics to admit that, in contrast to their earlier drinking days, they now can become intoxicated on just a few beers, or mixed drinks. As the toxic effects of chronic alcohol exposure accumulate, the liver becomes less efficient in biotransforming additional doses of that chemical. When clinicians evaluate such an individual, they will say that this individual's tolerance is "on the downswing." When chronic alcohol users become less and less tolerant to alcohol's effects, they have entered the later stages of alcohol dependence.

Dependence

Another warning sign that suggests addiction is the drinker's growing dependence on alcohol. There are two subforms of alcohol dependence. First, there is *psychological dependence.* In psychological dependence, the individual repeatedly self-administers alcohol because he/she finds it rewarding or believes it is a necessary "crutch." Such individuals believe that they cannot be sexual, sleep, relax, or socialize without first using alcohol. Often, alcohol-dependent persons believe they deserve to have a drink(s), for one reason or another.

The second form of dependence is *physical dependence.* Since the chronic use of alcohol forces the body to attempt to adapt to the constant presence of the chemical, in a very real sense the body might be said to now need the foreign chemical to maintain normal function. When the chemical is suddenly removed from the body, the body goes through a period of readjustment, as it relearns how to function without the foreign chemical. This period of readjustment is known as the *withdrawal syndrome.*

Like many drugs of abuse, alcohol has a characteristic withdrawal syndrome. This syndrome, however, is different from that of many drugs in that it involves not only some degree of subjective discomfort for the individual, but also the potential for life-threatening medical complications. For this reason, *all cases of alcohol withdrawal should be evaluated and treated by a physician.*

The severity of the withdrawal from alcohol depends on: (a) the intensity with which the individual used alcohol, (b) the duration of time during which the individual drank, and (c) the individual's state of health. Thus, the longer the period of alcohol use and the greater the amount ingested, the more severe the alcohol withdrawal syndrome. The symptoms of alcohol withdrawal for the chronic alcoholic will be discussed in more detail later in this chapter.

Craving

Often, the recovering alcoholic speaks of a craving for alcohol that continues long after he/she has stopped drinking. Some alcoholics talk of feeling "thirsty," or they find themselves preoccupied with the possibility of having a drink. It is not known why alcoholics crave alcohol. However, the fact that the individual becomes preoccupied with alcohol use, or craves a drink, is a sign that he/she has become dependent on it.

The TIQ Hypothesis

One theory for the phenomenon of craving was advanced by Trachtenberg and Blum (1987). The authors suggested that chronic alcohol use could significantly reduce the brain's production of opiatelike neurotransmitters known as the endorphins, the enkephalins, and the dynorphins. These neurotransmitters function in the brain's pleasure center to help moderate an individual's emotions and behavior.

Blum (1988) suggested that a by-product of alcohol metabolism and neurotransmitters normally found within the brain combine to form *tetrahydroisoquinoline* (TIQ). TIQ was thought to be capable of binding to opiatelike receptor sites within the brain's pleasure center. In theory, as this happens, the individual would experience a sense of well-being

(Blum & Payne, 1991; Blum & Trachtenberg, 1988). The authors suggested that this was the mechanism through which alcohol use was rewarding or pleasurable to the individual. However, TIQ's effects were thought to be short-lived, forcing the individual to drink more alcohol to regain or maintain the initial feeling of euphoria.

Further, the chronic use of alcohol was thought to cause the brain to reduce its production of enkephalins as the ever-present TIQ was substituted for these natural opiatelike neurotransmitters (Blum & Payne, 1991; Blum & Trachtenberg, 1988). The cessation of alcohol intake was thought to result in a neurochemical deficit that the individual would then attempt to relieve through further chemical use (Blum & Payne, 1991; Blum & Trachtenberg, 1988). This deficit was experienced as the craving for alcohol commonly reported by recovering alcoholics, according to the authors.

Although the TIQ theory had a number of strong adherents in the late 1980s and early 1990s, it has gradually fallen into disfavor. Several research studies have failed to find evidence to support the TIQ hypothesis. Few researchers in the field of alcohol addiction now believe that TIQ plays a major role in the phenomenon of alcohol craving.

Complications of Chronic Alcohol Use

The chronic use of alcohol may either directly or indirectly contribute to health problems for the drinker. Alcohol is a mild toxin, and chronic use often results in damage to one or more organ systems. It is also important to recognize that chronic alcohol use includes "weekend" or "binge" drinking. Repeated episodic alcohol abuse may bring about many of the same effects seen with chronic alcohol use.

There is no simple formula for calculating the risk of alcohol-related organ damage or for identifying the organs that will be affected (Segal & Sisson, 1985). As the authors noted:

> Some heavy drinkers of many years' duration appear to go relatively unscathed, while others develop complications early (e.g., after five years) in their drinking careers. Some develop brain damage; others liver disease; still others, both. The reasons for this are simply not known. (p. 145)

However, it is known that, depending on the individual, the chronic use of alcohol can have an impact on virtually every body system.

The Effects of Chronic Alcoholism on the Digestive System

As discussed in Chapter 4, during distillation many of the vitamins and minerals in the original wine are lost. Thus, whereas the original wine might have contributed something to the drinker's nutritional requirements, even this modest contribution is lost through distillation.

Further, when the body breaks down alcohol, it finds empty calories. The body obtains carbohydrates from metabolizing the alcohol, but does not get essential protein, vitamins, calcium, and other minerals. Also, the chronic use of alcohol may cause the drinker to experience diarrhea. These two factors may contribute to a state of vitamin depletion called *avitaminosis*, which is discussed later in this chapter.

One of the factors associated with an increased risk for the development of cancer is the chronic exposure to chemical toxins. Given this information, one would thus expect that chronic alcohol users are at increased risk for the development of cancer. This is indeed the case: it has been known for many years that chronic alcoholics have a higher risk of many forms of cancer than do nonalcoholics. The chronic use of alcohol is associated with higher rates of cancer of the upper digestive tract, the respiratory system, the mouth, pharynx, larynx, esophagus, and the liver (Garro, Espina, & Lieber, 1992). Alcohol use is associated with 75% of all deaths due to cancer of the esophagus (Rice, 1993). Further, although the research data is not clear at this time, there is also evidence suggesting a link between chronic alcohol use and cancer of the large bowel, and cancer of the breast (Garro et al., 1992).

The combination of cigarettes and alcohol is especially dangerous. Chronic alcoholics experience almost a sixfold increase in their risk of developing cancer of the mouth or pharynx, whereas cigarette smokers have slightly over a sevenfold increased risk of developing cancer of the mouth or pharynx (Garro et al., 1992, p. 83). However, alcoholics who also smoke have a *38-fold increased risk* of cancer in these regions, according to the authors.

Chronic exposure to alcohol has a profound impact on the liver, which is "the organ most commonly thought to be affected by alcohol" (Nace, 1987, p. 23). In humans, the liver is the primary site of alcohol biotransformation (Frezza et al., 1990; Schenker & Speeg, 1990). The chronic exposure to alcohol may result in alcohol-induced liver damage, even if the individual is not drinking in amounts that would be otherwise considered abusive (Lieber, 1996).

The first manifestation of alcohol-related liver problems is the development of a "fatty liver." In this condition, the liver becomes enlarged and does not function at full efficiency (Nace, 1987). There are few symptoms of a fatty liver that would be noticed by the average person. But a fatty liver can easily be detected by a medical examination. Blood tests designed to measure the health of the liver would detect characteristic abnormalities in the patient's liver enzymes (Schuckit, 1995a). A fatty liver is a common consequence of chronic alcohol use, and 100% of heavy alcohol users eventually will develop this condition (*Alcohol Alert*, 1993a; Sherman, Ward, Warren-Perry, Williams, & Peters, 1993).

The individual who continues to consume alcohol may develop another complication of alcoholism: *alcoholic hepatitis*. In alcohol-induced hepatitis, the cells of the liver become inflamed as a result of the body's continual exposure to alcohol. Symptoms of alcoholic hepatitis may include a low-grade fever, malaise, jaundice, an enlarged, tender liver, and dark urine (Nace, 1987). A medical examination may reveal characteristic changes in the blood chemistry (Schuckit, 1995b), and the patient might complain of abdominal pain (*Alcohol Alert*, 1993a).

For reasons that are not well understood, only between 10 and 35% of chronic drinkers develop this condition (*Alcohol Alert*, 1993a; Lieber, 1995). But in 20% to 65% of the cases that are severe enough to require hospitalization, the patient dies as a result of the alcohol-induced hepatitis (Bondesson & Saperston, 1996). It has been suggested that the individual's vulnerability to progressing from a fatty liver to alcoholic liver disease might be mediated by genetic factors (Achord, 1995; Sherman, 1993). Because of his/her genetic inheritance, the drinker would be more or less likely to develop alcohol-induced liver damage as a result of chronic alcohol use.

Individuals who suffer from alcohol-induced hepatitis should be avoid having surgery, if possible, as patients going through the acute states of alcohol withdrawal are poor surgical risks. If the patient were to be examined by a physician who was not aware of his/her history of alcoholism, the abdominal pain might be misinterpreted as a symptom of other conditions such as appendicitis, pancreatitis, or an inflammation of the gall bladder. As with any medical condition, proper diagnosis of alcoholic hepatitis is essential to provide for the appropriate care of the patient, and to arrive at this diagnosis, the physician must know about the patient's chronic use of alcohol.

Alcoholic hepatitis is "a slow, smoldering process which may proceed or coexist with" (Nace, 1987, p. 25) another form of liver disease, known as *cirrhosis of the liver*. In general, cirrhosis of the liver does not develop until after 10 to 20 years of heavy drinking (*Alcohol Alert*, 1993a). When this disorder does develop, the cells of the liver begin to die as a result of their chronic exposure to alcohol. Eventually, these dead liver cells are replaced by scar tissue. A physical examination of the patient with cirrhosis of the liver will reveal a hard, nodular liver, an enlarged spleen, spider angiomas on the skin, tremor, jaundice, mental confusion, signs of liver disease on blood tests, and possibly a number of other symptoms including testicular atrophy in males (Nace).

Although some researchers believe that alcoholic hepatitis precedes the development of cirrhosis of the liver, this has not been proven. Indeed, "alcoholics may progress to cirrhosis without passing through any visible stage resembling hepatitis" (*Alcohol Alert*, 1993a, p. 1). Thus, many chronic alcoholics never show symptoms of alcoholic hepatitis, and the first outward sign of serious liver disease is the development of cirrhosis of the liver.

Statistically, cirrhosis of the liver is the fourth leading cause of death for adults between the ages of 25 and 64 (Lieber, 1995). For reasons that are not fully understood, only 20% (*Alcohol Alert*, 1993a) to 30% (Hartman, 1995) of chronic drinkers develop cirrhosis of the liver. Nevertheless, alcohol-induced liver disease accounts for between 60 and 90% of all serious cases of liver disease seen in this country (American Medical Association, 1993a). The chronic use of alcohol is the primary cause of liver disease in the United States.

Scientists are not certain how alcohol causes, or contributes to, liver damage, and over the years different theories have been advanced (Achord, 1995). Repeated episodes of abusive drinking are thought to cause the destruction of liver cells, which are then replaced by scar tissue. As more and more tissue of the liver is damaged over time, large areas may be replaced by scar tissue. Because scar tissue is nonfunctional as the cells die, the liver is no longer able to effectively cleanse the blood. If too much of the liver is destroyed, various toxins, or poisons, build up in the individual's system. Some of these toxins, such as ammonia, are thought to then damage the cells of the central nervous system (Butterworth, 1995).

At one point, it was thought that malnutrition was a factor in the development of alcohol-induced liver disease. However, researchers have found that the individual's dietary habits do not seem to influence the development of alcohol-induced liver disease (Achord, 1995). Recently, scientists have developed blood tests capable of detecting one of the viruses known to infect the liver. The virus is known as "hepatitis virus-C" (or, Hepatitis-C or HVC) and is found in about 1.6% of the general population. This means that, under normal conditions, less than 2% of the population is infected with HVC. But, between 25 and 60% of chronic alcohol users have been found to be infected with HVC (Achord). This fact suggests that there may be a relationship between HVC infection, chronic alcohol use, and the development of liver disease.

Whatever its cause, cirrhosis itself can have severe complications, including liver cancer, and sodium and water retention (Nace, 1987; Schuckit, 1995a). Furthermore, the scar tissue and fat deposits prevent the liver from filtering the blood as efficiently as before, causing toxins to build up in the blood. This then adds to the damage being done to the brain by the alcohol (Willoughby, 1984). At the same time, the now enlarged liver puts a greater work load on the heart, as the swelling of the liver squeezes the blood vessels that pass through it, causing the blood pressure to build up within the vessels.

This condition, which is known as *portal hypertension*, in turn may contribute to a swelling of the blood vessels in the esophagus. When the blood vessels in the esophagus swell, weak spots form on the walls of the vessels much like weak spots form on an inner tube of a tire. These weak spots, which are called *esophageal varices*, may rupture. Ruptured esophageal varices constitute a medical emergency; even with the most advanced forms of medical treatment, estimates of the mortality rate for hemorrhage from esophageal varices range from between 30 and 60% (Huston, 1996) to between 40 and 70% (Jaffe, Chung, & Friedman, 1996).

As if that were not enough, alcohol has been implicated as one cause of *pancreatitis*, a painful inflammation of the pancreas. Approximately 35% of all known cases of pancreatitis are thought to be brought on by the chronic use of alcohol, and some research centers have found that alcoholism is the major cause of between 66 and 75% of the cases of pancreatitis treated at those facilities (McCrady & Langenbucher, 1996; Steinberg & Tenner, 1994). Pancreatitis develops slowly and usually requires a history of "10 to 15 years of heavy drinking" (Nace, 1987, p. 26) before symptoms appear. While pancreatitis can be caused by other toxic agents, such as the venom of scorpions or exposure to certain insecticides, ethyl alcohol is the most common cause (Steinberg & Tenner, 1994).

Alcohol is also irritating to the stomach lining. The ingestion of alcohol in concentrations of 10 to 20 "proof" (i.e., 5–10% pure alcohol) has been found to damage the lining of the stomach (Bode, Maute, & Bode, 1996). After examining bioposy specimens from 56 alcohol-dependent patients and from 66 control subjects, Bode et al. (1996) suggested that even low concentrations of alcohol might inhibit the stomach's ability to produce prostaglandins necessary to protect it from digestive fluids. This would account for the known fact that chronic alcohol use has been shown to cause *gastritis*, an inflammation of the lining of the stomach. This may result in bleeding from the stomach lining, or may even contribute to the formation of gastric ulcers (Willoughby, 1984).

It has been estimated that about 30% of heavy drinkers suffer from chronic gastritis (Matuschka, 1985). If an ulcer forms over a major blood vessel, the individual may experience a "bleeding ulcer," as the stomach acid eats through the stomach lining and blood vessel walls. This is a severe medical emergency that may, and frequently does, result in death. Although surgeons may use a laser beam to seal a bleeding ulcer, in extreme cases conventional surgery is necessary to save the patient's life. At times, the surgeon must remove the part of the stomach with the damaged section to stop the bleeding. This, in turn, will contribute to the body's difficulties in absorbing suitable amounts of vitamins from the food ingested (Willoughby, 1984). This, either by itself or in combination with further alcohol use, helps to bring about a chronic state of malnutrition in the individual.

The vitamin malabsorption syndrome that develops following the surgical removal of the majority of the individual's stomach makes the person a prime candidate for the development of tuberculosis (TB) if he/she continues to drink (Willoughby, 1984). The topic of TB is discussed in more detail in Chapter 33. At this point, however, it should be pointed out that upward of 95% of those alcoholics who have a portion of their stomach removed secondary to bleeding ulcers and who continue to drink ultimately will develop TB (Willoughby).

However, even without the trauma of surgery, alcohol can interfere with the ability of the body to absorb the chemicals needed for life. Chronic alcohol ingestion contributes to *malabsorption syndromes*, in which the individual's body is no longer able to absorb needed vitamins or minerals from food (Marsano, 1994). Beasley (1987) termed this condition a "leaky gut" and identified it as a common problem for chronic alcoholics. Some of the minerals that may not be absorbed by the body of the chronic alcoholic include zinc (Marsano, 1994), sodium, calcium, phosphorus, and magnesium (Lehman et al., 1994). The chronic use of alcohol also interferes with the body's ability to absorb or properly utilize vitamin A, vitamin D, vitamin B-6, thiamine, and folic acid (Marsano, 1994).

In some cases, the chronic use of alcohol contributes to *glossitis*, a painful inflammation of the tongue (Marsano, 1994). According to this author, alcoholism is also a factor that might cause stricture of the esophagus, making it harder for the individual to absorb adequate levels of food.

One of the eventual by-products of alcohol biotransformation is a carbohydrate. In cases of chronic alcohol use, the body substitutes the carbohydrates obtained from alcohol for those normally obtained from nutritious food (Charness, Simon, & Greenberg, 1989). The carbohydrates from alcohol provide only empty calories since the body will not be able to obtain the vitamins, protein, minerals, and amino acids that it needs from the alcohol.

Many chronic alcohol drinkers obtain up to one-half of their daily caloric intake from alcohol rather than from traditional food sources (Suter, Schultz, & Jequier, 1992). This factor contributes to the decline in the effectiveness of their immune system. In turn, the less-effective immune system helps to make these drinkers vulnerable to infectious diseases such as pneumonia and tuberculosis.

There are other consequences of heavy alcohol use for both the alcoholic and the heavy social drinker, such as the possible development of metabolic disorders. For example, chronic alcohol use interferes with the body's ability to adequately control blood glucose levels (*Alcohol Alert*, 1993c). Research has shown that between 45 and 70% of alcoholics with liver disease are also either glucose intolerant (a condition that suggests that the body is having trouble dealing with sugar in the blood) or diabetic (*Alcohol Alert*, 1994b). Many heavy drinkers experience episodes of abnormally high (*hyperglycemic*) or abnormally low (*hypoglycemic*) blood sugar levels. These conditions are caused by alcohol interfering with the secretion of digestive enzymes from the pancreas (*Alcohol Alert*, 1993c, 1994b).

Further, chronic alcohol use may interfere with the way the drinker's body metabolizes fats. When the individual reaches the point of obtaining 10% or more of his/her daily energy requirements from

alcohol rather than from nutritious foods, the person's body goes through a series of alcohol-induced changes (Suter, 1992). First, the chronic use of alcohol slows down the body's energy expenditure (metabolism). This, in turn, causes the body to store the unused lipids as fatty tissue. This is the mechanism responsible for the so-called beer belly commonly seen in the heavy drinker.

The Effects of Chronic Alcohol Use on the Cardiopulmonary System

Surprisingly, researchers have discovered that the moderate daily use of alcohol (i.e., one to two drinks), especially wine, has been found to have a beneficial effect on the cardiovascular system. The consumption of *no more than* two-and-a-half drinks per day seems to be associated with a significant reduction in the risk of heart attack in both men (Klatsky, 1990) and women (Doria, 1990). Although Kemm (1993) suggested that the safe limit was 21 "units" (p. 1373) of alcohol per week for men, and 14 units per week for women, the two drinks per day average still appears valid. Kemm defined a unit of alcohol as being ½ pint of beer, a 5-ounce glass of wine, or a standard mixed drink.

The ability of wine to reduce the risk of heart attack seems to be caused by alcohol's ability to inhibit the ability of blood platelets to "bind" together (Renaud & DeLorgeril, 1992). By inhibiting the action of blood platelets to start the clotting process, the moderate use of alcohol may result in a lower risk of heart attack and certain kinds of strokes. This should not be surprising, since wine contains salicylic acid, the active ingredient of aspirin ("Gallic Hearts," 1994). As discussed in Chapter 12, aspirin has been found to inhibit the ability of blood platelets to form clots.

However, there is a fine line between "just enough" alcohol, and too much (R. Herman, 1993). The issue of possible health benefits from moderate alcohol use is controversial, and the World Health Organization (WHO) denounced *any* claims of health benefits from moderate alcohol use on the grounds that this may result in people drinking more alcohol (Craft, 1994). It has also been discovered that, while moderate alcohol use might provide some degree of protection against some forms of coronary artery disease, it also increases the individual's risk of developing alcohol-related brain damage (Karhunen, Erkinjuntti, & Laippala, 1994). Further, for women, drinking even one drink per day significantly increases the risk of breast cancer (Brody, 1993). Thus, the role of alcohol in reducing the risk of heart attack is limited at best and carries with it other health risks.

When the individual exceeds the safe limit of alcohol use on a chronic basis, alcohol not only loses its protective action, but may actually harm the cardiovascular system. The excessive, chronic use of alcohol results in the suppression of normal red blood cell formation, and both blood-clotting problems and anemia are common complications of alcoholism (Nace, 1987). Further, excessive alcohol use is thought to be a factor in the development of cerebral vascular accidents (strokes, or CVAs). Sacco (1995) estimated that chronic alcohol use causes 23,500 strokes each year in the United States.

Bacterial pneumonia is at least twice as common in alcoholics as in nonalcoholics (Nace, 1987). As noted, the chronic use of alcohol reduces the effectiveness of the immune system. This increases the chances that the alcohol-dependent person will develop infections. Another reason chronic alcohol users are at risk for the development of pneumonia is a process known as *aspirative pneumonia*. Alcohol's relationship with aspirative pneumonia is an indirect one. Remember that alcohol is a toxin. When the individual ingests too much of a toxin, the body may try to expel it through vomiting. But alcohol use also interferes with the vomiting reflex. Thus, it is possible for the drinker to aspirate (inhale) some of the material vomited. If the lungs are then unable to cleanse themselves of this foreign material, it will decompose there setting the stage for bacterial growth. The bacteria then cause a form of pneumonia. (An additional danger is that an individual who is unconscious when vomiting may suffocate in the material aspirated.)

Alcohol is also implicated in damage to the cardiovascular system itself. In large amounts, defined as more than the one or two drinks per day identified earlier, alcohol is known to be *cardiotoxic*, that is, toxic to the muscle tissue of the heart. Chronic alcohol use is considered the most common cause of

heart muscle disease (Rubin & Doria, 1990). Prolonged exposure to alcohol (i.e., 6 beers/day or a pint whiskey/day for 10 years) may result in permanent damage to the heart muscle tissue, resulting in hypertension (or high blood pressure) and inflammation as well as a general weakening of the heart muscle known as *alcohol-induced cardiomyopathy* (Figueredo, 1997).

Alcoholic cardiomyopathy appears to be a special example of a more generalized process in which chronic alcohol use results in damage to *all* striated muscle tissue (Fernandez-Sola et al., 1994). The authors examined a number of men who were, and were not, alcoholic. They found that alcoholic men in general had less muscle strength and greater levels of muscle tissue damage, than did the nonalcoholic men in this study. The authors concluded that alcohol is toxic to muscle tissue, and that the chronic use of alcohol will result in a loss of muscle tissue throughout the body.

Cardiomyopathy develops in 25% (Schuckit, 1995a) to 40% of chronic alcoholic users (Figueredo, 1997). But even this figure might not reflect the true scope of alcohol-induced heart disease. Rubin and Doria (1990) suggest, "the majority of alcoholics" (p. 279), which they defined as those individuals who obtained between 30 and 50% of their daily caloric requirement through alcohol, will ultimately develop "pre-clinical heart disease" (p. 279). Because of the body's compensatory mechanisms, many chronic alcoholics do not show evidence of heart disease except on special tests designed to detect this disorder (Figueredo, 1997; Rubin & Doria, 1990). However, about 50% of those individuals with alcohol-induced cardiomyopathy will die within four years, if they continue to drink (Figueredo).

Although many individuals take comfort in the fact that they drink to excess only occasionally, binge drinking is not without its dangers. Binge drinking may result in a condition known as the "holiday heart syndrome" (Figueredo, 1997; Lange, White, & Robinson, 1992). Episodic drinkers, such as those who go on binges only around the holidays, are prone to develop an irregular heartbeat known as *atrial fibrillation*. Not every case of atrial fibrillation is caused by alcohol abuse. However, the condition may be fatal, if it is not diagnosed and properly treated by a physician. Thus, even episodic alcohol use is not without some degree of risk.

The Effects of Chronic Alcoholism on the Central Nervous System

Alcohol is toxic to the cells of the central nervous system (CNS), and will prevent it from working properly. One example of the toxic effects of alcohol is the way that alcohol interferes with memory formation. Neuropsychological testing has revealed that alcohol may begin to affect memory trace formation after as little as one drink. On average, however, one needs to consume more than five drinks in an hour's time for alcohol to significantly impact memory formation (Browning, Hoffer, & Dunwiddie, 1993). Thus memory problems are seldom apparent in the casual or social drinker.

On the other hand, memory disturbance is one of the most frequent symptoms experienced by the heavy drinker. The individual may find it impossible to remember events that took place while intoxicated, a condition that is commonly known as a *blackout*. These periods of alcohol-induced amnesia may last several days although, for the most part, they involve shorter periods (Segal & Sisson, 1985; Willoughby, 1984). During a blackout, the individual may *appear* to be conscious to others and is able to carry out many complex tasks. However, afterward, the drinker will not have any memory of what he/she did during the blackout. In a sense, the alcohol-induced blackout is similar to another condition known as *transient global amnesia* (Kaplan et al., 1994; Rubino, 1992).

Scientists do not understand the mechanism behind either an episode of transient global amnesia, or the alcoholic blackout. However, in general, it is believed that alcohol prevents the individual from being able to form (encode) memories during the period of acute intoxication (Browning et al., 1993). The alcohol-induced blackout is "an early and serious indicator of the development of alcoholism" (Rubino, 1992, p. 360). The majority of individuals who use alcohol on a chronic basis admit to having alcohol-induced blackouts, when asked. For example, Schuckit, Smith, Anthenelli, and Irwin (1993) found that 521 men of the 636 male alcoholics in their sample (or 82% of the sample group) admitted

they had experienced alcohol-related blackouts at some point in their drinking history.

The chronic use of alcohol may contribute to other, more serious forms of neurological dysfunction in addition to blackouts. While it was once thought that alcohol-induced central nervous system damage did not appear until after relatively late in the individual's drinking career, recent research indicates that this might not be true. Strong evidence suggests that 15% of alcohol-dependent individuals will show signs of alcohol-induced brain damage before showing overt signs of alcohol-related liver damage (Berg, Franzen, & Wedding, 1994; Bowden, 1994). The research conducted by the team of Volkow et al. (1992) would support this theory. The authors used the technique of positron emission tomography (PET scan) to measure the metabolism of different regions of the brains of normal and alcoholic males. The alcoholic male subjects used in this study had at least a 15-year history of alcohol abuse, and had only recently completed alcohol withdrawal. The men in both groups were free from major illness, and there was no evidence of major neurological impairment on standard neuropsychological tests for any of the men in the study.

The PET scan results demonstrated significantly reduced levels of brain metabolism in the left parietal and right frontal cortex regions of the brains of the alcohol-dependent volunteers, areas of the brain that are known to be affected by chronic alcohol use. On the basis of their research, the authors concluded that the effects of alcohol on the brain last well beyond the stage of acute withdrawal. Further, Volkow et al. (1992) found that the PET scan was able to identify evidence of alcohol-induced neurological dysfunction at a stage *before* the development of brain damage severe enough to be measured using standard neuropsychological tests. These findings point the way for further research and suggest that the PET scan might be a tool that could identify individuals who are at risk for alcohol-induced brain damage if they keep drinking.

Although the chronic use of alcohol has been called the single most preventable cause of dementia in this country (Beasley, 1987), researchers still do not agree as to the mechanism by which alcohol contributes to brain damage (Roehrs & Roth, 1995).

Research has suggested that up to 75% of chronic alcohol users will show evidence of alcohol-induced cognitive impairment following detoxification (Butterworth, 1995; Hartman, 1995; Tarter, Ott, & Mezzich, 1991), and between 15 and 30% of all nursing home patients are there because of permanent alcohol-induced brain damage (Schuckit, 1995a). Further, it has been estimated that alcohol-induced dementia is the "second most common adult dementia after Alzheimer's disease" (Nace & Isbell, 1991, p. 56).

While evidence suggests that a limited degree of improvement in cognitive function is possible in alcoholics who remain abstinent from alcohol for extended periods, this does not mean that every alcoholic who abstains from alcohol will achieve a complete recovery (Grant, 1987; Loberg, 1986). Research also indicates that, following abstinence, only 20% of chronic alcohol users may return to their previous level of intellectual function (Nace & Isbell, 1991). Some limited degree of recovery is possible in perhaps 60% of the cases, and virtually no recovery of lost intellectual function is seen in 20% of the cases, according to the authors.

It is not known how the chronic use of alcohol contributes to the death of nerve cells. One theory suggests that the observed neurological damage is another consequence of alcohol-induced avitaminosis (Willoughby, 1984). Another central nervous system complication seen as a result of chronic alcohol abuse is *vitamin deficiency amblyopia*. This condition will cause blurred vision, a loss of visual perception in the center of the visual field known as central scotomata and, in extreme cases, atrophy of the optic nerve (Mirin, Weiss, & Greenfield, 1991). The alcohol-induced damage to the visual system may be permanent.

Wernicke-Korsakoff's Syndrome

Perhaps the most serious complication of chronic alcohol use is a form of brain damage once known as *Wernicke's encephalopathy* (Charness et al., 1989). Wernicke's encephalopathy develops in about 20% of chronic alcohol users (Bowden, 1994). Alcohol-induced avitaminosis is again thought to be a major factor in the development of Wernicke's encephalopathy. As a result of the lack of adequate vita-

min intake by the individual's body, the individual's body will gradually be depleted of thiamine, one of the "B" family of vitamins. Even with the best of medical care, the mortality rate during the acute phase of Wernicke's encephalopathy is 15% to 20% (Ciraulo, Shader, Ciraulo, Greenblatt, & von Moltke, 1994b; Zubaran, Fernandes, & Rodnight, 1997).

Chronic thiamine deficiency results in characteristic patterns of brain damage, which is often detected on physical examination of the brain following death. The patient who is suffering from Wernicke's encephalopathy often appears confused, possibly to the point of being delirious and disoriented. He/she also is apathetic and unable to sustain physical or mental activities (Victor, 1993). A physical examination reveals a characteristic pattern of abnormal eye movements known as *nystagmus* and such symptoms of brain damage as gait disturbances and ataxia (Lehman et al., 1994).

Before physicians developed a method to treat Wernicke's encephalophy, up to 80% of the patients who developed this condition went on to develop a condition known as *Korsakoff's psychosis* or *syndrome*. Another name for Korsakoff's syndrome is the *alcohol amnestic disorder* (Charness et al., 1989; Victor, 1993). Even when Wernicke's encephalophy is properly treated through the most aggressive thiamine replacement procedures known to modern medicine, fully 25% of the patients who develop Wernicke's disease will go on to develop Korsakoff's syndrome (Sagar, 1991).

For many years, scientists thought that Wernicke's encephalopathy and Korsakoff's syndrome were separate disorders. It is now known that Wernicke's encephalopathy is the acute phase of the Wernicke-Korsakoff syndrome. One of the most prominent symptoms of the Korsakoff phase of this syndrome is that the patient is unable to remember the past accurately. In addition, the individual will also have difficulty learning new information. Despite these problems, the patient frequently appears indifferent to his/her memory loss (Ciraulo et al., 1994b).

In the earlier stages, the person will be confused by his/her inability to remember the past clearly. He/she often "fills in" these memory gaps by making up answers to questions. This process is called *confabulation*. Confabulation is not always found in cases of Korsakoff's syndrome. But, when present, it is most common in the earlier stages (Parsons & Nixon, 1993; Victor, 1993). Later on, as the individual adjusts to the memory loss, he/she will not be as likely to use confabulation to cover up the memory problem (Blansjaar & Zwinderman, 1992; Brandt & Butters, 1986).

In rare cases, these individuals lose virtually all memories after a certain period of their lives and are almost "frozen in time." For example, Sacks (1970) offered an example of a man who, when examined, was unable to recall anything that happened after the late 1940s. The patient was examined in the 1960s, but when asked, he would answer questions as if he were still living in the 1940s. This example of confabulation, while extremely rare, can result from chronic alcoholism. More frequent are the less pronounced cases, where significant portions of the memory are lost, but the individual retains some ability to recall the past.

The exact mechanism of Wernicke-Korsakoff's syndrome is unknown. The characteristic nystagmus seems to respond to massive doses of thiamine, or vitamin B1. It is possible that victims of Wernicke-Korsakoff's syndrome possess a genetic susceptibility to the effects of the alcohol-induced thiamine deficiency (Parsons & Nixon, 1993). In other words, certain individuals might be more likely to develop a thiamine deficiency when they use alcohol on a chronic basis than others, because of their genetic heritage. While this is an attractive theory, in that it explains why some chronic alcoholics develop Wernicke-Korsakoff's syndrome and others do not, it remains just a theory.

Other researchers have suggested that the intellectual decline noted in Wernicke-Korsakoff's syndrome is caused by a different mechanism than the characteristic ocular nystagmus of this disorder. It has been suggested that the person with Wernicke-Korsakoff's syndrome is suffering from the neurotoxic effects of the long-term exposure to alcohol (Brandt & Butters, 1986). The authors pointed out that alcohol is a known neurotoxin, and that the chronic alcoholic may experience a gradual loss of the neurons necessary for intellectual performance.

Jensen and Pakkenberg (1993) offered a unique theory as to the effects of alcohol on the physical structure of the brain. The authors performed a postmortem examination of the brains of 55 individuals who had been active alcoholics prior to death. It was found that the chronic alcohol use did not cause the death of neurons so much as it caused them to become *disconnected* from their neighbors. The authors found evidence of degeneration *in specific regions of the nerve cells* known as the axons and dendrites, rather than evidence that entire nerve cells had died as a result of chronic alcohol exposure. The authors suggested that the loss of intellectual function seen in chronic alcohol use might reflect the disruption of established nerve pathways caused by the degeneration of the axons and dendrites of some of the brain cells.

These are only theories, which remain to be proven. It is known that, once Wernicke-Korsakoff's syndrome has developed, only a minority of its victims will escape without lifelong neurological damage. It is estimated that even with the most aggressive vitamin replacement therapy, only 20% (Nace & Isbell, 1991) to 25% (Brandt & Butters, 1986) of its victims will return to their previous level of intellectual function. The other 75% to 80% will experience greater or lesser degrees of neurological damage. Further, very little is known about the process of rehabilitation for the victims of Korsakoff's syndrome, or whether rehabilitation is even possible (Blansjaar & Zwinderman, 1992; Parsons & Nixon, 1993).

There is evidence that chronic alcohol abuse/addiction is a risk factor in the development of a movement disorder known as *tardive dyskinesia* (TD) (Lopez & Jeste, 1997). This condition may result from alcohol's neurotoxic effect, according to the authors. Although TD is a common complication in patients who have used neuroleptic drugs for the control of psychotic conditions for long periods, there are cases where an alcohol-dependent individual has developed TD despite having had no prior exposure to neuroleptic agents (Lopez & Jeste, 1997). The exact mechanism by which alcohol causes the development of tardive dyskinesia remains to be identified, and scientists have no idea why some alcohol abusers develop TD while others do not. According to the authors, TD usually develops in chronic alcohol users with a history of drinking for 10 to 20 years.

Alcohol's Effects on the Sleep Cycle

Alcohol is a CNS depressant, and while it may induce sleep, it interferes with the normal sleep pattern. Clinicians often encounter patients who complain of sleep problems, without revealing their alcohol abuse. For example, the staff of one sleep disorders clinic found that 12% of the patients who were seen because of insomnia were found to have a history of alcohol abuse or alcohol dependence (Frederickson, Richardson, Esther, & Lin, 1990). Alcohol also interferes with the normal dream cycle by suppressing what is known as the rapid eye movement (or REM) phase of sleep. There is a relationship between REM sleep and dreaming. The individual who stops drinking enters a period of abnormal sleep known as "REM rebound." This is a pattern of sleep where the person dreams more intensely and more vividly, often to the point of frequent nightmares. These rebound dreams may be so frightening that the individual may return to the use of alcohol to "get a decent night's sleep." The phase of "REM rebound" can last for up to six months after the person has stopped drinking, and, in rare cases, the effects of alcohol can interfere with the normal sleep cycle for between one and two years after detoxification (Frederickson et al., 1990; Satel, Kosten, Schuckit, & Fischman, 1993).

The Effects of Chronic Alcohol Use on the Peripheral Nervous System

The human nervous system is usually viewed as two interconnected systems. The brain and spinal cord make up the central nervous system, whereas the nerves found in the outer regions of the body are classified as the "peripheral" nervous system. The effects of alcohol-induced avitaminosis are sufficiently widespread to include the peripheral nerves, especially those in the hands and feet. This is a condition known as *peripheral neuropathy*. This condition is found in 10% (Schuckit, 1995b) to 33% of chronic alcohol users (Monforte et al., 1995).

Some of the symptoms of a peripheral neuropathy include feelings of weakness, pain, and a burning sensation in the afflicted region of the body (Lehman et al., 1994). Eventually, the person will

lose all feeling in the affected region. It should be noted that peripheral neuropathy is not only found in alcoholism. It is also a common complication in some forms of diabetes and, rarely, as a complication to other medical conditions. But fully 30% of all cases of peripheral neuropathy is thought to be alcohol-induced (Hartman, 1995).

The exact cause of alcohol-induced peripheral neuropathy is not known. Some researchers believe it is the result of a deficiency of the "B" family of vitamins in the body caused by either the poor eating habits commonly found in chronic alcohol use or the vitamin malabsorption syndrome that is a common complication of alcoholism, or a combination of these two factors (Beasley, 1987; Charness et al., 1989; Nace, 1987).

Monforte et al. (1995) suggested another theory: peripheral neuropathies might be the result of chronic exposure to either alcohol, which is a mild toxin, or its metabolites. As discussed in Chapter 4, some of the metabolites of alcohol are themselves toxic to the body. The authors failed to find evidence of a nutritional deficit for those hospitalized alcoholics who had developed peripheral neuropathies. But, they did find evidence of a dose-related relationship between the use of alcohol and the development of peripheral neuropathies.

Surprisingly, in light of alcohol's known neurotoxic effects, there is evidence to suggest that at some doses it may suppress the involuntary movements of Huntington's disease (Lopez & Jeste, 1997). While this is not to suggest that alcohol is an acceptable treatment for this disorder, this effect of alcohol might account for the authors' finding that patients with movement disorders such as essential tremor, or Huntington's disease, tend to abuse alcohol more often than close relatives who do not have a movement disorder.

The Effects of Chronic Alcoholism on the Person's Emotional State

The chronic use of alcohol can simulate the symptoms of virtually every form of neurosis, and even those seen in psychotic conditions. These symptoms are thought to be secondary to the individual's malnutrition, and the toxic effects of chronic alcohol use (Beasley, 1987). These symptoms include depressive reactions (Blondell et al., 1996; Schuckit, 1995a), generalized anxiety disorders, and panic attacks (Beasley, 1987).

There is a complex relationship between anxiety symptoms and alcohol use disorders. For example, without medical intervention, almost 80% of alcohol-dependent individuals will experience panic episodes during the acute phase of withdrawal from alcohol (Schuckit, 1995b). The chronic use of alcohol causes a paradoxical stimulation of the autonomic nervous system (ANS). Drinkers often interpret this ANS stimulation as a sign of anxiety and attempt to control it with alcohol or antianxiety medications. A cycle is then started where the chronic use of alcohol actually sets the stage for further anxietylike symptoms, resulting in the perceived need for more alcohol or medication. Stockwell and Town (1989) discussed this aspect of chronic alcohol use, and concluded: "Many clients who drink heavily or abuse other anixolytic drugs will experience substantial or complete recovery from extreme anxiety following successful detoxification" (p. 223). The authors recommend a drug-free period of *at least two weeks* in which to assess the need for pharmacological intervention for anxiety.

Evidence suggests that anxiety disorders are "more prevalent in alcohol abusers" than in the general population (Toneatto, Sobell, Sobell, & Leo, 1991, p. 91). However, of those patients diagnosed as having a generalized anxiety disorder (GAD), more than 20% are alcohol-dependent individuals whose "anxiety" is actually an early symptom of alcohol withdrawal (Beasley, 1987). Further, Decker and Ries (1993) estimated that 10% to 28% of patients who report that they suffer from anxiety symptoms will also have an alcohol use disorder. Stockwell and Town (1989) agreed with this observation, and warned that "many" (p. 223) of those who seek help for anxiety attacks are experiencing withdrawal-related rebound anxiety. The authors suggested that this rebound anxiety would clear up after the use of alcohol is discontinued.

The differentiation between "true" anxiety disorders, and alcohol-related anxietylike disorders is thus quite complex. The team of Kushner, Sher, and Beitman (1990) concluded that alcohol withdrawal symptoms may be "indistinguishable" (p. 692) from the symptoms of panic attacks and GAD. The authors also concluded that agoraphobia and social phobias usually predate alcohol use. Victims of these disorders usually attempt self-medication through the use of alcohol, and then develop problems associated with alcohol abuse. On the other hand, Kushner et al. (1990) concluded that the symptoms of simple panic attacks and generalized anxiety disorder are more likely to reflect the effects of alcohol withdrawal than a psychiatric disorder.

Social phobia frequently coexists with alcoholism (Marshall, 1994). Individuals with social phobias, who fear situations in which they are exposed to other people, tend to have alcohol-use problems twice as often as people from the general population, according to the author.

It is not uncommon for alcohol-dependent individuals to complain of anxiety symptoms when they see their physician, who may then prescribe a benzodiazepine to control the anxiety. This, in turn, allows chronic alcoholics to control their withdrawal symptoms during the day without having the smell of alcohol on their breath. (One alcohol-dependent individual explained, for example, that the effects of 10 mg of diazepam were similar to the effects of having had 3–4 quick drinks). Given this tendency for alcohol-dependent individuals to use benzodiazepines, it should not be surprising to learn that 25% to 50% of alcoholics are also addicted to these drugs (N. Miller & Gold, 1991b).

If the physician fails to obtain an adequate history and physical (or if the patient lies about his/her alcohol use), there is also a risk that the alcohol-dependent person might combine the use of antianxiety medication, which is a CNS depressant, with alcohol (which is also a CNS depressant). There is a significant potential for an overdose when two classes of CNS depressants are combined. Thus, the use of alcohol with CNS depressants such as the benzodiazepines or antihistamines presents a grave danger to the patient.

Also, as Beasley (1987) noted, the family of antianxiety agents known as benzodiazepines may, when combined with alcohol, bring about a *paradoxical rage reaction*. This condition results when a drug that is normally a depressant triggers an unexpected period of rage in the individual, who may then turn and lash out at others. During the paradoxical rage reaction, the individual might engage in assaultive or destructive behavior toward either themselves or others, while having no conscious memory of what he/she did during the paradoxical rage reaction (Lehman et al., 1994).

If antianxiety medication is needed, buspirone is thought to be effective (Kranzler et al., 1994). As discussed in Chapter 7, buspirone is not a benzodiazepine, and thus it does not present the potential for abuse seen with the latter family of drugs. The authors found that those alcoholic subjects in their study who suffered from anxiety symptoms, and who received buspirone, were more likely to both remain in treatment and consume less alcohol than those anxious subjects who did not receive buspirone. This suggests that buspirone might be an effective medication in treating anxious alcoholics.

Chronic alcohol use has been known to interfere with sexual performance for both men and women (Schiavi, Stimmel, Mandeli, & White, 1995). Although the chronic use of alcohol has been shown to interfere with the erectile process for men, the team of Schiavi et al. (1995) found that once the individual stopped drinking, the erectile dysfunction usually resolved itself. As noted in Chapter 32, however, there is evidence that disulfiram (often used in the treatment of chronic alcoholism) itself may interfere with a man's ability to achieve an erection.

There also is a relationship between alcohol use disorders and depression. Research has suggested that primary depression is actually quite rare in chronic alcohol users, with only between 2 and 3% (Powell, Read, Penick, Miller, & Bingham, 1987), to perhaps as many as 5% (Schuckit, 1995b) of the cases of depression seen in alcoholics actually being a primary depression. But it has been estimated that 10% to 15% of those individuals who are depressed will attempt to use alcohol to self-medicate their emotional distress (J. W. Campbell, 1992). Many people who are clinically depressed are unaware that, although alcohol initially numbs feelings of depression, ultimately it can contribute to the very depression that the person wishes to escape from. Willoughby (1984) noted that the depressant effects from one drink may last as long as 96 hours. The depressant effects of an alcohol binge of even one or

two days may linger for several weeks after abstinence (Segal & Sisson, 1985).

Thus, the use of alcohol as a self-medication for depression adds to the individual's feelings of depression over time. To further complicate the diagnostic picture, alcohol has been implicated as the cause of depressive reactions for chronic alcohol users. It has been suggested that during the first two weeks of treatment "most" (Wolf-Reeve, 1990, p. 72) chronic drinkers meet the diagnostic criteria for major depression.

In the vast majority of these cases, however, the individual is found to suffer from an alcohol-induced depression. Such alcohol-induced depressive episodes usually clear after 2 to 5 weeks of abstinence and usually do not require formal treatment (Decker & Ries, 1993; N. Miller, 1994; Satel et al., 1993). Experts in the field of alcoholism still do not agree on the minimum length of time to wait, for an alcohol-induced depressive reaction to clear. Decker and Ries noted that experts in the field of psychiatry suggest waiting periods of between four weeks and "several months" (p. 704) are necessary after the person stops drinking, to see if the alcohol-induced depression will resolve itself. Thus, there is no clear rule to suggest when antidepressant medication and/or psychiatric treatment might be needed to help the drinker recover from depression.

However, Blume (1994) issued a note of caution concerning the relationship between depression and alcohol use disorders. She noted that because most research into the effects of alcohol has been conducted using male subjects, there has been little understanding of the effects of alcohol on women. In her exploration of those few studies that have addressed the impact of alcoholism in women, Blume suggests that in 60% to 65% of the cases where an alcoholic woman is depressed, the woman is experiencing a major depression and should receive treatment.

It is known that active alcohol abuse has a negative effect on the recovery from depression. Mueller et al. (1994) examined the relationship between these two disorders and found that depressed individuals who were either (a) nonalcoholic or (b) abstinent alcoholics had twice the recovery rate from depression as did depressed active alcoholics. The authors also found evidence in their data to suggest that alcohol use did not cause the depressive disorder. Rather, the individual's depression appeared to be caused by other factors than alcohol use. But, once the depressive disorder was in place, the individual's alcohol use status was a major factor in whether he/she would recover from that depressive episode.

There is a strong relationship between depression and suicide (Hirschfield & Davidson, 1988). Since alcoholics tend to experience depressive symptoms either as a consequence of their drinking or because of a coexisting major depression, they are a high-risk group for suicide. The lifetime risk for suicide among alcoholics, whether their depression was primary to or secondary to their drinking, is almost 15% (Hirschfield & Davidson, 1988; Schuckit, 1986). Brent, Kupfer, Bromet, and Dew (1988) suggested that suicide is most likely to occur late in the course of alcoholism, when the individual begins to experience alcohol-related medical complications, such as cirrhosis of the liver.

The research team of Murphy, Wetzel, Robins, and McEvoy (1992) attempted to isolate the factors that seemed to predict suicide in the chronic male alcoholic. On the basis of their research, the authors identified seven factors that appeared to suggest suicide risk:

1. Drinking heavily in the days and weeks just prior to the act of suicide.
2. Talking about the possibility of committing suicide prior to the act.
3. Having little social support.
4. Suffering from a major depressive disorder.
5. Being unemployed at the time of the suicide.
6. Living alone.
7. Suffering from a major medical problem at the time of the act of suicide.

While the authors failed to find any single factor that seemed to predict a possible suicide in the suicidal chronic male alcoholic, they concluded, "As the number of risk factors increases, the likelihood of a suicidal outcome does likewise" (p. 461). Roy (1993) also identified several factors that seemed to be associated with an increased risk of suicide for adult alcoholics. Like Murphy et al. (1992), he failed to find a single factor that seemed to predict the possibility of suicide for the adult alcoholic. However, Roy did suggest that the following factors were potential indicators for an increased risk of suicide:

1. *Gender.* Men tend to commit suicide more often than women; the ratio of male:female suicides for alcoholics may be about 4:1.
2. *Marital status.* Single/divorced/widowed adults are significantly more likely to attempt suicide than are married adults.
3. *Coexisting depressive disorder.* Depression is associated with an increased risk of suicide.
4. *Adverse life events.* The individual who has suffered an adverse life event such as the loss of a loved one, a major illness, or legal problems is at increased risk.
5. *Recent discharge from treatment for alcoholism.* The first four years following treatment were found to be associated with a significantly higher risk for suicide, although the reason for this was not clear.
6. A *history of previous suicide attempts.* Approximately one-third of alcoholic suicide victims had attempted suicide at some point in the past.
7. *Biological factors.* Such factors as decreased levels of serotonin in the brain are thought to be associated with increased risk for violent behavior, including suicide.

Mental health professionals know that it is impossible to identify every potential suicide victim. However, it is known that some factors, including many of those identified here, are associated with an increased risk for suicide. Thus, substance abuse professionals should have a working knowledge of the risk factors that may alert health care providers to the possibility that a specific individual is at high risk for suicide in the near future.

Alcohol Withdrawal for the Chronic Alcoholic

Each year, "millions" (Yost, 1996, p. 657) of episodes of mild to moderate alcohol withdrawal take place. The symptoms of such alcohol withdrawal may subside quickly, without the need for medical intervention, and might not even be attributed by the individual to his/her use of alcohol. But in 200,000 to 450,000 cases each year in the United States, the individual's alcohol withdrawal is so severe that it requires medical intervention. In such cases, the individual is facing a medical emergency that may result in death.

The alcohol withdrawal syndrome is an acute brain syndrome. In 90% of the cases, the symptoms of withdrawal develop within 4 to 12 hours after either the individual's last drink or after a reduction in the level of drinking (APA, 1995). But in some cases, the withdrawal symptoms do not appear until 96 hours after the last drink or reduction in alcohol intake (Lehman et al., 1994; Weiss & Mirin, 1988). In extreme cases, the person will not begin to experience alcohol withdrawal symptoms until 10 days after his/her last drink (Slaby, Lieb, & Tancredi, 1981).

A standard rule is that the severity of the alcohol withdrawal symptoms experienced by the individual depends on the (a) intensity with which that individual used alcohol, (b) the duration of time during which the individual drank, and (c) the individual's state of health. Some of the symptoms of the alcohol withdrawal syndrome include agitation, anxiety, diarrhea, hyperactivity, exaggerated reflexes, insomnia, nausea, restlessness, sweating, tachycardia, vomiting, and vertigo (Lehman et al., 1994; Lieveld & Aruna, 1991).

In mild withdrawal cases, the patient may experience only few of these symptoms, and may not progress on to the next level of withdrawal. In more advanced cases, however, the symptoms may become more intense over the first 6 to 24 hours following the last use of alcohol. The patient may also begin to experience *alcoholic hallucinosis*. The hallmark of alcoholic hallucinosis are hallucinations (both visual and auditory) caused by the alcohol withdrawal process. These hallucinations are different than those seen in disorders such as schizophrenia, and while they usually do not indicate the onset of a schizophrenic disorder, they still may be quite frightening to the individual.

In extreme cases of alcohol withdrawal, these symptoms will continue to become more intense over the next 24 to 48 hours, and by the third day following the last drink the patient will start to experience

fever, incontinence, and/or tremors in addition to the above noted symptoms. Approximately 16% of those individuals experiencing severe alcohol withdrawal will experience a seizure as part of the withdrawal syndrome (Lehman, Pilich, & Andrews, 1994; Nace & Isbell, 1991). Alcohol-withdrawal seizures are seen both in individuals who do, and do not, develop alcoholic hallucinosis. However, about 5% (Lieveld & Aruna, 1991) to 10% (Weiss & Mirin, 1988) of alcohol-dependent individuals will develop the condition known as *Delirium Tremens* (DTs). The DTs are a manifestation of the most severe alcohol withdrawal syndrome and include symptoms such as: delirium, hallucinations, delusional beliefs that one is being followed, fever, and tachycardia (Lieveld & Aruna, 1991).

In some cases of DTs, the individual experiences a disruption of normal fluid levels in the brain (Trabert, Caspari, Bernhard, & Biro, 1992). This results when the mechanism in the drinker's body that regulates normal fluid levels is disrupted by the alcohol withdrawal process. The individual may become dehydrated or, in other cases, may retain too much fluid in his/her body. During the phase of alcohol withdrawal, some individuals become hypersensitive to the antidiuretic hormone (ADH). This hormone is normally secreted by the body to slow the rate of fluid loss through the kidneys, when the person is somewhat dehydrated. For reasons that are not understood, however, some patients retain *too much* fluid within their bodies rather than become dehydrated during the withdrawal process.

This excess fluid may contribute to the damage that the alcohol has caused to the brain, possibly by bringing about cerebral edema (Trabert et al., 1992). Researchers have found that only patients going through the DTs have the combination of higher levels of ADH and low body fluid levels. This finding suggests that a body fluid dysregulation process might somehow be involved in the development of the DTs (Trabert et al.).

Not every alcohol-dependent individual experiences the DTs. Rubino (1992) suggests that the alcohol withdrawal syndrome might be viewed as a continuum (see Figure 5.1). The least severe symptoms of alcohol withdrawal would be the tremulousness ("shakes") experienced by the individual when

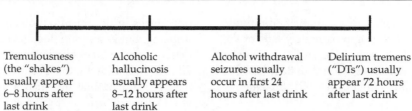

FIGURE 5.1 Continuum of alcohol withdrawal symptoms. Source: Chart suggested by Rubino, F. A. (1992). "Neurological Complications of Alcoholism." *Psychiatric Clinics of North America, 15,* 359–372.

the central nervous system must adjust to the absence of the alcohol that was present for so long. The syndrome of alcoholic hallucinosis might be viewed as a more severe manifestation of the alcohol withdrawal syndrome than the shakes, but would be less severe than withdrawal seizures. Finally, the most severe symptom of alcohol withdrawal would be the delirium tremens, or DTs, according to the author.

As useful as this continuum might be as a guide for judging the severity of the alcohol withdrawal syndrome, Rubino (1992) warns, "The syndrome may stop at any point spontaneously, however, or skip any part of the continuum for unknown reasons" (p. 360). Thus, this continuum must be viewed only as a rough guide as to the severity of the alcohol withdrawal syndrome. Further, there is some variation between individuals going through the alcohol withdrawal syndrome. There are cases on record of the person going into an alcohol withdrawal syndrome up to 10 days after the last drink (Slaby et al., 1981).

In the past, death from exhaustion resulted in 5% to 25% of individuals going through the most severe form of the alcohol withdrawal syndrome—the DTs (Lehman et al., 1994; Schuckit, 1995). However, improved medical care has decreased the mortality from DTs to about 1% (Milzman & Soderstrom, 1994) to 5% (Yost, 1996). The main causes of death for persons going through the DTs include sepsis, cardiac and/or respiratory arrest, or cardiac and/or circulatory collapse (Lieveld & Aruna, 1991). Persons going through the DTs are also a high-risk group for suicide as they struggle to come to terms with the emotional pain and terror associated with this condition (Hirschfield & Davidson, 1988; Weiss & Mirin, 1988).

Although a number of chemicals have been suggested as being of value in controlling the symptoms of alcohol withdrawal, the current medical practice is to use one of the benzodiazepines, usually chlordiazepoxide or diazepam, for this purpose. The use of pharmaceutical agents to control the alcohol withdrawal symptoms is discussed in Chapter 32.

Other Complications from Chronic Alcohol Use

Either directly, or indirectly, alcohol contributes to a large number of head injuries (Anderson, 1991; Sparadeo & Gill, 1989). It is not uncommon for the intoxicated individual to fall and strike his/her head on coffee tables, magazine stands, or whatever happens to be in the way. The chronic use of alcohol contributes to the development of three different bone disorders (Griffiths, Parantainen, & Olson, 1994):

1. *Osteoporosis.* Loss of bone mass.
2. *Osteomalacia.* A condition where new bone tissue fails to absorb minerals appropriately.
3. *Secondary hyperparathyroidism.* A hormonal disorder that develops when alcohol interferes with the body's ability to regulate calcium levels in the blood for extended periods, resulting in the calcium in the bones being reabsorbed into the blood, and the bones becoming weakened through calcium loss.

These bone disorders in turn contribute to the higher than expected level of injury and death seen when alcoholics fall or are involved in automobile accidents.

Alcohol is also a factor in traumatic brain injury. Researchers believe that approximately half of the estimated one million people who suffer a traumatic head injury each year have alcohol in their blood at the time of the injury (Anderson, 1991; Sparadeo & Gill, 1989).

Chronic alcohol use may reduce the individual's life expectancy by 15 years, with the leading causes of death being (in decreasing order of frequency) heart disease, cancer, accidents, and suicide (Schuckit, 1995b). Between 90,000 (Paulos, 1994) to 200,000 (Kaplan et al., 1994; Schuckit, 1995b) Americans die each year from alcohol-related accidents, diseases, or suicide.

In addition to this, women who drink while pregnant run the risk of causing alcohol-induced birth defects, a condition known as the *fetal alcohol syndrome*. This condition is discussed in detail in Chapter 20. It is important to be aware of a connection between alcohol use during pregnancy and birth defects.

Chronic alcoholism has been associated with a premature aging syndrome in which the individual appears much older than his/her actual age (Brandt & Butters, 1986). In many cases, the overall physical and intellectual condition of the alcoholic corresponds to that of someone 15 to 20 years older. One patient, a man in his 50s, was told by his physician that he was in good health—for a man about to turn 70.

Admittedly, every alcoholic will not suffer from every consequence reviewed in this chapter. Some chronic alcohol users will never suffer from stomach problems, for example, but may suffer from advanced heart disease as a result of their drinking. However, Schuckit (1995a) noted that, in one research study, 93% of alcohol-dependent individuals admitted to treatment had at least one important medical problem in addition to their alcoholism.

Research has demonstrated that, in most cases, the first alcohol-related problems are experienced when the person is in the late 20s or early 30s. The team of Schuckit, Smith, Anthenelli, and Irwin (1993) outlined a progressive course for alcoholism, based on their study of 636 male alcoholics. The authors admitted that their subjects experienced wide differences in the specific problems caused by their drinking, but as a group, the alcoholics began to experience severe alcohol-related problems in their late 20s. By their mid-30s, these individuals were likely to have recognized that they had a drinking problem, and to have experienced more severe problems as a result of their continued drinking. However, as the authors pointed out, there is a wide variation in this pattern, and some subgroups of alcoholics might fail to follow this pattern.

The issue of whether there is an addictive personality is discussed in Chapter 18. The only generalization that can be made about the risk factors for alcoholism is that compared with the general population the children of alcoholics appear to have between a threefold and a fourfold increased likelihood of becoming alcoholic (Ackerman, 1983; Schuckit, 1987; Vaillant, 1983). Researchers interpret this tendency as reflecting a genetic predisposition toward alcoholism that is passed from one generation to another, especially in males.

Evidence would suggest that this genetic predisposition also requires certain environmental factors to trigger the development of alcoholism. However, if the individual has ever had an addiction disorder, then this person should certainly be considered at risk for alcoholism.

Summary

This chapter explored the many facets of alcoholism. The scope of alcohol abuse/addiction in this country was reviewed including that alcoholism accounts for approximately 85% of the drug addiction problem in the United States.

In this chapter, the different forms of tolerance and the ways that the chronic use of alcohol can affect the body were discussed. The impact of chronic alcohol use on the central nervous system, the cardiopulmonary system, the digestive system, and the skeletal bone structure were reviewed. In addition, the relationship between chronic alcohol use and physical injuries, the effect of chronic alcohol use on the life span, and premature aging were examined. Finally, the process of alcohol withdrawal was discussed.

CHAPTER SIX

Barbiturates and Similar Drugs

Anxiety and insomnia have been problems for at least as long as physicians have been keeping records on their patients. The anxiety disorders are, collectively, the most common form of mental illness found in the United States (Blair & Ramones, 1996). Researchers believe that between 7% and 23% of the general population suffers from anxiety in one form or another (Baughan, 1995; Blair & Ramones, 1996). Over the course of their lives, approximately one-third of all adults will experience at least transient periods of anxiety intense enough to interfere with their daily lives (Spiegel, 1996). Further, scientists believe that in a year's time 35% or more of the adults in the United States experience some form of insomnia (Lacks & Morin, 1992). As these figures indicate, anxiety and insomnia cause a significant degree of distress to patients each year.

For thousands of years, alcohol was the only agent that could reduce anxiety levels or help people fall asleep. However, as was discussed in Chapter 5, alcohol's effectiveness as an antianxiety[1] agent (often called a "sedative") is limited. Thus, for many centuries, scientists have searched for effective antianxiety or hypnotic[2] medications. In this chapter, we review the medications that were used to control anxiety or promote sleep prior to the introduction of the

benzodiazepines in the early 1960s. In Chapter 7, the focus is on the benzodiazepine family of drugs, and on medications that have been introduced since the benzodiazepines first appeared.

Early Pharmacological Therapy of Anxiety Disorders and Insomnia

It was not until the year 1870 that *chloral hydrate* was introduced as a hypnotic. Researchers had found that chloral hydrate was rapidly absorbed from the digestive tract and that an oral dose of 1–2 grams would cause the typical person to fall asleep in less than an hour. Its effects usually lasted 8 to 11 hours, and since most people sleep around 8 hours at a time, it appeared to be ideal for use as a hypnotic.

However, physicians quickly discovered that chloral hydrate had several major drawbacks, the worst one being that chloral hydrate was irritating to the stomach lining. When used for extended periods, the drug was found to cause significant amounts of damage to the lining of the stomach. Also, physicians discovered that patients who used chloral hydrate for extended periods often became physically dependent on the drug. Finally, it was discovered that withdrawal from chloral hydrate after extended use was dangerous; many patients developed life-threatening withdrawal seizures.

Since its introduction, pharmacologists have discovered a great deal about chloral hydrate. Most importantly, after it is ingested, chloral hydrate is

[1] Occasionally, mental health professionals use the term *anxiolytic* instead of antianxiety. In this text, however, the term *antianxiety* is used.

[2] A "hypnotic" is a medication designed to help the user fall asleep.

65

rapidly biotransformed into *trichloroethanol*. It is this metabolite of chloral hydrate that causes the drug to be effective as a hypnotic. Despite its known dangers, chloral hydrate's relatively short biological half-life makes it of value in treating some elderly patients who suffer from insomnia. Thus, even with all the newer medications available to physicians, there are still patients who receive chloral hydrate to help them sleep.

Paraldehyde was first used as a hypnotic in 1882, although it had first been isolated in the year 1829. As a hypnotic, paraldehyde is quite effective. It produces little respiratory or cardiac depression, making it a relatively safe drug to use with patients who have some forms of pulmonary or cardiac disease. However, it tends to produce a noxious taste and odor, and users develop a strong odor on their breath after use. Paraldehyde is irritating to the mucous membranes of the mouth and throat, and must be diluted in a liquid before use.

The half-life of paraldehyde ranges from 3.4 to 9.8 hours, and about 70% to 80% of a single dose is biotransformed by the liver prior to excretion. From 11% to 28% of a single dose leaves the body unchanged, usually by being exhaled. This route of removal is the reason that users develop a characteristic unpleasant odor on their breath. Paraldehyde has an abuse/addiction potential similar to that of alcohol, and intoxication on paraldehyde resembles alcohol-induced intoxication. After the barbiturates were introduced, paraldehyde gradually fell into disfavor. However, it has a limited role in medicine, even today.

The *bromide salts* were first used for the treatment of insomnia in the mid-1800s. They were available without a prescription and were used well into the twentieth century. While bromides are indeed capable of causing the user to fall asleep, it was soon discovered that they tend to accumulate in the chronic user's body, causing a drug-induced depression after as little as just a few days of continuous use. The bromide salts have been totally replaced by newer drugs, such as the barbiturates.

Despite superficial differences in chemical structure, all these chemicals are central nervous system (CNS) depressants and share many characteristics. To a significant degree, the CNS depressants potentiate the effects of other CNS depressants. Further, as a group, they all have a significant potential for abuse. Even with these shortcomings, the CNS depressants were the treatment of choice for anxiety and insomnia, until the barbiturates were introduced.

History and Current Medical Uses of the Barbiturates

Late in the nineteenth century, chemists discovered the barbiturates. Experimentation quickly revealed that, depending on the dose, the barbiturates acted either as a sedative or, at a higher dosage level, as a hypnotic. In addition, it was discovered that the barbiturates were safer and less noxious than the bromides, chloral hydrate, or paraldehyde (Greenberg, 1993). In 1903, the first barbiturate—Veronal—was introduced for human use (Peluso & Peluso, 1988).

Since their introduction, some 2,500 different barbiturates have been isolated by chemists. Most of these barbiturates were never marketed and have remained only laboratory curiosities. Perhaps 50 barbiturates were marketed at one point or another in the United States, of which 20 are still in use (Nishino, Mignot, & Dement, 1995). After the introduction of the benzodiazepines in the 1960s, many barbiturates previously in use gradually fell into disfavor, and they now have no role in the routine treatment of anxiety or insomnia (Uhde & Trancer, 1995).

There are still areas of medicine, however, where certain barbiturates remain the pharmaceutical of choice (e.g., in some surgical procedures and the control of epilepsy). Surprisingly, although newer drugs have all but replaced the barbiturates in modern medicine, controversy still rages around the appropriate use of many of these chemicals. For example, although the barbiturates were once thought to be effective in the control of pressure levels within the brain following trauma, physicians now question the effectiveness of barbiturates in the control of intracranial hypertension (Lund & Papadakos, 1995).

In some states, a form of barbiturate is used to execute criminals by lethal injection (Truog, Berde, Mitchell, & Grier, 1992). Another equally controversial use of the barbiturates is in the sedation of terminally ill cancer patients (Truog et al., 1992). The authors suggest that extremely large doses of select barbiturates be used to sedate patients in excruciating pain from the terminal stages of some forms of cancer. While doses at this level might speed the patient's death through respiratory depression, the authors argue that the ability of the barbiturates to provide some freedom from pain make it an attractive adjunct to the treatment of at least some terminal cancer patients.

Thus, even today, more than a century after their discovery, the barbiturates remain controversial drugs.

The Abuse Potential of Barbiturates

The barbiturates have a considerable abuse potential. In the period between 1950 and 1970, the barbiturates were, as a group, second only to alcohol as drugs of abuse (Reinisch, Sanders, Mortensen, & Rubin, 1995). Although for the most part they have been replaced by newer drugs, the barbiturates are still abused. For example, in years past, heroin addicts would use barbiturates to boost the effects of low-potency heroin by mixing the barbiturate with the heroin prior to injection (Kaminski, 1992). However, in this era of high-potency heroin (see Chapter 11), it is not known whether heroin addicts still add barbiturates to their heroin to increase the drug's effects.

Among individuals over the age of 40, there is a subgroup of people who became addicted to the barbiturates when they were younger. For people of this generation, the barbiturates were the most effective treatment for anxiety and insomnia, and many users became—and remain—addicted (Kaplan et al., 1994). Thus, although they have a limited role in modern medicine, the barbiturates continue to represent a significant part of the drug abuse problem.

Finally, there is evidence to suggest that, with the increasing restrictions on the prescribing of benzodiazepines in many states, the number of prescriptions for barbiturates might even be on the increase (American Society of Hospital Pharmacists, 1993).

The Pharmacology of Barbiturates

Even now, more than a century after their introduction, the exact mechanism by which the barbiturates work is still not entirely known (American Society of Hospital Pharmacists, 1993; Nishino et al., 1995). Chemically, the barbiturates are remarkably similar. The only major difference between the various members of the barbiturate family of drugs is the length of time that it takes the individual's body to absorb, biotransform, and then excrete the specific form that has been used.

One factor that influences the absorption of barbiturates is the specific chemical's lipid solubility. Different barbiturates vary in this respect. Those forms of barbiturate that are easily soluble in lipids are rapidly distributed to all blood-rich tissues, including the brain itself. Thus, pentobarbital, which is highly lipid-soluble, may have an onset of effect in 10 to 15 minutes. In contrast to this, phenobarbital is poorly lipid-soluble and does not begin to have an effect until 60 minutes or longer after the user has ingested the medication.

While neuropharmacologists understand why different forms of barbiturates might have a different duration of effect and speed of action, the exact mechanism by which barbiturates work is still not known. It is known, however, that the barbiturates can be grouped into four classes,[3] using the *duration of action* as the criterion:

1. *Ultrashort-acting barbiturates*. When injected, the effects of the ultrashort-acting barbiturates begin in a matter of seconds, and last for less than one hour. Examples include Pentothal and Brevital. The ultrashort barbiturates are extremely lipid-soluble and thus pass through the blood-brain barrier quickly and have an effect on the brain in just a few seconds. These medications are often utilized in surgical procedures where a rapid onset of effects and a short duration of action are desirable (Snyder, 1986).

2. *Short-acting barbiturates*. When injected, the effects of the short-acting barbiturates begin in a matter of minutes, and last between 4 and 8 hours. Barbiturates in this classification include Nembutal, among others (Kaplan et al., 1994). In terms of

---

[3] Other classification systems also are in use. For example, some researchers classify barbiturates by using their chemical structures as the defining criteria. This text follows the classification system suggested by Snyder (1986).

lipid solubility, the short-acting barbiturates fall between the ultrashort-acting barbiturates and the intermediate-acting barbiturates.

3. *Intermediate-acting barbiturates.* The effects of the intermediate acting barbiturates begin within an hour, and last some 6 to 8 hours. Included in this group are such drugs as Amytal (amobarbital) and Butisol (butabarbital) (Schuckit, 1995a).

4. *Long-acting barbiturates.* The long-acting barbiturates are absorbed slowly, and their effects last for a prolonged period. When taken orally, it may take more than an hour for a long-acting barbiturate to begin to have an effect, and the drug continues to be active in the individual's body for 10 to 12 hours (Snyder, 1986). Phenobarbital is perhaps the most commonly encountered drug in this class.

One point of confusion is that the short-acting barbiturates do *not* have extremely short half-lives. As discussed in Chapter 3, the biological half-life of a drug provides only a rough estimate of the time that a specific chemical will remain in the body. The short-acting barbiturates might have an effect on the user only for a few hours and still have a half-life of 8 to 12 hours, or even longer. This is because their effects are limited not by the speed at which they are biotransformed by the liver, but by the speed with which they are removed from the blood, and distributed to the organs in the body.

Significant levels of the shorter-acting barbiturates can be stored in different organs of the body, long after the drug has stopped having a biological effect. As discussed later in this chapter, barbiturate molecules stored in different body organs will slowly be released back into the general circulation. Thus, even short-acting barbiturates may cause significant "hangover" effects (Uhde & Trancer, 1995).

Overall, the chemical structures of the various barbiturates are quite similar, and once in the user's body, they all tend to have similar effects. Table 6-1 provides an overview of the normal dosage levels of some of the commonly used barbiturates.

There are few significant differences in the relative potency of the barbiturates; as a group, they tend to have remarkably similar effects on the human body.

But, as a general rule, the shorter-term barbiturates are usually biotransformed by the liver before being excreted from the body (Nishino et al., 1995). In contrast, a significant proportion of the longer-term barbiturates are eliminated from the body essentially unchanged.

Thus, between 25% and 50% of phenobarbital, which has a half-life of 2 to 6 days, is excreted by the kidneys virtually unchanged. In contrast, methohexital has a half-life of only 3 to 6 hours, and virtually all of it is biotransformed by the liver before it is excreted from the body (American Society of Hospital Pharmacists, 1993). Another difference between the members of the barbiturate family is the degree to which the drug molecules become protein-bound. As a general rule, the longer the drug's half-life, the stronger the degree of protein binding for that form of barbiturate.

When used on an outpatient basis, the barbiturates are typically administered orally. On occasion, especially in a medical setting, an ultrashort-acting barbiturate is administered intravenously, such as when it is used as an anesthetic in surgery. On rare occasions, the barbiturates are administered rectally, through suppositories.

When taken orally, the barbiturate molecule is rapidly and completely absorbed from the small intestine (Julien, 1992; Winchester, 1990). Once it

TABLE 6-1 Normal Dosage Levels of Commonly Used Barbiturates

Barbiturate	Sedative dose*	Hypnotic dose**
Amobarbital	50–150 mg/day	65–200 mg
Aprobarbital	120 mg/day	40–60 mg
Butabarbital	45–120 mg/day	50–100 mg
Mephobarbital	96–400 mg/day	not used as hypnotic
Pentobarbital	60–80 mg/day	100 mg
Phenobarbital	30–120 mg/day	100–320 mg
Secobarbital	90–200 mg/day	50–200 mg
Talbutal	30–120 mg/day	120 mg

Source: Table based on information provided in Uhde & Trancer (1995).
* Administered in divided doses.
** Administered as a single dose at bedtime.

reaches the blood, the barbiturates are distributed throughout the body, but the concentrations will be highest in the liver and the brain (American Society of Hospital Pharmacists, 1993). The barbiturates are all lipid-soluble, but they vary in their ability to form bonds with blood lipids. As a general rule, the more lipid-soluble a barbiturate is, the more highly protein-bound that chemical will also be (Winchester, 1990).

The behavioral effects of the barbiturates are similar to those of alcohol ("Sleeping Pill," 1988). Thus, like alcohol, once a barbiturate reaches the bloodstream, it is distributed throughout the body and will affect all body tissues to some degree. At normal dosage levels, the barbiturates depress not only the activity of the brain, but also to a lesser degree the activity of the muscle tissues, the heart, and respiration (Matuschka, 1985). However, the barbiturates have their strongest effect within the central nervous system (Rall, 1990).

In the brain, the barbiturates are thought to simulate the effects of the neurotransmitter gamma-aminobutyric acid (GABA) (Hobbs et al., 1995). At the same time, the barbiturates are thought to block the effects of another neurotransmitter, *glutamate*. Scientists believe that GABA is the most important inhibitory neurotransmitter in the brain, whereas glutamate has an stimulating effect on the neurons of the brain (Bohn, 1993; Nutt, 1996; Tabakoff & Hoffman, 1992). At the level of the neuron, the barbiturates reduce the frequency which the GABA receptor site opens, but increases the period of time that it remains open. This action reduces the electrochemical potential of the cell, reducing the frequency with which that neuron can fire (Cooper, Bloom, & Roth, 1996). Thus, on a cellular level, the barbiturates block the effects of the neurotransmitter involved in activation while simulating the effects of the inhibitory neurotransmitter.

At the regional level within the brain, the barbiturates have their greatest impact on the cortex, the reticula activating system (RAS), which is responsible for awareness, and the medulla oblongata, which controls respiration (American Society of Hospital Pharmacists, 1993). At low dosage levels, the barbiturates will reduce the function of the nerve cells in these regions of the brain, bringing on a state of relaxation and, at slightly higher doses, a drug-induced sleep. At extremely high dosage levels, the barbiturates will interfere with the normal function of the neurons of the central nervous system to such a degree that death is possible.

The therapeutic dose of the typical barbiturate is relatively close to the level necessary to bring about an overdose. Some of the barbiturates have a therapeutic dosage to lethal dosage level ratio of only 1 : 3, suggesting that they have little safety margin. This low safety margin, and the significantly higher safety margin offered by the benzodiazepines is one reason the barbiturates have, for the most part, been replaced by the benzodiazepines.

Subjective Effects of Barbiturates at Normal Dosage Levels

At low doses for the occasional user, the barbiturates reduce feelings of anxiety, or, possibly, bring on a sense of euphoria. The individual might also report a feeling of sedation, or fatigue, possibly to the point of drowsiness. At low dosage levels, the barbiturates may also decrease motor activity. Thus, the individual's reaction time will increase, and he/she might have trouble coordinating muscle movements.

The physical sensations brought about by low doses of barbiturates are very similar to those of alcohol, and the subjective effects are "practically indistinguishable from alcohol's" (Peluso & Peluso, 1988, p. 54; "Sleeping Pills," 1988). This is to be expected, since both alcohol and the barbiturates affect the cortex of the brain through a similar pharmacological mechanism. Thus, on occasion, the disinhibition effects of the barbiturates, like alcohol, may cause a state of paradoxical excitement.

Complications of the Barbiturates at Normal Dosage Levels

For almost 60 years, the barbiturates were the treatment of choice for insomnia. Because the barbiturates were so extensively prescribed to help people sleep, it is surprising to learn that research has shown that tolerance rapidly develops to the hypnotic effects of barbiturates. Research suggests that they are not effective as hypnotics after just a few days of regular use (Rall, 1990; Ray & Ksir, 1993).

Further, despite their traditional use as a treatment for insomnia, the sleep that one achieves through the use of barbiturates is not the same as a normal state of sleep. The barbiturates suppress a portion of the sleep cycle known as the Rapid Eye Movement (or REM) state of sleep (Peluso & Peluso, 1988). Scientists who study sleep believe that the individual needs to experience REM sleep for his/her emotional well-being. A reflection of the importance of REM sleep might be found in the observation that about one-quarter of a young adult's total sleep time is normally spent in REM sleep (Kaplan et al., 1994). Barbiturate-assisted sleep results in a reduction in the total amount of time that the individual spends in REM sleep (Rall, 1990). Thus, through the interference of the normal sleep pattern, barbiturate-induced sleep may affect the emotional and physical health of the individual.

When the barbiturates are repeatedly used as a sleep aid and then discontinued, the person will enter a state known as "REM rebound." During this period, the person will dream more intensely and more vividly, as the body tries to catch up on lost REM sleep time. These dreams have been described by individuals as being nightmares that were strong enough to tempt the individual to return to the use of drugs in order to get a "good night's sleep again." This rebound effect might last for one to three weeks, although in rare cases it has been known to last for up to two months (Tyrer, 1993).

Another drawback of the barbiturates is the possibility of a drug hangover the following day (Shannon et al., 1995). In a sense, the physical experience of the barbiturate hangover is similar to that of an alcohol hangover. Subjectively, the individual simply feels "not quite awake" or "unable to get going" the next day. This occurs because many of the barbiturates have extended biological half-life periods. As discussed in Chapter 3, in general, it takes five half-life periods to completely eliminate a single dose of a chemical from the blood. Thus, small amounts of a barbiturate might remain in the person's bloodstream for hours, or even days, after just a single dose, and in some cases, the effects of the barbiturates on judgment, motor skills, and behavior might last for several days (Kaminski, 1992).

If the person continually adds to this reservoir of unmetabolized drug by ingesting additional doses of the barbiturate, there is a greater chance of experiencing a drug hangover. However, whether because of a single dose or repeated doses, the hangover is caused by the same mechanism: traces of unmetabolized barbiturates remaining in the bloodstream for extended periods after the individual stops taking the medication.

The elderly, or those with impaired liver function, are especially likely to have difficulty with the barbiturates because the liver's ability to metabolize many drugs, such as the barbiturates, declines with age. In light of this fact, Sheridan, Patterson, and Gustafson (1982) advised that older individuals who receive barbiturates be started at one-half the usual adult dosage, and that the dosage level gradually be increased until the patient reaches the point where the medication is having the desired effect.

Another consequence of barbiturate use, even in a medical setting, is that this class of pharmaceuticals can cause sexual performance problems such as decreased desire for either partner, and both erectile problems and delayed ejaculation for the male (Finger, Lund, & Slagel, 1997). Also, hypersensitivity reactions have been reported with the barbiturates. Such hypersensitivity reactions are most common in (but not limited to) individuals with asthma. Other complications occasionally seen at normal dosage levels include nausea, vomiting, diarrhea, and, in some cases, constipation. Some patients have developed skin rashes while receiving barbiturates, although the reason for this is not clear. Finally, patients who are prescribed barbiturates often develop an extreme sensitivity to sunlight known as *photosensitivity*. Thus, patients who receive barbiturates must take special precautions to avoid sunburn, even limited exposure to the sun's rays. Because of these problems, and because medications are now available that do not share the dangers associated with barbiturate use, they are not considered to have any role in the treatment of anxiety or insomnia (Tyrer, 1993).

Children with attention-deficit/hyperactivity disorder (ADHD) (or, what was once called "hyperactivity") who also receive phenobarbital are likely to experience a resurgence of their ADHD symptoms. This effect would seem to reflect the ability of the barbiturates to suppress the action of the reticula activating system (RAS) in the brain. It is thought that the RAS of children with ADHD is underactive, so any medication that further reduces the effectiveness of this neurological system will contribute to the development of ADHD symptoms.

Drug Interactions between the Barbiturates and Other Medications

Research has found that the barbiturates interact with numerous other chemicals, increasing or decreasing the amount of these drugs in the blood through various mechanisms. The mixture of barbiturates with any of the CNS depressants (e.g., alcohol, narcotic-based analgesics, phenothiazines, benzodiazepines) is especially dangerous and may result in death (Barnhill, Ciraulo, Ciraulo, & Greene, 1995). Each drug potentiates the effects of the other, by interfering with the biotransformation of the other chemical by the liver. This allows the toxic effects of each drug to continue with greater intensity than one would expect from either chemical alone.

The antihistamines are another class of CNS depressants that might cause a potentiation effect in the patient using a barbiturate (Rall, 1990). Since many antihistamines are available without a prescription, there is a very real danger of unintentional potentiation effects if the patient taking a barbiturate ingests an over-the-counter cold or allergy medicine.

Patients who are taking barbiturates should not use antidepressants known as monoamine oxidase inhibitors (MAOIs, or MAO inhibitors) as the MAOI may inhibit the biotransformation of the barbiturates (Ciraulo, Creelman, et al., 1995). Patients using barbiturates should not take the antibiotic doxycycline, except under a physician's supervision. The barbiturates will reduce the effectiveness of this antibiotic, which may have serious consequences for the patient (Meyers, 1992). If the patient is using barbiturates and tricyclic antidepressants concurrently, the barbiturate will cause the blood plasma levels of the tricyclic antidepressant to drop by as much as 60% (Barnhill, Ciraulo, Ciraulo, & Greene, 1995). The barbiturates in such cases increase the speed with which the antidepressants are metabolized by activation of the liver's microsomal enzymes.

This is the same process through which the barbiturates speed up the metabolism of many oral

contraceptives, corticosteroids, and the antibiotic Flagyl (metronidazole) (Kaminski, 1992). When used concurrently, barbiturates reduce the effectiveness of these medications, according to the author. Women who are taking both oral contraceptives and barbiturates should be aware of the potential for barbiturates to reduce the effectiveness of oral contraceptives (Graedon & Graedon, 1995, 1996).

Individuals who are taking the anticoagulant medication warfarin should not use a barbiturate, except under a physician's supervision. Barbiturate use can interfere with the normal biotransformation of warfarin, resulting in abnormally low blood levels of this anticoagulant medication (Graedon & Graedon, 1995). Further, if the patient should stop taking barbiturates while on warfarin, it is possible for the individual's warfarin levels to rebound to dangerous levels. Thus, these two medications should not be mixed, except under a physician's supervision.

When the barbiturates are biotransformed, they activate a region of the liver that also is involved in the biotransformation of the asthma drug theophylline (sold under a variety of brand names). Patients who use a barbiturate while taking theophylline may experience abnormally low blood levels of the latter drug, a condition that could result in less than optimal control of the asthma. Thus, patients should not use these two medications at the same time, except under a physician's supervision (Graedon & Graedon, 1995).

Finally, in one research study, five of seven patients on pentobarbital who smoked marijuana began to hallucinate (Barnhill et al., 1995). This would suggest that individuals who use barbiturates should not risk possible interactions between these medications and marijuana.

As is obvious from this list of potential interactions between barbiturates and other pharmaceuticals, the barbiturates are a powerful family of drugs. A physician should carefully supervise every case where a patient is using two different chemicals concurrently.

Effects of the Barbiturates at Above-Normal Dosage Levels

When used above the normal dosage levels, barbiturates may cause a state of intoxication similar to that seen with alcohol intoxication. Patients who are intoxicated by barbiturates will demonstrate such behaviors as slurred speech and unsteady gait, without the characteristic smell of alcohol (Jenike, 1991). These individuals will not test positive for alcohol on blood or urine toxicology tests (unless they also have alcohol in their systems). Specific blood or urine toxicology screens must be carried out to detect barbiturate intoxication, if the patient has used these drugs.

Because barbiturates can cause a state of intoxication like that induced by alcohol, some users will ingest more than the normal dose of the drug. The barbiturates have only a narrow "therapeutic window"—the difference between a dosage level high enough to cause sleep is only a little lower than the level necessary to cause an overdose. If the dosage level is increased beyond that normally necessary to induce sleep, or if the individual has used more than one CNS depressant, several different things may happen. As the increasing blood levels of barbiturate interfere with the normal function of the medulla oblongata (the part of the brain that maintains respiration), there is a reduction in respiratory response. There is also a progressive loss of reflex activity, and, if the dose were large enough, coma and, ultimately, death (Jenike, 1991).

In past decades, prior to the introduction of the benzodiazepines, the barbiturates accounted for more than three-fourths of all drug-related deaths in the United States (Peluso & Peluso, 1988). Even now, intentional or unintentional barbiturate overdose continues to be one of the most common causes of drug-related deaths. The estimated death rate in England and Wales for barbiturates is calculated to be 69–176 deaths for each million prescriptions written (Serfaty & Masterton, 1993). Mendelson and Rich (1993), in their study of successful suicides in the San Diego, California, area, found that approximately 10% of those individuals who committed suicide with a drug overdose used barbiturates either exclusively or at least as one of the chemicals that were ingested.

Thus, the barbiturates present a danger of either intentional or unintentional overdose. They do not, however, directly cause any damage to the central nervous system. If the overdose victim reaches

medical support before developing shock or hypoxia, he or she may recover completely from a barbiturate overdose (Sagar, 1991). For this reason, *any suspected barbiturate overdose should be treated by a physician immediately.*

Tolerance of and Dependence on Barbiturates

The primary uses for barbiturates today are limited, as for the most part newer, safer, and more effective drugs have replaced them. Nevertheless, barbiturates continue to have a limited range of medical applications, including the control of epilepsy and the treatment of some forms of severe head injury (Julien, 1992).

An unfortunate characteristic of the barbiturates is that, with regular use, tolerance to many of their effects develops rapidly. Tolerance does not develop to all the effects of these drugs, however. For example, when the barbiturates are used for the control of seizures, tolerance may not be a significant problem. A patient taking phenobarbital for the control of seizures will eventually become somewhat tolerant to its sedative effect, but will not become tolerant to the anticonvulsant effect of the medication. But if a patient takes a barbiturate for its *sedating or hypnotic* effects, then over time he/she will become tolerant to this drug-induced effect, and the barbiturate may become less and less effective.

Patients have been known to try to overcome the process of neuroadaptation to the barbiturates by increasing their dosage of the drug without consulting with their physician. Unfortunately, this attempt at self-medication has resulted in a large number of unintentional barbiturate overdoses, some of which have been fatal. This is because, unlike the narcotic family of drugs, while the individual might experience some degree of neuroadaptation to the barbiturates, there is no concomitant increase in the lethal dose (Jenike, 1991).

A similar process is observed in barbiturates abusers, who use the chemical for its ability to bring about a drug-induced feeling of euphoria. As the user becomes tolerant to the euphoric effects of barbiturates, he/she will experience less and less euphoria from the drug. In such cases, it is not uncommon for the abuser to increase the dose in order to maintain the drug-induced euphoria. Unfortunately, as stated earlier, the lethal dose of barbiturates remains relatively stable, in spite of the growing tolerance/neuroadaptation to the drug. Thus, as a barbiturate abuser increases his or her daily dosage level in order to continue to experience the drug-induced euphoria, he/she will come closer and closer to the lethal dose.

In addition to the phenomenon of tolerance to the barbiturate family of drugs, *cross-tolerance* is also possible between barbiturates and other, similar, chemical agents. Cross-tolerance occurs when a person who has become tolerant to one family of chemicals also becomes tolerant to the effects of other, similar drugs. Cross-tolerance between alcohol and the barbiturates is common, as is some degree of cross-tolerance between the barbiturates and the opiates, and barbiturates and the hallucinogen PCP (Kaplan et al., 1994).

The United States went through a wave of barbiturate abuse and addiction in the 1950s. Thus, physicians have long been aware that *once the person is addicted, withdrawal from barbiturates is potentially life-threatening, and should be attempted only under medical supervision* (Jenike, 1991). The barbiturates should never be abruptly withdrawn; to do so could bring about an organic brain syndrome with such symptoms as confusion, seizures, possible brain damage, and even death. Approximately 80% of barbiturate addicts who abruptly discontinue the drug experience withdrawal seizures, according to the author.

There is no set formula to estimate the danger period for barbiturate withdrawal problems. The exact period during withdrawal when the barbiturate addict is most at risk for such problems as seizures depends on the specific barbiturate being abused (Jenike, 1991). As a general rule, however, the longer-lasting forms of barbiturates tend to have longer withdrawal periods. If a person abruptly stops taking a short- to intermediate-acting barbiturate, withdrawal seizures usually begin on the second or third day. Barbiturate-withdrawal seizures are rare after the 12th day following cessation of the drug. An individual who stops taking one of the longer-acting barbiturates might not have a withdrawal seizure

until as late as the 7th day after the last dose of the drug (Tyrer, 1993).

A person physically dependent on the barbiturates experiences a number of symptoms during the withdrawal process. Virtually every barbiturate-dependent patient experiences a feeling of apprehension that lasts for the first 3 to 14 days of withdrawal (Shader, Greenblatt, & Ciraulo, 1994). Other symptoms that the patient experiences during this period include muscle weakness, tremors, anorexia, muscle twitches and a possible state of delirium, according to the authors.

Physicians can prescribe medications to minimize these symptoms; however, the patient should be warned that there is no such thing as a symptom-free withdrawal.

Barbituratelike Drugs

Because of the many adverse side effects of the barbiturates, pharmaceutical companies have long searched for substitutes that might be effective, yet safe to use. During the 1950s, several new drugs were introduced to treat anxiety and insomnia including Miltown (meprobamate), Quaalude and Sopor (both brand names of methaqualone), Doriden (glutethimide), Placidyl (ethchlorvynol), and Noludar (methyprylon). Table 6-2 provides dosage equivalencies of these drugs and phenobarbital.

Although these drugs were thought to be nonaddicting when first introduced, research has shown that barbituratelike drugs have an abuse potential similar to that of barbiturates. This should not be surprising since the chemical structure of some of

TABLE 6-2 Dosage Equivalencies for Barbiturate like Drugs

Generic name of drug of abuse	Dose equivalent to 30 mg of phenobarbital
Chloral hydrate	500 mg
Ethchlorvynol	350 mg
Meprobamate	400 mg
Methyprylon	300 mg
Glutethimide	250 mg

the barbituratelike drugs such as glutethimide and methyprylon are much like that of the barbiturates themselves (Julien, 1992). And like the barbiturates, glutethimide and methyprylon are metabolized mainly in the liver.

Both Placidyl (ethchlorvynol) and Doriden (glutethimide) are considered to be especially dangerous, and neither drug should be used for a number of reasons (Schuckit, 1995b). For example, the prolonged use of ethchlorvynol may result in a drug-induced loss of vision known as *amblyopia*. Fortunately, this drug-induced amblyopia is not permanent, but will gradually clear when the drug is discontinued (Michelson, Carroll, McLane, & Robin, 1988).

Since its introduction, the drug glutethimide has become ". . . notorious for its high mortality associated with overdose" (Sagar, 1991, p. 304). The high mortality associated with glutethimide overdose is a result of the drug's narrow therapeutic range. The lethal dose of glutethimide is only 10 grams, a dose that is only slightly above the normal dosage level (Sagar).

Meprobamate was a popular sedative in the 1950s, when it was sold under at least 32 different brand names including "Miltown" or "Equanil" (Lingeman, 1974). It is considered "obsolete" by current standards (Rosenthal, 1992) and although it is still popular among older patients, older physicians often continue to prescribe it. Meprobamate is addictive, although this potential was not clearly recognized when it was first introduced. It has been little used since the early 1970s, but some patients who have been using this medication continuously since that period or before remain addicted as a result of their initial prescription(s) (Rosenthal).

Surprisingly, despite its reputation and history, meprobamate still has a minor role in medicine, especially for patients who are unable to take benzodiazepines (Cole & Yonkers, 1995). The peak blood levels of meprobamate following an oral dose are seen in 1 to 3 hours, and the half-life is 6 to 17 hours following a single dose. The chronic use of meprobamate may result in the half-life being extended to 24 to 48 hours (Cole & Yonkers). The LD_{50} of meprobamate is estimated to be about 28,000 mg. However, some deaths have been noted following overdoses of

12,000 mg, according to the authors. Physical dependence to this drug is common when patients take 3200 mg/day or more.

Methaqualone was a drug that achieved significant popularity among illicit drug abusers in the late 1960s and early 1970s. It was originally intended as a nonaddicting substitute for the barbiturates in the mid-1960s. Depending on the dosage level being used, physicians prescribed it both as a sedative, and as a hypnotic (Lingeman, 1974). Illicit drug users quickly discovered that when one resisted the sedative/hypnotic effects of methaqualone, he or she would experience a sense of euphoria.

Methaqualone is rapidly absorbed from the gastrointestinal tract following an oral dose, and the individual begins to feel its effects in 15 to 20 minutes. The usual dose for methaqualone, when used as a sedative, was 75 mg, and the hypnotic dose was between 150 and 300 mg. Tolerance to the sedating and hypnotic effects of methaqualone developed rapidly, and many abusers gradually increased their daily dosage levels in an attempt to reachieve the initial effect. Some individuals who abused methaqualone were known to use upwards of 2000 mg in a single day (Mirin et al., 1991), a dosage level that was quite dangerous for the individual. Indeed, the lethal dose of methaqualone was estimated to be approximately 8000 mg for a typical 150-pound user (Lingeman, 1974).

Shortly after the drug was introduced, reports began to appear suggesting that methaqualone was being abused. It was purported to have aphrodisiac properties (which has never been proven) and was said to provide a mild sense of euphoria for the user (Mirin et al., 1991). Persons who have used methaqualone report feelings of euphoria, well-being, and behavioral disinhibition. As with the barbiturates, however, tolerance to the drug's effects quickly develops, but the lethal dosage of methaqualone remains the same. Death from methaqualone overdose was common, especially when the drug was taken with alcohol. The typical cause of death was heart failure, according to Lingeman (1974).

In the United States, methaqualone was withdrawn from the market in the mid-1980s, although it is still manufactured by pharmaceutical companies in other countries. It is often smuggled into this country or is manufactured in illicit laboratories and sold on the street. Thus, the substance abuse counselor must have a working knowledge of methaqualone and its effects.

Summary

For thousands of years, alcohol was the only chemical that was even marginally effective as an antianxiety or hypnotic agent. Although a number of chemicals with hypnotic action were introduced in the mid-1800s, each was of limited value in the fight against anxiety or insomnia. Then, in the early 1900s, the barbiturates were introduced. The barbiturates, which have a mechanism of action similar to that of alcohol, were found to have an antianxiety and a hypnotic effect. The barbiturates rapidly became popular and were widely used both for the control of anxiety and to help people fall asleep.

Like alcohol, however, the barbiturates were found to also have a significant potential for addiction. This resulted in a search for nonaddictive medications that could replace the barbiturates. In the post-World War II era, a number of synthetic drugs with chemical structures similar to those of the barbiturates were introduced. Although the manufacturers often claimed that these drugs were "nonaddicting," they were ultimately found to have an addiction potential similar to that of the barbiturates. Since the introduction of the benzodiazepines, the barbiturates and similar drugs have fallen into disfavor. However, there is evidence to suggest that they might be making a comeback.

CHAPTER SEVEN

Benzodiazepines and Similar Agents

In 1960, the first of a new class of antianxiety[1] drugs, chlordiazepoxide, was introduced in the United States. Chlordiazepoxide is a member of a family of chemicals known as the *benzodiazepines*. The benzodiazepines were found to be effective in the treatment of a wide range of disorders, such as the control of anxiety symptoms, insomnia, muscle strains, and seizures, without many of the risks inherent in the barbiturates. Since the first benzodiazepine was introduced, they have become the most frequently prescribed psychotropic medication in this country (Gonzales, Stern, Emmerich, & Rauch, 1992). Each year, approximately 13% of the population of the United States will use a benzodiazepine at least one time (Blair & Ramones, 1996).

The benzodiazepines were initially viewed as nonaddicting substitutes for the barbiturates or barbituratelike drugs. However, in the 35 years since their introduction, serious questions have been raised about the abuse potential of the benzodiazepines. Misuse and abuse of benzodiazepines results in hundreds of millions of dollars in unnecessary medical costs each year in the United States (Benzer, 1995). This chapter reviews the history of the benzodiazepines, their medical applications, and the problem of abuse/addiction to benzodiazepines and similar agents in the United States.

Medical Uses of the Benzodiazepines

Initially, the benzodiazepines were introduced as antianxiety agents. This remains a major use for this group of medications. But several benzodiazepines have also been found to be of value in treating other medical problems such as seizure disorders and muscle strains (Ashton, 1994; Shader & Greenblatt, 1993). Because the effects of the benzodiazepines are more selective than that of the barbiturates, they are able to reduce anxiety without causing the same degree of sedation and fatigue seen with barbiturates. This is the major reason the benzodiazepines have become the drugs-of-choice for the treatment of anxiety. Some benzodiazepines used in this country for the treatment of anxiety include diazepam (Valium), chlordiazepoxide (Librium), clorazepate (Tranxene), alprazolam (Xanax), and lorazepam (Ativan).

In addition to this, some benzodiazepines have been found useful in the control of seizures. At least one benzodiazepine, diazepam (Valium) has been found to be useful in treating many forms of human suffering: It is an antianxiety medication, can be used in the control of seizures, and, helps damaged muscles recover (American Psychiatric Association, 1990). Another benzodiazepine, clonazepam (Clonopin),[2] also is effective in the long-term control of seizures and is an antianxiety agent (Shader & Greenblatt, 1993).

---

[1] Some authors use the term *anxiolytic* in place of antianxiety. In this text, the term *antianxiety* is used.

[2] Some authors spell the name of this medication "Klonopin."

Some other members of the benzodiazepine family of drugs have been found useful as a *short-term* treatment for insomnia. Such benzodiazepines include temazepam (Restoril), triazolam (Halcion), flurazepam (Dalmane), and quazepam (Doral) (Gillin, 1991; Hussar, 1990). Two benzodiazepines, alprazolam (Xanax) and adinazolam (Deracyn) are reportedly of value in the treatment of depression. Although it does not have antidepressant effects, alprazolam is reportedly of value in treating the anxiety often found in cases of depression, and thus would indirectly help the patient feel better.

However, adinazolam appears to have a direct antidepressant effect, a feature that makes it unique among the benzodiazepines. Researchers believe that adinazolam works by increasing the sensitivity of certain neurons within the brain to serotonin (Cardoni, 1990). A deficit of, or insensitivity to, serotonin is thought to be the cause of at least some forms of depression. Thus, by increasing the sensitivity of the neurons of the brain to serotonin, adinazolam would seem to have a direct antidepressant effect that is lacking in most benzodiazepines.

Benzodiazepines and Suicide Attempts

The possibility of suicide through a drug overdose is a serious concern for the physician, especially when the patient is depressed. Because of their high Therapeutic Index (discussed in Chapter 3), the benzodiazepines have traditionally held the reputation of being "safe" drugs to use with potentially suicidal patients. Unlike the barbiturates (see Chapter 6), the benzodiazepines have a Therapeutic Index of $1:200$ (Kaplan & Sadock, 1990).

Animal research suggests that the LD_{50} for diazepam alone is around 720 mg per kilogram of body weight for mice, and 1240 mg/kg for rats (Medical Economics Company, 1993). Although the LD_{50} for humans is not known, these figures suggest that diazepam is an exceptionally safe drug.

This is not to say, however, that the benzodiazepines are totally safe. In the past decade, approximately 5.9 deaths were recorded for each million prescriptions written for a benzodiazepine in England and Wales (Serfaty & Masterton, 1993). Because of differences in pharmacological characteristics, some members of this family of pharmaceuticals carry more risk than others of causing death in an overdose situation (Buckley, Dawson, Whyte, & O'Connell, 1995). For example, the authors concluded that Restoril (temazepam) was much more dangerous than Serax (oxazepam) in the suicidal patient. Thus, while the authors suggest that benzodiazepines not be prescribed for the patient who is at high risk for suicide, they also note that the prescribing physician should use one of the benzodiazepines found less likely to cause death in an overdose situation if a benzodiazepine is necessary.

For many years after their introduction, physicians could do little beyond provide supportive treatment for patients who had overdosed on a benzodiazepines. However, they now are able to administer a medication that blocks the same receptor site within the brain that is utilized by benzodiazepines. This medication, Mazicon (flumazenil) occupies the benzodiazepine receptor site without causing any sedation, thus protecting the individual from the effects of a benzodiazepine overdose. However, physicians must administer flumazenil in a hospital setting. Because multiple agents are often ingested in suicide attempts, and because flumazenil is effective only in blocking the effects of benzodiazepines, *any suspected drug overdose should be treated by a physician.*

Pharmacology of the Benzodiazepines

The benzodiazepines are similar in their effects, differing mainly in their duration of action ("Sleeping Pills," 1988). Table 7-1 reviews the relative potency and biological half-lives, of some of the benzodiazepines in use in the United States.

Like many pharmaceuticals, the benzodiazepines can be classified on the basis of their pharmacological characteristics. Tyrer (1993), for example, adopted a classification system based, not on the duration of the effects of the benzodiazepines, but on the duration of their elimination half-lives (discussed in Chapter 3), separating the benzodiazepines into four groups:

1. *Very short half-lives* (4 hours or less).
2. *Short half-lives* (4–12 hours).

3. *Intermediate half-life* (12–20 hours).
4. *Long half-life* (20 or more hours).

The benzodiazepines in use range from moderately to highly lipid-soluble (Ayd, 1994). Lipid-solubility is important because the more lipid-soluble a chemical is, the faster it is absorbed through the small intestine after being taken by mouth (Roberts & Tafure, 1990). Also, highly lipid-soluble drugs are able to easily pass through the blood-brain barrier (Ballenger, 1995).

Once in the general circulation, the benzodiazepines are all protein-bound. However, there is some degree of variation in the percentage of the medication that is protein-bound. Diazepam, for example, is more than 99% protein-bound (APA, 1990), while 92% to 97% of chlordiazepoxide is protein-bound (Ayd, Janicak, Davis, & Preskorn, 1996) and alprazolam is only about 80% protein-bound (Medical Economics Company, 1997). This variability is one factor that influences the duration of effect for benzodiazepines after a single dose (American Medical Association, 1994).

As a general rule, the benzodiazepines are almost completely absorbed when administered orally (American Medical Association, 1994) but are poorly absorbed from intramuscular or subcutaneous injection sites. Since it is difficult to predict the degree of bioavailability when benzodiazepines are injected, they are usually administered orally. One exception to this rule is that when the patient is experiencing uncontrolled seizures, intravenous injections of diazepam or a similar benzodiazepine might be used.

Most members of the benzodiazepine family must be biotransformed before elimination can proceed. This task is carried out mainly in the liver, and in the process of biotransformation metabolites are produced that have biological effects of their own. These biologically active metabolites may contribute to the duration of a drug's effects, and these may be far different than the elimination half-life of the parent compound (Hobbs et al., 1995).

Many benzodiazepine metabolites require extended periods of time before being eliminated from the body. Further, there is some variation between individuals in terms of how fast benzodiazepines might be biotransformed. For example, during the process of biotransformation the benzodiazepine flurazepam will produce five different metabolites with psychoactive effects of their own. In some individuals, the half-life of the original dose of flurazepam, and its metabolites, might continue to have an effect on the user for as long as 280 hours after the original dose.

The exceptions to this rule are lorazepam, oxazepam, and temazepam. These benzodiazepines are either eliminated without biotransformation or produce metabolites that have minimal physical effects on the patient. As discussed later in this chapter, these benzodiazepines are often preferred for older patients, who may experience oversedation as a result of the long half-lives of some benzodiazepine metabolites.

Although the benzodiazepines are often compared with the barbiturates, they actually are far different than the barbiturates in the way they function in the brain. Because the barbiturates simulate the action of the neurotransmitter gamma-aminobutyric acid (GABA), they nonselectively depress the *entire* range of activity of neurons in many different parts of the brain, including the cortex. This results

TABLE 7-1   Selected Pharmacological Characteristics of Some Benzodiazepines

Generic name	Equivalent dose	Half-life (hours)
Alprazolam	0.5 mg	6–20
Chlordiazepoxide	25 mg	30–100
Clonazepam	0.25 mg	20–40
Clorazepate	7.5 mg	30–100
Diazepam	5 mg	30–100
Flurazepam	30 mg	50–100
Halazepam	20 mg	30–100
Lorazepam	1 mg	10–20
Oxazepam	15 mg	5–21
Prazepam	10 mg	30–100
Temazepam	30 mg	9.5–12.4
Triazolam	0.25 mg	1.7–3.0

in significant degrees of sedation along with the desired effect of a reduction in anxiety levels.

The benzodiazepines, on the other hand, are more selective in their action. Clinical research has suggested that the benzodiazepines enhance the action of GABA. This neurotransmitter is found in many regions of the brain, and so any drug that increases the effect of GABA would have an effect on many different parts of the brain. Thus, it is not surprising to learn that the benzodiazepines have a psychoactive effect in both the limbic system and the cortex of the brain (American Medical Association, 1994).

Scientists believe that GABA is the most important inhibitory neurotransmitter in the brain (Bohn, 1993; Nutt, 1996; Tabakoff & Hoffman, 1992). It is thought that by binding to one of the GABA receptor sites, and also to a chloride channel on the neuron surface, benzodiazepines make the receptor site on the neuron more sensitive to GABA. But the neuron still requires that the receptor site be activated by GABA to have an effect on that nerve cell (Hobbs et al., 1995).

Neurons that utilize GABA are especially common in the *locus ceruleus* (Cardoni, 1990; Johnson & Lydiard, 1995). Nerve fibers from the locus ceruleus connect with other parts of the brain thought to be involved in fear and panic reactions. Further, animal research has demonstrated that stimulation of the locus ceruleus region of the brain causes behaviors similar to those seen in humans who are having a panic attack (Johnson & Lydiard). Thus, by reducing the level of activity of the neurons in the locus ceruleus, the benzodiazepines are thought to reduce the individual's anxiety level. But, scientists believe that the process by which benzodiazepines might reduce anxiety is far different than the mechanism by which these medications achieve their muscle relaxant and anticonvulsant effects (Hobbs et al., 1995). Thus, there is still a lot that remains to be discovered about how these drugs work.

All the benzodiazepines have a sedative effect on the user (Ballenger, 1995). However, when *excessive* sedation is observed with a benzodiazepine, it is usually a result of too large a dose being used for that particular person (Ayd et al., 1996). Advancing age

is one factor that may make the individual more susceptible to the phenomenon of benzodiazepine-induced oversedation (Ashton, 1994; Ayd, 1994). There are two reasons for this. First, because of an age-related decline in blood flow to the liver and kidneys, the elderly require more time than younger adults to biotransform and/or excrete many drugs, (Bleidt & Moss, 1989). Consequently, many older patients become oversedated, or, in some cases, experience a paradoxical excitement, as their bodies struggle to adjust to the effects of a dose of a benzodiazepine. To put the impact of these age-related changes on benzodiazepine metabolism into some perspective, the elderly may require *three times as long* as a young adult to fully metabolize diazepam and chlordiazepoxide (L. Cohen, 1989).

Many physicians recommend that for older patients who require a benzodiazepine, lorazepam or oxazepam might be the best choice (Ashton, 1994; Graedon & Graedon, 1991). This is because lorazepam and oxazepam have a shorter half-life and are more easily biotransformed than diazepam and similar benzodiazepines.

Both Deracyn (adinazolam) and Doral (quazepam) are exceptions to the rule that the older patient is more likely to experience excessive sedation than a younger patient. It is not uncommon for patients to experience sedation from adinazolam. As many as two-thirds of those who receive this medication may experience some degree of drowsiness, at least until their bodies adapt to the drug's effects (Cardoni, 1990). Further, since the active metabolites of Doral (quazepam) have a half-life of 72 hours, there is a strong possibility that the user will experience a hangover effect from the drug the next day (Hartmann, 1995).

Benzodiazepines, as well as barbiturates, induce hangovers, especially some of the longer-lasting benzodiazepines (Ashton, 1992, 1994). The data in Table 7-1 suggest that, for some individuals, the half-life of some benzodiazepines may be as long as 100–280 hours. Further, as discussed in Chapter 3, it usually requires five half-life periods before virtually all of a drug is biotransformed/eliminated from the body. If that patient were to take a second, or even a third dose of the medication before fully biotransforming the first dose, he/she would begin to accumulate unmetabolized medication in body tissues. The unmetabolized medication would continue to have an effect well past the time that the patient thought the drug's effects had ended.

It is surprising to learn that although they are most often prescribed as antianxiety agents, there is little information about the long-term effectiveness of benzodiazepines as antianxiety agents (Ayd, 1994). Some researchers believe that the antianxiety effects of the benzodiazepines last about 1 or 2 months, and that these drugs are not useful in treating anxiety continuously over a long period of time (Ashton, 1994; Ayd et al., 1996). It has been suggested that the manufacturer of the benzodiazepine Xanax (alprazolam) did not inform physicians that, after 8 weeks of continuous use, patients who received Xanax in one research study had just as many panic attacks as the patients who received only a placebo (S. Walker, 1996). This report casts considerable doubt as to the effectiveness of this benzodiazepine as a long-term antianxiety agent.

Other researchers, however, believe that the benzodiazepines are an effective agent in the long-term control of anxiety. The *Harvard Medical School Mental Health Letter* ("Sleeping Pill," 1988) stated that while patients might develop some tolerance to the sedative effects of benzodiazepines, they did not become tolerant to the antianxiety effects. Thus, within the medical community, there is some uncertainty as to the long-term effectiveness of benzodiazepines in the control of anxiety symptoms.

Benzodiazepine Tolerance, Abuse, and Addiction

Within a few years of benzodiazepine's introduction, reports of abuse and addiction began to surface. Even patients who were taking the benzodiazepines only at recommended dosage levels appeared to experience what is known as a *discontinuance* syndrome after using these medications for just a few months. These observations fueled reports in the media that suggested the benzodiazepines had a significant abuse potential. In reality, physicians remain undecided as to the actual abuse potential of the benzodiazepines.

It is known that when a person takes a benzodiazepine for an extended period, his/her brain will go through a process of neuroadaptation (Sellers et al., 1993, p. 65). During this process, the central nervous system becomes tolerant to the drug's effects. If that person were to then suddenly discontinue the medication, he/she would experience rebound or discontinuance symptoms, as his/her brain began to adapt to the absence of the benzodiazepine. Some researchers believe that this state of pharmacological tolerance to the benzodiazepines is evidence that the patient has become addicted to the medication.

Remember that two signs of addiction are a state of physical dependence and tolerance to the drug's effects. Some physicians believe that the discontinuance syndrome is clear evidence that users become tolerant to benzodiazepines and also physically dependent on them "within a few weeks, perhaps days" (N. Miller & Gold, 1991b, p. 28). Other researchers view the rebound or discontinuance symptoms as a natural consequence of benzodiazepine use. Sellers et al. (1993) argued, for example, that evidence "of neuroadaptation is not sufficient to define drug-taking behavior as dependent" (p. 65). Thus, although patients who discontinue the medication may experience a discontinuance syndrome, this is seen as a natural process. Advocates of this position point out that the body must go through a period of adjustment whenever *any* medication is discontinued.

Researchers disagree as to the percentage of patients who will develop a discontinuance syndrome after using the benzodiazepines for an extended period. Ashton (1994) suggested that approximately 35% of those patients who take a benzodiazepine continuously for 4 or more weeks will become physically dependent on the medication. These individuals will experience withdrawal symptoms when they stop taking the medication, according to the author. In rare cases, pharmacological dependence on the benzodiazepines might develop in just days (APA, 1990; N. Miller & Gold, 1991b; "Sleeping Pills," 1988).

On the other hand, Blair and Ramones (1996) suggested that in most cases where the benzodiazepines are used at normal dosage levels for less than 4 months, the risk of a patient becoming dependent on a benzodiazepine is virtually nonexistent. But after 4 months of continuous use, the picture is even more confusing. The *Harvard*

Medical School Mental Health Letter ("Sleeping Pills," 1988) suggested that after 4 to 6 months of daily use, the majority of patients would become physically dependent on benzodiazepines. After 8 months of daily use, "most" (p. 3) patients would experience benzodiazepine withdrawal symptoms when they discontinued the drug, and ". . . after a year almost all . . ." (p. 3) patients would experience some symptoms during withdrawal, according to the author.

In contrast to the preceding estimate, Blair and Ramones (1996) suggested that only 25% to 45% of those patients who had used a benzodiazepine continuously for 2 years would be dependent on these drugs. Even after 6 to 8 years of continuous use at normal dosage levels, only 75% of the patients who used a benzodiazepine would be dependent on the drug, according to the authors. Nevertheless, while researchers disagree as to the percentage of the patients who become addicted to a benzodiazepine after extended use, they do not suggest that these drugs can be used for longer than 4 months without causing physical dependence in at least some patients.

Some factors that influence the development of pharmacological dependence on the benzodiazepines include (a) the frequency with which that individual has used a benzodiazepine (b) the total period of time during which the individual has used benzodiazepines, (c) the individual's unique biochemistry, (d) the individual's history of prior addiction to chemicals, and (e) the pharmacological characteristics (potency, biological half-life, etc.) of the specific benzodiazepine being used.

Abuse Potential

Until now, we have been talking about the discontinuance syndrome that develops after a patient has been using a benzodiazepine daily, at recommended dosage levels. What about the actual abuse potential of these drugs? Researchers disagree — some have concluded that the benzodiazepines have a rather low "reward potential." In contrast to heroin, cocaine, or the other drugs of abuse, most drug users do not find that the benzodiazepines provide them with a "buzz" or a "high." These findings are similar to that of clinical research evidence,

which suggests that most people do not find benzodiazepine use pharmacologically rewarding. Thus, there is little incentive for most people to increase the daily dosage level above what was prescribed.[3]

On the other hand, S. Walker (1996) stated that the benzodiazepines are as addictive as "hard core drugs" (p. 79), and Spiegel (1996) also suggested that the risk of benzodiazepine abuse is quite high. To explain this apparent contradiction, Cole and Kando (1993) suggest that the vast majority of those who abuse benzodiazepines do so as part of a pattern of polydrug abuse. "Patients taking only benzodiazepine in large doses to get 'high' are quite rare" (p. 58), according to the authors. However, they also accepted that an exception to this rule might be the medical patient who has increased his/her daily dosage level above what was prescribed, in an attempt to overcome chronic feelings of dysphoria. However, overall, it was rare for a patient to be abusing only benzodiazepines (Cole & Kando, 1993; Wesson & Ling, 1996).

This conclusion seems difficult to defend, in light of the results of clinical field research. Substance abuse workers have long been aware that, at least some drug users find the benzodiazepines are attractive recreational drugs. The pharmacological characteristics of alprazolam, for example, might make it a prime drug of abuse (Juergens & Morse, 1988; Sellers et al., 1993; S. Walker, 1996). Alprazolam reaches peak blood levels in 1–2 hours and in the healthy individual is fully metabolized in between 6–16 hours. When abused, these characteristics allow the user to experience an intense high, followed by a rapid dropoff of the drug's effects.

Some researchers maintain that in the vast majority of cases the benzodiazepines are both appropriately prescribed and used according to the physician's instructions (Appelbaum, 1992; Woods, Katz, & Winger, 1988). Other researchers maintain that the benzodiazepines present the user with a strong potential for abuse.

---

[3] On the other hand, Graedon and Graedon (1991) concluded that one reason BuSpar (discussed later in this chapter) has not won wide acceptance as an antianxiety medication is that, unlike the benzodiazepines, it does not produce a "buzz" for the user.

In either case, once a person has become physically dependent on benzodiazepines, withdrawal from these drugs can be difficult. The research team of Schweizer, Rickels, Case, and Greenblatt (1990) worked with a group of 63 benzodiazepine-dependent individuals, and attempted to carry out a 25% per week reduction program in their dosage benzodiazepine levels. Despite this slow withdrawal schedule, the authors found that one-third of those individuals addicted to benzodiazepines with long half-lives, and 42% of those addicted to short half-life forms of benzodiazepines were unable to complete the withdrawal program. The authors attributed their findings to the patient's personality structure, suggesting that some patients may have greater difficulty during withdrawal than others.

Factors Influencing the Benzodiazepine Withdrawal Process

The research team of Rickels, Schweizer, Case, and Greenblatt (1990) examined the phenomenon of withdrawal from benzodiazepines, to identify factors that might influence the withdrawal process. The authors concluded that the severity of benzodiazepine withdrawal was dependent on five different drug treatment factors, plus several patient factors.

According to the authors, the drug treatment factors were (a) the total daily dose of benzodiazepines being used, (b) the total time during which benzodiazepines had been used, (c) the half-life of the benzodiazepine being used (short half-life benzodiazepines tend to produce more withdrawal symptoms than do long half-life benzodiazepines), (d) the potency of the benzodiazepine being used, and (e) the rate of withdrawal (gradual, tapered withdrawal, or abrupt withdrawal).

According to the authors, several patient factors also influenced the withdrawal from benzodiazepines: (a) the patient's premorbid personality structure, (b) expectations for the withdrawal process, and (c) individual differences in the neurobiological structures within the brain thought to be involved in the withdrawal process. Interactions between these two sets of factors were thought to determine the severity of the withdrawal process, according to Rickels et al. (1990). Thus, for the person addicted to these medications, withdrawal can be a complex, difficult process.

Complications Caused by Benzodiazepine Use at Normal Dosage Levels

The benzodiazepines are not perfect drugs. As a group, the benzodiazepines have a number of drawbacks. For example, although some benzodiazepines are of value in the control of seizures, they are of only limited value in the long-term control of epilepsy (Morton & Santos, 1989). This is because tolerance to the anticonvulsant effects is possible when these drugs are used for extended periods.

Another shortcoming of the benzodiazepines at normal dosage levels was discussed earlier. Although these medications are not general neuronal depressants, as are the barbiturates, excessive sedation is still occasionally seen even at normal dosage levels. This effect is most often noted in the older patient or in the patient with significant levels of liver damage. The fact that the elderly are most likely to experience excessive sedation is unfortunate because two-thirds of those who receive prescriptions for benzodiazepines are above the age of 60 years (Ayd, 1994).

One should remember that different benzodiazepines will have slightly different side effect profiles, based on small differences in their chemical structure, and individual differences in the biochemistry of the user. Some of the side effects of benzodiazepines include hallucinations, euphoria, irritability, tachycardia, sweating, and disinhibition (Hobbs et al., 1995). One benzodiazepine, Dalmane (flurazepam), tends to cause confusion and oversedation, especially in the elderly. This medication is often used as a treatment for insomnia. One of the metabolites of flurazepam is desalkyflurazepam, which, depending on the individual might have a half-life of between 40 and 280 hours (Gillin, 1991). Thus, the effects of a single dose might last *up to 12 days* in some patients. As noted, the elderly are especially vulnerable to this side effect.

With such an extended half-life, the use of flurazepam for even a few days might cause a person to experience significant levels of CNS depression for some time after the last dose of the drug. Further, if a person should ingest alcohol, or possibly even an over-the-counter cold remedy, before the flurazepam is fully metabolized, the unmetabolized drug could combine with the depressant effects of the alcohol or cold remedy to produce serious levels CNS depression.

Cross-tolerance between the benzodiazepines, alcohol, the barbiturates, and meprobamate is possible (Sands, Creelman, Ciraulo, Greenblatt, & Shader, 1995; Snyder, 1986). The benzodiazepines may also potentiate the effects of other CNS depressants such as antihistamines, alcohol, or narcotic analgesics, presenting a danger of over sedation or death (Barnhill et al., 1995).[4] Many of the benzodiazepines have been found to interfere with normal sexual function, even at normal dosage levels (Finger et al., 1997). When used for extended periods, even at normal dosage levels, and then discontinued, the withdrawal symptoms may mimic the symptoms of anxiety or sleep disorders (N. Miller & Gold, 1991b). The authors noted that the benzodiazepine withdrawal symptoms were "virtually indistinguishable from" (p. 34) the symptoms of the anxiety or sleep disorder for which the medication was first prescribed. The danger is that the patient might begin to take benzodiazepines again, in the mistaken belief that the withdrawal symptoms from benzodiazepines indicated that the original problem still existed.

Even at normal dosage levels, the benzodiazepines may occasionally cause irritability, hostility, rage, or outright aggression (Ashton, 1994; Hobbs et al., 1995; Juergens, 1993; S. Walker, 1996). This paradoxical rage reaction in a person who has used a benzodiazepine is thought to be the result of the disinhibition effects of this family of drugs. As the benzodiazepine lowers social inhibitions, the person is more likely to engage in behavior that was successfully controlled previously. A similar disinhibition effect is often seen in persons who drink alcohol. This effect is thought to be why the combination of alcohol and benzodiazepines occasionally results in a *paradoxical rage reaction* (Beasley, 1987). It is thought that the combination of the two chemicals lowers the individual's inhibitions to the point where he/she is unable to control repressed anger.

Another complication common to benzodiazepines is that, even at normal dosage levels, they seem to interfere with the formation of memory patterns (Ayd, 1994; Plasky, Marcus, & Salzman, 1988). Although in many cases the memory disturbance may be so subtle as to escape the notice of the individual (Juergens, 1993; O'Donovan & McGuffin, 1993), every benzodiazepine in use can result in some degree of memory loss. Thus, where Halcion (triazolam) has acquired a reputation for causing memory disturbance when used at therapeutic dosage levels, this effect would seem to be a characteristic common to all the benzodiazepines, not just triazolam (Hobbs et al., 1995; Juergens, 1993; O'Donovan & McGuffin, 1993). This effect is known as *anterograde amnesia*, a form of amnesia that involves the formation of memories after a specific event (Plasky et al., 1988). In this case, the person may be unable to remember information presented after the ingestion of the drug. The process seems to be similar to that of the alcohol-induced blackout (Juergens).

Even at normal dosage levels, the benzodiazepines may disrupt the normal psychomotor skills necessary to drive an automobile or work with dangerous power tools. Thus, tasks that require vigilance or speed of motor performance may be adversely affected by benzodiazepine use. Problems with psychomotor coordination can persist for several days following the initial use of benzodiazepines (Woods et al., 1988). Further, the benzodiazepines occasionally will produce mild respiratory depression, even at normal therapeutic dosage levels, especially in persons with pulmonary disease. Because of this, the benzodiazepines should be avoided in patients who suffer from sleep apnea, chronic lung disease, or other sleep-related breathing disorders, to avoid serious, possibly fatal, respiratory depression (Ashton, 1994; Hobbs et al., 1995). Doghramji (1989) has warned against the use of CNS depressants with patients who suffer from Alzheimer's disease. Such medications might potentiate preexisting sleep apnea problems, according to the author, which would place the patient's life at risk.

Even at therapeutic dosage levels, the benzodiazepines have been found to interfere with normal sexual functioning. Further, although clinical depression is not commonly encountered as a side

---

[4] When in doubt about whether two or more medications should be used together *always* consult a physician, pharmacist, or the local poison control center. For example, the movie star Judy Garland, reportedly died as a result of the combined effects of alcohol and the benzodiazepine diazepam (Snyder, 1986).

effect of benzodiazepine use, rare cases of drug-induced depression have been reported (Ashton, 1992, 1994; Juergens, 1993; B. Smith & Salzman, 1991). The exact mechanism by which the benzodiazepines could cause, or at least contribute to, depressive episodes is not clear at this time. Suicide is a possible outcome of the benzodiazepine-induced depressive episode. To further complicate matters, there is evidence to suggest that benzodiazepine use might contribute to actual thoughts of suicide on the part of the user (Ashton, 1992, 1994; Juergens, 1993). Thus, it is often difficult to determine whether the patient's suicidal thoughts reflect this benzodiazepine-induced complication.

Although it is not possible to list every reported side effect of the benzodiazepines, the preceding review illustrates that these medications are both extremely potent and, have a significant potential to cause harm to the user.

The Trials of Halcion

Since the benzodiazepine Halcion (triazolam) was first introduced, it has been a controversial drug. Intended as a hypnotic, Halcion is the subject of at least 100 lawsuits against the manufacturer by individuals who believe that they have been harmed by their own (or another person's) use of this drug (C. Dyer, 1992). Further, at least 2300 adverse reactions have been reported to the manufacturer, Upjohn Pharmaceuticals, from the United States alone (Hand, 1989). At least 1100 additional reports of adverse reactions were filed by physicians in Holland before the drug was banned in that country (*60 Minutes*, 1994).

Some of the side effects of therapeutic doses of Halcion (triazolam) include: periods of confusion and disorientation (Gillin, 1991; Salzman, 1990), behavioral disinhibition, hyperexcitability, daytime anxiety, amnesia, and confusion (Gillin, 1991; O'Donovan & McGuffin, 1993). As this list of side effects suggests, Halcion (triazolam) is "a very, very dangerous drug" (Kayles, quoted in *60 Minutes*, 1994, p. 2). It has even been suggested that:

> . . . compared with other benzodiazepines, triazolam causes more agitation, confusion, amnesia, hallucinations, and bizarre or abnormal behavior. Suicides, attempted suicides, deaths, and violent crimes have been associated with triazolam administration. In most of the adverse reaction reports, the drug was taken as recommended. (Hand, 1989, p. 3)

Evidence has come to light suggesting that, for reasons that are still unclear, the manufacturer *under*reported some of the side effects associated with Halcion during at least one early study into the drug's safety (Cowley, 1992; *60 Minutes*, 1994). Both in the United States and in a number of other countries, government agencies have reviewed the side effects of triazolam and reconsidered whether this drug meets their safety standards. As a result of their review, the British government banned the sale of Halcion (triazolam) in England as of October 1991 (C. Dyer, 1992). Since then, triazolam has also been banned in 12 other countries, including Norway, Finland, Brazil, and Jamaica (C. Dyer, 1993).

In the United States, the Food and Drug Administration (FDA) set up a special review panel to determine whether the drug is safe. After a yearlong study, the FDA panel concluded that Halcion is safe, but recommended that stronger warnings be issued by the manufacturer about potential side effects (C. Dyer, 1992). However, there are questions as to how objective the FDA review panel might have been and whether the manufacturer presented all the facts to the panel for its consideration.

When Upjohn Pharmaceuticals' representatives met with the FDA review panel, they claimed that there were no studies substantiating the reports of adverse Halcion-induced effects. They presented the results of one study, known as "Protocol 321," to the FDA as evidence that the drug was safe (*60 Minutes*, 1994). However, the true findings of this study were apparently not provided to the FDA review panel. The study actually found that 70% of the subjects experienced major side effects from the drug (*60 Minutes*, 1994). But this information was "either missing or minimized when Upjohn sent this official summary of the test to the FDA" (*60 Minutes*, 1994, p. 3). Thus, there appear to be serious questions as to the safety of the drug Halcion (triazolam). It may take many years for the numerous lawsuits against the manufacturer of Halcion (triazolam) to be settled, and it would appear that Halcion will remain a most controversial drug for some time to come.

Drug Interactions Involving the Benzodiazepines

There have been a "few ancedotal case reports" (Sarid-Segal, Creelman, & Shader, 1995, p. 193) of patients who have suffered adverse effects from the use of benzodiazepines while taking lithium. The authors reviewed a single case report of "profound hypothermia resulting from the combined use of lithium and diazepam" (p. 194). In this case, lithium was implicated as the agent that caused the individual to suffer a progressive loss of body temperature. Further, the authors noted that diazepam and oxazepam appear to cause increased levels of depression in patients who are also taking lithium. The reason for this increased level of depression in patients who are using both a benzodiazepine and lithium is not known at this time.

Patients who are on Antabuse (disulfiram) should use benzodiazepines with caution, since disulfiram reduces the speed at which the body can metabolize benzodiazepines such as diazepam and chlordiazepoxide (Zito, 1994). The author recommended that, when a patient must use both medications concurrently, the physician should choose a benzodiazepine that does not produce any biologically active metabolites (e.g., oxazepam, lorazepam).

There is evidence that blood levels of Halcion (triazolam) may be as high as double when the patient also takes the antibiotic erythromycin (sold under several brand names) (Graedon & Graedon, 1995). Further, there is evidence that probenecid may slow the biotransformation of the benzodiazepine lorazepam, thus causing excess sedation in some patients (Sands et al., 1995).

Patients taking a benzodiazepine should not use the antipsychotic medication clozapine (Zito, 1994). There have been reports of severe respiratory depression caused by the combination of these two medications, possibly resulting in several deaths. Patients with heart conditions who are taking the medication digoxin as well as a benzodiazepine should have frequent tests to check the digoxin level in their blood (Graedon & Graedon, 1995). There is some evidence that benzodiazepine use might cause the blood levels of digoxin to rise, possibly to the level of digoxin toxicity, according to the authors.

Further, the use of benzodiazepines might cause higher than normal blood levels of such benzodiazepines as diazepam when combined with anticonvulsant medications such as phenytoin, mephenytoin, and ethotoin; the antidepressant fluoxetine; or medications for the control of blood pressure such as propranolol, and metoprolol (Graedon & Graedon, 1995). Thus, it is unwise for patients to use these medications at the same time.

Women using oral contraceptives should discuss her use of a benzodiazepine with a physician prior to taking one of these medications. Zito (1994) noted that oral contraceptives reduce the rate at which the body metabolizes some benzodiazepines, thus making it necessary to reduce the dose of these medications. Patients taking antitubercular medications such as isoniazid might need to adjust their benzodiazepine dosage (Zito). Further, there is evidence that suggests patients who take antacids have trouble absorbing chlordiazepoxide as quickly as they might normally if they had taken the chlordiazepoxide without an antacid (Ciraulo, Shader, Greenblatt, & Barnhill, 1995).

Because of the possibility of excessive sedation, the benzodiazepines should *never* be intermixed with medications classified as a CNS depressant, except under the supervision of a physician. Such medications include alcohol, narcotic analgesics, and the antihistamines (Graedon & Graedon, 1995). The combined effects of the two classes of medications may result in excessive, if not dangerous, levels of sedation.

Although this list is not exhaustive, it illustrates that there is a potential for an interaction between the benzodiazepines and a number of other medications. A physician or pharmacist should always be consulted prior to taking two or more medications at the same time, to rule out the possibility of an adverse interaction.

Subjective Experience of Benzodiazepine Use

As a class, the antianxiety agents have similar effects on the user. The person using an antianxiety agent at normal dosage levels experiences a gentle state of relaxation. In addition to their effects on the cortex, the benzodiazepines have an effect on the spinal cord, which contributes to muscle relaxation through some unknown mechanism (Ballenger, 1995). When used in the treatment of insomnia, the benzodiazepines initially reduce the sleep latency period, which is the length of time between when the individual first goes to bed, and when he or she finally falls asleep. At first, persons who utilize one of the benzodiazepines to help them sleep often report a sense of deep and refreshing sleep.

However, drugs in the benzodiazepine family also interfere with the normal sleep cycle, reducing rapid eye movement (REM) sleep (Ballenger, 1995). It is during the REM phase that we dream, and experimental research would suggest that dreaming is necessary for mental health (Hobson, 1989). Alcohol, the barbiturates, and the benzodiazepines have all been noted to interfere with the amount of REM sleep that the user achieves.

When a person who has used a CNS depressant such as alcohol, the barbiturates, or the benzodiazepines then discontinues the use of this chemical, he/she will experience "REM rebound" (Ashton, 1994; Hobbs et al., 1995). REM rebound is a phenomenon in which the individual, apparently to "catch up" on lost REM sleep, experiences an increase in the amount of sleep time spent in REM sleep after stopping the use of a CNS depressant.

After protracted periods of benzodiazepine use, the individual may experience significant levels of REM rebound with vivid, and possibly frightening, dreams. There are cases on record where these nightmares have motivated the person to resume drug use to "get a good night's sleep" again. But note that *protracted* is a relative term. In some cases, an individual used a benzodiazepine as a hypnotic for only 1 or 2 weeks, yet still experienced significant rebound symptoms ("Sleeping Pills," 1988; Tyrer, 1993).

REM rebound is not the only rebound symptom that the user might experience after stopping the use of a benzodiazepine. Patients who have used a benzodiazepine for daytime relief from anxiety have reported symptoms such as anxiety, agitation, tremor, fatigue, difficulty concentrating, headache, nausea, gastrointestinal upset, a sense of paranoia, depersonalization, impaired memory, and insomnia after

stopping the drug (Graedon & Graedon, 1991). The individual may experience rebound insomnia for 3 to 21 days after discontinuing benzodiazepine use.

The benzodiazepines with shorter half-lives are most likely to cause rebound symptoms when the patient experiences an abrupt drop in medication blood levels (Ayd, 1994; O'Donovan & McGuffin, 1993; Rosenbaum, 1990). For example, alprazolam has a short half-life, and the blood levels drop rather rapidly just before it is time for the next dose. During this period, the individual is most likely to experience an increase in anxiety levels, a phenomenon known as "clock watching" (Rosenbaum, 1990, p. 1302) by the patient, who waits with increasing anxiety until it is time for another dose.

The author recommended that the patient being withdrawn from alprazolam gradually be switched to clonazepam, which is a long-acting medication. Clonazepam is about twice as potent as alprazolam, but has a longer half-life. The transition between alprazolam and clonazepam takes about one week, after which time the patient should be taking only clonazepam. This medication may then be gradually withdrawn, resulting in a slower decline in blood levels. However, the patient still should be warned that there will be some rebound anxiety symptoms.

Although the patient might believe otherwise, these symptoms are not a sign that the original anxiety is still present, rather, are simply a sign that the body is adjusting to the gradual reduction in clonazepam blood levels.

Long-Term Consequences of Chronic Benzodiazepine Use

Although introduced as safe and nonaddicting substitutes for the barbiturates, it has been found that the benzodiazepines do indeed have a significant abuse potential. Dietch (1983) explored benzodiazepine abuse and outlined several criteria to aid in the recognition of benzodiazepine abuse: (a) taking the drug after the medical/psychiatric need for its use has passed, (b) showing symptoms of physical or psychological dependence on one of the benzodiazepines, (c) taking the drug in amounts greater than the prescribed amount, (d) taking the drug to obtain an euphoriant effect, and (e) using the drug to decrease self-awareness, or the possibility of change.

During withdrawal, the benzodiazepine-dependent individual might experience symptoms of anxiety, insomnia, dizziness, nausea and vomiting, muscle weakness, tremor, confusion, convulsions (seizures), irritability, sweating, and a drug-induced withdrawal psychosis (Juergens, 1993). There have been rare reports of depression, manic reactions, and obsessive-compulsive symptoms as a result of benzodiazepine withdrawal (Juergens). In extreme cases, patients have been known to experience transient feelings of depersonalization, muscle pain, and a hypersensitivity to light and noise during benzodiazepine withdrawal (Spiegel, 1996).

Psychological Dependence

In addition to the problems of physical dependence, Dietch (1983) noted that it is possible to become *psychologically* dependent on benzodiazepines: "Psychological dependence on benzodiazepines appears to be more common than physical dependence" (p. 1140). Such persons might take the drug either continuously or intermittently because of their *belief* that they need benzodiazepines, despite their actual medical requirements.

For example, research has demonstrated that tolerance to the sleep-inducing (or, hypnotic) effect of the benzodiazepines develops after a few days of continual use (Ashton, 1994), although Ayd (1994) and the American Psychiatric Association (1990) suggested that tolerance to the hypnotic effects of the benzodiazepines might take perhaps 2 to 4 weeks to develop. In either case, tolerance to the hypnotic effects of benzodiazepines develops after only a short period of continuous use. Yet many people continue to take benzodiazepines as a sleep aid for extended periods, possibly as long as several years, because they believe the medication is still helping them get a good night's sleep.

There is a tendency, at least among some users of the benzodiazepines, to increase their dosage levels above that prescribed by their physician. This phenomenon is not well understood. Although the benzodiazepines do cause tolerance (Snyder, 1986), "the magnitude of such increases appears to be small" (Dietch, 1983, p. 1141), and in general "subjects

tended to titrate their dose according to the level of environmental stress." The limited information on this phenomenon is based on patients who were prescribed one of the benzodiazepines for medical/psychiatric reasons. There is virtually no information on how drug abusers may utilize this class of drugs, or what dosage level addicts prefer. Woods et al. (1988) postulated that the person who was most likely to abuse benzodiazepines was one who had a history of polydrug abuse.

All the CNS depressants, including the benzodiazepines, are capable of producing a *toxic psychosis*, especially in overdose situations. Some professionals also call this condition an "organic brain syndrome." Some of the symptoms seen with a benzodiazepine-related toxic psychosis include visual and auditory hallucinations, and/or paranoid delusions. This drug-induced psychosis will usually clear in 2 to 14 days (Miller & Gold, 1991b).

As with the barbiturates, *withdrawal from benzodiazepines should only be attempted under the supervision of a physician*. In addition to drug-induced psychosis, severe withdrawal symptoms may include hyperthermia, delirium, convulsions, and possible death (Jenike, 1991). Detoxification may be necessary on an inpatient basis in some cases. Although most patients can be slowly withdrawn from benzodiazepines with few or no side effects by the physician in charge of the detoxification program (Woods et al., 1988), some patients may experience discomfort during withdrawal.

Benzodiazepines as a Substitute for Other Drugs of Abuse

Juergens (1993) reported that many individuals who abuse the amphetamines and cocaine often also abuse benzodiazepines. Such polydrug abuse is done either to control some of the side effects of the stimulant use, or to "come down" from the stimulants in order to sleep. Because of the similarity in the effects of alcohol and benzodiazepines, alcohol-dependent persons often substitute a benzodiazepine for alcohol in situations where they cannot drink. The author of this text has met a number of recovering alcoholics who reported that 10 mg of diazepam had the same subjective effect for them as 3 or 4 "stiff" drinks. Further, the long half-life of diazepam often is sufficient to allow these individuals to work the entire day, without starting to go into alcohol withdrawal. Finally, the benzodiazepine allows alcoholics to continue the day's activities without the telltale smell of alcohol on their breath.

Opiate addicts in methadone maintenance programs often take a single, massive dose of a benzodiazepine (the equivalent of 100–300 mg of diazepam) to boost the effect of their daily methadone dose (APA, 1990; Juergens, 1993). There is evidence to suggest that the experimental narcotic buprenorphine may, when mixed with benzodiazepines, offer the user less of a "high," thus reducing the incentive for the narcotics user to try to mix medications (Sellers et al., 1993).

Buspirone: The First Decade

In 1986, a new medication named "BuSpar" (buspirone) was introduced. Buspirone is a member of a new class of medications known as the *azapirones*, which are chemically different from the benzodiazepines. Buspirone was found as a result of a search by pharmaceutical companies for antipsychotic drugs that did not have the harsh side effects of the phenothiazines or similar chemicals (Sussman, 1994).

Buspirone was found to have an antianxiety effect, with a clinical picture of fewer side effects than the benzodiazepines, while being "comparable with that of both diazepam and clorazepate" in terms of its ultimate effectiveness (Feighner, 1987, p. 15; Manfredi et al., 1991). As an additional advantage, buspirone only rarely caused sedation or fatigue for the user (Rosenbaum & Gelenberg, 1991; Sussman, 1994), and there was no evidence of potentiation between buspirone and select benzodiazepines, or alcohol and buspirone (Feighner, 1987; Manfredi et al., 1991).[5]

However, clinical trials of buspirone suggested that some patients would experience gastrointestinal problems, drowsiness, decreased concentration, dizziness, agitation, headache, feelings of lightheadedness, nervousness, diarrhea, excitement, sweating/

clamminess, nausea, depression, and some feelings of fatigue (Cardieuz, 1996; Cole & Yonkers, 1995; Feighner, 1987; Graedon & Graedon, 1991; Manfredi et al., 1991; Newton, Marunycz, Alderdice, & Napoliello, 1986). Buspirone has also been found to cause decreased sexual desire in some users, as well as sexual performance problems in some men (Finger et al., 1997).

In contrast to the benzodiazepine family of drugs, buspirone has no significant anticonvulsant action. It also lacks the muscle relaxant effects of the benzodiazepines (Cardieuz, 1996; Eison & Temple, 1987). Buspirone has been found to be of little value in those cases of anxiety that involve insomnia, which is a significant proportion of anxiety cases (Manfredi et al., 1991). It has been found to be of value in the control of the symptoms of general anxiety disorder, but, not the anxiety of panic attacks.

On the positive side, buspirone was found to be effective in the treatment of many patients who suffered from an anxiety disorder with a depressive component (Cardieuz, 1996; Cohn, Wilcox, Bowden, Fisher, & Rodos, 1992). There is evidence to suggest that buspirone might be of value in the treatment of some forms of depression, both as the primary form of treatment and as an agent to potentiate the effects of other antidepressants (Sussman, 1994). In addition, buspirone has been found to be of value in the treatment of obsessive-compulsive disorder, social phobias, posttraumatic stress disorder, and possibly alcohol withdrawal symptoms (Schweizer & Rickels, 1994; Sussman, 1994). Physicians who treat geriatric patients have found that buspirone is effective in controlling aggression in anxious, confused older adults, without adding to psychomotor instability that can contribute to the patient falling (Ayd et al., 1996). It has also been found to reduce the frequency of self-abusive behaviors (SAB) in mentally retarded subjects, according to the authors.

Researchers have found that the addition of buspirone to antidepressant medications seems to bring many resistant or nonresponsive cases of depression under control (Cardieuz, 1996). Finally, there is some evidence that buspirone may be able to control the craving that many cigarette smokers report when they try to stop smoking, especially if the smoker

[5] This is not, however, a suggestion that the user try to use alcohol and buspirone at the same time. The author does *not* recommend the use of alcohol with any prescription medication.

tends to be anxious (Ayd et al., 1996; Schweizer & Rickels, 1994).

The Pharmacology of Buspirone

The mechanism of action for buspirone is different from that of the benzodiazepines (Eison & Temple, 1987). Where the benzodiazepines tend to bind to receptor sites that utilize the neurotransmitter GABA, buspirone tends to bind to one of the many serotonin receptor sites known as the $5\text{-}HT_{1A}$ site (Ayd et al., 1996; Cardieuz, 1996; Sussman, 1994). Buspirone appears to function in a manner that moderates the level of serotonin within the brain (Cardieuz, 1996). If there is a deficit of serotonin, as there is in depressive disorders, buspirone seems to stimulate the production of more of this neurotransmitter (Anton, 1994; Sussman, 1994). If there is an excess of serotonin, as there is in many forms of anxiety disorders, buspirone lowers the serotonin level (Cardieuz, 1996). Thus, depending on dosage level being used, individual differences in the distribution of $5\text{-}HT_{1A}$ receptor sites in the brain, and the individual's normal level of serotonin in the brain, buspirone might either enhance, or decrease, the production of serotonin as a neurotransmitter.

Whereas the benzodiazepines are effective almost immediately, buspirone must be used for as long as 2 to 4 weeks before its maximum effects are seen (Graedon & Graedon, 1991; Sussman, 1994; Thornton, 1990). The half-life of buspirone is only 1 to 10 hours (Cole & Yonkers, 1995). This short half-life requires that the individual take 3 to 4 divided doses of buspirone each day; on the other hand, the half-life of benzodiazepines like diazepam makes it possible for that drug to be used only 1 or 2 times a day (Schweizer & Rickels, 1994). Finally, unlike many other sedating chemicals, there does not appear to be any cross-tolerance between buspirone and the benzodiazepines, alcohol, the barbiturates, or meprobamate (Sussman, 1994).

To further illustrate the differences between buspirone and the benzodiazepines, BuSpar has been found to bind to dopamine and serotonin type 1 receptors in the hippocampus, a different portion of the brain than the area where the benzodiazepines exert their effect (Manfredi et al., 1991). Research into the abuse potential of buspirone is mixed at this time. Lader (1987) concluded that buspirone "failed to demonstrate any abuse liability in either animal or human studies" (p. 25), a conclusion supported by a number of other researchers (Anton, 1994; Rosenbaum & Gelenberg, 1991; Thornton, 1990).

Most certainly, there is no evidence of a withdrawal syndrome from buspirone such as that seen in chronic benzodiazepine abuse, according to Sussman (1994):

> Recreational users (of chemicals) rated buspirone as no more attractive than placebo with regard to "stimulant/euphoria" (potential) and buspirone was not sought in self-administration studies. (Sussman, 1994, p. 14)

In contrast to these conclusions, Murphy, Owen, and Tyrer (1989) found evidence of both an addictive effect and a characteristic withdrawal syndrome from buspirone. Thus, at this point in time, the potential for buspirone abuse/addiction remains unclear.

Side Effects

As noted earlier, a side effect of benzodiazepine use is occasional memory problems. Buspirone has failed to demonstrate any impact on memory in a sample of 39 subjects suffering from generalized anxiety disorder, as measured by psychological tests (Rickels, Giesecke, & Geller, 1987). These results suggest that buspirone does not cause amnesia, as do many benzodiazepines.

Buspirone has not been shown to lessen the intensity of withdrawal symptoms experienced by patients who were addicted to benzodiazepines (Rickels, Schweizer, Csanalosi, Case, & Chung, 1988). There is, in fact, evidence suggesting that patients currently taking a benzodiazepine might be slightly *less* responsive to buspirone than patients without benzodiazepine experience (Cardieuz, 1996). But, unlike the benzodiazepines, there is no evidence of tolerance to buspirone's effects, nor any evidence of physical dependence or a withdrawal syndrome from buspirone when the medication is used as directed for short periods (Cardieuz, 1996; Rickels et al., 1988).

A rare complication of buspirone use is the development of a drug-induced neurological condition known as the *serotonin syndrome* (Mills, 1995).

Approximately 11% of those patients who develop the serotonin syndrome die despite the best medical care. Some of the symptoms of the serotonin syndrome include irritability, confusion, an increase in anxiety, drowsiness, hyperthermia (increased body temperature), sinus tachycardia, dilation of the pupils, nausea, muscle rigidity, and seizures. Although the serotonin syndrome may develop as long as 24 hours after the patient ingests a medication that affects the serotonin neurotransmitter system, in 50% of the cases in this study the patient developed the syndrome within 2 hours of starting the medication (Mills, 1995).

There have been a limited number of cases in which patients who were taking buspirone and a monoamine oxidase inhibitor (MAOI) developed abnormally high blood pressure (Ciraulo, Creelman, et al., 1995). However, there are countless other cases where patients have taken these two medications at the same time, without apparent ill effect. Thus, the possible role of either medication in the development of the observed hypertension is still unknown.

The manufacturer's claim that buspirone offers many advantages over the benzodiazepines in the treatment of anxiety states has not been totally fulfilled. Rosenbaum and Gelenberg (1991) cautioned, "Many clinicians and patients have found buspirone to be a generally disappointing alternative to benzodiazepines" (p. 200). Nevertheless, the authors recommended a trial of buspirone for "persistently anxious patients" (p. 200). Further, buspirone would seem to be the drug of choice in the treatment of anxiety states in the addiction-prone individual.

Zolpidem

The drug zolpidem was used as a sleep-inducing (hypnotic) drug in Europe for 5 years before it was introduced to the United States in 1993 (Hobbs et al., 1995). It is sold as an orally administered hypnotic, available only with a physician's prescription, in the United States.

Technically, zolpidem is not a member of the benzodiazepine family of drugs. Rather, it is the first of a new family of sleep-inducing chemicals known as *imidazopryidines*. Zolpidem binds to just one of the receptor sites in the brain used by the benzodiazepines and thus is more selective than the agents that bind to a number of related receptor sites in the brain. Because zolpidem binds to only one of the benzodiazepine receptor sites, it has only a minor anticonvulsant effect. Under normal conditions, the biological half-life of zolpidem is about 1.5–2.4 hours (Kryger, Steljes, Pouliot, Neufeld, & Odynski, 1991). Most of a single dose of zolpidem is biotransformed into inactive metabolites, before excretion by the kidneys.

Hartman (1995) suggested that there is little evidence of tolerance developing to zolpidem's hypnotic effects, even after as long as one year. However, Ayd (1994) suggested that there were some rare reports of patients who have developed some degree of tolerance to the hypnotic effects of zolpidem. Thus, it would appear that tolerance to zolpidem's effects is possible, but that the majority of patients do not seem to develop significant tolerance to the drug's hypnotic effects.

Unlike older hypnotics, at therapeutic dosage levels zolpidem causes only a minor reduction in REM sleep (Hobbs et al., 1995). Further, it does not interfere with the other stages of sleep, allowing for a more natural and restful night's sleep by the patient (Hartmann, 1995). However, patients who suffer from sleep apnea should not take this medication, since zolpidem tends to worsen the apnea (Hartmann, 1995).

Some of the reported adverse reactions at therapeutic dosage levels include nightmares, headaches, gastrointestinal upset, agitation, and some daytime drowsiness (Hartmann, 1995). There have also been a few isolated cases of a zolpidem-induced psychosis (Ayd, 1994; Ayd et al., 1996). Side effects are more often encountered at higher dosage levels, and it is for this reason that the recommended dosage level of zolpidem should not exceed 10 mg/day (Evans, Funderburk, & Griffiths, 1990; Merlotti et al., 1989). Zolpidem has been found to cause some cognitive performance problems similar to those seen with the benzodiazepines (Ayd et al., 1996).

At dosage levels of 20 mg/day or above, zolpidem has been found to significantly reduce REM sleep. Also, at dosage levels of 20 mg/day or more, zolpidem was found to cause rebound insomnia when the drug is discontinued. At dosage levels of 50 mg/day, volunteers who received zolpidem reported such symptoms as visual perceptual disturbances, ataxia, dizziness, nausea, and/or vomiting. Patients who have ingested up to 40 times the maximum recommended dosage have recovered, although the effects of zolpidem will combine with those of other CNS depressants if the patient has ingested more than one medication in an overdose attempt, and such multiple-drug overdoses might prove fatal. As with all medications, *any suspected overdose of zolpidem either by itself, or in combination with other medications, should be treated by a physician.*

There is evidence that zolpidem "may have some abuse potential in people with histories of sedative-hypnotic abuse" (Evans et al., 1990, p. 1254). However, the authors suggested that the abuse potential of zolpidem was less than that of a commonly prescribed benzodiazepine: triazolam. Thus, the prescribing physician must balance the potential for abuse against the medication's potential benefit to the patient.

Rohypnol: A New Drug of Abuse

In the mid-1990s, a "new" drug of abuse appeared first in Florida, and later, across the southern United States. This drug was Rohypnol (flunitrazepam) a member of the benzodiazepine family of drugs that had been in clinical use as a presurgical medication, a muscle relaxant, and a hypnotic, in 60 other countries around the world. Each day, more than 2.3 million doses of flunitrazepam are sold around the world (Saum & Inciardi, 1997). But because it is not manufactured as a pharmaceutical in the United States, substance abuse rehabilitation professionals in this country had limited experience with flunitrazepam when people began to bring it into this country.

Legally, flunitrazepam was classified as a controlled substance by the United States government in October 1996. Individuals convicted of trafficking or distributing this drug may be incarcerated for up to 20 years ("Rohypnol," 1997). In the press, flunitrazepam has gained a reputation as a "date rape" drug (Saum & Inciardi, 1997) because it is thought to induce a period of amnesia in the user, a trait that some men reportedly have used to their advantage

to have unwanted sex with their dates. However, the actual frequency of this occurrence is not known ("Rohypnol," 1997).

Chemically, flunitrazepam is a derivative of the benzodiazepine chlordiazepoxide (Eidelberg, Neer, & Miller, 1965) and is reportedly 10 times as powerful as diazepam ("Rohypnol Use Spreading," 1995). The usual method of administration is by mouth. Flunitrazepam is well absorbed from the gastrointestinal tract, with between 80 and 90% of a single 2 mg dose being absorbed by the user's body (Mattila & Larni, 1980). Peak blood levels following a single oral dose are reached 1 to 2 hours after the drug is ingested (Saum & Inciardi, 1997). Once in the blood, 80% to 90% of the flunitrazepam is briefly bound to plasma proteins, but the drug is rapidly transferred from the plasma to body tissues. Because of this characteristic, flunitrazepam has an elimination half-life that is significantly longer than its duration of effect. Indeed, the elimination half-life is approximately 20 hours (Mattila & Larni, 1980).

During the process of biotransformation, flunitrazepam produces a number of different metabolites, some of which are themselves biologically active (Mattila & Larni, 1980). Less than 1% of the drug is excreted unchanged. About 90% of a single dose is eliminated by the kidneys after biotransformation, while about 10% is eliminated in the feces. Because of this characteristic elimination pattern, patients in countries where flunitrazepam is legal who have kidney disease require modification of their dosage level, since the main route of elimination is through the kidneys.

The usual pharmaceutical dose of flunitrazepam is 1–2 mg, but illicit users will often take 4 mg of the drug in one dose, which will begin to produce sedation in 20 to 30 minutes. The drug's effects normally last for 8 to 12 hours. Some users will mix flunitrazepam with ketamine (discussed in Chapter 13), nitrous oxide (discussed in Chapter 14), or fentanyl (discussed in Chapter 11) to enhance the effect ("Rohypnol Use Spreading," 1995). Illicit users may also use flunitrazepam while smoking marijuana and while using alcohol (Lively, 1996). The combination of flunitrazepam and marijuana is said to produce a "floating" effect on the user. In Europe, cocaine users have been known to ingest flunitrazepam to control the agitation often seen with cocaine abuse, and it is often used to enhance the effect of low-potency heroin (Saum & Inciardi, 1997). Adolescents often see the mixture of alcohol and flunitrazepam as a cheap drunk, because the effects of these two CNS depressants combine to bring about a state of intoxication after the individual has ingested just one beer and the drug (Saum & Inciardi).

Although the drug is used as a sedative, flunitrazepam, like the other benzodiazepines, is capable of inducing a state of paradoxical excitement or aggression. Flunitrazepam has an anticonvulsant effect (Eidelberg et al., 1965) and is capable of bringing about pharmacological dependence. Chronic users report that flunitrazepam can cause excessive sedation, headaches, tremor, and drug-induced amnesia (Office of National Drug Control Policy, 1996). For chronic users, withdrawal from flunitrazepam is potentially serious, and should only be carried out under the care and supervision of a medical professional. There have been reports of withdrawal seizures taking place as late as 7 days after the last use of flunitrazepam ("Rohypnol Use Spreading," 1995).

Summary

Since their introduction in the 1960s, the benzodiazepines have become one of the most frequently prescribed medications. As a class, the benzodiazepines are the treatment of choice for the control of anxiety and insomnia as well as many other conditions. They have also become a significant part of the drug abuse problem. Although many of the benzodiazepines were introduced as nonaddicting and safe substitutes for the barbiturates, there is evidence to suggest that they have an abuse potential similar to that of the barbiturate family of drugs.

A new series of pharmaceuticals, including buspirone (sold under the brand name BuSpar) and zolpidem, have been introduced in the past decade. Buspirone is the first of a new class of antianxiety agents, which works through a different mechanism than the benzodiazepines. While buspirone was introduced as nonaddicting, this claim has been challenged by at least one team of researchers. Zolpidem has an admitted potential for abuse; however, research at this time suggests that this abuse potential is less than that of a benzodiazepine commonly used as a hypnotic: triazolam. Researchers are actively discussing the potential benefits and liabilities of these new medications.

Amphetamines and CNS Stimulants

The use of central nervous system (CNS) stimulants dates back more than two thousand years. Historical evidence suggests that gladiators in ancient Rome used CNS stimulants to help them overcome the effects of fatigue, so they could fight longer (Wadler, 1994). Not surprisingly, people still use chemicals that act as CNS stimulants to fight off the effects of fatigue so they can work or, in times of conflict, fight longer.

There are several different families of chemicals that might be classified as CNS stimulants including: cocaine, the amphetamines, amphetaminelike drugs such as Ritalin (methylphenidate), and over-the-counter agents such as ephedrine. Because all these agents act as CNS stimulants, the behavioral effects of many of these drugs are remarkably similar (Gawin & Ellinwood, 1988). For this reason, the amphetaminelike drugs are discussed only briefly, whereas the amphetamines are reviewed in greater detail. Cocaine is discussed in Chapter 9.

The Amphetaminelike Drugs

Ephedrine

This chemical is produced by plants of the *Ephedra* genus. Historical evidence suggests that the Chinese were using this plant for its medicinal value at least five thousand years ago (Graedon & Graedon, 1991). The active agent, ephedrine, was first isolated by chemists in 1897 (Mann, 1992). But there was little interest in ephedrine by Western medicine until 1930, when the first report of its effectiveness

in treating asthma appeared in a medical journal (Karch, 1996). Ephedrine quickly became the treatment of choice for the treatment of asthma, and demand for ephedrine raised concern whether the demand might not exceed the supply of plants in the 1930s. The importance of this fear is discussed in the following section of this chapter.

Scientists have found that ephedrine's primary effects are strongest in the peripheral regions of the body rather than in the central nervous system. Ephedrine's ability to act as a bronchodilator made it useful in opening airways constricted by conditions such as asthma. Over the years, ephedrine has been found to be useful in the short-term treatment of allergic rhinitis, sinusitis, and hay fever, as well as an adjunct to the treatment of myasthenia gravis (Shannon et al., 1995). It also has a limited use in some surgical procedures (Karch, 1996).

Within the body, ephedrine stimulates the sympathetic nervous system, in a manner similar to that of adrenaline (Laurence & Bennett, 1992; Mann, 1992). The drug may be taken orally, but also may be injected. Peak blood levels from a single dose are achieved in 15 minutes to 1 hour (Shannon et al., 1995). The biological half-life of ephedrine is about 4 to 6 hours (Karch, 1996). There is little research into the way that ephedrine is distributed within the body, but it is known that very little of the drug is biotransformed before it is eliminated from the body by the kidneys.

The side effects of a normal dose of ephedrine include anxiety, insomnia, urinary retention, and heart palpitations (Graedon & Graedon, 1991). Because tolerance to its bronchodilator action develops rapidly, physicians recommend using ephedrine only for short periods. When abused, ephedrine can cause a drug-induced psychosis, hypertension, coronary artery spasm, and intracranial hemorrhage (Karch, 1996).

Ephedrine was once available over-the-counter as a treatment for asthma and nasal congestion. But the drug was often abused by cross-country truckers, who used it to ward off the effects of fatigue. It has also become common for "street" chemists to use ephedrine for the manufacture of illicit amphetamines, or methkathinone ("Ephedrine is Used Illegally," 1995). Because of its potential for abuse, and the fact that newer, more effective, pharmaceuticals are available for the control of asthma symptoms, the federal government placed restrictions on the over-the-counter sale of ephedrine in 1994.

Methylphenidate

Ritalin is a brand name for the chemical *methylphenidate*. Some researchers classify methylphenidate as a true amphetamine because of its actions and chemical structure. In this text, it is considered to be an amphetaminelike drug. Methylphenidate has been found to function as a CNS stimulant and is of value in the treatment of a rare neurological condition known as *narcolepsy*. Methylphenidate also has been found to be of value in the treatment of Attention-Deficit/Hyperactivity Disorder (ADHD) (to be discussed in more detail in the following section). It is also of occasional use in the treatment of depression (Shannon et al., 1995).

When used orally, methylphenidate is rapidly absorbed from the gastrointestinal tract. It is thought to be approximately half as potent as D-amphetamine (Wender, 1995). Peak blood levels are achieved in 1.9 hours, although extended-release forms of the drug might not reach peak blood levels for 4 to 7 hours after the medication was ingested (Shannon et al., 1995). The half-life of methylphenidate is from 1 to 3 hours, and the effects of a single oral dose last for between 3 and 6 hours, according to the authors. The effects of a single dose of an extended-release form of methylphenidate might continue for 8 hours.

When used in the treatment of attention-deficit/hyperactivity disorder, patients take 15–90 mg of methylphenidate per day, in divided doses (Wender, 1995). About 80% of a single dose of methylphenidate is biotransformed into ritalinic acid, which is then excreted by the kidneys. Side effects of methylphenidate include anorexia, insomnia, weight loss, failure to gain weight, nausea, heart palpitations, angina, anxiety, liver problems, dry mouth, hypertension, headache, upset stomach, enuresis, skin rashes, dizziness, or exacerbation of the symptoms of Tourette's syndrome (Maxmen & Ward, 1995; Shannon et al., 1995). Methylphenidate may lower the seizure threshold in patients with a seizure disorder, and if the patient should have a seizure, it is recommended that the drug be discontinued. Abusers report that the drug causes them to experience a high or feeling of euphoria, which is the main reason this drug is abused. There are case reports suggesting that in rare cases methylphenidate can cause damage to the liver (Karch, 1996).

The Amphetamines

History of the Amphetamines

The amphetamines are, essentially, *analogs* of ephedrine (Lit, Wiviott-Tishler, Wong, & Hyman 1996). The amphetamines were first discovered in 1887, but it was not until 1927 that these drugs were found to have medicinal value (Kaplan & Sadock, 1990; Lingeman, 1974). Following the introduction of ephedrine for the treatment of asthma, questions began to be raised as to whether the demand for it might exceed the supply. Pharmaceutical companies began to search for synthetic alternatives and found that the amphetamines had a similar effect on asthma patients. In 1932, an amphetamine product called "Benzedrine" was introduced for the treatment of asthma and rhinitis (Derlet & Heischober, 1990; Karch, 1996). The drug was contained in an inhaler similar to the kind used for "smelling salts." The ampule, which could be purchased over the counter, would be broken, releasing the concentrated amphetamine liquid into the surrounding cloth. The Benzedrine ampule would then be held under the nose and the fumes inhaled, much like smelling salts are, to reduce the symptoms of asthma.

It was not long, however, before it was discovered that these ampules of Benzedrine could be unwrapped, carefully broken open, and the concentrated drug used for injection.[1] Street drug users quickly discovered that the effects were similar to that of cocaine. The amphetamines were introduced in an era when the dangers of cocaine were well-known, and they came to be viewed by many as a "safe" substitute.

Researchers quickly discovered that the amphetamines had a stimulant effect on the central nervous system, and they were often used to ward off fatigue. During World War II, the amphetamines were used by American, British, German, and Japanese armed forces to counteract fatigue and heighten endurance (Brecher, 1972). During World War II, United States Army Air Corps crew members stationed in England took an estimated 180,000,000 Benzedrine pills to help them stay awake and work longer (Lovett, 1994). It is rumored that Adolf Hitler was addicted to amphetamines (Witkin, 1995). President John F. Kennedy, during his term of office, is rumored to have used methamphetamine, another member of the amphetamine family of chemicals (Witkin, 1995). In 1991 during the "Operation Desert Storm" campaign, some 65% of United States pilots questioned admitted to having used an amphetamine at least once during combat operations (Emonson & Vanderbeek, 1995).

It is possible to excuse the use of amphetamines during World War II, or Operation Desert Storm, as being necessary to meet the demands of the war. But, for reasons that are not well understood, there were waves of amphetamine abuse in both Sweden and Japan immediately following World War II (Snyder, 1986). In the United States, amphetamine use reached "epidemic proportions" (Kaplan & Sadock, 1990, p. 305) by the year 1970. Physicians would prescribe amphetamines for patients who

wished to lose weight or who were depressed, while illicit amphetamine users would take the drug because it helped them to feel good. In just the year 1970, before the government imposed strict controls on the prescription and manufacture of amphetamines, pharmaceutical companies in the United States produced some 10 billion amphetamine tablets. This figure is a measure of how popular amphetamines were both as a prescription medication and as a drug of abuse (a large percentage of these pills were diverted to illicit users).

However, at the same time that the amphetamines were so popular as drugs of abuse, they were falling into disfavor within the medical community. Researchers had discovered that the amphetamines were of minimal value in weight loss programs. Further, new types of antidepressant medications had replaced the amphetamines as the treatment of choice for depressive disorders. Although the amphetamines remained the medication of choice for the treatment of some neurological disorders, these conditions were quite rare.

The amphetamines have a unique position in history, for medical historians now believe that it was the arrival of large amounts of amphetamines, especially methamphetamine, that contributed to an outbreak of drug-related violence, putting an end to San Francisco's "summer of love" of 1967 (D. Smith, 1997). By the mid-1970s it was common knowledge among illicit users that high doses of the amphetamines would cause agitation, and its effects on the cardiovascular system could result in death. Further, even if it did not kill the user, many people experienced a severe, drug-induced depression that could last for days or weeks when the drug was discontinued. Finally, users came to understand that the chronic use of amphetamines would dominate the user's life. In San Francisco, physicians at the Haight-Ashbury free clinic coined the slogan "Speed kills" to warn the general public of the dangers of amphetamine abuse.

In the United States, amphetamine use peaked in the late 1960s and early 1970s, and then waned as the drug declined in popularity. At this same time, cocaine became the preferred stimulant of abuse. With the decline of cocaine, there is now evidence that the amphetamines are again becoming popular

---

[1] Needless to say, the amphetamines are no longer sold without a prescription.

drugs of abuse (Baberg, Nelesen, & Dimsdale, 1996; Witkin, 1995).

Scope of the Problem of Stimulant Abuse and Addiction

After peaking in the late 1960s or early 1970s, amphetamine abuse in the United States reached its lowest point in the late 1980s or early 1990s. It has been gradually increasing since then. The team of Baberg, Nelesen, and Dimsdale (1996) found that, in the San Diego area, amphetamine abuse reached its lowest levels in the year 1992; between 1992 and 1993, deaths involving amphetamine use increased between 61 and 73%. Other researchers have found that hospital emergency room visits involving the use of methamphetamine have increased by several orders of magnitude in the first half of this decade (Witkin, 1995).

The problem of CNS stimulant abuse/addiction in the United States has long been overshadowed by cocaine use/abuse (Jaffe, 1995a). However, at least 4 million people in the United States are thought to have used the most potent form of amphetamine, methamphetamine, at least once in their lives (Office of National Drug Control Policy, 1996). Further, there is information that suggests methamphetamine might be the most commonly abused *intravenous* drug in the United States (Norton, Burton, & McGirr, 1996). About 800,000 people in the United States are thought to use some form of amphetamine each month (Nash & Park, 1997).

In the United States, the average age at which a person begins to use CNS stimulants is 18.8 years (G. Cohen et al., 1996). Users typically use amphetamines manufactured in clandestine laboratories. During the 1960s and 1970s, the government imposed a number of controls on the legitimate manufacture and use of amphetamines. These controls made the diversion of legally manufactured amphetamines to the illicit market more difficult. But, since the amphetamines are easily manufactured with common chemicals, illicit users simply turned to drugs from illegal laboratories. Most of the amphetamine now being used in the United States comes either from illicit drug laboratories in California or from Mexican drug dealers, who manufacture

the drug, then smuggle it across the border (Lovett, 1994; Witkin, 1995).

Medical Uses of Amphetamines and CNS Stimulants

The amphetamine family of drugs is one of the more powerful groups of CNS stimulants (Jaffe, 1990). In addition to their effects on the CNS, the amphetamines and similar drugs (e.g., Ritalin) improve the action of the smooth muscles of the body (Hoffman & Lefkowitz, 1990). These drugs thus have potential for improving athletic performance, at least to some degree, and are often abused for this purpose. However these effects are not uniform, and overuse of the CNS stimulants can actually *decrease* athletic abilities in some users.

The amphetamines have an *anorexic* side effect,[2] and at one time this side effect of the amphetamines was thought to be useful in the control of weight. Subsequent research, however, has demonstrated that the amphetamines are only minimally effective as a weight control agent. Tolerance to the appetite-suppressing side effect of the amphetamines develops in only 4 weeks (Snyder, 1986). After the user becomes tolerant to the anorexic effect of amphetamines, it is not uncommon for the user to regain the weight initially lost. At the end of a 6-month period, there is no significant difference between the amount of weight lost by patients using amphetamines and patients who simply try to reduce their weight by dieting (Maxman & Ward, 1995).

Amphetamines were once thought to be antidepressants. But researchers have since discovered that the antidepressant effect of the amphetamines is short-lived, and they are now rarely used in the treatment of depression (Potter, Rudorfer, & Goodwin, 1987). The amphetamines and related compounds do have a limited medical value, however. First, in a limited number of cases, these drugs have been found to be useful in the control of the symptoms of hyperactivity in children (Kaplan & Sadock, 1990). Surprisingly, although the amphetamines are CNS

---

[2] Anorexia means that the individual has lost his/her desire to eat. A drug with an anorexic effect thus causes the individual to lose his/her desire to eat as often.

stimulants, they have a calming effect on individuals who have Attention-Deficit/Hyperactivity Disorder (ADHD). Researchers think that Ritalin and the amphetamines achieve this effect by enhancing the function of the reticular activating system (RAS) of the brain. This is the portion of the brain thought to be involved in focusing one's attention (Gold & Verebey, 1984). The RAS is thought to screen out extraneous stimuli, so that the person can concentrate on a specific task. In children who suffer from hyperactivity, an underactive RAS may allow the children to be easily distracted. The amphetamines are believed to stimulate the RAS to the point where the child is able to function more effectively.

Further, the amphetamines have been found to be the treatment of choice for a rare neurological condition known as *narcolepsy*. Narcolepsy is a lifelong neurological condition that causes the person to be subject to sudden spells of falling asleep during waking hours ("Amphetamines," 1990; Mirin et al., 1991). Doghramji (1989) described narcolepsy as an incurable disorder which is thought to reflect a chemical imbalance within the brain. One of the chemicals involved, dopamine, is the neurotransmitter that the amphetamines cause to be released from neurons in the brain. The amphetamines may at least partially correct the dopamine imbalance that causes narcolepsy.

Pharmacology of the Amphetamines

The amphetamine family of chemicals consists of several variations of the parent compound. Each variation yields an amphetamine molecule that is similar to the others except for minor variations in potency and pharmacological characteristics. The most common forms of amphetamine are dextroamphetamine (*d*-amphetamine sulfate), which is considered twice as potent as the other common form of amphetamine (Lingeman, 1974) and methamphetamine (*d*-desoxyephedrine hydrochloride). For reasons that are not well understood, illicit amphetamine abusers seem to prefer methamphetamine over dextroamphetamine. Collectively, these compounds are often simply called *amphetamines*, a practice followed in this chapter except when a specific form is being discussed.

Illicit amphetamines can be introduced into the body by several routes. The drug molecule tends to be basic, and when taken orally, it is easily absorbed through the lining of the small intestine (Laurence & Bennett, 1992). As a general rule, an oral dose of amphetamine will begin to have an effect on the user within 20 (Siegel, 1991) to 30 minutes (Mirin et al., 1991). The amphetamines are also easily absorbed into the body when injected. The speed with which the amphetamines begin to have an effect on the user who injects the drug depends on several factors, including whether the chemical is injected directly into a vein, into muscle tissue, or, just under the skin. Although there has been a great deal of discussion about smokable forms of methamphetamine (see "Ice," later in this chapter), the most common methods of methamphetamine abuse are the oral ingestion of tablets or injection of methamphetamine powder (Karch, 1996).

The amphetamine molecule is easily absorbed through the tissues of the nasopharynx, and thus amphetamine powder can be "snorted." While it is common for illicit users to snort amphetamine powder, this method of administration is never used in medical practice. The amphetamine molecule is also able to easily cross over from the lungs to the general circulation when smoked, and this is also a common method of amphetamine abuse ("'Meth's' Reach to Addicts," 1995; Shields, 1990). When smoked, the amphetamines are absorbed into the circulation through the lungs, and reach the brain in seconds.

In the normal patient who has received a single oral dose of an amphetamine, the peak plasma levels are achieved in 1 to 3 hours. The biological half-life of the different forms of amphetamine vary, as a result of the different chemical structure of the specific form of amphetamine being used. For example, the biological half-life of dextroamphetamine is 10.25 hours, while the half-life of methamphetamine is only 4 to 5 hours (Derlet & Heischober, 1990; Medical Economics Company, 1993; Shannon et al., 1995).

The chemical structure of the basic amphetamine molecule closely resembles that of two different neurotransmitters: norepinephrine and dopamine. The effects of amphetamines in the peripheral regions of the body are caused by its ability to stimulate norepi-nephrine release, while its CNS effects are the result of its impact on the dopamine-using regions of the brain (Lit et al., 1996). Once in the brain, the amphetamine molecule is absorbed into those neurons that use dopamine as a neurotransmitter. Within these neurons, the amphetamine molecule then stimulates the neuron to release its stores of dopamine, which in turn stimulates nearby neurons (Hyman & Nestler, 1996).

One of the regions of the brain that uses dopamine as a neurotransmitter is the mesolimbic region of the brain. This region of the brain seems to be part of the pleasure center of the brain, and the release of dopamine that is stimulated by the omphet-amines causes a sense of euphoria. Another region in the brain where the amphetamines have an effect is the medulla (which is involved in the control of respiration), causing the individual to breathe more deeply and more rapidly. At normal dosage levels, the cortex is also stimulated, which reduces feelings of fatigue and possibly increases concentration (Kaplan & Sadock, 1990).

There is considerable variation in individual sensitivity to the effects of the amphetamines. There have been rare reports of toxic reactions to amphetamines at dosage levels as low as 2 mg (Hoffman & Lefkowitz, 1990). While the estimated lethal dose of amphetamines for a nontolerant individual is 20–25 mg/kg (Chan, Chen, Lee, & Deng, 1994), there is one clinical report of a case where the person ingested a dose of only 1.5 mg/kg, with fatal results. There are also case reports where amphetamine-naive individuals (that is to say individuals who have not developed tolerance to the amphetamines) have survived a total single dose of 400–500 mg (or 7.5 mg/kg body weight for a 160-pound person). However the patients who ingested these dosage levels required medical support to overcome the toxic effects of the amphetamines. Individuals who are tolerant to the effects of the amphetamines may use massive doses "without apparent ill effect" (Hoffman & Lefkowitz, 1990, p. 212).

Some of the amphetamine in the body is biotransformed by the liver. During the process of amphetamine biotransformation, a number of metabolites are formed as the biotransformation process progresses from one step to the next. The exact number of metabolites varies, depending on the specific form of amphetamine being used. For example, during the process of methamphetamine biotransformation, seven different metabolites are formed at various stages in the process of biotransformation, before the drug is finally eliminated from the body.

While some of the amphetamines are biotransformed by the liver, a significant percentage is excreted from the body essentially unchanged. Researchers have found that in the first several days following a single oral dose of an amphetamine, between 35 and 45% is excreted unchanged by the kidneys (Karch, 1996). If the individual's urine is quite acidic, up to 60% of a dose of amphetamine will be filtered from the blood, and be excreted unchanged (Shields, 1990). However, if the individual's urine is extremely alkaline, perhaps as little as 5% of a dose of amphetamine will be filtered out of the blood by the kidneys, and excreted unchanged, according to the author. This is because the drug molecules tend to be reabsorbed by the kidneys when the urine tends to be more alkaline. Thus, the speed at which a dose of amphetamines is excreted from the body varies in response to how acidic the individual's urine is at the time that the drug passes through the kidneys.

Neuroadaptation/Tolerance to Amphetamines

The steady use of an amphetamine by a patient will result in an incomplete state of neuroadaptation. For example, when a physician prescribes an amphetamine in the treatment of narcolepsy, it is possible to maintain the person on the same regimen for years, without any modification of the original dosage (Jaffe, 1995a).

But, amphetamine abusers find that they quickly become tolerant to amphetamine-induced euphoria. There are two basic ways that amphetamine abusers try to overcome their tolerance to the euphoric effects of these drugs. First, over time there is a tendency for the person to use higher and higher dosage levels of amphetamines (Peluso & Peluso, 1988) in an attempt to reachieve the initial sense of euphoria. Some chronic amphetamine users, for example, have reached the point where they must use 5,000–15,000 mg in a day's time, repeatedly injecting small doses of amphetamines over the course of the day in order to try and overcome their tolerance to the effects of smaller doses (Chan et al., 1994; Derlet & Heischober, 1990).

The second method is to substitute intravenously administered amphetamines for the oral or the intranasal methods of amphetamine use. The intravenous form of drug administration delivers a large amount of concentrated drug to the body in a relatively short amount of time. This may allow the user to reachieve the sense of euphoria that was lost when he/she became tolerant to the drug. Thus, it is not uncommon for users to "graduate" to the intravenous use of amphetamines when they are no longer able to achieve the desired effects through oral or intranasal use of the drug.

Interactions between the Amphetamines and Other Medications

Patients who are taking amphetamines should avoid taking them with fruit juices or ascorbic acid, as these substances decrease the absorption of amphetamines (Maxman & Ward, 1995). Patients should avoid mixing amphetamines with opiates, as these drugs increase the anorexic and analgesic effects of narcotic analgesics. Further, patients who are taking the class of antidepressants known as monoamine oxidase inhibitors (MAOIs, or MAO inhibitors) should avoid amphetamines as the combination can result in dangerous elevations in the person's blood pressure (Barnhill et al., 1995). *Always consult with a physician or pharmacist before taking two or more medications at the same time, to make sure that there is no danger of harmful interactions between the chemicals being used.*

Methods of Amphetamine Abuse

The amphetamines are often ingested in pill form. Amphetamine powder may be used intranasally, or methamphetamine crystals may be smoked. The methods of amphetamine abuse that result in the highest blood levels of the chemical are smoking and, intravenous injection. An extreme pattern of intravenous amphetamine abuse is seen when the user embarks on what is known as a "speed run."

A speed run is an extended period when the user repeatedly uses amphetamines to try to capture, and maintain, a drug-induced feeling of euphoria.

During such speed runs, the individual uses larger and larger doses of the drug over time, often using amphetamines until his/her supply is exhausted. As noted earlier, long-term users of amphetamines have been known to repeatedly inject small doses of the drug over the course of a day, until the total amount reaches anywhere from 5,000 to 15,000 mg. Such dosage levels would be fatal to the naive (inexperienced) drug user.

Subjective Experience of Amphetamine Use

The amphetamine experience is, to a large degree, similar to that seen with cocaine or adrenaline (Kaminski, 1992). However, there are some major differences between the effects of cocaine and that of the amphetamines: (a) whereas the effects of cocaine last from a few minutes to an hour at most, the effects of the amphetamines last many hours; (b) unlike cocaine, the amphetamines are effective when used orally; and (c) unlike cocaine, the amphetamines have only a very small anesthetic effect (Weiner, 1985).

The effects of the amphetamines on any given individual depend on that individual's mental state, the dosage level utilized, the relatively potency of the specific form of amphetamine, and the manner in which the drug is used. The usual oral dosage level is 15–30 mg per day (Lingeman, 1974); however, this depends on the potency of the amphetamine or amphetaminelike drug being used (Julien, 1992).

At low to moderate oral dosage levels, the individual will experience feelings of increased alertness, an elevation of mood, a feeling of mild euphoria, less mental fatigue, and an improved level of concentration (Kaplan & Sadock, 1990; Weiner, 1985). Like many drugs of abuse, the amphetamines stimulate the pleasure center in the brain. Thus, both the amphetamines and cocaine produce "a neurochemical magnification of the pleasure experienced in most activities" (Gawin & Ellinwood, 1988, p. 1174) when initially used. The authors went on to note that the initial use of amphetamines or cocaine would:

> . . . produce alertness and a sense of well-being . . . lower anxiety and social inhibitions, and heighten energy, self-esteem, and the emotions

aroused by interpersonal experiences. Although they magnify pleasure, they do not distort it; hallucinations are usually absent. (p. 1174)

At high dosage levels, such as when methamphetamine is injected or smoked, the user might initially experience an intense sense of euphoria, which has been called a "rush" or a "flash." This sensation was described as "instant euphoria" by the author Truman Capote (quoted in R. K. Siegel, 1991, p. 72). Other users have compared the flash to sexual orgasm. Researchers have not studied the rush in depth, but it appears to last for only a short period (Jaffe, 1995a). Following the initial rush, the user may experience a warm glow, or gentle euphoria, that may last for several hours.

Side Effects of Amphetamine Use at Normal Dosage Levels

Patients who are taking amphetamines under a physician's supervision may experience such side effects as dryness of the mouth, anorexia, headache, insomnia, and periods of confusion (Fawcett & Busch, 1995). The patient's systolic and diastolic blood pressure will both increase, and the heart rate will reflexively slow down. Other potential side effects at normal dosage levels include dizziness, agitation, a feeling of apprehension, flushing, pallor, muscle pains, excessive sweating, and delirium, according to the authors. When the medication wears off, it is not uncommon for the patient to experience a sense of fatigue, or lethargy, and mild depression, that may last for a few hours, or days.

Consequences of Amphetamine Abuse

In addition to causing the user to experience a sense of euphoria and cheerfulness, the amphetamines cause some unwanted side effects. Because they are powerful chemicals, the amphetamines affect many different body systems. Some complications of the amphetamine abuse include all the side effects seen when these medications are used by patients under a physician's supervision. However, amphetamine abuse also can cause a wide range of other problems in many different organ systems.

Chapter Eight

Central Nervous System

A common side effect of the amphetamines is a drug-induced state of anxiety, or irritability. It is not uncommon for illicit drug users to try to counteract the anxiety and tension often experienced as side effects of amphetamine abuse through the use of alcohol, marijuana, or benzodiazepines. Peluso and Peluso (1988) estimated that *half* of all regular amphetamine users may also be classified as heavy drinkers. These individuals attempt to control the side effects of the amphetamines through the use of alcohol, which is a CNS depressant. Another form of polydrug abuse is seen when alcoholics use amphetamines to counteract the sedating effects of the alcohol, so that they can drink for longer periods. Thus, polydrug abuse is a common characteristic of amphetamine abusers.

Amphetamine users also might experience periods of drug-induced confusion, irritability, fear, suspicion, drug-induced hallucinations, and/or a drug-induced delusional state (Julien, 1992; King & Ellinwood, 1992). Other possible consequences of amphetamine abuse include assaultiveness, irritability, weakness, insomnia, panic states, suicidal, and homicidal tendencies (Derlet & Heischober, 1990; "'Meth's' Reach to Addicts," 1995). Physicians faced with patients who are experiencing an amphetamine-induced state of agitation or delusional thinking may want to use either haloperidol or diazepam to help the individual calm down (Derlet & Heischober, 1990).

The chronic use of amphetamines seems to contribute to the user's development of extreme sensitivity to anxiety states (Satel et al., 1993). The drug-induced anxiety and panic attacks may persist for months, or even years, after the last actual use of amphetamines. The authors suggest that these drug-related anxiety and panic attacks may be intensified if the individual should again start to abuse CNS stimulants such as the amphetamines.

Further, the authors cited research that suggests chronic amphetamine users may experience sleep disturbances for up to 4 weeks after the last use of the drug. The authors also cited evidence that suggests that chronic amphetamine users may have abnormal EEG tracings (a measure of the electrical activity in the brain) for up to 3 months after their last use of the drug. Thus, the effects of chronic amphetamine abuse on the individual's emotions may continue long after the last actual use of the drug.

It is not uncommon for both new and chronic amphetamine abusers to experience a psychotic reaction. This side effect of the amphetamines was first reported in a journal article that appeared in 1938 (Karch, 1996). In its earlier stages, the amphetamine-induced psychosis is often indistinguishable from schizophrenia (Kaplan & Sadock, 1990). This drug-induced state often includes confusion, suspiciousness, hallucinations, and delusional thinking, as well as episodes of violence. In contrast to actual schizophrenia, the hallucinations experienced by an individual who is suffering from an amphetamine psychosis tend to be mainly visual (Kaplan & Sadock, 1991). Further, the amphetamine-induced hyperactivity and absence of a thought disorder help to distinguish an amphetamine psychosis from actual schizophrenia, according to the authors.

Under normal conditions, this drug-induced psychosis clears up within days after the drug is discontinued (Kaplan & Sadock, 1990). In some cases, however, this drug-induced psychosis may require weeks or months to clear up. Researchers in Japan following World War II noted that in 15% of the cases of amphetamine-induced psychosis, it took up to 5 years following the last amphetamine use before the drug-induced psychotic condition eased (Flaum & Schultz, 1996). On occasion, the amphetamine-induced psychosis seems to become permanent.

As recently as the mid-1980s, it was thought that the amphetamines could bring on a latent schizophrenia in a person vulnerable to this condition. It was thought that the psychosis would have manifested itself at some point even if the person had not used amphetamines. But the amphetamines are now known to be able to cause a drug-induced psychosis in essentially normal people (Kaplan & Sadock, 1990). The ability of chronic amphetamine abuse to alter the normal function of the brain seems to make the user vulnerable to the development of a drug-induced paranoid psychosis (Flaum & Schultz, 1996).

Prolonged use of the amphetamines may also result in the individual experiencing a condition known as *formication*, which is the sensation of having unseen bugs crawling either on, or just under, the skin ("Amphetamines," 1990; R. K. Siegel, 1991). Victims have been known to scratch or burn the skin, in an attempt to rid themselves of these unseen bugs. Also, following prolonged periods of amphetamine abuse, many individuals become fatigued and/or depressed. It is not uncommon for the individual's depression to reach suicidal proportions (Fawcett & Busch, 1995). These amphetamine-induced feelings of depression could last for extended periods, possibly for months, following cessation of amphetamine use.

A rare complication of amphetamine use is the development of a drug-induced neurological condition known as the *serotonin syndrome* (Mills, 1995). Approximately 11% of those patients who develop this condition die despite receiving the best medical care. Some of the symptoms of the serotonin syndrome include irritability, confusion, an increase in anxiety, drowsiness, hyperthermia (increased body temperature), sinus tachycardia, dilation of the pupils, nausea, muscle rigidity, and seizures. Although the serotonin syndrome may develop as long as 24 hours after the patient ingested a medication that affects the serotonin neurotransmitter system, in 50% of the cases studied, the patient developed the syndrome within just two hours of starting the medication (Mills, 1995). This condition constitutes a medical emergency that should be treated by a physician.

Research evidence now exists suggesting that the chronic use of amphetamines brings about actual physical damage to the cells of the brain, which in turn affects how the brain functions. Researchers are still not sure how chronic amphetamine use can cause a "sustained neurophysiologic change" in the brain of the user (Gawin & Ellinwood, 1988, p. 1178). Animal research suggests that the chronic use of amphetamines can cause permanent changes in the blood flow patterns within the brain. King and Ellinwood (1992) warned that ". . . chronic amphetamine users are at high risk for cerebrovascular damage" (p. 255).

The exact mechanism through which the amphetamines bring about changes in the blood flow pattern within the brain is not clear. However, one possibility is that, since amphetamine abuse can result in hypertensive episodes on the part of the user, the rapid changes in blood pressure levels may damage the blood vessels in the brain. Most certainly, this is the mechanism through which the individual might experience a cerebral hemorrhage ("stroke") (Brust, 1993; King & Ellinwood, 1992). Such strokes result in the destruction of some blood vessels within the brain, which may contribute to brain damage or even death.

There also is evidence that the amphetamines are emotionally, and possibly physically, addictive for at least some users. Admittedly, *most* amphetamine users do not become addicted (Gawin & Ellinwood, 1988), but there is no way, at present, to determine who is at risk for becoming addicted to amphetamines. Another possible complication of amphetamine use is that the periods of drug-induced euphoria experienced in the amphetamine binge might create "vivid, long-term memories" (Gawin & Ellinwood, 1988, p. 1175) of the drug experience for the user. These memories, in turn, form part of the foundation of the craving that many amphetamine users experience when they stop using the drug. The recovery process from prolonged amphetamine use follows the same pattern seen for cocaine, and this euphoric recall is a very real problem for recovering abusers.

The Digestive System

There have been a few reports of liver damage associated with amphetamine abuse (Jones, Jarvie, McDermid, & Proudfoot, 1994). However, the exact mechanism(s) by which illicit amphetamines cause damage to the liver is still not clear. The consequences of prolonged amphetamine use, like that of cocaine, include the complications seen in persons who have neglected their dietary requirements. Vitamin deficiencies are common consequences of chronic amphetamine abuse (Gold & Verebey, 1984). Prolonged use of the amphetamines may result in the user vomiting, becoming anorexic, or developing diarrhea (Kaplan & Sadock, 1990).

The Cardiovascular System

Overall, the amphetamines appear to have less potential for causing cardiovascular damage than does cocaine abuse (discussed in Chapter 9) (Karch, 1996). However, this does not mean that amphetamine abuse does not carry some risk of cardiovascular damage. Despite their lower potential for cardiovascular damage, amphetamine abuse can result in hypertensive reactions, especially at high dosage levels (Wender, 1995).

Further, the amphetamines have the potential to cause a number of cardiac problems, including chest pain (angina), atrial and ventricular arrhythmias, myocardial ischemia (Derlet & Heischober, 1990; Lange et al., 1992), cardiomyopathy (Brent, 1995; Fawcett & Busch, 1995), and myocardial infarction (Fawcett & Busch, 1995; Packe, Garton, & Jennings, 1990). When abused, the amphetamines may cause a spasm in the coronary arteries at a time when the heart's workload is increased by the drug's effects on the rest of the body (Hong, Matsuyama, & Nur, 1991; Packe et al., 1990). Often, the result is what is commonly called a "heart attack," which may prove fatal to the amphetamine abuser. Amphetamine abuse may also cause sudden episodes of congestive heart failure, again, a potentially fatal condition (Derlet & Horowitz, 1995).

The Pulmonary System

There has been very little research into the impact of amphetamine abuse and lung function (Albertson, Walby, & Derlet, 1995). But, since a common method of amphetamine abuse is for the user to smoke the drug and inhale the fumes, it is reasonable to expect the side effects of smoked amphetamine to resemble those found when the user smokes cocaine. Thus, amphetamine abuse might result in sinusitis, pulmonary infiltrates, pulmonary edema, exacerbation of asthma, pulmonary hypertension, and pulmonary hemorrhage/infarct (Albertson et al., 1995).

Other Consequences of Amphetamine Abuse

There is evidence that amphetamine use/abuse can exacerbate the symptoms of some medical disorders such as Tourette's syndrome and tardive dyskinesia (Lopez & Jeste, 1997). In both men and women, amphetamine abuse may result in sexual performance problems (Finger et al., 1997). High doses or the chronic use of amphetamines can cause an inhibition of orgasm in the user, according to the authors, as well as delayed or inhibited ejaculation in men. The practice of smoking methamphetamine has caused the formation of corneal ulcers on the eyes of some users (Chuck, Williams, Goldberg, & Lubniewski, 1996). The chronic use of amphetamines may cause a toxic condition within the body that might prove to be fatal. As noted earlier, however, there is a wide variation in what might be considered a "toxic" dose of amphetamine (Julien, 1992).

"Ice"

In the late 1970s, a new form of methamphetamine known as "ice" was reported as having been abused on the mainland United States for the first time. Historical evidence suggests that ice was brought to Hawaii from Japan by Army troops following World War II, where its use remained endemic to Hawaii for many years ("Drug Problems," 1990). Although police and drug abuse professionals believe that ice reached the mainland United States in the late 1970s ("Ice Overdose," 1989), this form of methamphetamine did not gain much notoriety until the news media on the West Coast began to give the drug a certain prestige by reporting its effects and dangers. Potential users on the mainland began to ask about the drug, creating a market for ice, and its use began to spread from a few isolated areas on the West Coast to other regions of this country.

Nobody can predict the future of ice in this country. Most certainly, it has not spread as quickly as had once been anticipated. The feared "ice storm," or epidemic of ice use, that was predicted to take place in the early 1990s never materialized ("Asiatic Amphetamine Abuse," 1994; Brent, 1995; "Whatever Happened to Ice?" 1994). But, ice does appear to be slowly spreading across this country. Today, the greatest concentration of ice abusers is still on the West Coast (Johnston, O'Malley, & Bachman, 1994), but there is evidence that ice has become available in Texas and Florida (Gold, 1990b; "Ice Overdose," 1989).

Ice is a colorless, odorless, form of concentrated crystal methamphetamine that resembles a chip of ice, or clear rock candy. Some samples of ice sold on the street have been 98% to 100% pure amphetamine (Kaminski, 1992). Since its introduction, ice has become quite popular in some regions of this country (Kaminski, 1992; "Raw Data," 1990). It is often sold on the streets as a "safe" alternative to crack cocaine (*Mayo Clinic Health Letter*, 1989), and there are many different street names for ice.

How Ice Is Used

Ice is smoked in a manner similar to crack. Like crack, the drug crosses into the blood through the lungs, and reaches the brain in a matter of seconds. However, where the "high" from crack lasts perhaps 20 minutes, the high from ice lasts significantly longer. Estimates as to the duration of the effects of ice vary from 8 hours ("Raw Data," 1990) to 12 ("New Drug 'Ice'," 1989; "Drug Problems," 1990), to 14 ("Ice Overdose," 1989) or 18 (McEnroe, 1990), up to 24 hours (Evanko, 1991). Kaminski suggested that the effects of ice last as long as 30 hours (1992). The long duration of its effect, while in some dispute, is consistent with the pharmacological properties of the amphetamines compared with those of cocaine. The stimulant effects of the amphetamines in general last for hours, whereas cocaine's stimulant effects usually last for a shorter period.

How Ice Is Produced

Like crack, this form of methamphetamine is manufactured in clandestine laboratories. However, unlike crack, which must be processed from cocaine smuggled into the country, methamphetamine can be manufactured from chemicals legally purchased from any chemical supply store (R. K. Siegel, 1991).

The Effects of Ice

In addition to the physical effects of methamphetamine, reviewed earlier in this chapter, users have found that ice has several advantages over crack cocaine. First, although it is more expensive than crack on the basis of weight, ice is actually cheaper dose for dose. Second, because of its duration of effect, it *seems* to be more potent than crack. Third, since ice melts at a lower temperature than crack; it does not require as much heat to use. This means that ice can be smoked without the elaborate equipment needed for crack.

Fourth, because it is odorless, ice may be smoked in public without any characteristic smell alerting passersby that it is being used. Finally, another advantage is that, if the user decides to stop smoking for a moment or two, ice will cool and reform as a crystal. This makes it highly transportable and offers an advantage over crack because the user can use only a small piece of the drug at any given time.

Complications of Ice Abuse

Many complications of ice use are the same as those seen with other forms of methamphetamine abuse. This is understandable, since ice is simply a different form of methamphetamine than the powder or pills sold on the street for oral or intravenous use. But many problems are associated with ice. Although it is often sold as a safe alternative to crack, this is hardly true. The typical amount of methamphetamine admitted into the body when the user smokes ice is between *150 and 1,000 times the maximum recommended therapeutic dosage* for that drug (Hong et al., 1991). This level of methamphetamine may be toxic to the user and may prove fatal.

Ice has been known to cause extreme elevations in the user's blood pressure, which may contribute to a heart attack or cerebrovascular accident (stroke) and/or chest pain. Other known side effects of ice include confusion, seizures, cardiac arrhythmias (disruption of the normal rhythm of the heart, which may prove fatal), periods of aggressive acting out, and cardiovascular collapse (Beebe & Walley, 1995). The vasoconstrictive effects of methamphetamine have been suggested as the reason some users develop potentially dangerous elevations in body temperature (Beebe & Walley, 1995). When the body temperature passes above 104°F, the prognosis for recovery is quite poor.

The chronic use of ice can result in feelings of paranoia, hallucinations, delusional thinking, and, periods of aggression (Beebe & Walley, 1995). There have been reports that female patients who have had anesthesia to prepare them for caesarean sections have suffered cardiovascular collapse because of the interaction between the anesthesia and ice. Methamphetamine abuse has been known to cause kidney and/or lung damage, as well as permanent damage to the structure of the brain itself, pulmonary edema, vascular spasm, cardiomyopathy, drug-induced psychotic reactions, acute myocardial infarctions (i.e., heart attack), and cerebral arteritis (Albertson et al., 1995; "Drug Problems," 1990; Hong et al., 1991). As these findings suggest, ice is hardly a safe drug.

It now appears that the addiction potential of ice is at least as great as that of crack, if not greater ("Drug Problems," 1990). But ice is not the last word in CNS stimulants. A new CNS stimulant has been gaining in popularity in this country even as ice spreads outward from the West Coast to the rest of the United States. In the section that follows, we discuss this latest arrival, methkathinone.

"Kat"

A recent arrival here in the United States is a CNS stimulant known as methkathinone, or "Kat" (sometimes spelled "Cat" or "Khat"). Kat is a member of the kathinone family of chemicals, which are found naturally in several species of plants from Africa (Goldstone, 1993; Monroe, 1994). The chemical structure of methkathinone is similar to that of the amphetamines and ephedrine (Karch, 1996).

The Legal Status of Kat

Kat was classified a Schedule I controlled substance in 1992. Schedule I drugs are those with a limited medical use, and a high addictive potential. Examples of Schedule I drugs include heroin and cocaine, and since it has been classified a Schedule I substance its manufacture in illicit laboratories is illegal (Monroe, 1994).

How Kat Is Produced

Kat is easily synthesized by illicit laboratories by using ephedrine and such compounds as drain cleaner, epsom salts, battery acid, acetone, toulene, various dyes, and hydrochloric acid to alter the basic ephedrine molecule. All these substances can be legally purchased in the United States (Monroe, 1994). These chemicals are mixed in such a way as to add an oxygen molecule to the original ephedrine molecule ("Other AAFS Highlights," 1995), to produce a compound with the chemical structure (2-methylamino-1-phenylpropan-1-one).

The Scope of Kat Use

The use of Kat was limited to the former Soviet Union for many years. In the early 1990s, however, the drug surfaced in parts of the United States, and illicit laboratories have been found producing Kat in Michigan, Wisconsin, Illinois, Missouri, Texas, and Ohio ("Other AAFS Highlights," 1995). Samples of the drug have been found in all these states, as well as Washington, Colorado, and Indiana (Monroe, 1994). There is evidence that most of those who are addicted to Kat make their own drug ("'Cat' Poses National Threat," 1993).

The Effects of Kat

Users typically either inhale or smoke Kat, although it can be injected (Monroe, 1994). The drug's effects are similar to those of the amphetamines. According to individual case reports offered by users, Kat produces a more intense high than does cocaine ("'Cat' Poses National Threat," 1993). In contrast to cocaine, the effects of Kat can last for up to 6 days (Monroe, 1994; Goldstone, 1993).

Once in the body, Kat is biotransformed into ephedrine ("Other AAFS Highlights," 1995). Thus, its effects are similar to those seen with the chronic use of ephedrine at high dosage levels. Following drug use, it is not uncommon for Kat users to fall into a deep sleep that might last for as long as several days (Monroe, 1994). Chronic users also have reported experiencing periods of depression following the use of Kat ("'Cat' Poses National Threat," 1993).

Adverse Effects of Kat Abuse

Because this is a "new" drug, much remains to be discovered about the effects of Kat on the user. Some reported adverse effects include the development of drug-induced psychotic reactions, agitation, hyperactivity, a strong, offensive body odor, sores in the mouth and on the tongue, and depression. Death has been known to occur as a result of Kat use, although the exact mechanism of death has not been identified. Monroe (1994) suggested that Kat users are at increased risk for heart attack, or stroke. Brent (1995) suggested that an overdose of Kat produces many of the same effects, and responds to the same treatment as an overdose of amphetamine.

It is still too early to tell how significant a role Kat will play in the recreational drug use trends of the 21st century. At this time, Kat seems to not so much have attracted the casual user of chemicals so much as the hard-core stimulant user ("'Cat' Poses National Threat," 1993). However, in the past decade, Kat has slowly become more popular among illicit stimulant abusers.

Summary

Although they had been discovered in the 1880s, the amphetamines were first introduced as a treatment for asthma some 50 years later, in the 1930s. The early forms of amphetamine were sold over the counter in cloth-covered ampoules that were used in much the same way as smelling salts are today. Within a short time, however, it was discovered that the ampoules were a source of concentrated amphetamine that could be injected. The resulting high was found to be similar to that of cocaine (which had gained a reputation as being a dangerous drug) and had the added "benefit" of lasting much longer.

The amphetamines were used extensively both during and after World War II. After the war, American physicians prescribed amphetamines for the treatment of depression and as an aid for weight loss. By the year 1970, amphetamines accounted for 8% of all prescriptions written. Since then, however, physicians have learned that the amphetamines present a serious potential for abuse. The amphetamines have come under increasingly strict controls that limit the amount of amphetamine manufactured and the reasons for prescribing it.

Because the amphetamines are easily manufactured, there has always been an underground manufacture and distribution system for these drugs. In the late 1970s and early 1980s, street drug users drifted away from the amphetamines to the supposedly safe stimulant of the early 1900s: cocaine. Recent evidence suggests that the pendulum has started to swing back in the opposite direction. A new generation has discovered the amphetamines, and use of this class of drugs is increasing as illicit drug abusers move away from the known dangers of cocaine back to the amphetamines. This new generation of amphetamine addicts have not learned the dangers of amphetamine abuse so painfully discovered by amphetamine users of the late 1960s: "Speed" kills.

CHAPTER NINE

Cocaine

As we discussed in Chapter 8, the central nervous system (CNS) stimulants include the amphetamines, and amphetaminelike drugs such as ephedrine and Ritalin. Although cocaine shares many characteristics with the CNS stimulants, it is also a unique drug of abuse in many ways. In this chapter, we discuss both the ways that cocaine resembles and is different from the CNS stimulants.

A Brief Overview of Cocaine

Cocaine is obtained from the coca bush *Erythroxylon coca*, which grows naturally in the higher elevations of Peru, Bolivia, and Java (DiGregorio, 1990). The high mountains of South America are barely habitable, in part because the thin atmosphere makes it difficult to work for extended periods of time. However, thousands of years ago, natives learned that if they chewed the leaves of the coca plant, they could reduce their feelings of fatigue, thirst, and hunger, making it possible for them to work longer (P. White, 1989). Cocaine use rapidly became a part of everyday life in South America.

Prior to the invasion of Peru by the Spanish conquistadores in the 16th century, cocaine was used by the Incas in their religious ceremonies, as a medium of exchange (Ray & Ksir, 1993), and as part of the burial ritual (Byck, 1987). However, its use was generally reserved for the upper classes until the Spanish conquistadores overpowered the Incas (Mann, 1994). After that, the practice of chewing cocaine became widespread throughout South America, especially after the Spanish landlords discovered that native workers were more productive when allowed to use cocaine leaves.

The practice of chewing coca leaves, or drinking a tea brewed from the leaves, has continued until this time. People of the mountain regions of Peru chew the leaves mixed with lime, which is obtained from seashells (White, 1989). The lime works with saliva to release the cocaine from the leaves and helps reduce the bitter taste of the coca leaf. Also, chewing coca leaves is thought to actually help the chewer absorb some of the phosphorus, vitamins, and calcium in the mixture (P. White). Thus, although its primary use is to help the workers perform more efficiently at high altitudes, some small nutritional benefit may be obtained from chewing coca leaves.

There is some dispute as to whether the stimulant effect of chewing coca leaves is addictive. Jaffe (1990, 1995b) noted that the mountain dwellers of Peru who chew cocaine on a regular basis "appear to have little difficulty in discontinuing use of the drug when they move to lower altitudes" (1990, p. 541). This may be because chewing the leaves is a rather inefficient method of abusing cocaine, according to the author. The individuals in this study who chewed cocaine were not thought to have obtained a significant level of the drug in the blood, according to Jaffe.

Karch (1996) reported that, at most, the blood level of cocaine that users achieve from chewing coca leaves scarcely enters the lower range of blood levels achieved by those who snort cocaine and therefore is barely enough to have a psychoactive effect. Thus, the question of whether natives who chew coca leaves are addicted to the cocaine they absorb has not been answered.

What *is* clear is that the reason coca plants are grown in South America has changed in the past few decades. Since cocaine became a popular drug of abuse in the 1970s, most of the Erythroxylon coca plants in South America have been grown for the international cocaine trade (Mann, 1994). Only a small minority of the coca bushes are cultivated for native use or, since the introduction of synthetic agents like Novocain, to meet the needs of medicine.

Cocaine in Recent U.S. History

Although cocaine had been in use for thousands of years in South America, the active agent of cocaine was only isolated in 1859,[1] by Albert Neiman (Scaros, Westra, & Barone, 1990). Following the isolation of the drug, European researchers began to concentrate large amounts of relatively pure cocaine for human use. The extracts from the coca leaf were used to make a wide range of popular drinks, wines, and elixirs (Martensen, 1996). For example, in response to the decision by the city of Atlanta to prohibit the use of alcohol, John Stith-Pemberton developed a new product that he thought would serve as a "temperance drink" (Martensen, 1996, p. 1615). In time, the world would come to know Stith-Pemberton's product by another name: "Coca-Cola."

The newly developed hypodermic needle made it possible to introduce cocaine directly into the bloodstream for the first time, and physicians began to experiment with the new drug to determine its uses. No less a figure than Sigmund Freud experimented with cocaine, at first thinking it might be a cure for depression[2] (Rome, 1984) and, later, a possible "cure" for narcotic withdrawal symptoms (Byck, 1987; Lingeman, 1974). However, when Freud discovered

the drug's previously unsuspected addictive potential, he discontinued his research on cocaine.

In the late 1800s and early 1900s, cocaine, like most medicines, was easily available without a prescription and was used in a wide variety of products and medicines. All too often, the presence of cocaine in the mixture was not mentioned on the labels of patent medicines. This factor contributed to the epidemics of cocaine abuse that developed in Europe between 1886 and 1891, in both Europe and the United States between 1894 and 1899, and again in the United States between 1921 and 1929. These waves of cocaine abuse/addiction and the use of cocaine in so many patent medicines, along with fears that it had narcotic qualities and was corrupting Southern blacks, prompted the passage of the Pure Food and Drug Act of 1906 (Mann, 1994) and the classification of cocaine as a narcotic in 1914 (Martensen, 1996).

The Pure Food and Drug Act of 1906 required makers to list the ingredients of a patent medicine or elixir on the label. As a result of this law, cocaine was removed from many patent medicines. With the passage of the Harrison Narcotics Act of 1914, nonmedical cocaine use in the United States was prohibited (Derlet, 1989). This, combined with the isolation of the United States in World War I and World War II, and the introduction of the amphetamines in the 1930s, served to virtually eliminate cocaine use in this country. It did not resurface as a major drug of abuse in the United States until the late 1960s. By then, cocaine had the reputation of being the "champagne of drugs" (P. White, 1989, p. 34) for those who could afford it. Those who could not afford it were interested in learning more about this "wonder drug," and cocaine again became popular as a recreational stimulant.

There were many reasons for cocaine's rising popularity in the late 1960s. First, cocaine had been all but forgotten since the Harrison Narcotics Act of 1914. Physicians either were unaware of or dismissed as "moralistic exaggerations" the bitter lessons about cocaine's dangers that had been learned in the late 1800s and early 1900s (Gawin & Ellinwood, 1988, p. 1173).

Second, during the late 1960s, there was a growing disillusionment with the amphetamines as

---

[1] Schuckit (1995) reported that cocaine was isolated in 1857, rather than 1859.

[2] Surprisingly, recent research (Post, Weiss, Pert, & Uhde, 1987) has cast doubt on the antidepressant properties of cocaine.

recreational drugs. The amphetamines had acquired a reputation as known killers. Drug users would warn each other that "speed kills," a reference to the many hazards of taking amphetamines. Cocaine had the reputation of safely bringing about many of the same sensations produced by amphetamine use. Further, as noted, the addictive potential of cocaine had been forgotten (Gawin & Ellinwood, 1988). Users viewed it as a "nonaddicting" substitute for the amphetamines, and it acquired a mystique as a special, glamorous drug. In addition, government restrictions on amphetamine production by legitimate pharmaceutical companies helped focus attention on cocaine as a recreational drug in the late 1960s.

Cocaine became increasingly popular in the 1970s and the first half of the 1980s, both in the United States and elsewhere around the world. Although we tend to overlook drug use trends outside the United States, the truth is that cocaine use was on the increase in other parts of the world long before it reached this country. By the mid-1970s, the practice of smoking coca paste was popular in parts of South America, but had only started to gain popularity in this country.

In the 1970s, cocaine dealers were eager to find new markets in the United States. It was well-known that cocaine "freebase," or "base" (discussed later in this chapter), provided an intense sense of euphoria, but this use required elaborate equipment that would provide only a small amount of base for smoking. ("The Men Who Created Crack," 1991). They came up with "crack," a form of cocaine that could be smoked without elaborate preparations, and it became popular in the 1980s.

Thus, in the United States, the process during the 1970s and early 1980s was the reverse of what had happened just a half century earlier. In the 1930s, cocaine was replaced by the amphetamines as the stimulant of choice. Just four decades later, cocaine replaced the amphetamines as the preferred CNS recreational stimulant. The popularity of cocaine as a drug of abuse appears to have peaked sometime around 1986, and casual cocaine use has continued to decline since then (Kleber, 1991). Cocaine has by no means disappeared, however, and it remains a significant part of the drug abuse problem in the United States.

Current Medical Uses of Cocaine

Cocaine is not just a drug of abuse. Although it is a potent central nervous system stimulant, it also functions as an effective local anesthetic. This property of cocaine was discovered approximately 100 years ago (Byck, 1987; Mann, 1994). Cocaine appears to function as a local anesthetic by blocking the nerve signals, or impulses, of the peripheral nerves. The application of cocaine at the proper point will change the electrical potential of these peripheral nerves, preventing them from passing on pain impulses to the brain.

Because of this effect, cocaine was once commonly used by physicians as a topical analgesic for procedures involving the ear, nose, throat, rectum, and the vagina. The onset of cocaine's action when used as a local analgesic is approximately 60 seconds, with a duration of effect as long as 2 hours (Shannon et al., 1995). Cocaine was also included in a mixture called Brompton's cocktail, which was used to control the pain of cancer. However, this mixture has fallen out of favor and is rarely, if ever, used today (Scaros et al., 1990).

As a pharmaceutical, cocaine's usefulness was limited by its often undesirable side effects. Physicians have found a number of other chemicals that offer the advantages of cocaine without its side effects or potential for abuse. Today, cocaine "has virtually no clinical use" (House, 1990, p. 41), although on rare occasions it is still used by physicians to control pain.

Scope of the Problem of Cocaine Abuse and Addiction

The United States is still the world's largest consumer of cocaine, an "honor" that this country has held for many years (Sabbag, 1994). The Washington-based research group Abt Associates, Inc. (1995a) advanced what they termed a "high-range estimate" (p. 3) of 340 *metric tons*[3] of pure cocaine being imported into the United States each year to

---

[3] A metric ton is equal to 1000 kilograms, or 2204.6 pounds. The figure of 340 metric tons would equal 374.78 standard tons, or 749,560 *pounds* of pure cocaine.

meet the demand of domestic users. The television news program *60 Minutes* (1997a), citing data released by the Drug Enforcement Administration (DEA), reported that 1000 to 1200 tons of cocaine are smuggled into the United States each year. The average sample of cocaine purchased on the street through illicit sources is approximately 61% pure ("South American Drug," 1997). To obtain this cocaine, users in the United States spend an estimated $90 billion (Abt Associates, Inc., 1995a) to $100 billion (Will, 1993) each year.

One would expect that since casual cocaine abuse in the United States peaked in the mid-1980s, the total amount of cocaine used in this country would have declined since then. Surprisingly, however, the amount of cocaine consumed each year in the United States has remained at about the mid-1980 level (Abt Associates, Inc., 1995a; Gold & Palumbo, 1991). This apparent contradiction is explained by the fact that while there are fewer casual cocaine users, there has been an increase in the number of heavy users. This theory is consistent with the data uncovered by Cornish et al. (1995), who found that the number of regular cocaine users (individuals who used cocaine at least once a week) increased from 647,000 in 1985, to 855,000 just a decade later.

Estimates vary as to the scope of cocaine abuse and addiction. The Office of National Drug Abuse Policy (1996) reported that two-thirds of the cocaine consumed in the United States was used by just 25% of those who use it. This suggests that there is a small group of heavy cocaine users and a larger group of casual users. It is estimated that between 23 and 24 million people in the United States have used cocaine at least once (Hollander, Hoffman, Burnstein, Shih, & Thode, 1995; O'Brien, 1996). Estimates of the number of people who use cocaine as often as once a month in the United States range from 1.5 million (Nash & Park, 1997) to 5 million (Hollander et al., 1997). Jaffe (1995b) offered a different estimate of 3 million Americans who use cocaine less than once a month, 800,000 people who use cocaine at least once a month, and 500,000 who use cocaine at least once a week. This estimate was in addition to the estimated 500,000 crack cocaine users, according to the author.

The team of Haverkos and Stein (1995) suggested that 2 million people use cocaine in the United States, of which 600,000 use the drug at least once a week, and 300,000 use it daily. Abt Associates, Inc. (1995a), suggested that there were between 1.5 and 2.5 million "hardcore" (p. 15) cocaine users, but did not define their use of the term. The amount of cocaine consumed by each user varies. For example, hard-core cocaine users in the United States are thought to have spent $23.3 billion on cocaine in 1993, while occasional users spent $7.5 billion (Abt Associates, Inc., 1995a).

Since there is no clear picture as to the true scope of cocaine abuse in this country, about all that researchers agree on is that casual use seems to have peaked in the mid-1980s and has been declining ever since. But, as these figures suggest, cocaine remains a significant part of the drug abuse problem in the United States.

Pharmacology of Cocaine

Cocaine hydrochloride is a water-soluble drug that quickly diffuses into the general circulation after entering the body. From the bloodstream, it is rapidly transported to the brain and other blood-rich organs such as the heart. Despite its rapid distribution, the level of cocaine varies from one organ to another. For example, because it easily crosses the blood-brain barrier (see Chapter 3), the level of cocaine in the brain is usually higher than it is in the blood plasma, especially in the first 2 hours following use of the drug ("Cocaine in the Brain," 1994).

The effects of cocaine on the central nervous system are not well understood (Hollander, 1995). Researchers have identified at least five different subtypes of receptors in the brain that react to the neurotransmitter *dopamine*. One of these dopamine receptor sites, which scientists call the dopamine D_3 receptor site, seems to be where cocaine causes at least some of its CNS effects. On the basis of their work with rats, Caine and Koob (1993) found that the dopamine D_3 receptor site was activated by cocaine. When the authors administered a drug that selectively blocked the dopamine D_3 receptor site to the rat, the animal's use of cocaine dropped significantly. Indeed, when the authors experimented with compounds that were very selective, which is to say that the compounds would block *only* the dopamine D_3 receptor site, the animal's use of cocaine would decrease more than when they used a drug that blocked two or more of the subtypes of dopamine receptors.

It is of interest to note that, in the rat's brain, the dopamine D_3 receptors are concentrated in the so-called limbic system, especially those regions of the rat brain associated with emotional, cognitive, and endocrine functions (Caine & Koob, 1993). When human cocaine users were examined using the positron emission tomographic (PET) scan, researchers discovered that cocaine molecules tend to bind most strongly to the dopamine-rich regions of the brain known as the *basal ganglia* (Nutt, 1996). In some unknown manner, cocaine is then able to stimulate the so-called pleasure center located in the mesolimbic and mesocortical regions of the limbic system of the brain (Jaffe, 1995b).

Some researchers believe that cocaine seems to cause a massive discharge of the neurotransmitter dopamine along the nerve pathways that connect the ventral tegmentum region of the brain with the nucleus accumbens (Beitner-Johnson & Nestler, 1992; Restak, 1994). But cocaine does not just cause the release of dopamine. It also blocks a process known as *reabsorption* or *reuptake* (Leshner, 1996). Neurotransmitter reuptake is a method by which the individual neuron deactivates a neurotransmitter once it has been released. Normally, the process of neurotransmitter release and reabsorption results in a pattern of "on-off" firing of the neurons along the nerve pathway. But, as stated, once the dopamine supplies have been released, cocaine blocks their reabsorption; it also blocks the reabsorption of the neurotransmitters noradrenaline and serotonin in the brain (Henry, 1996).

Thus, cocaine is able to cause a biphasic response by the neurons in the brain of the user. First, the neurons in the ventral tegmentum region release their stores of dopamine in response to the arrival of cocaine. Then, cocaine blocks the reabsorption of the dopamine after it has been released. Through this mechanism, cocaine is thought to "flood" the nerve pathways in the nucleus accumbens, which helps to generate our pleasure response by sending chemical messages to the pleasure center of the brain.

Another of the brain subunits affected by cocaine is the *diencephalon*, which is the region of the brain responsible for temperature regulation. This results in a higher than normal body temperature for the user. At the same time that cocaine is altering the brain's temperature regulation system, it also causes the constriction of surface blood vessels. This combination of effects results in hyperthermia: excess body heat. The individual's body will conserve body heat at just the time when it needs to release the excess thermal energy caused by the cocaine-induced dysregulation of body temperature. This is the mechanism through which cocaine-induced hyperthermia can prove dangerous, or even fatal, to the user (Hall, Talbert, & Ereshefsky, 1990).

After periods of chronic abuse, the neurons within the brain will have released virtually all their stores of the neurotransmitter dopamine. Low dopamine levels are thought to be involved in the development of depressive disorders. Thus, pharmacologically, chronic cocaine use may induce a state of depression by depleting the dopamine levels in the brain. Further, tolerance to cocaine's euphoric effect may develop within "hours or days" (Schuckit, 1995a, p. 122). As tolerance develops, the individual requires more and more cocaine to achieve the same euphoric effect initially experienced at a lower dosage level. This urge to increase the dosage and continue using the drug can reach the point where it "may become a way of life and users become totally preoccupied with drug-seeking and drug taking behaviors" (R. K. Siegel, 1982, p. 731).

When used as a pharmaceutical, cocaine's effects are very short-lived. This is also true when cocaine is abused. For example, when cocaine is injected intravenously, the peak plasma levels are reached in just 5 minutes, and the effects begin to diminish after 20 to 40 minutes (Weddington, 1993). One reason the effects of intravenously administered cocaine are so short-lived is that the half-life of intravenously administered cocaine is only between 30 and 90 minutes (Jaffe, 1995b; Julien, 1992; Marzuk et al., 1995; Mendelson & Mello, 1996).

There are about a dozen known metabolites of cocaine (Karch, 1996). About 90% to 95% of a dose of intravenously administered cocaine is biotransformed into one of two different metabolites: *benzoylecgonine* (BEG) and *ecogonine methyl ester* (Cone, 1993; Kerfoot, Sakoulas, & Hyman, 1996). The other metabolites are of minor importance and need not be considered further in this text. Only about 5% to 10% of a single dose of cocaine is excreted from the body unchanged. Neither of these metabolites has any known biological activity in the body. BEG has a half-life of 7.5 hours (Marzuk et al., 1995). Because the half-life of BEG is longer than that of the parent compound and it is stable in frozen urine, this is the chemical that laboratories usually test for when they test a urine sample for evidence of cocaine use.

Surprisingly, cocaine will "autometabolize" (i.e., the body will continue to biotransform the cocaine in the blood after the user has died). Thus, a postmortem blood sample might not reveal any measurable amount of cocaine in the blood, even if the user was known to have used cocaine prior to death.

Drug Interactions Involving Cocaine

Cocaine is a potent chemical, and thus has the potential to interact with a wide range of both pharmaceuticals and illicit drugs. For example, when a person uses both cocaine and alcohol, some of the cocaine is biotransformed into a metabolite known as *cocaethylene* (Karch, 1996). Cocaethylene is toxic to the body and has a longer half-life than that of cocaine itself. Because it functions as a powerful calcium channel blocker, cocaethylene might exacerbate the cardiovascular side effects of cocaine (discussed later in this chapter) (Barnhill et al., 1995; Karch, 1996; Mendelson & Mello, 1996).

Barnhill et al. (1995) discussed a number of isolated cases in which a person abusing cocaine had also ingested alcohol, only to die of a condition known as *pulmonary edema* a little later. Unfortunately, cocaethylene may lengthen the cocaine-induced euphoria, making it more likely that the person will combine these two chemicals in the future despite the increased cardiovascular risk.

Some abusers inject a combination of cocaine and an opiate, a process known as "speedballing." However, for reasons that are not well understood, cocaine actually enhances the respiratory depressive effect of the opiates, possibly resulting in episodes of respiratory arrest in extreme cases (Kerfoot et al., 1996). As discussed later in this chapter, cocaine abuse often results in a feeling of irritation, or anxiety. To control the agitation and anxiety that are often side effects of cocaine use, it is often used in conjunction with alcohol, tranquilizers, or marijuana. The combination of marijuana and cocaine appears capable of increasing the heart rate by almost 50 beats per minute in individuals using both substances (Barnhill et al., 1995).

There is a case report of a patient who was abusing cocaine, who took an over-the-counter cold medication that contained phenylpropanolamine. This person developed what seems to have been a drug-induced psychosis that included homicidal thoughts (Barnhill et al., 1995). It is not clear whether this is an isolated incident, or, if the interaction between cocaine and phenylpropanolamine can precipitate a psychotic reaction, but the concurrent use of these chemicals is not recommended.

How Illicit Cocaine Is Produced

Byrne (1989b) outlined the steps involved in producing cocaine for sale on the streets in the United States. First, the cocaine leaves are harvested. In some parts of Bolivia, this may be done as often as once every three months, as the climate is well suited for the plant's growth. Second, the leaves are dried, usually by letting them sit in the open sunlight for a few hours or days. Byrne reported that, although technically illegal, cocaine is openly set out to dry in some parts of Bolivia.

In the third step of production, the dried leaves are put in a plastic-lined pit, and mixed with water and sulfuric acid (White, 1989). The mixture is crushed by workers who wade into the pit in their bare feet. After the mixture has been crushed, diesel fuel and bicarbonate are added to the mixture. After a period of time, during which workers reenter the pit several times to continue to stomp through the mixture, the liquids are drained off. Lime is then mixed with the residue, forming a paste (Byrne, 1989b) which is cocaine base. It takes 500 kilograms of leaves to produce one kilogram of cocaine base (P. White, 1989).

The fourth step involves adding water, gasoline, acid, potassium permanganate, and ammonia to the cocaine paste obtained in the previous step. This forms a reddish brown liquid, which is then filtered. A few drops of ammonia are added to the mixture producing a milky solid that is filtered and dried. The fifth step begins when the dried cocaine base is dissolved in a solution of hydrochloric acid and acetone. A white solid forms, which settles to the bottom of the tank (Byrne,1989b; P. White, 1989). This solid material is the compound cocaine hydrochloride.

In the sixth step, the cocaine is filtered and dried under heating lights. This will cause the mixture to form a white, crystalline powder. This is gathered up, packed, and shipped, usually in kilogram packages (there are 2.2046 pounds in a kilogram). Before each kilogram is repackaged for sale on the street, it is diluted either with mannitol or local anesthetics such as lidocaine (Byrne, 1989b). The cocaine is then packaged in 1-gram units, and sold to individual users. For more information about how street drugs are adulterated, see Chapter 34.

How Cocaine Is Abused

Cocaine may be used in several ways. First, cocaine hydrocloride powder may be inhaled through the nose ("intranasal" use, or "snorting"). Second, it may be injected directly into a vein (an "intravenous" injection). Cocaine hydrochloride is a water-soluble form of cocaine well adapted to either intranasal or intravenous use (Sbriglio & Millman, 1987). Third, cocaine "base" may be smoked. Fourth, cocaine may be used orally ("sublingual"). We will examine each of these methods of cocaine abuse in detail.

Intranasal Cocaine Abuse

Historical evidence suggests that the practice of snorting cocaine began around 1903, which is the year that case reports of septal perforation began to appear in medical journals (Karch, 1996). Snorting cocaine powder is currently the most common method of cocaine abuse. Between 77 and 95% of those individuals who abuse cocaine snort it, that is, use the drug intranasally (L. Boyd, 1995; Hatsukami & Fischman, 1996). To snort it, cocaine powder is usually arranged on a piece of glass, in

thin lines 3–5 cm long. Each "line" contains 25–100 mg of cocaine (Karch, 1996; Strang, Johns, & Caan, 1993). The powder is diced up, usually with a razor blade, on the piece of glass or mirror, to make the particles as small as possible. The powder is then inhaled through a drinking straw, or rolled paper.

When it reaches the nasal passages, which are richly supplied with blood vessels, the cocaine is quickly absorbed. This allows some of the cocaine to gain rapid access to the bloodstream, usually in 30 to 90 seconds (House, 1990), where it is carried to the brain. The peak effects of snorted cocaine are reached within 10 minutes, and the effects wear off in about 45 to 60 minutes (Strang et al., 1993; Weiss, Greenfield, & Mirin, 1994).

Because cocaine functions as a vasoconstrictor, scientists question whether it might not limit its own absorption when it is snorted. For example, the team of Strang et al. (1993) concluded that when it is used intranasally, only 5% of the cocaine is actually absorbed. The authors suggested that the cocaine reduced the blood flow to the nasal tissues it came in contact with, limiting its absorption. In contrast to this estimate, Hatsukami and Fischman (1996) estimated that between 25 and 94% of a 32-milligram dose of cocaine would be absorbed when snorted. The authors also suggested that the actual amount of cocaine absorbed varies as a result of the total dose, with higher doses having greater absorption rates. Karch (1996) took a middle-of-the-road position on this issue, suggesting that because of its vasoconstrictive effect, it takes longer for cocaine to be absorbed when it is snorted. Thus the question of whether intranasally administered cocaine might limit its own absorption has not been fully answered.

Intravenous Cocaine Abuse

It is possible to introduce cocaine directly into the body through intravenous injection. Cocaine hydrochloride powder is mixed with water, then injected into a vein. This is the least common method of using cocaine; only 7% of those individuals who abuse cocaine inject it (Hatsukami & Fischman, 1996). Intravenously administered cocaine will reach the brain in just 3 to 5 seconds according to Restak (1994) and 15 to 20 seconds according to R. T. Jones

(1987). Intravenous administration of cocaine results in 20 times more drug reaching the brain as through intranasal cocaine use (Strang et al., 1993).

Intravenous cocaine abusers have often reported a rapid, intense feeling of euphoria called the "rush" or "flash," which is similar to a sexual orgasm. Following the rush, the user will experience a feeling of euphoria that lasts 10 to 15 minutes. Intravenously administered cocaine is biotransformed quickly, which is one reason its effects last only about 15 minutes (Weiss et al., 1994).

Sublingual Cocaine Use

This form of cocaine abuse is becoming increasingly popular, especially when the hydrochloride salt of cocaine is utilized (R. T. Jones, 1987). The tissues in the mouth, especially under the tongue, are richly supplied with blood, allowing large amounts of the drug to enter the bloodstream quickly. After reaching the brain, the cocaine is transported to the brain, with results similar to those seen in the intranasal administration of cocaine.

Cocaine Smoking

Especially since the introduction of crack, the practice of smoking cocaine has arguably become the most widely recognized method of cocaine abuse. However, researchers believe that only about 36% of cocaine users in the United States actually smoke the drug (Hatsukami & Fischman, 1996).

The practice of burning or smoking different parts of the coca plant dates back to at least 3000 B.C., when the Incas would burn coca leaves at religious festivals (R. K. Siegel, 1982). The practice of smoking cocaine resurfaced in the late 1800s, when coca cigarettes were used to treat hay fever and opiate addiction. By the year 1890, cocaine smoke was being used in the United States for the treatment of whooping cough, bronchitis, asthma, and other conditions (R. K. Siegel, 1982).

However, smoking cocaine for recreational purposes is apparently a relatively new phenomenon. This is because it is not possible to smoke cocaine hydrochloride, the most popular form of cocaine. The high temperatures needed to vaporize cocaine hydrochloride also destroy it, making it of limited value to those who want to smoke it.

Cocaine abusers had long known that it is possible to smoke the alkaloid base of cocaine, but transforming cocaine hydrochloride into the alkaloid base was a long, dangerous process. First, cocaine powder had to be mixed with a solvent such as ether, and a base such as ammonia (Warner, 1995). The cocaine will then form an alkaloid base that can be smoked. This form of cocaine is called "freebase" (or, simply, "base"). Then the precipitated cocaine freebase is passed through a filter, which effectively increases the concentration of the obtained powder. But this process of filtration does not remove all of the impurities from the original sample of cocaine (R. K. Siegel, 1982). Some of the impurities found in the original cocaine will still remain in the alkaloid base.

When the cocaine powder obtained through this process is smoked, the cocaine "freebase" powder vaporizes, and the person can inhale the fumes. This process allows the cocaine to reach the brain in just 7 *seconds* (Beebe & Walley, 1991). When cocaine is smoked, between 60 and 90% of the cocaine crosses over into the general circulation from the lungs (Beebe & Walley, 1991; Hatsukami & Fischman, 1996). Thus, when cocaine is smoked, a high concentration of the chemical quickly reaches the general circulation. So potent are the effects of smoked cocaine that Gold and Verebey (1984) called it "tantamount to intravenous administration without the need for a syringe" (p. 714). Indeed, there is evidence that when cocaine is smoked, it reaches the brain more quickly than when it is injected (Hatsukami & Fischman, 1996).

The process of preparing cocaine freebase is long, dangerous, and complicated. The chemicals used to separate cocaine freebase from its hydrochloride salt are volitile, and there is a danger of explosion. As a result, smoking cocaine freebase never became popular in the United States. In the early 1980s, a new form of cocaine known as "crack" began to appear on the streets. Crack is a solid chunk of cocaine base that has been prepared for smoking. Unlike cocaine freebase, however, crack is prepared for smoking before reaching the user. Cocaine hydrochloride is mixed with baking soda and water in illicit factories or laboratories, then heated until the cocaine crystals begin to precipitate at the bottom of the container (Warner, 1995). Breslin (1988) provided an insight into how one crack factory worked:

> Curtis and his girlfriend dropped the cocaine and baking soda into the water, then hit the bottle with the blowtorch. The cocaine powder boiled down to its oily base. The baking soda soaked up the impurities in the cocaine. When cold water was added to the bottle, the cocaine base hardened into white balls. Curtis and Iris spooned them out, placed them on a table covered with paper, and began to measure the hard white cocaine. (p. 212)

The crack produced is sold in small, ready-to-use pellets, usually in containers that allow the user one or two inhalations for a relatively low price (Beebe & Walley, 1991; Gawin, Allen & Humblestone, 1989). For example, the price of one piece of crack, known as a "rock," is as low as two dollars in some parts of the country ("Feds Say Heroin," 1994). The low cost of crack is one reason it is so attractive to the under-eighteen crowd and in low-income neighborhoods. (Bales, 1988; Taylor & Gold, 1990)

In 1996, substance abuse rehabilitation professionals noted a disturbing new trend among some crack users in both England and isolated cities of the United States. In these areas, limited numbers of users were dissolving the pellets of crack in alcohol, lemon juice, vinegar, or water, and then injecting it into their bodies through large-bore needles ("Crack Injection," 1996). Apparently, intravenous-cocaine abusers were resorting to this practice when their traditional sources of cocaine hydrochloride were unable to provide them with the powder for injection. It is not known how popular this practice will become, but it represents a distressing new twist to the ongoing saga of cocaine abuse and addiction.

Over the years, a class distinction has evolved in terms of the *form* of cocaine being abused by different people. Cocaine hydrochloride, which is most often sold as a *powder* is thought to be abused mainly by middle-class users, whereas *crack* is found most often in the ghetto areas, according to some rehabilitation counselors. Federal sentencing guidelines require that a first-time offender with 5 grams of crack be sentenced to prison for 5 years, while a first-time offender needs to possess 500 grams of cocaine hydrochloride to be sentenced to 5 years in prison

(Hatsukami & Fischman, 1996). This legal distinction between cocaine hydrochloride and crack, has resulted in 22 times as many African Americans as whites being convicted and sentenced for possession of cocaine (Hatsukami & Fischman). The distinction between cocaine hydrochloride and cocaine freebase is a legal one and is not based on the pharmacological effects of these different forms of the same chemical (Hatsukami & Fischman).

Subjective Effects of Cocaine When It Is Abused

As with many drugs of abuse, two factors influence the individual's subjective experience from cocaine. First, the individual's *expectancies* for cocaine play a role in how the user interprets the drug's effects. Second, there are the actual physiological effects of the drug. These two factors interact to shape the individual's experience from cocaine, and, how it is abused.

Schafer and Brown (1991) found that experienced cocaine users anticipate both positive (e.g., euphoria) and negative (e.g., depression) effects from cocaine. Further, experienced cocaine users expect (a) a generalized feeling of arousal as a result of their cocaine use, (b) some feelings of anxiety, and (c) feelings of relaxation and a reduction in tension.

When cocaine is smoked, or injected, the user might experience a feeling of intense euphoria called the "rush" or "flash" (Jaffe, 1995b). This feeling bursts on the user in just seven seconds when cocaine is injected or smoked. The rush has been compared with the sexual orgasm in intensity and pleasure by at least some cocaine users who state that "it alone can replace the sex partner of either sex" (Gold & Verebey, 1984, p. 719). Some male users have reported having a spontaneous ejaculation without direct genital stimulation after either injecting or smoking cocaine. There also appears to be a link between chronic cocaine use and compulsive acting-out behavior for both men and women (Washton, 1995).

The speed with which cocaine activates the brain's reward system when it is injected or smoked makes it a powerful reinforcer. Further, the intensity of the drug's effects also make it a powerful reinforcer. Within seconds of injecting or smoking cocaine, the initial rush is replaced by a period of excitation or euphoria that lasts for between 10 (Strang et al., 1993) and 20 minutes (Weiss et al., 1994). During this period, the individual will feel an increased sense of competence, energy (Gold & Verebey, 1984), or extreme self-confidence (Taylor & Gold, 1990). Some users of cocaine feel powerful, "energized." While there is no objective evidence that a person under the effects of cocaine actually is stronger, the user is likely to *feel* more powerful because of the effects of cocaine on the nervous system, (Schuckit, 1995). This is one of the positive effects that experienced cocaine users anticipate.

The experience of snorting cocaine powder is less intense than smoking or injecting it. Still, intranasal use of cocaine results in a sense of euphoria and well-being. This euphoria may last only a few minutes for the individual who smokes cocaine (Byck, 1987), to an estimated 20 minutes to an hour for the individual who snorts cocaine powder; then the effects begin to wane. To regain the drug-induced pleasure, the user must again use cocaine.

Tolerance to the euphoric effects of cocaine develops quickly. To overcome their tolerance, many users have been known to engage in a cycle of continuous cocaine use known as "coke runs." The usual cocaine run lasts about 12 hours, although there have been cases where they have lasted up to 7 days (Gawin, Khalsa, & Ellinwood, 1994). During this time, the user is smoking or injecting additional cocaine every few minutes, until the total cumulative dose may reach levels that would kill the inexperienced (i.e., "cocaine-naive") user. This is a similar pattern to that seen when animals are given unlimited access to cocaine. Animal research has demonstrated that rats who are given intravenous cocaine for pushing a bar set in the wall of their cage will do so repeatedly, ignoring food or even sex, until they die from convulsions or infection (Hall et al., 1990).

Complications of Cocaine Abuse/Addiction

Cocaine has the distinction of being the illicit drug that causes the most visits to hospital emergency rooms (Shih & Hollander, 1996). Cocaine abuse is potentially fatal, and in some cases death occurs so rapidly that "the victim never receives medical attention other than from the coroner" (Estroff, 1987, p. 25). In addition, cocaine abuse can cause a wide range of other problems including addiction; respiratory dysfunction; damage to the cardiovascular system, liver, and central nervous system; emotional disorders, and traumatic injury or death.

Addiction

In the 1960s and early 1970s, there were those who believed that cocaine was not addictive. The belief that cocaine was not addictive was fueled by the observation that few users in the late 1960s could afford enough cocaine to allow them to use it long enough to become addicted. But, as has been discussed, cocaine has a potential to cause physical and psychological addiction.[4]

Physical dependence on cocaine does not develop instantly. Depending on the method by which the individual uses the drug, there appears to be a difference in the speed with which cocaine addiction will develop. Individuals who snort cocaine may take as along as 3 to 4 years to become fully addicted to the drug (Lamar, Riley, & Staghabadi, 1986), while those who smoke crack can be fully addicted in only 6 to 10 *weeks*.

There also appears to be a progression in the methods by which cocaine abusers utilize the drug, as their addiction to cocaine grows in intensity. As the user's need for the drug becomes more intense, he/she switches from the intranasal method of cocaine use, to those methods that introduce greater concentrations of the drug into the body. For example, 79% to 90% of those who admitted to the use of crack cocaine started to use the drug intranasally (Hatsukami & Fischman, 1996).

Respiratory System Dysfunctions

The cocaine user who smokes the drug may experience chest pain, cough, and damage to the bronchioles of the lungs (O'Connor, Chang, & Shi, 1992). There have been reports that, in some cases, the alveloli of the user's lungs have ruptured, allowing

[4]While it is true that not everybody who uses cocaine becomes addicted, it is not possible to determine at this time *who* will become addicted when experimenting with this drug. If only for this reason, cocaine abuse should be discouraged.

the escape of air (and bacteria) into the surrounding tissues. This will establish the potential for infection to develop, while the escaping gas may contribute to the inability of the lung to fully inflate (a "pneumothorax"). Other complications of cocaine smoking include the development of an asthmalike condition, chronic bronchiolitis (also known as "crack lung"), pulmonary hemorrhage, and chronic inflammation of the throat (Albertson et al., 1995; House, 1990; Taylor & Gold, 1990). There is evidence suggesting that cocaine-induced lung damage may be irreversible.

There is also evidence that at least some of the observed increase in fatal asthma cases may be caused by unsuspected cocaine abuse ("Asthma Deaths," 1997). While cocaine abuse may not be the cause of all asthma-induced deaths, it may induce asthma attacks in at least some individuals, and these asthma attacks may prove to be fatal.

The chronic intranasal use of cocaine can result in sore throats, inflamed sinuses, hoarseness, and, on occasion, a breakdown of the cartilage of the nose. Damage to the cartilage of the nose may develop after as little as three weeks' intranasal cocaine use (O'Connor et al., 1992). Other medical problems caused by intranasal cocaine use include bleeding from the nasal passages and the formation of ulcers in the nasal passages, according to the authors.

Cardiovascular System Damage

Researchers have known for some time that cocaine can damage the heart and cardiovascular system. Cocaine use can result in severe hypertension, sudden dissection of the coronary arteries, sudden death, tachycardia, cardiac ischemia, angina pectoris, pericardial chest pain, and myocarditis (Albertson et al., 1995; Brent, 1995; Decker, Fins, & Frances, 1987; Derlet, 1989; Derlet & Horowitz, 1995; Hollander, 1995; Jaffe, 1990; O'Connor et al., 1992). In addition, cocaine abuse can cause, or at least speed up, the development of atherosclerotic plaques in the user (Hollander et al., 1997).

At one time, researchers believed that cocaine abuse could cause increased platelet aggregation, that is, somehow cause the user's blood cells to form clots more easily. Such a side effect of cocaine would account for reports that cocaine abusers were at risk for many of the cardiovascular problems noted in the previous paragraph. In 1996, this theory was tested by the team of Heesch et al. The authors used a sample of 12 men, who were nonsmokers and were not drug abusers. To control for possible confounding medication effects, the volunteers also did not use aspirin or any other medication for two weeks before participation in the study. At the end of this "washing out" period, each man received an intranasal dose either of 2 mg/kg of cocaine or a placebo, while the researchers monitored his blood chemistries. At a later time, the subjects received a second dose of either 2 mg/kg of cocaine or a placebo, so that each man received one dose of cocaine, and one placebo, in a random order. The team of Heesch et al. (1996) failed to find any evidence that cocaine was able to cause platelet aggregation.

Researchers *have* discovered that cocaine can increase the heart rate, while simultaneously decreasing the blood flow through the coronary arteries. The team of Moliterno et al. (1994) administered a 2mg/kg intranasal dose of cocaine to volunteers who had agreed to participate in their study. Although this dosage level of cocaine is smaller than that typically used on the street, the authors found a temporary 7% decrease in coronary artery diameter in the volunteers who had no known coronary artery disease. For those individuals with coronary artery disease, however, even this limited dose of cocaine resulted in a 9% reduction in coronary artery diameter for a period of time. When the coronary artery diameter is reduced, its ability to carry adequate levels of blood to the heart is also reduced.

The authors then administered the same dose of cocaine to volunteers who were cigarette smokers and who had known coronary artery disease. Their results suggest that, for this subgroup, the combined effects of the tobacco and cocaine resulted in a 19% reduction in coronary artery diameter. This is a significant decrease in diameter. The authors concluded that this might be one mechanism through which cocaine is able to cause damage to the heart of the user. In effect, the results of the study by Moliterno et al. (1994) suggest that cocaine causes a reduction in the supply of blood to the heart muscle, at the very time when the cocaine is also causing an increase in the performance demand on this same muscle tissue.

In theory, the outcome of this process, even in individuals with no known coronary artery disease, is that the heart muscle is unable to obtain an adequate supply of blood. This condition is known as *myocardial ischemia*, and, if not corrected, holds the potential to damage the heart muscle. Research has shown that cocaine-induced myocardial ischemia may develop up to 18 hours after the individual's last use of cocaine (Kerfoot et al., 1996). In a medical setting, drugs known as beta-adrenergic antagonists are often used to treat myocardial ischemia. But these drugs contribute to cocaine-induced constriction of blood vessels, placing the patient's life at added risk (Shih & Hollander, 1996). Thus, it is imperative that the physician be informed whether the patient being treated for a possible myocardial ischemia has recently used cocaine.

Scientists have long known that cocaine can interfere with the ability of the heart to regulate its own rhythm (an "arrhythmia"), a condition that may prove fatal to the user. However, researchers have not identified the exact mechanism by which cocaine causes cardiac arrhythmias. One theory is that cocaine impacts cardiac function through its ability to alter the release of one or more members of the *catecholamine* family of chemicals. The catecholamine family of chemicals includes epinephrine, which is a chemical normally produced in the adrenal glands. In the body, epinephrine functions as a vasoconstrictor. Other members of the catecholamine family include the neurotransmitters norepinephrine and dopamine. There is evidence that the chronic use of cocaine will interfere with the normal production and utilization of the catecholamines in the body (Beitner-Johnson & Nestler, 1992). In addition to being a neurotransmitter in the brain, norepinephrine is also found in the heart tissue. Beitner-Johnson and Nestler (1992) suggested on the basis of their research that cocaine might block the normal function of norepinephrine in the heart, causing the individual's death.

A variation of the catecholamine hypothesis suggested by Beitner-Johnson and Nestler (1992) was advanced by the *Forensic Drug Abuse Advisor* ("How Cocaine Causes," 1994). According to this journal, the chronic use of cocaine causes increased levels of norepinephrine in the blood. Over time, the above-normal norepinephrine levels place an increased workload on the heart, especially the left ventricle. Eventually, the heart weakens, and becomes enlarged. Such enlargement of the heart is a known risk factor for sudden death, even for individuals who do not use cocaine. In this manner, the chronic use of cocaine is thought to contribute to the risk of sudden death for the user.

Thus, although researchers are still not sure about the exact mechanism, there is little doubt that cocaine use is often associated with a number of cardiac problems. As if this list were not frightening enough, some scientists believe that in addition to the massive damage seen in a major heart attack, cocaine abuse might also cause "microinfarcts," or microscopic areas of damage to the heart muscle (Gawin et al., 1994). These microinfarcts ultimately reduce the heart's ability to function effectively and may lead to further heart problems later on. Further, there is evidence that the former cocaine user may experience "silent" episodes of cardiac ischemia while going through withdrawal from this drug of abuse (Kerfoot et al., 1996).

As these research studies suggest, the problem of cocaine-induced heart problems is not a minor one. At one point, it was thought that only a small percentage of the patients with chest pain who seek admission to hospital emergency treatment centers were there because of cocaine-induced angina. But the team of Hollander, Todd, et al. (1995) discovered that this belief is not always correct. On the basis of their research on a sample of 359 patients seen in urban or suburban hospitals for evaluation and treatment of chest pain, the authors concluded that fully 17% of the patients under the age of 60 seen in hospital emergency rooms for chest pain had cocaine metabolites in their urine. Further, 28% of the patients who had cocaine metabolites in their urine had denied its use. Since the treatment of cocaine-induced angina differs from the treatment of chest pain caused by other factors, the authors recommended that physicians routinely consider the possibility that patients seen for evaluation of chest pain may have used cocaine.

There does not seem to be any pattern to cocaine-induced cardiovascular problems, and both first-time users and long-term cocaine users have suffered heart attacks. In a hospital setting, between 56 and 84% of those patients with cocaine-induced

chest pain are found to have abnormal electrocar-
diograms (Hollander, 1995). Cocaine users who experience chest pain but do not seek medical help
may be ignoring symptoms of potentially fatal cocaine-related cardiac problems.

Another rare, but potentially fatal complication
of cocaine abuse is a condition known as *acute aortic dissection* (Brent, 1995). This condition, which is
occasionally seen in individuals other than cocaine
users, develops when the wall of the main artery of
the body, the aorta, suddenly develops a weak spot.
The exact mechanism by which cocaine can cause
an acute aortic dissection is not known, but it is a
medical emergency that may require surgical intervention to save the patient's life.

Peripheral Circulatory Problems

Male cocaine abusers run the risk of developing
erectile dysfunctions, including a painful, potentially
dangerous, condition known as priapism (Finger
et al., 1997). In contrast to the intravenous injection
of opiates, however, it is not common for intravenous
cocaine abusers to develop scar tissue at the injection
site. This is because the adulterants commonly found
in powdered cocaine are mainly water-soluble and
thus less irritating to the body than the adulterants
found in opiates (Karch, 1996).

Cocaine Abuse as a Cause of Liver Damage

There is evidence that cocaine metabolites, especially cocaethylene, are toxic to the liver (Karch,
1996). Medical research has also discovered that a
small percentage of the population simply cannot
biotransform cocaine, no matter how small the
dosage level used. In such cases, the liver is unable
to produce an essential enzyme necessary to break
down the cocaine, a condition known as *pseudo-
cholinesterase deficiency* (Gold, 1989b). For people
with this condition, the use of even a small amount
of cocaine could result in serious, if not fatal, complications.

Cocaine Abuse as a Cause of Central
Nervous System Damage

Although virtually nothing is known about the effects of either intentional or accidental cocaine
abuse by children (Mott, Packer, & Soldin, 1994),
the authors found evidence that cocaine abuse by
children might be the cause of seizures, possibly by
lowering the threshold for children predisposed to
seizures. Further, the authors found evidence of
neurological damage in almost half of the children
studied. The relationship between cocaine abuse
and seizures in children was so strong that the authors recommended that all children/adolescents
brought to the hospital for a previously undiagnosed
seizure disorder be tested for cocaine abuse.

Research has suggested that chronic use of cocaine might result in brain damage in adults. As
noted earlier, cocaine is a potent vasoconstrictor. The
vasoconstriction properties of cocaine is suspected to
be one mechanism by which cocaine can cause brain
damage (Pearlson et al., 1993). The authors used the
single photon emission computed tomography technique (or, SPECT), a new scanning device that allows scientists to study blood flow patterns in living
tissues. They documented evidence of altered blood
flow patterns within the frontal cortical and basal
ganglia regions of the brains of chronic cocaine users.

To uncover this evidence, the authors administered a 48-mg intravenous dose of cocaine to 8 volunteers, and then performed a SPECT analysis on
their subjects. They found that the frontal and basal
ganglia regions of the brain developed reduced blood
flow rates. Further, the authors found that the subjective experience of the rush or high was related to
the degree of blood flow reduction. In other words,
the greater the measured reduction in blood flow, the
better the drug use experience was rated by the individual. The authors could not determine whether
these blood flow pattern changes reflect temporary or
permanent changes in the vasculature of the brain,
or, the degree to which changes in blood flow patterns result in physical changes in the brain's structure. However, the possibility exists that this might be
one mechanism through which chronic cocaine use
causes neurological dysfunctions.

One very rare complication of cocaine use is the
drug-induced neurological condition known as the
serotonin syndrome (Mills, 1995). Although rare, approximately 11% of those patients who develop the
serotonin syndrome die, despite the best medical
care. Some of the symptoms of the serotonin syndrome include irritability, confusion, an increase in

anxiety, drowsiness, hyperthermia (increased body temperature), sinus tachycardia, dilation of the pupils, nausea, muscle rigidity, and seizures. Although the serotonin syndrome can develop as long as 24 hours after the patient ingests a medication that, affects the serotonin neurotransmitter system, in 50% of the cases in this study, the patient developed the syndrome within 2 hours of starting the medication (Mills). This condition constitutes a medical emergency that should be treated by a physician.

A number of studies have contrasted the test performance of chronic cocaine users against normal subjects on a series of psychoneurological tests. In one such study, O'Malley, Adamse, Heaton, and Gawin (1992) found that 50% of those who abused cocaine on a regular basis showed evidence of cognitive impairment on the test battery used in this study, compared with only 15% of the control subjects. The authors suggested that cocaine, when abused for a long time, might function as a neurotoxin. It was not clear whether this neurological impairment was permanent; however, studies have found that cocaine abuse seems to be the cause of neurological dysfunction.

Cocaine may cause brain damage in other ways. The vasoconstriction that is a side effect of cocaine use may result in elevated blood pressure. If the blood pressure rises to a high enough level, or if the person has a weak spot in the lining of a blood vessel, a "cerebrovascular accident" (also known as a "CVA," or "stroke") may result. This is the mechanism through which cocaine seems to cause strokes in both the brain, and the spinal cord (Derlet, 1989; Derlet & Horowitz, 1995; Jaffe, 1990; Mendoza & Miller, 1992). Depending on where the stroke occurs, it may kill the victim, result in blindness, or simply cause permanent neurological impairment.

Cocaine-induced strokes are not a consequence of only chronic cocaine abuse. The person using cocaine for the first time may have a cocaine-related stroke. Cocaine abusers may also experience transient ischemic attacks (TIAs), and seizures as an unwanted side effect of the drug use (Derlet, 1989; O'Connor et al., 1992). For reasons that are still not clear, cocaine-induced seizures may not occur until up to 12 hours after the last use of the drug, according to the authors.

Further, animal research has suggested that, after repeated exposures to cocaine, it is possible to develop seizures at a dose that previously had not brought on such convulsions. This process was termed a "pharmacological kindling" (Post et al., 1987). While cocaine itself might have a short half-life "the sensitization effects are long lasting" (p. 113). The authors believe that the sensitizing effects of cocaine might thus lower the seizure threshhold, at least in some individuals, and went on to observe:

> Repeated administration of a given dose of cocaine without resulting seizures *would in no way assure the continued safety of this drug even for that given individual* [italics added]. (p. 159)

Thus, while the *immediate effects* of cocaine might last only a short time, the body might become hypersensitive to cocaine for long periods of time. If this should happen, the person might suffer serious—possibly fatal—side effects from a dosage level of cocaine that was once easily tolerated.

The process of kindling would seem to be a side-effect of cocaine's effects on the region of the brain known as the *amygdala*. The amygdala is part of the temporal lobe of the brain, and is known to be vulnerable to the kindling phemonenon (M. Taylor, 1993). Thus, cocaine's effects on the amygdala can make this region of the brain hypersensitive, causing the user to experience cocaine-induced seizures even at dosage levels that he/she once easily tolerated.

Cocaine's Effects on the User's Emotional State and Perceptions

It has been suggested (Hamner, 1993) that cocaine abuse might exacerbate the symptoms of posttraumatic stress disorders (PTSD). The exact mechanism by which cocaine seems able to add to the emotional distress of PTSD is not clear. However, evidence suggests that individuals who suffer from PTSD find that their distress is made worse by the psychobiological interaction between the effects of the drug, and their traumatic experiences.

Cocaine use may exacerbate the symptoms of some medical disorders such as Tourette's syndrome, and tardive dyskinesia (Lopez & Jeste, 1997). Further, after periods of extended use, some people have experienced the so-called cocaine bugs, a hallucinatory experience of bugs crawling on, or just under, the skin of their bodies. The technical term for this is *formication* ("Amphetamines," 1990). Patients who have experienced cocaine-induced formication have been known to have burned their arms or legs with matches or cigarettes, or scratched themselves repeatedly, in an attempt to rid themselves of these unseen bugs (Lingeman, 1974).

Cocaine has also been implicated as causing the user to experience anxiety, or even panic reactions (DiGregorio, 1990). Louie (1990) reported that *one-fourth* of the patients seen at a panic disorder clinic eventually admitted to the use of cocaine. Further, up to 64% of cocaine users experienced some degree of anxiety as a side effect of the drug, according to the author. As noted earlier, there is a tendency for cocaine users to try to self-medicate this side effect through the use of marijuana. Other chemicals that cocaine abusers often use to control the drug-induced anxiety include the benzodiazepines, narcotics, barbiturates, and alcohol.

The cocaine-induced anxiety and panic attacks may not immediately stop after the individual has discontinued the drug. These cocaine-induced panic attacks may continue for "months or years into the period of abstinence" (Satel et al., 1993, p. 700). This seems to be a result of the ability of cocaine to make the user sensitive to anxiety states. Thus, the drug-induced anxiety reaction may last for a long time after the last period of cocaine use.

Chronic use of cocaine has been implicated in the development of a drug-induced psychosis very similar to paranoid schizophrenia. However, there are often subtle differences between the symptoms of paranoid schizophrenia, and those of a cocaine-induced psychosis, according to Rosse et al. (1994). The authors compared the symptoms of individuals in a cocaine-induced psychosis with those of other patients who were diagnosed as having paranoid schizophrenia, and found that the patients with a cocaine-induced psychosis tended to be more suspicious, and to be profoundly afraid of being discovered or harmed while under the influence of cocaine. Further, cocaine-induced psychosis was often marked by hypervigilance.

Estimates of the scope of cocaine-induced psychotic reactions range from 53% (Decker & Ries, 1993) to 65% (Beebe & Walley, 1991). This condition is sometimes called "coke paranoia" by illicit cocaine users. It usually clears within a few hours (Davis & Bresnahan, 1987) to a few days (Kerfoot et al., 1996; Schuckit, 1995) after the person stops using cocaine. Gawin et al. (1994) suggested that the delusions found in a cocaine-induced psychotic reaction usually clear after the individual's sleep pattern has returned to normal. Occasionally, however, the cocaine-induced paranoid state seems to become permanent (Maranto, 1985).

The mechanism by which chronic cocaine abuse might contribute to the development of a drug-induced psychosis remains unknown. One possibility is that those individuals who develop a cocaine-induced paranoid state might possess a biological vulnerability for schizophrenia, which is then activated by chronic cocaine abuse (Satel & Edell, 1991). However, another possibility is that in certain susceptible individuals the biological vulnerability is not for the chronic use of cocaine to result in schizophrenia, but in a short-lived paranoid state as an unwanted drug side effect (Satel, 1992).

Approximately 20% of the chronic users of crack cocaine in one study were reported to have experienced drug-induced periods of rage, or outbursts of anger and violent assaultive behavior (Beebe & Walley, 1991). Finally, as noted earlier, either a few hours after snorting the drug, or within 15 minutes if the person has injected it, the person slides into a state of depression. After periods of prolonged use, the individual's postcocaine depression can reach suicidal proportions (Maranto, 1985). Cocaine-induced depression is thought to be the result of cocaine's depleting the nerve cells in the brain of two neurotransmitters—norepinephrine and dopamine. After a period of abstinence, the neurotransmitter levels usually return to normal, and the cocaine-induced depressive episode gradually ends.

However, suicide is a common consequence of depression (whether cocaine-induced or not), and thus there is a danger that the cocaine user will attempt, or actually commit, suicide prior to recovering from a cocaine-induced depression. Indeed, one study in New York City found that *one-fifth* of all suicides involving a victim under the age of 60 were cocaine related (Marzuk et al., 1992).

Cocaine Use as an Indirect Cause of Death

In addition to its potential to cause death by a variety of mechanisms, cocaine use may indirectly cause, or at least contribute to, the user's premature death. In the last paragraph, we discussed how cocaine abuse might cause the user to experience a depressive reaction so severe that he/she committed suicide. Cocaine was also found to be a factor in 26.7% of all deaths for people between the ages of 15 and 44 in New York City (Marzuk et al., 1995). The authors carried out a program of testing body fluids for 14,843 residents of New York City who died as a result of trauma between 1990 and 1993. They found either cocaine itself, or the metabolite benzoylecgonine, in 26.7% of these individuals.

While this does not mean that cocaine use caused these individuals to suffer some form of traumatic injury that resulted in death, the authors concluded that cocaine use, like alcohol use, increased the risk that the individual would participate in aggressive or risky behaviors that might result in death.

Withdrawal and Recovery from CNS Stimulant Abuse

Although the treatment process is discussed in more detail in later chapters of this text, brief mention of the treatment of addiction to CNS stimulants should be made here. Although a great deal is known about the manifestations of cocaine addiction, very little is known about the natural history of cocaine dependence (Jaffe, 1990). Thus a great deal remains to be discovered about cocaine abuse and its effects on the user.

Although cocaine has a reputation of being exceptionally addictive, the truth is that not everybody who abuses cocaine becomes addicted. Researchers disagree as to the exact percentage of those who use cocaine and then go on to become addicted. The National Institute on Drug Abuse (quoted in Kotulak, 1992) suggested that only about 10 percent of

those who use cocaine actually go on to become heavy users. Restak (1994) gave a higher estimate of between 25 and 33% of users becoming addicted. However, this is not to deny the reality that many people do become addicted to cocaine, with terrible consequences for themselves and their families. The truth is that there is simply no way of predicting who is, or is not, at risk for becoming addicted to cocaine. If for no other reason that this, cocaine abuse should be avoided.

For those who do abuse cocaine, or who might become addicted to it, hospital-based detoxification is rarely necessary ("Amphetamines," 1990). Since cocaine-induced depression may reach suicidal proportions, however, hospital-based observation and treatment may be necessary to protect the individual who is depressed as a result of cocaine abuse. The decision to hospitalize/not hospitalize a cocaine abuser should be made on a case-by-case basis by qualified physicians. Some of the factors that must be considered in making the decision to recommend hospitalization for a cocaine abuser include the individual's current state of mind, his/her medical status, and whether he/she has adequate resources and social support to deal with the withdrawal process on an outpatient basis.

There is little research into the factors that bring about addiction to the CNS stimulants. In contrast to the research into the genetics of alcoholism, "research on genetic factors in stimulant abuse has not been pursued" (Gawin & Ellinwood, 1988, p. 1177). Thus, there is no information into possible genetic markers that might identify the person who is vulnerable to cocaine addiction.

Researchers believe that protracted cocaine abuse may result in a withdrawal syndrome (Hazleton, 1984; Satel et al., 1991). Gawin and Ellinwood (1988) characterized the cocaine-withdrawal syndrome as being "comparable to the acute withdrawal of the alcohol hangover" (p. 1176). Although the cocaine withdrawal syndrome does not include "severe . . . symptoms such as those seen in opiate withdrawal" (Gold & Verebey, 1984, p. 720), research has shown that it is marked by such complaints as paranoia, depression, fatigue, craving for cocaine, agitation, chills, insomnia, nausea, changes in sleep patterns, ravenous hunger, muscle tremors, headache, and vomiting (DiGregorio, 1990). These symptoms begin 24 to 48 hours after the last dose of cocaine, and persist for 7 to 10 days, according to the author.

Stages of Recovery

A triphasic model for the postcocaine binge recovery process has been proposed (Gawin et al., 1994; Gawin & Kleber, 1986). In the early part of the first stage, which lasts from 1 to 14 days, the person experiences feelings of agitation, depression, and anorexia (loss of desire to eat), as well as a strong craving for cocaine. As the person progresses through the second half of the first phase, they lose the craving for cocaine, but experience insomnia and exhaustion, combined with a strong desire for sleep. The second half of the first phase lasts from the 4th until the 7th day of recovery, according to the authors.

The second phase of recovery begins after the 7th day of abstinence. The person returns to a normal sleep pattern and gradually experiences stronger cravings for cocaine and higher levels of anxiety. Conditioned cues may exacerbate the individual's craving for stimulants, drawing the person back to chemical use. If the person can withstand the environmental and intrapersonal cues for further drug use, he/she moves into the "extinction" phase and gradually returns to a more normal level of function.

The third stage of recovery, the extinction phase, begins after 10 weeks of abstinence. If the person cannot maintain sobriety and again goes on a stimulant binge, the cycle repeats itself. If the person withstands the craving, there is a good chance of achieving sobriety. Hall, Havassy, and Wasserman (1991) concluded that approximately 80% of those cocaine addicts who were able to abstain from cocaine use for 12 weeks after treatment were still drug-free after 6 months.

However, this does not mean that the individual has fully recovered from cocaine addiction. Cocaine and amphetamine addicts may suddenly experience craving for these drugs "months or years after its last appearance" (Gawin & Ellinwood, 1988, p. 1176), and long after the last period of chemical use.

The research team of Satel, Price, Palumbo, McDougle, Krystal, Gawin, Charney, Heninger,

and Kleber (1991), examined the cocaine withdrawal process, and concluded that their data failed to support the model advanced by Gawin and Kleber (1986). The authors found that, for their sample, the cocaine withdrawal process was marked by mild withdrawal symptoms that declined over the first 3 weeks of inpatient treatment. The symptoms they noted were much milder than had been anticipated and failed to follow the triphasic model suggested by earlier research.

Researchers have acknowledged that a withdrawal syndrome appears to follow prolonged cocaine use. But, they have not determined the exact nature of this syndrome, and are exploring theoretical models to better understand what happens when a cocaine addict stops using chemicals. Further, as part of the process of exploring different ways of working with cocaine addicts, a number of pharmacological agents are being investigated in the hopes of finding a drug, or combination of drugs, that will control the postcocaine craving that complicates the treatment of cocaine addiction for many of those who are recovering. These agents are discussed in Chapter 32.

The treatment of stimulant addiction involves more than just helping the addict stop using the drug. A common complication of stimulant addiction is that the addict has often forgotten what a drug-free life is like (R. K. Siegel, 1982). Further, Gold and Verebey (1984) pointed out that cocaine addiction may lead to vitamin deficiencies, especially of the B complex and C vitamins. Since the stimulant effects of the amphetamines are so similar to that of cocaine, one would expect that the amphetamines would also lead to vitamin deficiencies in a pattern similar to that seen in chronic cocaine abuse.

The authors found that 73% of a sample of cocaine abusers tested had at least one vitamin deficiency. The authors concluded that these vitamin deficiencies reflected the malnutrition found in cocaine abuse, since cocaine may cause anorexia. The authors recommended vitamin replacement therapy as part of the treatment of cocaine addiction.

Total abstinence from drugs of abuse is essential in the treatment of cocaine or amphetamine addiction, and follow-up treatment should include behavior modification and psychotherapy (Gold & Verebey, 1984). Hall et al. (1991) found that those cocaine addicts who made a commitment to full abstinence following treatment were more likely to avoid further cocaine use, than addicts who did not desire abstinence as a treatment goal. Social support and self-help group support (e.g., Alcoholics Anonymous, Narcotics Anonymous, Cocaine Anonymous) are often of great help. As with the other forms of drug addiction, the recovering individual is at risk for cross-addiction to other chemicals, and needs to avoid other drug use for the rest of his/her life.

Summary

Although humans have used cocaine for hundreds, if not thousands, of years, it has only been in the past 150 years that the active agent of the coca bush has been isolated and identified. By coincidence, the ability to concentrate large amounts of cocaine took place at about the same time as the development of the intravenous needle. This allowed users to inject large amounts of the relatively pure cocaine, directly into the circulatory system, where it was rapidly transported to the brain. Users quickly discovered that intravenously administered cocaine brought on a sense of euphoria, which immediately made it a popular drug of abuse.

At the turn of the century, government regulations limited the availability of cocaine, which was mistakenly classified as a narcotic at that time. The development of the amphetamine family of drugs in the 1930s, along with increasingly strict enforcement of the laws against cocaine use, allowed drug-addicted individuals to substitute legally purchased amphetamines for the increasingly rare cocaine. In time, the dangers of cocaine use were forgotten by all but a few medical historians.

In the late 1960s and early 1970s, government regulations began to limit the availability of amphetamines. Cocaine emerged as a substitute for the difficult-to-obtain amphetamines in the late 1970s and early 1980s. To entice users, new forms of cocaine were introduced, including concentrated "rocks" of cocaine, known as crack. To the cocaine user of the 1980s, cocaine seemed to be a harmless drug, although historical evidence suggested otherwise.

In the 1980s, users rediscovered the dangers associated with cocaine abuse, and the drug gradually has fallen into disfavor. It appears that the most recent wave of cocaine addiction peaked around 1986 and that fewer and fewer people are becoming addicted to this drug. A disturbing new trend among drug abusers and addicts is to smoke a combination of crack cocaine and heroin. This new form of cocaine use seems to have come about in response to the growing threat of HIV infection and the growing availability of heroin in this country. When cocaine is smoked, either alone, or in combination with heroin prepared for smoking, the danger of HIV transmission is effectively avoided. Cocaine smokers do not share intravenous needles.

In the past few years, the reported number of cocaine and heroin related emergency room visits has significantly increased in this country. Thus, cocaine probably will remain a part of the drug abuse problem well into the next century.

CHAPTER TEN

Marijuana

For many generations, marijuana has been a most controversial substance of abuse, and misperceptions surrounding this substance abound. People talk about marijuana as if it were a chemical in its own right. Actually, marijuana is not a chemical or a drug: it is a plant. Over the years, people have discovered that some of the chemicals in this plant seem to have beneficial properties. Through experimentation, people have learned that if they smoke parts of the plant, or, less often, consume it, some of the chemicals in the plant will enter their bodies.

But, unlike recreational substances such as alcohol, cocaine, or the amphetamines, marijuana is not in itself a recreational substance in the technical sense. It is only a plant, which happens to contain some chemicals that may be used for recreational purposes. In this sense, marijuana is similar to tobacco.

History of Marijuana Use in the United States

It has only been in the 20th century that marijuana has gone through a number of transformations. Prior to this century, physicians considered marijuana as a medicinal substance, and used it to treat a number of different disorders. The first historical references to marijuana date back to the reign of the Chinese Emperor Shen Nung (2737 B.C.), when it was used as a medicine (Scaros et al., 1990). Thus, the use of marijuana in medicine has been documented to go back "at least 5,000 years" (Denis Petro, quoted in *Health Facts*, 1991, p. 4).

As recently as the 19th century, physicians in the United States and Europe used marijuana as an analgesic, hypnotic, as a treatment for migraine headaches, and as an anticonvulsant (Grinspoon & Bakalar, 1992, 1993, 1995). An example of the use of marijuana in the treatment of disease is an 1838 case, where physicians used hashish to completely control the terror and "excitement" (Elliott, 1992, p. 600) of a patient who had contracted rabies. Then, during the early part of this century, researchers found that marijuana was either ineffective, or at least less effective, than many other pharmaceuticals being introduced as part of the fight against disease. This, along with increasingly strict federal regulations, caused marijuana to fall into disfavor as a pharmaceutical (Grinspoon & Bakalar, 1993, 1995). By the 1930s, marijuana was removed from the doctor's pharmacopoeia.

The practice of smoking marijuana cigarettes for their psychoactive effects was apparently introduced into the United States by Mexican immigrants who had come north to find work in the 1920s (Mann, 1994). Recreational marijuana smoking was quickly adopted by others, especially jazz musicians (Musto, 1991). With the start of Prohibition in 1920, the working class turned to growing or importing marijuana as a substitute for alcohol (Gazzaniga, 1988).

Its use declined with the end of Prohibition, when alcohol could once more be easily obtained. But, a small minority of the population continued to use it as a recreational substance.

The passage of the Marijuana Tax Act of 1937 certainly drove marijuana use underground but did not eliminate its use entirely.[1] In the 1960s, marijuana again became a popular substance of abuse, and has retained that status ever since. Marijuana is the most frequently used illicit substance in the world (Woody & MacFadden, 1995). In North America, it is "the most frequently used drug in the United States" (Nahas, 1986, p. 82), and in Canada (Russell et al., 1994).

Medicinal Marijuana

Although marijuana is illegal in the United States, since the 1970s a small number of physicians have again started to wonder if one or more of the chemicals in the marijuana plant may be of value in the fight against disease and suffering. A number of physicians have used the marijuana plant, or selected chemicals found in that plant, to control the nausea sometimes caused by cancer chemotherapy. The drug Marinol (dronabinol) was introduced as a synthetic version of one of the chemicals found in marijuana, THC (discussed later in this chapter), to control severe nausea. Marinol has met with mixed success, possibly because marijuana's antinausea effects are caused by a chemical other than THC (D. Smith, 1997).

Some researchers claim that marijuana might be as useful in the control of certain forms of glaucoma (Grinspoon & Bakalar, 1993; Jaffe, 1990; Voelker, 1994). There is also limited evidence that suggests marijuana might also be of value in the treatment of multiple sclerosis, rheumatoid arthritis, and possibly chronic pain conditions (Grinspoon & Bakalar,

1997; "Medical Benefits," 1991). Finally, some physicians believe that marijuana might help control the weight loss often seen in patients with late-stage AIDS (discussed in Chapter 32) (Hearn, 1995).

The possible use of marijuana in the treatment of disease has resulted in considerable controversy in the medical field. Some physicians point out that there is no evidence to suggest that marijuana is of value in the treatment of these, or other, disorders (Dr. Janet Lapey, quoted in Voelker, 1994). On the other hand, advocates of the possible medicinal value of marijuana continue to point to anecdotal reports that suggest marijuana seems to be effective in treating at least some of the previously listed disorders. One study conducted in 1991 found that 44% of oncologists (physicians who specialize in the treatment of cancer) who responded to a survey admitted to having instructed patients to use marijuana, on occasion (Hearn, 1995). Many health care professionals now advocate its use, at least with certain patients, or recommend conducting further research on its potential as a pharmaceutical.

In 1996, the United States Drug Enforcement Administration (DEA) began a series of administrative hearings to determine the status of marijuana as a possible medicinal agent. An administrative law judge ruled in 1988 that marijuana should be reclassified as a Schedule II substance (a chemical with some medical uses, but potentially addictive). The DEA overruled its own judge, and ruled that marijuana would remain prohibited (Kassirer, 1997).

Despite this ruling, by 1996 the legislature of the state of California had passed three separate bills making the use of marijuana legal for cancer and AIDS patients. Each time, the governor of California vetoed the bill presented to him. But, by the summer of 1996, 750,000 residents of the state of California signed a petition demanding that the state consider the medical use of marijuana, and the Medical Marijuana Initiative passed in the November 1996 elections (Grinspoon & Bakalar, 1997). A similar, but more restrictive, law was passed in Arizona at the same time, according to the authors. Similar proposals are being suggested in a number of other states. Thus, marijuana may remain a controversial recreational substance for many years to come.

---

[1] Contrary to popular belief, the Marijuana Stamp Act of 1937 did not make *possession* of marijuana illegal, but *did* impose a small tax on it. A person who paid the tax received a stamp verifying payment of the tax to the authorities. Since the stamp also alerts authorities to the fact that the owner has marijuana in their possession, illegal users of marijuana do not apply for the forms to pay the tax. The stamps are of interest to stamp collectors, however, and a few collectors have actually paid the tax to obtain the stamp for their collection.

Marijuana Is Technically a Plant, Not a Drug

Although people speak of marijuana as if it were a single substance, it is actually a plant, whose scientific name is *Cannabis sativa*. The cannabis plant grows wild in the countryside of much of the United States, and is often known by such names as "ditchweed." This wild marijuana is of very low potency and rarely is used as a recreational substance. Marijuana intentionally grown for recreational purposes is more potent, and evidence suggests that marijuana may be the biggest cash crop in the United States (Guttman, 1996; D. C. Lewis, 1996).[2]

There is some question whether the marijuana most commonly used in this country is more potent now than it was in the 1960s and early 1970s. Some researchers believe that the marijuana sold on the streets is now up to *10 times as potent* as the marijuana sold just a few decade ago ("How Much Marijuana," 1995). However, this assertion has been challenged by other researchers (Woody & MacFadden, 1995). Indeed, because so many factors can influence the potency of a given sample of marijuana, it is difficult to determine its relative potency. As a general rule, however, the typical marijuana sample has a THC[3] content of between 6 and 8%.

THC is found throughout the plant, but the highest concentrations are in the small upper leaves and flowering tops (Mirin et al., 1991). Technically, the term *marijuana* refers to the relatively weak preparations of the cannibis plant that are used for smoking or eating. The term *hashish* means the thick resin obtained from the flowers. The resin is dried, forming a brown or black substance that has a high concentration of THC. This is subsequently either ingested orally (often mixed with some sweet substance) or smoked. In this chapter, however, we use the generic term marijuana for any part of the plant that is smoked or ingested.

Scope of the Problem

Globally, an estimated 200–300 million people are regular users of marijuana (Woody & MacFadden, 1995). It is the most popular illicit substance used in the United States (Abood & Martin, 1992; "Blunts and Crude," 1993; Millman & Beeder, 1994). Nationally, some 46% of the population between the ages of 15 and 54 years of age has used marijuana at least once (Anthony, Arria, & Johnson, 1995). An estimated 68 million people in the United States admit to having used marijuana at least once in their lives (Grinspoon & Bakalar, 1995b; Woody & MacFadden, 1995).

Ten million people in the United States are thought to use marijuana on a regular basis, while another 20 million Americans are occasional users ("How Much Marijuana," 1995). The team of Nash and Park (1997) estimated that 10 million people in the United States use marijuana at least once each month. The annual consumption of marijuana in this country is about 1,476 metric tons, 75% of which is imported into this country through illicit channels and 25% of which is grown in the United States ("How Much Marijuana").

Marijuana is especially popular as a substance of abuse among the young. The average age at which marijuana users begin to use it is estimated to be 18.2 years (G. Cohen et al., 1996). Perhaps 15 million "young people" (Mirin, Weiss, & Greenfield, 1991, p. 301) use marijuana at least once a month, 9 million use it weekly, and 6 million use it daily. The popularity of marijuana rests on the fact that a "few puffs on a joint is this generation's social martini" (Peluso & Peluso, 1988, p. 110). It has, in a real sense, become an accepted part of the social scene. Because of this, both the legal and the social sanctions against marijuana use have repeatedly changed in the past 30 years. In some states, possession of a small amount of marijuana was decriminalized, only to be *recriminalized just a few years later (Woody & MacFadden, 1995). The legal status of marijuana varies from one state to another.

Researchers believe that most of those who use marijuana will experiment with the substance briefly, and then discontinue further use. Only a minority of

---

[2] The estimated value of the marijuana being raised in the United States, not the amount being cultivated, makes it the most valuable cash crop in this country.

[3] As discussed later in this chapter, THC is the active agent of marijuana.

those who try marijuana go on to use the substance on a regular basis for an extended period.

Pharmacology of Marijuana

The *Cannabis sativa* plant contains over 400 different identified compounds, of which an estimated 61 have some psychoactive effect (Restak, 1994; University of California, Berkeley, 1990b). Only one of these chemicals, delta-9-tetrahydro-cannabinol, or "THC" as it is often called, is thought to account for most of marijuana's observed effects on humans. THC was first identified as the main active ingredient of marijuana in 1964 (Bloodworth, 1987; Mirin et al., 1991; Restak, 1994; Schwartz, 1987).

THC is a lipid-soluble chemical, which means that it is able to pass from the blood into the brain quickly (Woody & MacFadden, 1995). In August 1990, after a search that has taken more than a generation, a team of researchers from the National Institute of Mental Health discovered one receptor site within the brain that is used by the THC molecule (Matsuda, Lolait, Brownstein, Young, & Bonner, 1990). These researchers were attempting to isolate certain neuropeptides that transmit pain signals between cells, but stumbled upon a process through which THC inhibits the function of the enzyme *adenylate cyclase*. This enzyme is also involved in the transmission of pain messages. Thus, by accident, researchers identified at least one of the sites within the brain where THC carries out its effects.

Since this discovery, researchers at the Hebrew University in Jerusalem have identified a molecule within the brain that binds to the same receptor that THC was found to use (Restak, 1993). The researchers named this molecule *anandamide*. Although researchers are not sure of anandamide's function within the brain, it is assumed that THC binds to the same receptor sites normally occupied by anandamide (Nutt, 1996). In addition to its impact on anandamide, marijuana use has been found to affect the synthesis and turnover of the neurotransmitter *acetylcholine* in the limbic region of the brain (Hartman, 1995). Acetylcholine is a neurotransmitter involved in the process of alertness, and this may be one reason marijuana users tend to feel

somewhat sedated and relaxed while under the influence of the drug. It is not known if this effect is caused by THC or by one of the other psychoactive compounds found in marijuana.

The primary site of THC biotransformation is in the liver. The half-life of THC appears to vary as a result of whether metabolic tolerance has developed or not. However, the liver is not able to biotransform THC very quickly. Thus, in experienced users, marijuana has a half-life of about 3 days (Schwartz, 1987), to a week (Bloodworth, 1987). About 65% of the metabolites of THC are excreted in the feces, and the rest are excreted in the urine (Schwartz, 1987; Woody & MacFadden, 1995). Unmetabolized THC binds to fat cells in the body, and with repeated episodes of marijuana use over a short period, significant amounts of THC may be stored in the body's fat reserves. In between periods of active marijuana use, the fat-bound THC is slowly released back into the blood (Schwartz, 1987).

This process can account for the phenomenon in which a heavy marijuana user might test positive for THC in urine toxicology screens for weeks after his/her last use (Schwartz, 1987). However, this happens only with *very* heavy marijuana users. In the casual user, urine toxicology tests will usually detect evidence of THC for only about 3 days after he/she last used it.

Tolerance to the effects of THC develop rapidly. Once tolerance has developed, the user must either wait a few days until his/her tolerance for marijuana begins to diminish, or, alter the manner in which he/she uses marijuana. For example, after tolerance to marijuana has developed, the chronic marijuana smoker must use "more potent cannabis, deeper, more sustained inhalations, or larger amounts of the crude drug" (Schwartz, 1987, p. 307) to overcome his/her tolerance to marijuana.

Interactions between Marijuana and Other Chemicals

There has been relatively little research into the possible effects of marijuana use on other chemicals. It was suggested that when patients taking lithium used marijuana, it would cause their blood lithium levels to increase (Ciraulo et al., 1995). The reason for this increase in blood lithium level is not clear. However, because lithium is quite toxic and has only a narrow therapeutic window between the optimal level of lithium and toxicity, this interaction between marijuana and lithium is potentially dangerous to the person who uses both substances.

There also has been a case report of a patient who smoked marijuana while taking Antabuse (disulfiram). The patient developed a hypomanic episode that subsided when he stopped using marijuana (Barnhill et al., 1995). When the patient again resumed the use of marijuana while taking Antabuse, he again became hypomanic, according to the authors, suggesting that the episode of mania was due to some unknown interaction between these two chemicals.

For reasons that are not clear, adolescents who use marijuana while taking an antidepressant medication such as Elavil (amitriptyline) run the risk of developing a drug-induced delirium. Thus, individuals who are taking antidepressants should not use marijuana.

Methods of Administration

In the United States, the primary method of marijuana use is smoking. Occasionally users will ingest marijuana by mouth, usually after it has been baked into a product such as cookies or brownies. But, for the most part, users smoke homemade cigarettes made out of marijuana. The marijuana may be smoked either alone or mixed with other substances. Most commonly, the marijuana is smoked by itself, in the form of cigarettes. These "joints" usually contain between 500 mg and 750 mg of marijuana, and provide an effective dose of approximately 5 to 20 mg of THC per joint. The marijuana in the average joint weighs about 0.014 ounces, and the typical user consumes about 18 joints a month (Abt Associates, Inc., 1995a).

A variation on the marijuana cigarette is the blunt. Blunts are made by removing one of the outer leaves of a cigar, unrolling it, filling it with high potency marijuana mixed with chopped cigar tobacco, and then rerolling the mixture into what is, essentially, a marijuana "cigar" ("Blunts and Crude," 1993). Users report some degree of stimulation, possibly from the nicotine in the cigar tobacco entering the lungs along with the marijuana smoke.

The technique by which marijuana is smoked is somewhat different than the normal smoking technique used for cigarettes or cigars (Schwartz, 1987). Users must inhale the smoke deeply into their lungs, then hold their breath for 20 to 30 seconds, to get as much THC into the blood as possible (Schwartz). Researchers disagree as to the amount of THC that will be absorbed by the marijuana smoker. Scaros et al. (1990) suggested that about 18% of the available THC is absorbed through the lungs into the blood by smoking. But Jaffe (1990) suggested that 2% to 50% of the THC might be absorbed, depending on the individual, and, the exact method of smoking marijuana used. The team of Loskin, Maviglia, and Friedman (1996) suggested that 50% of the available THC was absorbed into the blood when the person smoked marijuana.

When smoked, the effects begin almost immediately, usually within seconds (Weiss & Mirin, 1988) to perhaps 10 minutes (Bloodworth, 1987). It has been estimated that to produce a sense of euphoria, the user must inhale approximately 25–50 micrograms per kilogram of body weight when marijuana is smoked, and between 50–200 micrograms per kilogram of body weight if the marijuana is ingested orally (Mann, 1994). Doses of 200–250 micrograms per kilogram when smoked, or 300–500 micrograms when taken orally, may cause the user to hallucinate, according to the author.

As these figures suggest, it takes an extremely large dose of THC before the individual will begin to hallucinate. Marijuana users in other countries often have access to high-potency sources of THC, and thus may achieve hallucinatory doses. But, it is extremely rare for marijuana users in this country to have access to such potent forms of the plant. Thus, for the most part, the marijuana being smoked in this country will not cause the individual to hallucinate, although in many parts of the country marijuana is classified as a hallucinogenic by law enforcement officials.

The marijuana in use in the United States *will* cause the individual to achieve a sense of euphoria, however. When it is smoked, the effects of marijuana reach peak intensity within 30 minutes, and begin to decline in an hour (Weiss & Mirin, 1988). Estimates of the duration of the subjective effects of marijuana range from 2 or 3 hours (Brophy, 1993), on to 4 hours (Bloodworth, 1987; Grinspoon & Bakalar, 1992).

When ingested by mouth, the user absorbs only 4% to 12% of the available THC (Jaffe, 1990). Also, the oral user does not experience the immediate effects found by smoking marijuana, but usually requires 30 to 60 minutes (Mirin et al., 1991), to perhaps 2 hours (Schwartz, 1987), before beginning to feel the euphoric effects of THC. Estimates of the duration of marijuana's effects when ingested orally range from 3 to 5 hours (Mirin et al., 1991; Weiss & Mirin, 1988) upward to 5 to 12 hours (Kaplan et al., 1994).

Proponents of the legalization of marijuana point out that in terms of *immediate* lethality, marijuana appears to be a "safe" drug. Animal research suggests that the LD_{50} of THC is about 125 mg/kg (Nahas, 1986). A 160-pound person weighs about 72.59 kilograms. If, as stated earlier, the typical marijuana cigarette contains 20 mg of THC, then the estimated LD_{50} for this person would be the equivalent of smoking 453 marijuana cigarettes at once. But this estimate assumes that 100% of the available THC in a marijuana cigarette would be absorbed. Since only 2% to 50% of the THC in a marijuana cigarette is actually absorbed, the person in our hypothetical example would need to smoke *more* than 450 marijuana cigarettes at once to theoretically reach the LD_{50}. If we take the high estimate of 50% of the THC in the average marijuana cigarette being absorbed, then the estimated number of marijuana cigarettes that a typical 160-pound person would have to smoke to reach the LD_{50} is just over 900 marijuana cigarettes at once. To express this in other terms, it has been suggested that a person would have to smoke *40 pounds* of marijuana in a 20-minute span of time, to die as a result of a marijuana overdose (Graff, Rivera, Simmons, & Willerth, 1996).

In contrast to the estimated 434,000 deaths each year in this country from tobacco use, and the total of 125,000 yearly fatalities from alcohol use, there are only an estimated 75 marijuana-related deaths each year. Unlike the various diseases caused by either alcohol or tobacco, most marijuana-related deaths are caused by accidents that take place while the individual is under the influence of this substance rather than as a direct result of any toxic effects of THC (Crowley, 1988).

There has never been a documented case of a marijuana overdose (Grinspoon & Bakalar, 1993, 1995, 1997; Nahas, 1986). In terms of its immediate toxicity, marijuana appears to be "among the least toxic drugs known to modern medicine" (Weil, 1986, p. 47). The effective dose of THC is estimated to be approximately 1/20,000 and 1/40,000 the lethal dose (Grinspoon & Bakalar, 1993, 1995; Kaplan et al., 1994).

Subjective Effects of Marijuana

At moderate dosage levels, marijuana will bring about a two-phase reaction (Brophy, 1993). The first phase begins shortly after the drug enters the bloodstream, when the individual will experience a period of mild anxiety, followed by a sense of well-being, or euphoria, as well as a sense of relaxation and friendliness (Kaplan et al., 1994). These subjective effects are consistent with the known physical effects of marijuana. Research has found that marijuana causes "a transient increase in the release of the neurotransmitter dopamine" (Friedman, 1987, p. 47), a neurochemical thought to be involved in the experience of euphoria.

As with many drugs of abuse, the individual's expectations influence how he/she interprets the effects of marijuana. Marijuana users tend to anticipate that the drug will (a) impair cognitive function as well as the user's behavior, (b) help the user relax, (c) help the user interact socially and enhance sexual function, (d) enhance creative abilities and alter perception, (e) bring with it some negative effects, and (f) bring about a sense of craving (Schafer & Brown, 1991). Individuals who are intoxicated on marijuana frequently report an altered sense of time, as well as mood swings (Kaplan et al., 1994), and feelings of well-being and happiness (Abood & Martin, 1992). Marijuana also seems to bring about a splitting of consciousness, in which users may experience the sensation of observing themselves while under the influence of the drug (Grinspoon & Bakalar, 1995; Kaplan et al., 1994).

Marijuana users have often reported a sense of being on the threshold of a significant personal insight, but are unable to put this insight into words. These reported drug-related insights seem to come about during the first phase of the marijuana reaction. The second phase begins when the individual becomes sleepy, which takes place following the acute intoxication caused by marijuana (Abood & Martin, 1992; Brophy, 1993).

Adverse Effects of Occasional Marijuana Use

There are few immediate adverse reactions to marijuana ("Deglamorising," 1995; Mirin et al., 1991). When marijuana is smoked, some of the smaller blood vessels in the body will dilate. It is not clear whether this effect is caused by THC itself, or by one of the other chemicals found in the cannabis plant. However, this is the mechanism that causes marijuana users to often have bloodshot eyes: the small blood vessels in the eyes have dilated and are thus more easily seen.

One of the most common adverse reactions to marijuana use is that of drug-related anxiety, or even panic attacks (Kaplan et al., 1994; Millman & Beeder, 1994). Factors that seem to influence the development of marijuana-related panic reactions are the individual's prior experience with marijuana, expectations for the drug, the dosage level being used, and the setting in which the drug is used. Such panic reactions are most often seen in the inexperienced marijuana user (Bloodworth, 1987; Mirin et al., 1991). Usually simple reassurance is the only treatment needed (Kaplan et al., 1994; Millman & Beeder, 1994).

A more serious, but rare, adverse reaction is the development of a marijuana-induced psychotic reaction, often called a *toxic psychosis*. The effects of a marijuana-induced toxic psychosis are usually short-lived and will clear up in a few days to a few weeks (Millman & Beeder, 1994). If the drug-induced psychotic reaction should last longer than a few days, it may very well reflect an underlying psychotic condition rather than a drug-induced condition. Research has suggested that marijuana use is unlikely to trigger a psychotic reaction in a person unless he/she (a) has suffered a previous psychotic

episode, or (b) is predisposed to psychosis (Linszen, Dingemans, & Lenior, 1994; Mathers & Ghodse, 1992; Nahas, 1986). Fortunately, researchers think that marijuana-induced psychotic reactions result only from extremely heavy marijuana use (Abood & Martin, 1992; Kaplan et al., 1994; Mathers & Ghodse, 1992). Thus, for the casual user, the danger of a marijuana-induced psychosis is thought to be quite low.

Linszen et al. (1994) noted that THC functions as a dopamine agonist in the nerve pathways of the region of the brain known as the *medial forebrain bundles*, which use dopamine as the primary neurotransmitter. Dopamine is also the neurotransmitter implicated in schozophrenia, suggesting that this might be the mechanism through which marijuana contributes to the emergence of psychotic symptoms in schizophrenia.

Marijuana is known to reduce sexual desire in the user, and, for male users, may contribute to erectile problems, and, delayed ejaculation (Finger et al., 1997). Finally, an extremely rare consequence of marijuana use is the development of an acute depressive reaction (Grinspoon & Bakalar, 1992). This marijuana-related depression is most common in the inexperienced user, and may reflect the activation of an undetected depression on the part of the user. The depressive episode is usually mild and does not require professional intervention except in rare cases, according to the authors. It usually clears up in less than 24 hours (Millman & Beeder, 1994).

Consequences of Chronic Marijuana Use

The hemp plant from which marijuana is obtained has been shown to contain some 400 different chemicals. More than 2,000 separate metabolites of these 400 chemicals may be found in the body after the individual has smoked marijuana (Jenike, 1991). Many of these metabolites may remain present in the body for weeks after a single episode of marijuana smoking; however, the long-term effects of these chemicals on the human body have not been studied in detail (University of California-Berkeley, 1990b). In addition to this, if the marijuana is adulterated (as it frequently is), the various adulterants will add their own contribution to the flood of chemicals being admitted to the body when the person uses marijuana. Again, there is little research into the long-term effects of these adulterants or their metabolites on the user.

The active agent of marijuana, THC, has been demonstrated to cause lung damage and reduce the effectiveness of the body's immune system. Research suggests that marijuana smokers absorb four times as much tar as do cigarette smokers (Tashkin, 1993). Smoking marijuana can also cause increased levels of carbon monoxide in the blood (Oliwenstein, 1988). It has been reported that the marijuana smoker will absorb five times as much carbon monoxide per joint as would the smoker of a single regular cigarette (Oliwenstein, 1988; Polen et al., 1993; University of California-Berkeley, 1990b). Smoking just 4 marijuana joints appears to have the same negative impact on lung function as smoking 20 regular cigarettes (Tashkin, 1990).

Furthermore, chronic marijuana users who smoke just a few marijuana joints a day seemed to develop the same type of damage to the cells lining the airways as do cigarette smokers who go on to develop lung cancer (Oliwenstein, 1988; Tashkin, 1993; University of California-Berkeley, 1990b). Research has shown that marijuana smoke contains 5 to 15 times the amount of a known carcinogen, benzpyrene, as does tobacco smoke (Bloodworth, 1987; Tashkin, 1993) The heavy use of marijuana was suggested as a cause of cancer of the respiratory tract and the mouth (tongue, tonsils, etc.) in a number of younger individuals who would not be expected to have cancer (Tashkin).

There are several reasons for the observed relationship between heavy marijuana use and lung cancer. In terms of absolute numbers, marijuana smokers tend to smoke fewer joints than smokers of cigarettes. However, they also smoke unfiltered joints, a practice that allows more of the particles from the joint into the lungs than is the case for cigarette smokers. Marijuana smokers also smoke more of the joint than cigarette smokers do cigarettes. This increases the individual's exposure to microscopic contaminants in the joint. Finally, marijuana smokers inhale more deeply than cigarette smokers, and retain the smoke in the lungs for a longer time (Polen et al., 1993). Again, this increases the individual's exposure to the potential carcinogenic agents in marijuana smoke.

An example of marijuana's ability to irritate the lungs is that, like tobacco smokers, marijuana users have an increased frequency of bronchitis and other upper respiratory infections (Mirin et al., 1991). The chronic use of marijuana also may contribute to the development of obstructive pulmonary diseases, similar to those seen in cigarette smokers (University of California-Berkeley, 1990b). Another observed effect of marijuana use is drug-induced suppression of the immune system. Researchers still do not understand the mechanism through which marijuana might reduce the effectiveness of the immune system. Although for the normal person, this immunosupressant effect is usually quite minor, even a weak immunosuppressant effect could have ". . . a devastating effect on AIDS patients" (Bloodworth, 1987, p. 180) or other patients who suffer from a disorder of the immune system.

Marijuana use has been implicated as the cause of a number of reproductive system dysfunctions. There is evidence suggesting that marijuana causes reduced sperm counts in men (Brophy, 1993). Further, male chronic marijuana users have been found to have 50 percent lower blood testosterone levels as compared with men who do not use marijuana (Bloodworth, 1987). Chronic female marijuana users have experienced abnormal menstruation, and/or a failure to ovulate (Brophy, 1993; *Mayo Clinic Health Letter*, 1989).

There is mixed evidence suggesting that chronic marijuana use could result in fertility problems in the woman. Wray and Murthy (1987) suggested that chronic marijuana use could cause fertility problems in women. However, Grinspoon and Bakalar (1992) pointed out that research studies into the effects of marijuana on the reproductive potential of women has been flawed, in that few studies have utilized proper control groups. Thus, it is not clear whether the woman's marijuana use was responsible for the observed changes in reproductive health found in some studies.

Persons who have previously used hallucinogenics may also experience marijuana-related "flashback" experiences (Jenike, 1991). Such flashbacks are usually limited to the six-month period following the last marijuana use (Jenike, 1991) and will eventually stop if the person does not use any further mood-altering chemicals (Weiss & Mirin, 1988).

The flashback experience is discussed in more detail in Chapter 13.

For years, researchers believed that marijuana did not cause any physical damage to the brain. Researchers have now uncovered evidence, however, suggesting that the chronic use of marijuana may result in physical damage to a region of the brain known as hippocampus (Friedman, 1987; Kaufman & McNaul, 1992; Loskin et al., 1996; Schuster, 1990). This is a portion of the brain that is thought to be involved in the processing of sensory information. Chronic exposure to THC "damages and destroys nerve cells and causes other pathological changes in the hippocampus" (Friedman, 1987 p. 47). These findings suggest that the chronic use of marijuana might actually cause structural changes to this region of the brain (Loskin, et al., 1996).

This would make sense, since there is evidence that chronic marijuana use may cause memory problems (American Academy of Family Physicians, 1990a; Wray & Murthy, 1987). This seems to be because marijuana interferes with the retrieval mechanisms of memory (Wray & Murthy, 1987). This may only be a temporary effect of marijuana that clears up in a few weeks after the last marijuana use (American Academy of Family Physicians, 1990a). Thus, there appears to be evidence that the chronic use of marijuana can cause at least temporary brain dysfunction.

The team of Pope and Yurgelun-Todd (1996) compared the performance of 65 heavy marijuana users (who had used marijuana at least 22 of the preceding 30 days) with light users (who had used marijuana only 1 day out of the preceding 30) on a battery of standard neuropsychological tests. The authors excluded volunteers with evidence of a current or past psychiatric disorder, or evidence of severe head injury in the past, to avoid contamination of their results with the effects of these conditions. They found that heavy marijuana users had reduced scores on those tests that tapped the "attentional/executive system" (p. 526) of the brain. Based on their findings, the authors concluded that marijuana affects a number of different regions in the brain, including those involved in sustained attention (a brain stem function), and the capacity to shift attention (which is controlled by prefrontal cortical

areas of the brain). While the results of this investigation were suggestive, the authors cautioned that they were not conclusive, and that further research into the effects of marijuana are needed.

Another team that explored the impact of chronic marijuana use on neuropsychological function was that of Fletcher et al. (1996). The authors compared the test performance of two groups of marijuana users—a young adult group and a middle-age group—with that of nonusers of the same age. They found that the older marijuana-using subgroup performed significantly worse on two tests of short-term memory than did their nonusing counterparts, a finding that the authors interpreted as evidence that chronic marijuana use might interfere with memory function.

Marijuana use also contributes to impaired reflexes at least in the period immediately after the use of the drug (Jenike, 1991). Automobile drivers under the influence of marijuana will frequently misjudge the speed and length of time required for braking, factors that may contribute to accidental death while using marijuana (Mirin et al., 1991). Schwartz (1987) reported that marijuana use may impair coordination and reaction time for 12 to 24 hours after the euphoria from the last marijuana use ended. The author also noted that teenagers who smoked marijuana as often as six times a month "were 2.4 times more likely to be involved in traffic accidents" (p. 309) as were nonusers.

Meer (1986) tested 10 private airplane pilots on a flight simulator 24 hours after they had smoked one marijuana cigarette. Although their performance had improved over their simulator performance one to four hours after smoking the marijuana cigarette, these pilots still demonstrated significant impairment on flight simulation testing. For example, one pilot's simulation performance would have landed the plane off the runway. The exact significance of these findings is not clear, but this study suggests that marijuana's effects on coordination may last longer than was once thought.

Marijuana use can cause a significant increase in heart rate, a side effect that may be of some consequence to persons who suffer from heart disease (Barnhill et al., 1995; Bloodworth, 1987; Schuckit, 1995). Cocaine users often smoke marijuana concurrently with cocaine, to use the sedative effects of marijuana for counteracting the excessive stimulation caused by the cocaine. The combination of marijuana and cocaine can increase heart rate above that seen from either drug alone, raising the heart rate an additional 50 beats per minute (Barnhill et al., 1995).

Researchers have found that chronic marijuana users have been found to have changes in the electrical activity of the brain, as measured by electroencephalographic (EEG) studies for up to 8 months after their last use of this substance. Again, in addition to its potential to indirectly contribute to cardiovascular problems, there is evidence of possible brain damage as a result of marijuana use.

Amotivational Syndrome

There is conflicting evidence as to whether chronic marijuana use might bring about an "amotivational syndrome." Some researchers have described a marijuana related amotivational syndrome, consisting of decreased drive and ambition, short attention span, easy distractibility, and a tendency not to make plans beyond the present day (Mirin et al., 1991). However, there are also many researchers who do not believe that marijuana can cause this so-called amotivational syndrome (Abood & Martin, 1992).

It has been suggested that the amotivational syndrome might be a research artifact. Individuals who tend to use marijuana on a regular basis are also likely to be those individuals who are typically bored, depressed, listless, alienated from society, and cynical. These are some of the very same characteristics thought to be a result of the marijuana-induced amotivational syndrome (Grinspoon & Bakalar, 1992), and thus might predate the individual's marijuana use rather than be a result of the chemical use.

It is not clear whether marijuana causes these observed personality characteristics, or, if people with these personality traits are most likely to use marijuana on a regular basis. Further research is necessary to determine once and for all whether the amotivational syndrome does indeed exist and the role that chronic marijuana use plays in its development (Schwartz, 1987).

Although marijuana is, in terms of immediate lethality, quite safe, there is significant evidence that chronic use can contribute to, or is the primary cause of, a number of potentially serious medical problems. Thus, it appears that marijuana use is not as benign as advocates of this substance would have us believe.

The Myth of Marijuana-Induced Violence

In the 1930s and 1940s, it was widely believed that marijuana use would cause the user to become violent. Researchers no longer believe that marijuana is likely to induce violence. In fact, the sedating and euphoric effects of marijuana would be more likely to reduce the tendency toward violence while the user is intoxicated, rather than to bring it about. Thus, few clinicians now believe that marijuana use is associated with an increased tendency for violent acting out.[4]

The Addiction Potential of Marijuana

As stated in earlier chapters, two of the cardinal symptoms of addiction to any chemical are the development of tolerance to that chemical, and the existence of a withdrawal syndrome when that drug is discontinued. In this sense, marijuana meets the criteria for a potentially addictive substance, since smoking as few as three marijuana cigarettes a week may result in tolerance to the effects of marijuana (Bloodworth, 1987).

Chronic marijuana use may also result in a very mild withdrawal syndrome. Because of its long half-life in the human body, the THC withdrawal symptoms are not as severe as those seen in cases of narcotic or barbiturate withdrawal (Bloodworth, 1987). However, heavy, chronic marijuana use can result in a withdrawal syndrome that includes irritability, anxiety, insomnia, nausea, and a loss of appetite (Abood & Martin, 1992; Bloodworth, 1987; Group for the Advancement of Psychiatry, 1990). Other possible symptoms of withdrawal include sweating and vomiting (Nahas, 1986). Thus, despite claims to the contrary, marijuana meets the criteria necessary to be classified as an addictive drug.

---

[4] However, if the marijuana is adultrated with any other chemical(s), then the effects of that chemical(s) must be considered as a possible cause of drug-induced violent behaviors. For example, the hallucinogen PCP is known to trigger violent behaviors in some users.

The Treatment of Marijuana Abuse/Addiction

Although marijuana use has been popular in this country since the Prohibition era, and most certainly after the "hippie" generation "discovered" marijuana in the 1960s, virtually nothing is known about the treatment of marijuana abuse/dependence (Stephens, Roffman, & Simpson, 1994; "Treatment Protocols," 1995).

In the short term, acute reaction to marijuana does not require any special intervention (Brophy, 1993). Thus, marijuana-induced feelings of anxiety or panic reactions usually respond to "firm reassurance in a nonthreatening environment" (Mirin et al., 1991, p. 304). However, the patient should be watched to ensure that no harm comes to either the marijuana user or to others.

There are a number of problems associated with working with marijuana abusers. First, it is rare for a person to be abusing *only* marijuana. Thus, treatment usually must focus on the abuse of several chemicals, rather than just marijuana alone. Second, marijuana users usually do not present themselves for treatment, unless there is some form of coercion, in part because they usually do not view themselves as being addicted to a recreational chemical ("Treatment Protocols," 1995).

Third, even when the marijuana user *does* enter treatment, the specific therapeutic methods for working with the chronic marijuana user are not well developed (Mirin et al., 1991). It is known that marijuana users often use it as a way to cope with negative feelings, especially anger ("Treatment Protocols," 1995). Thus, rehabilitation professionals must help the client identify specific problem areas in his/her life, and then help the individual identify non-drug-related coping mechanisms for these trigger situations.

Total abstinence from *all* psychoactive drugs is required if treatment is to work (Bloodworth, 1987). A treatment program that identifies the individual's reason/s for continue drug use and that helps the individual find alternatives to further drug use, is thought to be most effective. Supplemental groups that focus on vocational rehabilitation and socialization skills are also of value in the treatment of the chronic marijuana user (Mirin et al., 1991). Jenike (1991) reported that treatment efforts should focus on understanding the abuser's disturbed psychosocial relationships.

Bloodworth (1987) concluded that "family therapy is almost a necessity" (p. 183). Group therapy as a means of dealing with peer pressure to use chemicals was necessary in this author's opinion, and self-help support groups such as Alcoholics Anonymous (AA) or Narcotics Anonymous (NA) "cannot be overemphasized" (Bloodworth, 1987, p. 183).

Summary

Marijuana has been the subject of controversy for the past several generations. Despite its popularity as a drug of abuse, surprisingly little is actually known about marijuana. Indeed, after a 25-year search, researchers have identified what appears to be one specific receptor site that the THC molecule uses to cause at least some of its effects on perception and memory.

Although little is known about marijuana, some groups have called for its complete decriminalization. Other groups maintain that marijuana is a serious drug of abuse with a high potential for harm. Even the experts differ as to the potential for marijuana to cause harm. Where Weil (1986) classified marijuana as one of the safest drugs known, Oliwenstein (1988) termed marijuana a dangerous drug.

The available evidence suggests that marijuana is not as benign as it was once thought. Marijuana, either alone or in combination with cocaine, increases the heart rate, a matter of some significance to those with cardiac disease. There is evidence that chronic use of marijuana can cause physical changes in the brain, and the smoke from marijuana cigarettes has been found to be even more harmful than tobacco smoke. Marijuana remains such a controversial drug that the U.S. government refuses to sanction research into its effects, on the grounds that they do not want to run the risk that researchers might find something about marijuana that proponents of its legalization could use to justify their demands (D. Smith, 1997).

CHAPTER ELEVEN

Opiates

The opiates are a source of endless confusion not only for health care professionals, but for the general public. Narcotic analgesics are derived from the opiate family of chemicals. But because of the history of opiates as drugs of abuse, both the general public and physicians view them with distrust. For example, research has found that more than 50% of physicians are afraid to prescribe narcotic analgesics because of the mistaken belief that they might cause the patient to become "addicted" to them (60 Minutes, 1996a). As a result of this fear, only a minority of patients in pain receive adequate doses of a narcotic analgesic to control pain (Paris, 1996).

While the narcotic analgesics do have a significant abuse potential, they also remain potent and extremely useful medications. Thus, to try to clear up some of the confusion that surrounds the legitimate use of narcotic analgesics, this chapter is split into two sections. Section I focuses on the role and applications of narcotic analgesics as pharmaceutical agents. In Section II, the narcotic analgesics are considered as drugs of abuse.

I. THE MEDICAL USES OF NARCOTIC ANALGESICS

A Short History of the Narcotic Analgesics

At some point in what has been called the "Stone Age," early humans discovered that if you made an incision at the top of the *Papaver somniferum* plant during a brief period in its life cycle, the plant would extrude a thick resin. It was discovered that the dried resin, which is known by the name *opium,* could then be ingested by mouth to control pain. Archaeologists do not know when this discovery was made. Much of the early history of opium took place before the invention of written records. However, researchers have found the residue of the opium poppy plant in Stone Age dwellings in what is now northern Italy and Switzerland (Restak, 1994). Further, there is archaeological evidence suggesting that the opium poppy was being cultivated as a crop in certain regions of Europe by the latter part of the Neolithic Age (Spindler, 1994).

One of the earliest written records concerns the use of opium. In a document known as the Ebers Papyri, dating back to approximately 7000 B.C., there is a reference to the use of opium as a treatment for children who suffer from colic (Thomason & Dilts, 1991). By the 16th and 17th centuries, opium was used for virtually every ailment that European physicians encountered (Melzack, 1990). Through experimentation, it had been discovered that opium was useful in the control of mild to severe levels of pain. Further, it had been discovered that opium could be used to treat diarrhea, especially that of dysentery.[1] The ability of opioids to control anxiety and their limited antipsychotic

---

[1] Dysentery is an infection of the lower intestinal tract that results in severe pain as well as massive diarrhea, often mixed with blood and mucus. It is caused by contaminated water and was found in crowded army camps where sanitation was primitive. Unless the fluid loss is controlled, dysentery can prove rapidly fatal.

effect made them marginally effective in controlling the symptoms of psychotic disorders (Beeder & Millman, 1995; Woody, McLellan, & Bedrick 1995). Indeed, opium was used to treat so many different disorders that, until recently, it was perhaps the only medicine that physicians could prescribe with predictable results (Ray & Ksir, 1993; Reisine & Pasternak, 1995).

Although opium was long recognized as being effective, it was not until the year 1803[2] that Friedrich W. A. Serturner first isolated a pure alkaloid base from opium that was recognized as its active agent. This chemical was later called *morphine* after the Greek god of dreams, Morphius. With the discovery of morphine, researchers were one step closer to understanding how narcotic analgesics helped to control pain. As chemists explored the chemical compounds in the sap of the opium poppy, they discovered that a total of 20 distinct alkaloids in addition to morphine could be obtained from that plant (Gold, 1993; Kaplan & Sadock, 1990; Reisine & Pasternak, 1995). After these alkaloids were isolated, medical science found uses for many of the chemicals. Unfortunately, most of these alkaloids also have an abuse potential. For example, codeine, which is also obtained from the opium poppy, has a modest, but very real, abuse potential.

In 1857, about a half century after morphine was first isolated, Alexander Wood invented the hypodermic needle. This invention made it possible to quickly and relatively painlessly inject drugs directly into the body. Thus, by the middle of the 19th century, chemists were able to produce large amounts of relatively pure morphine from raw opium, while the invention of the hypodermic needle made it possible to introduce this chemical directly into the body. This invention, combined with the mistaken belief that injected morphine was not addicting, the tendency for many people to treat their own ailments with patent medicines, and the liberal use of morphine, or its parent compound opium, in battlefield hospitals in the latter half of the 1800s, resulted in a severe outbreak of opiate addiction in the United States.

It is hard to remember that in the latter half of the 19th century the world of medicine was far different than it is today. The vast majority of the people in the United States had little faith in what medical science had to offer. It was not unusual for the patient to rely on time-honored folk remedies, and patent medicines, rather than those recommended by a physician (Norris, 1994). Both cocaine and morphine were included in the remedies that were sold throughout the United States during the latter part of the 19th century, spreading the use of these medications.

All too often, the user of a patent medicine was unaware of its contents or that it was potentially addictive. In this way, large numbers of civilians became addicted to the narcotic in the patent medicine. In many other cases, the individual had started to use either opium or morphine for the control of pain, or to treat diarrhea, only to become physically dependent on the chemical. In either case, since opiates were freely available, it was not uncommon for the user to unknowingly become addicted to the opiate in the medicine. When the user tried to stop, he/she would begin to experience withdrawal symptoms. Like magic, the medicine also was effective in treating this new disorder, which went into remission for as long as the individual resumed its use. This pattern was so common that, by the year 1900, *more than 1% of the entire population of the United States* was addicted to opium or to narcotics (Restak, 1994).

In addition to addiction to narcotics through patent medicines, many people had become addicted to smoked opium. The practice of smoking opium was brought to the United States by Chinese immigrants, many of whom came to work on the railroad in the era following the Civil War. Opium smoking became somewhat popular, especially on the Pacific Coast, and by the year 1900 fully a quarter of the opium imported into this country was for smoking (Jonnes, 1995; Ray & Ksir, 1993).

Thus, by the early years of the 20th century, opiates were not only highly valued pharmaceutical agents, but drugs of abuse. Faced with an epidemic of unrestrained opiate use, the United States Congress passed the Pure Food and Drug Act of 1906. This law required manufacturers to list the ingredients of their product on the label, revealing for the first time that

---

[2] Restak (1994) gave the year in which morphine was first isolated as 1805, not 1803.

many a trusted remedy contained narcotics. Other provisions in the law, especially the Harrison Narcotics Act of 1914, prohibited the use of narcotics without a prescription signed by a physician.

Since then, the battle against narcotic abuse/addiction has waxed and waned; however, it has never disappeared. Even now, a century after the first laws were passed in an effort to control the use of narcotic analgesics, they remain a significant part of the drug abuse problem.

The Classification of Analgesics

To understand the role that narcotic analgesics play in modern medicine, it is necessary to understand something about the nature of pain. Pain is the most common, and least understood, complaint encountered by physicians (Fishman & Carr, 1992). Thus, there is a demand for medications that can control a patient's suffering. To meet this demand, researchers have developed a group of medications that collectively are known as *analgesics*. An analgesic is a chemical that is able to bring about the "relief of pain without producing general anesthesia" (Abel, 1982, p. 192).

There are two different groups of analgesics. The first are those agents that cause *local anesthesia*. Cocaine is the prototype local anesthetic. When used properly, cocaine blocks the transmission of nerve impulses from the site of the injury to the brain. In so doing, cocaine (or any of the other local anesthetics developed after cocaine) prevents the brain from receiving the nerve impulses that would otherwise transmit the pain message from the site of the injury to the brain.

The second group of analgesics are more global in nature. These drugs alter the individual's perception of pain within the central nervous system (CNS) itself. This group of analgesics was further divided into two subgroups by Abel (1982). The first of these is the *narcotic* family of drugs, which have both a central nervous system depressant capability as well as an analgesic effect. The second subgroup of global analgesics are nonnarcotic analgesics such as aspirin, acetaminophen, and similar agents. The nonnarcotic analgesics are discussed in Chapter 12. In this chapter, the narcotic analgesics are examined.

Many of the narcotic analgesics may be traced either directly or indirectly to opium. The term *opiate* was once used to designate those drugs actually derived from opium (Jaffe & Martin, 1990). Recently, a number of either synthetic or semisynthetic opiatelike painkillers have been introduced. Current terminology utilizes the term *opioid* in a generic sense, to refer to any drug that is similar to morphine in its actions. Some authors, however, utilize the terms opiate and opioid interchangeably (Jaffe & Martin). For the purpose of this text, the traditional terms opiate and narcotic will be utilized.

Where Opium Is Produced

Because the synthesis of morphine in the laboratory is difficult, most of the morphine used by physicians is still obtained from the opium poppy (Reisine & Pasternak, 1995). Thus, there is a legitimate need for the continued cultivation of the opium poppy to meet the needs of medicine. Currently, most of the legally produced opium comes from India (Sabbag, 1994). The opium raised in this one country is sufficient to meet the medical needs for narcotic analgesics for the entire world. However, illegal crops of opium poppies are raised in Southeast Asia, including Afghanistan, which is the second largest producer of illicit opium in the world. Other countries involved in the illicit opium trade include Iran, Pakistan, China, Burma, Laos, Thailand, Colombia, and Mexico (Karch, 1996; Sabbag, 1994). Thus, the supply of opioids obtained from poppies far exceeds the supply necessary to meet the world's needs for morphine. Most of this excess opium finds its way to the illicit narcotics market.

Current Medical Uses of the Narcotic Analgesics

Since the introduction of aspirin, narcotics are no longer utilized to control only mild levels of pain. As a general rule, the opiates are most commonly utilized to control acute, severe pain (Bushnell & Justins, 1993). They are occasionally used to control severe, chronic pain as well (*60 Minutes*, 1996a). In addition, they are of value in the control of severe diarrhea and control of the cough reflex in some forms of disease. Several different forms of opiates have been developed over the years, with various potencies and duration of effects. The generic and brand names of some of the more commonly used narcotic analgesics are provided in Table 11-1.

Codeine, which is an alkaloid contained in the same milky sap from the plant *Papaver somniferum* from which opium is obtained, was first isolated in 1832 (Jaffe, 1995b; Melzack, 1990). It has a mild analgesic effect, and like its chemical cousin, morphine, it is able to suppress the cough reflex. Because of these properties, codeine is frequently prescribed by physicians to help control coughing and for control of mild to moderate levels of pain. When used as an analgesic, codeine is usually administered in combination with aspirin or acetaminophen (Cherny & Foley, 1996).

Pharmacology of the Narcotic Analgesics

Although morphine was first isolated almost 200 years ago, it is still the standard against which

TABLE 11-1   Some Common Narcotic Analgesics[1]

Generic name	Brand name	Approximate equianalgesic parenteral dose
Morphine	—	10 mg every 3–4 hours
Hydromorphone	Dilaudid	1.5 mg every 3–4 hours
Meperidine	Demerol	100 mg every 3 hours
Methadone	Dolophine	10 mg every 6–8 hours
Oxymorphone	Numorphan	1 mg every 3–4 hours
Fentanyl	Sublimaze	0.1 mg every 1–2 hours
Pentazocine	Talwin	60 mg every 3–4 hours
Buprenorphine	Buprenex	0.3–0.4 mg every 6–8 hours
Codeine	—	75–130 mg every 3–4 hours[2]
Oxycodone	Perdocet, Tylox	Not available in parenteral dosage forms

Source: This chart is based on information contained in Medical Economics Company (1995), and Cherny and Foley (1996).
[1] This chart is intended for comparison use only. It is not intended to serve as, nor should it be used for, a guide to patient care.
[2] It is not recommended that doses of codeine above 65 mg be used, because doses above this level do not result in significantly increased analgesia, and may result in increased risk of unwanted side effects.

other analgesics are measured (Bushnell & Justins, 1993; Murray, DeRuyter, & Harrison, 1995). Although scientists have studied the process of pain perception for hundreds of years, up until recently they did not understand *how* the brain translated nerve impulses from an injured region of the body into the experience of pain. It has only been since the 1970s that researchers were able to unravel some of the mystery of how experience of pain is formed.

In the brain, the narcotic analgesics mimic the actions of a family of closely related chemicals known as the *opioid peptides* (Simon, 1992). There are at least 18 opioid peptides that function as neurotransmitters in the brain and spinal cord (Hirsch, Paley, & Renner, 1996). The known opioid peptides are grouped into three families known as the *endorphins*, the *enkephalins*, and the *dynorphins*.

Researchers are still trying to understand the ability of the opioid peptides to function as neurotransmitters. It is known that the opioid peptides are involved in such diverse functions as the perception of pain, moderation of emotions, the perception of anxiety, the feeling of sedation, appetite suppression, anticonvulsant activity within the brain, smooth muscle motility, regulation of a number of body functions (e.g., temperature, heart rate, respiration, blood pressure), and perhaps even the perception of pleasure (Hawkes, 1992; Restak, 1994; Simon, 1992).

As this list suggests, the opioid peptides are powerful chemicals. In contrast, morphine and its chemical cousins are only crude copies of the opioid peptides. For example, the opioid peptide known as *beta endorphin* is thought to be 200 times as potent an analgesic as morphine. Researchers believe that despite their relative weakness, narcotic analgesics have the ability to occupy receptor sites in the central nervous system normally utilized by the opioid peptides and thus simulate the action of these naturally occurring neurotransmitters.

In the past decade, researchers have identified a number of receptor sites within the brain that are utilized by the opioid peptides (Foley, 1993). There is some disagreement as to the exact number of receptor sites. However, the different receptor sites are identified by letters from the Greek alphabet. Table 11-2 summarizes what we know about the different receptor sites in the brain utilized by narcotic analgesics, and the function controlled by each receptor subtype.

One of the areas within the brain where the opioids seem to work is the medial portion of the thalamus (Restak, 1994). The thalamus seems to be involved in the perception of pain. Narcotic analgesics appear to mimic the action of the opioid peptide(s) normally found in this region of the brain, thus controlling the experience of pain. On the other hand, the experience of euphoria often reported by narcotic abusers seems to be caused by the effects of the opioids on the ventral tegmental region of the brain (Kaplan et al., 1994). This area of the brain uses dopamine as its major neurotransmitter and connects the cortex of the brain with the limbic system.

Another region of the brain rich in opioid peptide receptors is the *amygdala* (Reeves & Wedding, 1994). This region of the brain functions as a halfway point between the senses and the hypothalamus, which is the "emotion center" of the brain, according to the authors. It is thought that the amygdala will release opioid peptides in response to sensory data. By releasing opioid peptides in response to sensory inputs, the amygdala is able to influence the formation of memory. For example, the sense of pleasure that one feels on solving an

intricate mathematics problem is caused by the amygdala's release of opioid peptides. This pleasure, in turn, makes it more likely that the student will remember the solution to that problem if he/she encounters it again.

By mimicking the actions of opioid peptides in the brain, narcotic analgesics reduce the individual's awareness of pain. A further advantage of the narcotic analgesics is that analgesia is achieved without a significant loss of consciousness, although at first the patient may experience a degree of sedation (American Medical Association, 1994; Jaffe, 1992). As a result of this sedating side effect, the opiates reduce the individual's anxiety level, promote drowsiness, and allow sleep despite severe pain (Restak, 1994; Shannon et al., 1995). These latter effects seem to reflect the impact of the morphine molecule on the locus coeruleus region of the brain (Gold, 1993; Jaffe, 1992). As stated in Chapter 7, this is a region of the brain that is thought to play a role in the perception of anxiety. The locus coeruleus is also involved in the perception of pain (Miller & Gold, 1993).

Morphine

To simulate the effects of neurotransmitters found in the brain, morphine (and its chemical cousins) must be transported there from the site of administration. Morphine is well absorbed from the gastrointestinal tract. However, for reasons to be discussed, orally administered morphine is only of limited value in the control of pain. Morphine is also easily absorbed from injection sites, and because of this characteristic, it is often administered through intramuscular or intravenous injections. Finally, morphine is also easily absorbed through the mucous membranes of the body, and it is occasionally administered in the form of rectal suppositories.

The peak effects of a single dose of morphine are seen in about 60 minutes after an oral dose, and in 30 to 60 minutes when the drug is administered through intravenous injection (Shannon et al., 1995). After absorption into the circulation, morphine goes through a two-phase process of distribution throughout the body (Karch, 1996). In the first phase, which lasts only a few minutes, the morphine is distributed to various blood-rich tissues, including

TABLE 11-2 Opioid Receptors and Their Functions

Opioid receptor	Biological activity associated with opioid receptor
Mu	Analgesia, euphoria, respiratory depression, suppression of cough reflex
Delta	Analgesia, euphoria, endocrine effects, psychomotor functions
Kappa	Analgesia in spinal cord, sedation, miosis
Sigma	Dysphoria, hallucinations, increased psychomotor activity, respiratory activity
Epsilon	Unknown
Lambda	Unknown

Source: Based on information provided in Ashton (1992), and Jaffe (1989).

muscle tissue, the kidneys, liver, lungs, spleen, and the brain. In the second phase, which proceeds quite rapidly, the majority of the morphine is then biotransformed into a metabolite known as *morphine-3-glucuronide* (M3G), with a smaller amount being transformed into the metabolite *morphine-6-glucuronide* (M6G), or one of a small number of additional metabolites (Karch).

The process of morphine biotransformation takes place in the liver, and within 6 minutes of an intravenous injection, the majority of a single dose of morphine has been biotransformed into one of the two metabolites discussed in the preceding paragraph. Scientists have only recently discovered that M6G has biologically active properties, and it has been suggested that this metabolite might even be more potent than the parent compound, morphine (Karch, 1996). About 90% of morphine metabolites are eventually eliminated from the body by the kidneys (Shannon et al., 1995), while the other 10% will be excreted as unchanged morphine (Karch).

Morphine has a biological half-life of 2 to 3 hours, and approximately one-third of the morphine becomes protein-bound (Karch, 1996). The analgesic effects of a single dose of morphine last for approximately 4 hours (American Medical Association, 1994). Although it is well absorbed when administered through intramuscular or intravenous injection, morphine takes between 20 and 30 minutes to cross over through the blood-brain barrier to reach the target areas in the brain where it has its primary effect (Angier, 1990). Thus, there is a delay between the time that the narcotic analgesic is injected and when the patient begins to experience some relief from pain.

Codeine

Codeine has been found to have a number of applications in medicine. It has a mild analgesic potential and is often used in the control of mild to moderate levels of pain. About 10% of a dose of codeine is biotransformed into morphine, and it is this fraction of the total dose of codeine that reduces the individual's perception of pain (Reisine & Pasternak, 1995). Further, codeine, like many narcotic analgesics, is quite effective in the control of cough. This is accomplished through codeine's

ability to suppress the action of a portion of the brain known as the *medulla*, which is responsible for the maintenance of the body's internal state (Jaffe, 1992; Jaffe & Martin 1990). Except in extreme cases, codeine is the drug of choice for cough control (American Medical Association, 1994).

The Development of Tolerance to Narcotic Analgesics

Tolerance to the effects of the opiates develops unevenly: tolerance to the main effects and the side effects of narcotic analgesics develop at different rates. For example, tolerance to the analgesic action of opiates develops in as little as 1 to 2 weeks of regular use (Fulton & Johnson, 1993; McCaffery & Ferrell, 1994; Tyler, 1994). In contrast, however, the patient may never become fully tolerant to the ability of narcotics to affect the size of the pupil of the eyes.

As the patient gradually becomes tolerant to the analgesic effects of lower doses of a narcotic, his/her daily dosage level may be raised to levels that would literally kill a nontolerant patient. For example, a single intravenous dose of 60 mg of morphine in a single dose is potentially fatal to the opiate-naive person (Kaplan et al., 1994). In contrast, however, Fulton and Johnson (1993) gave an example of a patient whose daily morphine levels gradually increased from 60 mg/day to 3200 mg/day, before that patient died of cancer.

Drug Interactions Involving Narcotic Analgesics

The synthetic narcotic analgesic meperidine should not be used in patients who are taking, or have recently used, *monoamine oxidase inhibitors* (MAOIs, or MAO inhibitors) (Peterson, 1997). The effects of these two classes of medications could prove fatal to the patient, even if he/she stopped using MAOIs within the previous 14 days (Peterson, 1997). Patients who are taking narcotic analgesics should not use any other chemical classified as a CNS depressant, except under a physician's supervision, as there is a danger of excessive sedation from the combination of two or more CNS depressants (Ciraulo, Shader, et al., 1995).

Twenty-one of 30 methadone maintenance patients who started a course of antibiotic therapy with

Rifampin experienced opiate withdrawal symptoms that were apparently caused by an unknown interaction between the methadone and the antibiotic, according to Barnhill et al. (1995). The authors noted that the withdrawal symptoms did not manifest themselves until approximately the fifth day of Rifampin therapy, suggesting that the interaction between these two medications might require some time before symptoms are noted by the patient.

Subjective Effects of Narcotic Analgesics in Medical Practice

As stated earlier, narcotic analgesics are used for medical purposes to reduce the distress caused by pain (Thomason & Dilts, 1991). To understand how this is achieved, one must understand that pain is a multifaceted phenomenon. Melzack (1990) reported that there are actually two forms of pain. The first form, what the author termed *phasic* pain, is a sharp expression of discomfort that is experienced at the instant of injury.

Following the injury, the individual will begin to experience a steady, less intense, but more enduring form of pain known as *tonic* pain (Melzack, 1990). Not surprisingly, given the complexity of the central nervous system, there appear to be different neurological pathways for each form of pain. The neuropathways for phasic pain are naturally dampened quickly (Melzack), serving to warn the organism that injury has occurred without overwhelming it with needless pain messages. Tonic pain, on the other hand, seems to serve the function of warning the organism to rest, until recovery can take place. Where morphine is of little value in the control of phasic pain, it seems to be most suited for the enduring tonic form of pain (Fulton & Johnson, 1993; Melzack, 1990).

When therapeutic doses of morphine are given to a patient in pain, he/she will usually report that the pain becomes less intense, less discomforting, or perhaps disappears entirely (Jaffe, 1992; Reisine & Pasternak, 1995). Many factors affect the degree of analgesia achieved through the use of morphine: (a) the route by which the medication was administered, (b) the interval between doses, (c) the dosage level being used, and (d) the half-life of the specific medication being used (Fishman & Carr, 1992).

Other factors that influence the individual's experience of pain include the person's anxiety level, the person's expectations for the narcotic, the length of time the person has received narcotic analgesics, and his/her general state of tension. The more tense, frightened, and anxious a person is, the more likely he/she is to experience pain in response to a given stimuli. As discussed earlier, one effect of narcotic analgesics is to moderate some of the fear, anxiety, and tension that normally accompany pain states (Gold, 1993).

Complications Caused by Narcotic Analgesics in Medical Practice

Constriction of the Pupils

When used at therapeutic dosage levels, the opiates cause some degree of constriction of the pupils. Some patients experience constriction of the pupils even in total darkness (Shannon et al., 1995). Although this is a diagnostic sign that physicians often use to identify the opioid abuser (discussed later in this chapter), it is not *automatically* a sign that the patient is abusing his/her medication. Rather, this is a side effect of opioids that the physician expects in the patient who is using a narcotic analgesic for legitimate medical reasons, and which is unexpected in the patient who is not receiving such a medication.

Respiratory Depression

Another side effect seen at therapeutic dosage levels is some degree of respiratory depression. Although the degree of respiratory depression is not as significant when narcotics are given to a patient in pain (Bushnell & Justins, 1993), respiration may be affected for 4 or 5 hours even following a therapeutic dose of morphine (or a similar agent). For this reason, many experts advise that narcotic analgesics be used with caution in individuals who suffer from respiratory problems such as asthma, emphysema, chronic bronchitis, and pulmonary heart disease.

Some experts in the field have challenged the belief that morphine has a significant effect on respiration when used properly (Peterson, 1997; Supernaw, 1991). Peterson concluded that severe respiratory depression is uncommon in patients with no previous history of breathing problems. As these different reports suggest, physicians are still not sure how much respiratory depression can be caused by narcotic analgesics, or whether this is a problem for patients with respiratory disorders. Until a definitive answer to the question of whether narcotic analgesics cause respiratory depression, health care workers should anticipate that the narcotics will cause the respiratory center of the brain to become less sensitive to rising blood levels of carbon dioxide, and thus bring about some degree of respiratory depression (Bushnell & Justins, 1993; Thomason & Dilts, 1991).

Nausea and Vomiting

When used at therapeutic dosage levels, one common side effect of the narcotic analgesics is some degree of nausea and vomiting (Fishman & Carr, 1992). At normal dosage levels, approximately 10% to 40% of ambulatory patients experience some nausea, and approximately 15% actually vomit as a result of having received a narcotic analgesic (Cherny & Foley, 1996; Jaffe & Martin, 1990). Surprisingly, ambulatory patients seem to be most likely to experience nausea or vomiting after receiving a narcotic analgesic. Thus, patients should not walk around immediately after taking a narcotic analgesic, but should rest for a period of time.

These side effects are dose-related, that is, as the dosage level increases, these side effects are seen in a greater percentage of patients. Some individuals who are sensitive to the opiates may experience adverse reactions to narcotics at even low dosage levels. Melzack (1990) advanced the theory that the individual's response to the narcotics might be genetically mediated, and went on to hypothesize that a genetic mechanism might also account for the phenomenon of narcotics addiction.

At therapeutic dosage levels, morphine and similar drugs have been found to affect the gastrointestinal tract. One side effect of narcotic analgesics is that they can decrease the secretion of hydrochloric acid in the stomach. Also, the muscle contractions of peristalsis (which push food along the intestines) are also restricted (Shannon et al., 1995). Narcotic analgesics may actually cause spasm in the muscles involved in the process of peristalsis (Reisine & Pasternak, 1995). This is the side effect that makes

morphine so useful in the treatment of dysentery and severe diarrhea. But, for the patient who is not suffering from diarrhea, this side effect of narcotic analgesics may cause the individual to experience some degree of constipation. Indeed, constipation is the most common adverse side effect encountered when narcotic analgesics are used for extended periods (Cherny & Foley, 1996).

Other Side Effects

Another troublesome side effect of the narcotic analgesics is a stimulation of the smooth muscle tissue surrounding the bladder. This, plus a tendency for narcotic analgesics to reduce the voiding reflex, may result in a tendency for the patient to experience some degree of urinary retention (Jaffe, 1992; Tyler, 1994). Some patients who receive narcotic analgesics complain of excessive sedation and (in the case of morphine) of nightmares.

The Danger of Addiction

Many health care workers admit to being afraid that they will cause the patient to become addicted to narcotic analgesics by giving the patient too much medication. In reality, the odds that a patient with no prior history of alcohol/drug addiction will become addicted to narcotic analgesics when these medications are used for the short-term control of severe pain has been estimated at only 1:12-14,000 (Roberts & Bush, 1996). Most patients who develop a psychological dependence on opiates after receiving them for the control of pain seem to have a preexisting addictive disorder (Paris, 1996). The development of tolerance to the analgesic effects of opioids over time is a normal phenomenon and should not automatically be interpreted as a sign that the patient is becoming addicted to painkillers (Hirsch et al., 1996; McCaffery & Ferrell, 1994).

In large part because of the individual's high state of tolerance to opioids, physicians tend to *under*medicate opiate-tolerant patients prior to, and following, surgery (Imhof, 1995). Few physicians realize that those patients who have developed a tolerance to the analgesic effects of opiates, either through the legitimate use of narcotic analgesics or the abuse of opioids, will require higher-than-normal doses of opiates to control the pain of surgery. Fearing that they will bring about an overdose, or fearing that they are contributing to the patient's abuse of medications, physicians often undermedicate the patient, leaving him/her in needless pain.

Routes of Administration for Narcotic Analgesics in Medical Practice

Although the narcotic analgesics are well absorbed from the gastrointestinal tract when they are administered orally, orally administered narcotic analgesics are useful only in the control of mild to moderate levels of pain (Shannon et al., 1995). This is because the "first-pass metabolism" effect severely limits the amount of the drug that is able to reach the brain. For example, the liver biotransforms at least 80% of the morphine that is absorbed through the gastrointestinal tract *before* it reaches the brain (Tyler, 1994). Thus, orally administered narcotics are of limited value in the control of severe levels of pain. For example, to achieve the same degree of analgesia that can be accomplished by a single intramuscular injection of 10 mg of morphine, Cherny and Foley (1996) recommend that the patient receive 60 mg of morphine by mouth.

The intravenous administration of narcotics allows for the greatest degree of control over the amount of drug that actually reaches the brain. It is for this reason that the primary method of administration for narcotic analgesics is intravenous injection (Jaffe & Martin, 1990). However, there are exceptions to this rule. For example, there is a new transdermal patch, developed for the narcotic fentanyl. This is discussed in more detail in the following section.

Withdrawal from Narcotic Analgesics in Medical Practice

Most patients who receive narcotic analgesics for the control of pain, even when they do so for extended periods, are able to discontinue the medication without problems. A small number of patients develop a "discontinuance syndrome" similar to that seen in patients who receive benzodiazepines for an extended period. This syndrome is usually mild but may require that the patient gradually reduce his/her daily intake of narcotic analgesics rather than to stop using the medication all at once. Thus, narcotic

analgesics are relatively benign medications, when used properly.

Fentanyl

In 1968, a new synthetic narcotic known as *fentanyl* ("Sublimaze" is the brand name) was introduced. Because of its short duration of action, fentanyl has become an especially popular analgesic during and, immediately after, surgery (Shannon et al., 1995). It is well absorbed from muscle tissue, and a common method of administration is intramuscular (I.M.) injection. Fentanyl is also absorbed through the skin, and a transdermal patch has been developed on the theory that by slowly absorbing small amounts of fentanyl through the skin the patient can experience some relief from pain, without needing to receive repeated injections of the medication. The medication is only slowly absorbed through the skin, however, and therapeutic blood levels of fentanyl are not achieved for up to 12 hours after the individual first starts to use the patch (Tyler, 1994).

A new dosage form of fentanyl was recently introduced, fentanyl-laced candy, for use as a premedication for children about to undergo surgery ("Take Time to Smell," 1994). It is interesting to note that opium was once used in Rome to calm infants who were crying (Ray & Ksir, 1993). After thousands of years of medical progress, we have returned to the starting point of using opiates to calm the fears of children about to undergo surgery.

The Pharmacology and Subjective Effects of Fentanyl

Fentanyl is extremely potent, but there is some controversy over exactly how potent. For example, the journal *Forensic Drug Abuse Advisor* ("Take Time to Smell," 1994) suggested that fentanyl is 50 times as powerful as morphine. However, Karch (1996) suggested that fentanyl is 50 to 100 times as powerful as morphine, and Ashton (1992) suggested that fentanyl is 1,000 times as potent as morphine. Kirsch (1986) concluded that fentanyl is "approximately 3,000 times stronger than morphine, (and) 1,000 times stronger than heroin" (p. 18). According to Kirsch the active dose of fentanyl in man is one microgram. The author offered as a basis of comparison the observation that the average postage stamp weighs 60,000 micrograms. Thus, the average effective dose of fentanyl is 1/60,000 the weight of the typical postage stamp.

Fentanyl is highly lipid-soluble, and thus reaches the brain quickly after it is administered. This characteristic is of value when the drug is used in surgical procedures. The biological half-life of a single intravenous dose of fentanyl is rather short, perhaps on the order of 3 hours (Laurence & Bennett, 1992). Further, fentanyl's analgesic effect only persists for 30 to 120 minutes. The drug is rapidly biotransformed by the liver, and excreted from the body in the urine (Karch, 1996).

The effects of fentanyl on the individual's respiration might last longer than the analgesia produced by the drug (Shannon et al., 1995). This is a characteristic that must be kept in mind when the patient requires long-term analgesia. The primary reason fentanyl is so useful is that fentanyl produces a more rapid analgesic response than morphine in a medical setting. The analgesic effects of fentanyl are often seen just minutes after it was injected. This is a decided advantage when the physician seeks to control the pain of surgery or immediately after surgery.

Side Effects of Fentanyl

These may include blurred vision, a sense of euphoria, nausea, vomiting, dizziness, delirium, lowered blood pressure, constipation, possible respiratory depression, and, in extreme cases, respiratory arrest and cardiac arrest (Shannon et al., 1995). At high dosage levels, muscle rigidity is possible (Foley, 1993). Physicians have noted that, when fentanyl is administered to a patient, his/her blood pressure may drop by as much as 20% and heart rate may drop by as much as 25% (Beebe & Walley, 1991). Thus, the physician must balance the potential benefits to be gained by using fentanyl against the drug's potential to cause adverse effects. Although fentanyl is an extremely useful pharmaceutical, it is also a popular drug of abuse. This aspect of fentanyl is discussed later in this chapter.

Buprenorphine

Buprenorphine is a synthetic analgesic introduced in the 1960s that is estimated to be 25 to 40 times as potent as morphine (Singh, Mattoo, Malhotra, & Varma, 1992). Medical researchers quickly discovered that orally administered doses of buprenorphine are extremely useful in treating postoperative and cancer pain. Further, as discussed in Chapter 32, researchers have discovered that buprenorphine, when administered orally, appears to be at least as effective as methadone in blocking the effects of illicit narcotics.

Buprenorphine has a unique absorption pattern. The drug is well absorbed from intravenous and intramuscular injection sites, as well as when administered sublingually (J. Lewis, 1995). These methods of drug administration offer the advantage of rapid access to the general circulation, without the danger of first-pass metabolism. When administered orally, however, buprenorphine suffers extensive first-pass metabolism, a characteristic that limits the use of oral doses for analgesia.

On reaching the general circulation, approximately 95% of buprenorphine becomes protein-bound (Walter & Inturrisi, 1995). The drug is biotransformed by the liver, with 79% of the metabolites being excreted in the feces, and only 3.9% being excreted in the urine (Walter & Inturrise). Surprisingly, animal research suggests that the various drug metabolites are unable to cross the blood-brain barrier (BBB), according to the authors. This suggests that the drug's analgesic effects are achieved by the buprenorphine molecules that do cross the BBB to reach the brain rather than by any drug metabolites produced during the biotransformation process.

Once in the brain, buprenorphine binds to three of the same receptor sites in the brain that are utilized by morphine. Buprenorphine binds most strongly to the *Mu* and *Kappa* receptor sites, which is where narcotic analgesics tend to act to reduce the individual's perception of pain. For reasons that are still not clear, however, buprenorphine causes clinically significant levels of analgesia with a lower level of activation of the Mu receptor site than morphine causes (Negus & Woods, 1995).

Buprenorphine also tends to form weak bonds with the *Sigma* receptor site (J. Lewis, 1995). However, just because a drug is able to *bind* at a receptor site does not mean that it is always able to activate the receptor site. Buprenorphine is an excellent example of a drug that might bind to different receptor sites in the brain without having the same potential to activate these different receptor sites in the brain. In the human brain, buprenorphine easily binds to both the Mu and Kappa receptor sites. However, the drug has relatively little effect on the Kappa receptor site, while more strongly affecting the activity of the Mu receptor site (Negus & Woods, 1995).

Virtually all the drug's effects are achieved by buprenorphine's ability to bind at, and activate, the Mu opiate receptors in the brain (J. Lewis, 1995). Indeed, the drug effectively functions as a Kappa receptor site antagonist at the same dosage level that it activates the Mu opiate receptor sites in the brain to cause analgesia (Negus & Woods, 1995). Finally, buprenorphine molecules only slowly "disconnect" from their receptor sites, thus blocking large numbers of other buprenorphine molecules from reaching those same receptor sites. Thus, at high dosage levels, buprenorphine seems to act as its own antagonist, limiting its own effects.

As is obvious from this brief review of buprenorphine's pharmacology, it is a unique narcotic analgesic, which is more selective and more powerful than morphine. As discussed in the following section, however, it is slowly becoming more popular as a drug of abuse.

II. OPIATES AS DRUGS OF ABUSE

Many of the opiates are popular drugs of abuse. In this section, opiate abuse/addiction is discussed.

Overview

Why Do People Abuse Opiates?

Simply put, opiate-based analgesics are popular with illicit drug users because they make the user feel good. When they are used by people who are *not* experiencing any significant degree of pain, opioids reportedly cause the user to experience euphoria. When injected directly into the circulation, some opiates may cause the user to experience a rush or flash that is said to be similar to sexual orgasm (Bushnell & Justins, 1993; Hawkes, 1992; Jaffe, 1992, 1995b; Jaffe & Martin, 1990). Following the rush the user will experience a sense of euphoria that usually lasts for 1 to 2 minutes (Jaffe, 1995b). Finally, the user often experiences a prolonged period of blissful

drowsiness that may last several hours (Scaros, Westra, & Barone, 1990). These are characteristics that appeal to some drug users.

Neuropsychopharmacologists believe they have identified how narcotic analgesics bring about these effects. As discussed earlier in this chapter, narcotic analgesics seem to mimic the action of naturally occurring neurotransmitters. Two regions of the limbic system of the brain, the *nucleus accumbens* and the *ventral tegmentum* seem to be associated with the pleasurable response that many users report when they use opioids (Restak, 1994). Researchers believe that, by flooding these regions of the brain with narcotic analgesic molecules, the brain reacts as if massive amounts of endorphins were released.

The Mystique of Heroin

Heroin is, perhaps, the most commonly abused opiate in the United States, and it is perhaps the most destructive of the illicit drugs (Gold, 1993; Savage, 1993). Surprisingly, researchers are at a loss to explain why heroin *(diacetylmorphine)* is the preferred narcotic among opiate addicts in this country. But it is known that heroin-related deaths account for about half of all deaths from illicit drug use in the United States (Karch, 1996).

A Short History of Heroin

The drug was first developed by chemists at the Bayer pharmaceutical company of Germany, in 1898. Like morphine, heroin is obtained from raw opium. One ton of raw opium will, after processing, produce approximately 100 kilograms of heroin ("South American Drug," 1997). When the chemists who developed diacetylmorphine first tried it, they reported that the drug made them feel "heroic." Thus, the drug was given the brand name of "Heroin" (Mann & Plummer, 1991, p. 26).

Following the Civil War in the United States, there were large numbers of men who had become addicted to morphine and who used high doses of this drug to control their addiction. Because heroin was found to suppress the withdrawal symptoms of morphine addicts at low doses, physicians at the turn of the century thought it was nonaddicting, and it was initially sold as a cure for morphine addiction. It was not until 12 years later that the true addiction potential of heroin was finally recognized. By that time, many users had come to prefer heroin over morphine.

Pharmacology of Heroin

Heroin is more potent than morphine; a standard conversion formula is that 4 milligrams (mg) of heroin is as powerful as 10 mg of morphine (Brent, 1995; Lingeman, 1974). Further, because of differences in its chemical structure, heroin is much more lipid-soluble than morphine. This feature allows heroin to cross the blood-brain barrier 100 times faster than morphine (Angier, 1990). The speed with which it is able to reach the brain makes it an especially attractive drug of abuse.

In some countries, heroin is a recognized therapeutic agent, and it is manufactured by pharmaceutical companies under strict regulation and supervision for use as a medication. For example, physicians use it as an analgesic to control severe pain, especially cancer-related pain, in countries such as Canada and England. Even in these countries, however, its use is controversial (Parry, 1992). In the United States, heroin is *not* a recognized pharmaceutical, and its possession and manufacture are illegal.

Heroin in the United States Today

Although it is an illicit drug, the sale of heroin is estimated to be a $12 billion per year industry in this country (Abt Associates, 1995a). One reason for its popularity seems to be the user's *expectation* that heroin will produce a greater degree of euphoria than other opiates (Lingeman, 1974). Remember that the user's expectations play a role in the way the user interprets the drug's effect. Thus, the heroin addict's expectations help to shape his/her experience after injecting the drug. But, when injected into muscle tissue rather than directly into a vein, even experienced heroin users are unable to tell the difference between an injection of heroin and an injection of morphine.

Once in the body, the actions of heroin are similar to those of morphine. This makes sense, as morphine is a metabolite of heroin (Jaffe, 1992; Scaros et al., 1990). Once heroin is injected into the body, it is eventually biotransformed back into morphine by the liver. Surprisingly, it is not the heroin, but the

morphine that emerges from the process of biotransformation that has an analgesic potential (Reisine & Pasternak, 1995).

The main advantage of heroin for addicts is that it has only half the bulk of morphine, allowing it to be transported more easily (Lingeman, 1974). Heroin users also report that the rush they experience when they inject heroin is more intense than the rush from morphine injections. This may be because heroin is able to pass through the blood-brain barrier much faster than morphine.

Despite the introduction of new synthetic and semisynthetic opiates, heroin abuse accounts for approximately 90% of opiate abuse/addiction in the United States (Dygert & Minelli, 1993). Further, heroin is growing in popularity, especially with young users. It has been estimated that users begin to experiment with heroin at an estimated age of just over 20 years (G. Cohen et al., 1996). Heroin's popularity is such that younger drug users now prefer heroin over crack (*Addiction Letter*, 1994a; Ehrman, 1995; "Feds Say Heroin," 1994; Smolowe, 1993). However, the face of heroin abuse has changed over the past few years, as heroin users have explored new ways of abusing it.

In the mid-1980s, when the current "war on drugs" began, the average sample of heroin from the street was about 5% to 6% pure (Sabbag, 1994). Currently, researchers estimate that the heroin being sold on the street is between 65% (Gabriel, 1994) and 80% pure heroin (Office of National Drug Control Policy, 1995). The price of heroin on the street has declined by more than one-third since 1981, while the purity has increased more than 115% in that same time period ("Federal Drug Plans," 1996). These figures reflect the glut of heroin available to illicit users in the United States The high purity of heroin being sold, combined with its relatively low cost, its popularity among young adults, and the misperception that intranasal heroin is nonaddicting, all contribute to an increase in heroin use in the United States (Ehrman, 1995).

Buprenorphine

Another drug that is growing in popularity as an opiate of abuse is buprenorphine. As noted earlier, buprenorphine has been found to be a useful narcotic analgesic. Researchers are also considering oral doses of buprenorphine as an alternative to methadone (discussed in Chapter 32). Street addicts have discovered that *intravenously administered* buprenorphine has a significant abuse potential (Horgan, 1989; R. Moore, 1995). There have been reports of intravenous abuse of buprenorphine from New Zealand, Ireland, India (Singh et al., 1992), and the United States (Torrens, San, & Cami, 1993).

Researchers actually know very little about the abuse of buprenorphine (Fudala & Johnson, 1995). Apparently, the user injects either buprenorphine alone, or a mixture of buprenorphine and diazepam, cyclizine, or temazepam. While it is not clear how significant buprenorphine will be as a drug of abuse, the reader should be aware that there have been limited reports of intravenous buprenorphine abuse in this country.

Methods of Opiate Abuse

When opiates are abused, they may be injected under the skin (a subcuteaneous injection, or "skin popping"), injected directly into a vein ("mainlining"), smoked, or used intranasally. Opiates such as heroin are well absorbed through the lungs (as when it is smoked). The practice of smoking opium has not been common in the United States since the beginning of the 20th Century. Supplies of opium are limited in the United States, and opium smoking wastes much of the chemical. However, in parts of the world where supplies of opium are more plentiful, the practice of smoking opium remains common.

At this time, the practice of snorting heroin powder and smoking heroin have become popular ways of administering the drug. In some parts of the country, 60% of new heroin users snort the drug (Office of National Drug Control Policy, 1995). This change in heroin use patterns seems to reflect the attempt on the part of heroin abusers/addicts in this country to avoid exposing themselves to contaminated intravenous needles (Smolowe, 1993).

When heroin is smoked, the user heats heroin powder in a piece of aluminum foil, using a cigarette lighter or match as the heat source. The fumes are inhaled, allowing the individual to get "high" without exposure to contaminated needles ("Mixed Signals," 1991; Pinkney, 1990; Scaros et al., 1990). This practice, which is known as "chasing the dragon" (Strang, Griffiths, Powis, & Gossop, 1992), has been found in London and some isolated areas of the United States. Heroin smoking is not very effective, with approximately 80% of the heroin being destroyed by the process ("Heroin Smoking," 1996). Thus, heroin smoking is possible only when the drug is quite potent, as is the case with the heroin available on the streets at this time.

Another way that heroin is abused by smoking is the practice of smoking a combination of heroin and crack, rather than crack alone. The pellets that are smoked are called "speedball rock," "moon rock," or "parachute rock" (Dygert & Minelli, 1993). The combination of heroin and crack cocaine reportedly results in a longer high, and a less severe postcocaine use depression (Levy & Rutter, 1992). However, as discussed in Chapter 9, there is evidence that cocaine may exacerbate the respiratory depression produced by opiates.

The practice of snorting heroin is similar to the way that cocaine powder is inhaled. The user uses a razor blade or knife to dice the powder until it has a fine, talcumlike consistency. The powder then is arranged in a small pile, or a line, and inhaled through a straw.

Where Do Opioid Addicts Obtain Their Drugs?

Opiate abusers obtain their daily supply of the drug from many sources. Most street addicts buy street narcotics unless they have access to pharmaceuticals. The typical street narcotic is an opioid that has usually been smuggled into the United States, mixed with adulterants, then distributed for sale on the local level. The narcotics are usually sold in a powder form, in small individual packets. The powder is mixed with water, then heated in a small container (usually a spoon) over a flame (generally from a cigarette lighter or candle) to help dissolve the drug, and then is injected.

Health care professionals, with access to pharmaceutical supplies, may divert medications to themselves, although this is difficult because of the rigid controls on supplies of narcotics. Other users purchase pharmaceuticals that have been diverted to the illicit drug market. Pharmaceuticals are medications intended for legal use that have been diverted to the streets. Some opioid addicts have been known to befriend a person with a terminal illness, such as cancer, in order to steal narcotic analgesics from the suffering patient for their own use.

Users often inject the pharmaceutical, although some abusers ingest opioids. Those who inject a pharmaceutical usually either crush the tablet until it is a fine powder or take the capsule apart, and then mix the powder with water. This mixture is heated in the same manner as street drugs. The method of injection used by intravenous opiate abusers differs from the manner in which a physician or nurse injects medication into a vein. Lingeman (1974) observed that the technique used is called "booting" and described the process as one in which the narcotic is injected into the vein:

> a little at a time, letting it back up into the eye dropper, injecting a little more, letting the blood-heroin mixture back up, and so on. The addict believes that this technique prolongs the initial pleasurable sensation of the heroin as it first takes effect—a feeling of warmth in the abdomen, euphoria, and sometimes a sensation similar to an orgasm. (p. 32)

In the process, however, the hypodermic needle and the syringe (or the eye dropper attached to a hypodermic needle, a common substitute for a hypodermic needle) become contaminated with the individual's blood. When other addicts use the same needle, as is commonly done both by cocaine and opiate addicts, contaminated blood from one individual is passed to the next, and the next, and the next.... For this reason, many heroin addicts now choose to either smoke heroin or snort heroin powder, rather than to run the risk of exposing themselves to AIDS through an intravenous needle that may, or may not, be contaminated.

Sometimes, the narcotic analgesic abuser uses a pharmaceutical tablet or capsule originally intended for oral ingestion as the source of the drug to be injected. This practice inserts starch or other fillers not intended for intravenous use directly into the bloodstream (Wetli, 1987). Normally, fillers are mixed with oral medication to give it body and form. The chemical properties of these fillers are such that they are usually either destroyed by stomach acid when the medication is taken orally or at least

prevented from being absorbed into the body. In the latter case, the filler will harmlessly pass through the body and be excreted. But when tablets or capsules are used for intravenous use, the fillers cannot be inactivated by the body's defenses. Further, repeated exposure to pharmaceutical fillers, or the adulterants often found in street drugs, can cause extensive scarring at the point of injection. These scars form the famous "tracks" caused by repeated injections of illicit narcotics.

The Development of Tolerance

Over time, opiate abusers become tolerant to the euphoric effects of narcotics. As a result, they do not experience the rush or flash from opiates with the same intensity as they did when they first started to use these drugs. It is thought that the chronic use of narcotic analgesics causes the brain to reduce the amount of endorphines that it produces (Klein & Miller, 1986). Over time, the brain substitutes the chemical opiates for natural endorphines, and the effect of the narcotics becomes less intense.

Eventually, the user ceases to experience much euphoria at all from narcotic analgesics. There appears to be a "threshold effect" (Parry, 1992, p. 350) or a level after which the user will experience a "stable genial state" (p. 350) without becoming high on the narcotic. The chronic opioid user who reaches this state is no longer using the drug to get high. At this point, the individual is taking narcotics just to function in a normal state.

Both in the medical setting, and when abused, tolerance to each of the effects of the opiates develops at a different rate (Jaffe, 1989). For example, the individual can develop "remarkable tolerance" (Jaffe, p. 649) to both the analgesic and respiratory depressant effect of opiates, but still experience significant constipation as a result of opiate use/abuse. Thus, chronic abuse of narcotics can (and often does) cause significant constipation problems for the illicit narcotic user (Reisine & Pasternak, 1995).

Scope of the Problem of Opiate Abuse and Addiction in the United States

Although addiction to narcotic analgesics has been a problem for society for more than a century, researchers still know very little about the scope of opioid abuse and addiction. In the late 1960s, it was hypothesized that "the majority [of heroin abusers] go on to mainlining" (Lingeman, 1974, p. 106). Forty years later, researchers have come to believe that only a fraction of those who *briefly* experiment with opiates for recreational purposes become addicted (Jaffe, 1989).[3] The team of Anthony, Arria, and Johnson (1995) estimated that 1.5% of the population between the ages of 15 and 54 had used heroin at least once, but, that only 0.4% of this age group, or 26% of those who had tried heroin at least once, went on to become addicted to it. Jenike (1991), however, thought that approximately half of those who repeatedly use an opioid for recreational purposes become addicted.

For the typical heroin addict, there is a 2-year period between the initial use of opioids and, the development of physical addiction to the drug (Hoegerman & Schnoll, 1991). However, there are many variations on this pattern. Physical addiction to an opioid can develop quite rapidly. Indeed, an addiction to narcotics could develop in "less than two weeks" (p. 4), if the drugs were abused on a daily basis in regularly increasing doses. Thus, while opioids do not seem to be quite as addictive as the popular press portrays them as being, they have a significant addictive potential. Despite this potential, however, opiates are popular drugs of abuse.

Researchers have long been aware that some individuals apparently are able to occasionally abuse opiates, without becoming addicted (Shiffman, Fischer, Zettler-Segal, & Benowitz, 1990). These users are called "chippers," and may constitute 40% to 50% of the people who abuse heroin (Sabbag, 1994). Chippers seem to use opiates more in response to social stimuli than because of internal or pharmacological reasons and seem to have no trouble abstaining from opiates when they wish to do so.

Each year in the United States, between 10 and 15 metric tons of heroin are consumed (Leland, Katel, & Hager, 1996). Since heroin is, by definition, an illegal substance in the United States, all this heroin is consumed by illicit users. Estimates of the scope of heroin abuse/addiction in the United States vary. O'Brien (1996) estimated that there were between 750,000 and 1 million heroin users in the United States, but did not attempt to identify what percentage of this number were actually addicted to the drug. In contrast, Foley (1993) suggested that there were 1 million people in the United States who were intravenous heroin users, but were not addicted to the drug. The team of Nash and Park (1997) estimated that some 200,000 people in the United States had used heroin in the preceeding 30 days.

Dygert and Minelli (1993) gave an estimate of 3.5 million intravenous heroin abusers, who were not addicted to the drug. Finally, the Council on Addiction Psychiatry of the American Psychiatric Association (1994) estimated that there were "over 1 million chronic, hard-core intravenous heroin abusers" (p. 792) in the United States, but did not define the criteria by which they classified a person as being a "hard-core" heroin user.

The scope of heroin addiction in the United States is the subject of much controversy. The lowest estimates suggest that between 400,000 and 600,000 people in the United States are addicted to heroin (Kaplan et al., 1994; Kurtz, 1995). The highest estimate suggests that 1 million people in the United States are addicted to heroin (*Fighting Drug Abuse*, 1992). Researchers generally agree that the typical heroin addict is estimated to have to spend about $250 a week to buy the drugs necessary to support his/her habit (Abt Associates, 1995a). Further, researchers agree that males make up about three-fourths of the total number addicted to this drug (Kaplan & Sadock, 1990). But this ratio also suggests that of the estimated 600,000 heroin addicts in this country, perhaps 350,000 are males, and 150,000 are female. If the higher estimate of 1 million active narcotics addicts is used, then some 250,000 women are addicted to narcotics in this country.

Heroin-addicted persons are thought to be concentrated on the coasts. It is estimated that between 200,000 (Eisenhandler & Drucker, 1993; Ross, 1991) and 300,000 (Kaplan et al., 1994) heroin addicts live in New York City (Sabbag, 1994). Another 275,000 are thought to be concentrated in California (Pinkney, 1990). Despite the much publicized

[3] However, because it is not possible to predict who will become addicted, and who will not, the recreational use of narcotic analgesics is *not* recommended.

war on drugs of the past generation, heroin has again become a popular drug of abuse (Leland et al., 1996).

Virtually everything that we think we know about people who are addicted to narcotic analgesics is based on those people who utilize treatment programs in public hospitals (Kurtz, 1995). But, there are opiate addicts who hold stable jobs, with health insurance benefits, who receive health care through private health providers, and who do not support their chemical use through criminal activity (Eisenhandler & Drucker, 1993; Kurtz, 1995). Very little is known about this subpopulation of opiate addicts.

To examine the possibility that there was such an unknown subpopulation of people who were dependent on narcotic analgesics, Eisenhandler and Drucker (1993) examined the insurance records of 6.5 million hospital admissions over a 10-year period starting in 1982, and identified 31,810 cases where a patient hospitalized for treatment of opiate dependency had private health care insurance. The authors went on to estimate that 1% to 2% of those insured by private health care insurance were actually intravenous drug users. Since the majority of intravenous drug abusers inject narcotics, these findings suggest that a significant number of narcotics addicts are employed, have private health care coverage, and have never been identified as narcotics addicts by public service agencies. Virtually nothing is known about this subpopulation of addicted individuals, although they constitute part of the problem of opiate addiction in this country.

Do Some Factors Predispose One to Become a Narcotics Addict?

The traditional psychoanalytic view of addiction is that there is a dynamic interaction between the psychological distress that a person might experience, and the vulnerability of that person to develop an addiction. Psychoanalytic theorists have suggested, for example, that opiate addicts are drawn to narcotics because of the drug's ability to help them control powerful feelings of rage and anger.

However, clinical research data does not fully support the psychological vulnerability hypothesis central to the psychoanalytic model of narcotics addiction although it does suggest perhaps as many as 50% of those who abuse narcotics have suffered from periods of depression (Melzack, 1990). Further, those individuals who are actively using narcotics on a daily basis appear to be significantly more depressed than those who occasionally abuse opioids, and both groups are more depressed than those who do not use narcotics (Maddux, Desmond, & Costello, 1987).

However, the dysphoria so often seen in chronic opioid users seems to be a "pharmacological consequence" (Handelsman, Aronson, Ness, Cochrane, & Kanof, 1992, p. 284) of the chronic use of narcotics. The authors suggested that the depression and anxiety so often found in opioid addicts is a result of prolonged chemical use, not a cause of it. Support for this theory was provided by Kanof, Aronson, and Ness (1993). The authors of this study found that addicts who were gradually withdrawn from methadone after being part of a methadone maintenance program for extended periods experienced episodes of depression that sometimes lasted for several weeks after detoxification. They attributed this finding to the individual's prior use of narcotics, rather than to the process of withdrawal or a preexisting depressive state by the individual.

One consequence of the drug-related depression seen in narcotics addiction is that, for the recovering addict, feelings of dysphoria may serve as a cue that triggers further opiate use/abuse. Unless the individual is aware that dysphoric feelings are a consequence of prolonged heroin use, he/she may confuse the withdrawal-related dysphoria with "unhappy feelings that might have prompted experimentation with heroin in the first place" (Handelsman et al., 1992, p. 285). The question of whether narcotics addicts use opioids to self-medicate emotional pain or experience emotional pain as a pharmacological consequence of prolonged chemical use has yet to be answered to the satisfaction of all involved.

Withdrawal from Opioids for the Addicted Person

The hallmark sign of an addiction to opiates is the classic pattern of opioid withdrawal symptoms. These symptoms vary in intensity depending on three factors: (a) the dose of the opiate that was abused, (b) the length of time that the person has used the drug, and, (c) the speed with which withdrawal is attempted (Jaffe, 1989).

In other words, in theory an opiate addict who has been using the equivalent of 50 mg of morphine a day for 3 months will have an easier detoxification than would another individual who has been using the equivalent of 50 mg of morphine a day for 3 years. Also, an opiate addict who is gradually withdrawn from opiates at the rate of the equivalent of 10 mg of morphine a day will have an easier detoxification than would the opiate-dependent person who suddenly stops using the drug (goes "cold turkey").

The individual's perception of, and response to, the withdrawal process is influenced to a large degree by his/her cognitive set. This set is, in turn, influenced by the individual's knowledge, attention, motivation, and suggestibility. In the final analysis, the level of discomfort experienced by an individual during opiate withdrawal is a learned phenomenon. This phenomenon might be confirmed in real-life settings, where narcotics addicts are forced to go through the withdrawal process cold turkey. Individuals in a therapeutic community that actively discourages reports of withdrawal discomfort do not go through the dramatic withdrawal displays so often noted in methadone detoxification programs (Peele, 1985). Further, when the narcotics addict is incarcerated and denied further access to the drug, the individual is often able to go through withdrawal without the dramatic withdrawal seen at a detoxification center.

Acute Withdrawal

In general, opiate withdrawal symptoms begin 6 to 12 hours after the last dose of heroin (Gold, 1993; Jaffe, 1989; Weiss et al., 1994). To avoid these withdrawal symptoms, the addict must either inject the drug again or substitute the use of another drug. Withdrawal symptoms include a craving for more narcotics, tearing of the eyes, running nose, repeated yawning, sweating, restless sleep, dilated pupils, anxiety, anorexia, irritability, insomnia, weakness, abdominal pain, nausea, vomiting, gastrointestinal upset, chills, diarrhea, muscle spasms and muscle aches, irritability, and, in male addicts, possible ejaculation (Gold, 1993; Hoegerman & Schnoll, 1991; Scaros et al., 1990). Constipation is

a potential complication of narcotics withdrawal, which, in rare cases, can result in fecal impaction, and intestinal obstruction (Jaffe, 1989, 1990).

Some researchers believe that the withdrawal symptoms might make the person so uncomfortable as to reinforce the tendency toward continued drug use (Bauman, 1988). This is true even if the initial rush is no longer experienced because of drug tolerance (Jaffe, 1986, 1989). Research has suggested that perhaps 22% to 35% of opiate addicts have a pathological fear of detoxification that is almost phobic in intensity (Milby et al., 1994). Many opiate addicts may continue to use these drugs after they have developed tolerance to the chemical's euphoric effects because they are afraid of the possible discomfort of withdrawal.

Opiate addicts in a medical setting often emphasize the distress that they experience during withdrawal. While such displays are often quite dramatic, withdrawal from narcotics may be uncomfortable, but it is not fatal (Henry, 1996; Mattick & Hall, 1996). The only possible exception to this rule is for the infant who is born addicted to narcotics (Group for the Advancement of Psychiatry, 1990; Washton, 1995). For the average opiate-dependent adult, the level of withdrawal process causes about as much distress as an adult experiences during a bad case of influenza (Mattick & Hall, 1996).

Thus, the opiate withdrawal process is "seldom a medical emergency" (Kaplan & Sadock, 1990, p. 40).[4] However, opiate-dependent individuals often put on dramatic displays of their suffering while being detoxified from narcotics, to try to obtain more drugs from staff. Jenike (1991) gave several examples of the manipulativeness demonstrated by addicts in maintaining their drug habits. However, symptoms of the opiate withdrawal syndrome eventually abate in the healthy individual, even in the absence of treatment.

Extended Withdrawal Symptoms

There is evidence of a second phase of withdrawal from narcotics that lasts beyond the period of acute

---

[4]This assumes that the patient is using *only* opioids. A physician should supervise *any* drug withdrawal program to reduce potential danger to life that may exist if the patient is a polydrug user.

withdrawal. During this extended phase of withdrawal, which may last for several months, the individual may experience feelings of fatigue, heart palpitations, and a general feeling of restlessness (Satel et al., 1993). This phase of protracted abstinence may extend for up to 30 weeks after acute withdrawal (O'Brien, 1996; Satel et al., 1993).

During this stage of protracted abstinence, the physical functioning of the individual slowly returns to normal. The authors support this hypothetical phase of protracted abstinence by citing research studies that have found significant changes in respiration rate, size of the pupils of the eyes, blood pressure changes, and body temperature changes in recovering narcotics addicts for more than 17 weeks after the last dose of narcotics. However, Mattick and Hall (1996) suggested that the case for a protracted phase of withdrawal is quite weak, and that this phenomenon is not an accepted part of the recovery process from opiate addiction.

A rarely studied aspect of narcotics abuse is the tendency for addicts to attempt withdrawal on their own. Gossop, Battersby, and Strang (1991) examined a group of 47 narcotics addicts in England, and found that their sample had a total of 212 "informal" detoxification episodes. The most common method for self-detoxification was simply going "cold turkey," although a significant number of these attempts used either benzodiazepines or other narcotics to control the withdrawal symptoms. The authors concluded that very little is known about the phenomenon of self-detoxification, and suggested that written guidelines for the addict who wants to quit on his/her own might be of value.

Complications Caused by Opiate Abuse and Addiction

Surprisingly, in light of the reputation that narcotics have for wrecking lives, there is relatively little evidence to suggest permanent organ damage from the chronic administration of pharmaceutical opiates (Jaffe, 1992). Indeed, patients in extreme pain (e.g., as in some forms of cancer) receive massive doses of narcotic analgesics for extended periods, without showing evidence of opiate-induced damage to any of the body's organ systems.

This is consistent with historical evidence from earlier this century, where cases would come to light where a physician (or, less often, a nurse) had been addicted to morphine for years, or even decades. These incidents were not uncommon in the era prior to the development of strict government guidelines for the accountability of each dose of narcotic analgesic purchased by a physician or health care facility. The health care professional involved would take care to utilize proper "sterile" technique, thus avoiding the danger of infections inherent in using contaminated needles. With the exception of his/her opiate addiction, the addicted physician or nurse would appear to be in good health. For example, the famed surgeon William Halsted was addicted to morphine for 50 years, without suffering any apparent physical problems (T. Smith, 1994).

However, health care professionals have access to pharmaceutical quality narcotic analgesics, not a street drugs. The typical opiate addict must inject drugs purchased from illitic sources, of questionable purity. In addition to this, the lifestyle of the opioid addict carries with it serious health risks. Common health complications found in heroin abusers include cerebral vascular accidents (CVAs, or "strokes"), infectious endocarditis, liver failure, disorders of the body's blood clot formation mechanisms, malignant hypertension, heroin-related nephropathy, and uremia (Brust, 1993). Morphine abuse also has been implicated as a cause of decreased sexual desire for both men and women, as well as causing erectile problems in men (Finger et al., 1997).

It is not clear whether these effects are due directly to the abuse of heroin or to the fillers that are added to illicit opiates (for more information on drug fillers, see Chapter 34). However, one complication of intravenous heroin abuse/addiction that occasionally develops in some users is what is known as *cotton fever* (Brent, 1995). On occasion, heroin abusers try to "purify" the heroin by using wads of cotton as a crude filter. During times of hardship, users who cannot afford heroin supplies sometimes try to use the residual heroin in the cotton they previously used as a filter. When they inject the mixture, the microscopic cotton particles as well as the impurities filtered out by the cotton, often cause pulmonary arteritis (a serious medical condition involving inflammation of the pulmonary artery).

Medical researchers are still not sure whether prolonged exposure to narcotic analgesics is entirely harmless. Some researchers believe:

> Prolonged exposure to opioids induces, in some individuals, long-lasting adaptive changes that require continued administration of an opioid to maintain normal mood states and normal responses to stress. (Jaffe, 1992, p. 193)

As discussed later in this book, there are those who believe that even a single dose of narcotics brings about physical changes within the brain (Dole, 1988, 1989; Dole & Nyswander, 1965). After these physical changes supposedly take place, it is thought that the individual requires a constant supply of opioids to function on a normal level. This is the theory behind methadone maintenance programs. However, this theory has been challenged (Peele, 1989; Peele et al., 1991), and it is not universally accepted. For example, Hartman (1995) stated that opiates, including heroin, do not appear to have neurotoxic effects on human cognition.

When abused at high dosage levels, narcotics are capable of causing seizures (Foley, 1993). This rare complication usually responds to the effects of a narcotics blocker such as Narcan (naloxone), according to the author. One exception to this rule is seizures caused by the drug meperidine. Naloxone may actually reduce the patient's seizure threshold, making it more likely that he/she will continue to experience meperidine-induced seizures (Foley). Thus, the physician must identify the specific narcotic(s) being abused to initiate the proper intervention for opioid-induced seizures.

Despite these effects, however, there is little evidence to suggest that the narcotics are, by themselves, able to bring about the same level of toxic effects associated with other drugs of abuse.

Opiate Overdose

There are a number of reasons for overdoses by opiate abusers. For example, it is difficult to estimate the potency of illicit narcotics, and the user may miscalculate the amount of heroin that can safely be injected, bringing on an overdose. Some of these individuals die before they reach the hospital, but others survive long enough for health care professionals to intervene, and rescue them from the effects of the drug overdose.

An overdose of narcotics produces a characteristic pattern of reduced consciousness, pinpoint pupils, and respiratory depression (Henry, 1996). Death is often caused by respiratory arrest (Hirsch et al., 1996; Thomason & Dilts, 1991). Without medical intervention, death usually occurs 5 to 10 minutes following an intravenous injection of an opiate overdose, and 30 to 90 minutes following an intramuscular injection of an overdose of narcotic analgesics (Hirsch et al.). However, this data applies only for cases of overdose with pharmaceutical opiates. Medical experts are still not sure whether deaths from illicit narcotics are caused by the drugs themselves or by the multitude of other chemicals commonly added to street narcotics to dilute them.

Scaros et al. (1990) reported that a typical sample of street heroin also contains between 68 and 314 mg of quinine, which is a common adulterant. If the addict draws out the injection of heroin for a 10-second period, by slowly injecting the drug, then he/she will be injecting between 10 and 131 mg of quinine per second. This is a rate of injection *up to 182 times the maximum recommended rate of injection of quinine*. This rate of quinine injection is, in itself, capable of causing a fatal reaction in many individuals. Thus, some question exists as to whether deaths by "narcotics overdoses" are indeed caused by the narcotics, or, by other substances mixed in with narcotics sold on the streets.

Street Myths and Narcotics Overdose

There are several street myths about the treatment of opiate overdose. First, there is the myth that cocaine (or another CNS stimulant) helps in the control of an opiate overdose. Another myth is that it is possible to control the symptoms of an overdose by putting ice packs under the arms and on the groin of the overdose victim. A third myth concerning the narcotics overdose is that the person who had the overdose should be kept awake and walking around until the drug wears off.

The treatment of an opiate overdose is a complicated matter, that does not lend itself to such easy solutions. Even in the best equipped hospital, a narcotics overdose may result in death. The current treatment of choice for a narcotics overdose is a combination of respiratory and cardiac support, as well as a trial dose of *Narcan* (naloxone hydrochloride) (Henry, 1996). Naloxone hydrochloride is thought to bind at the receptor sites within the brain occupied by opiate molecules, displacing them from the receptors and reversing the effects of the opiate overdose.

Naloxone has a therapeutic half-life of only 60 to 90 minutes. Its effects are thus short-lived, and it may be necessary for the patient to receive several doses to fully recover from the opiate overdose (D. Roberts, 1995). Although naloxone-induced complications are rare, they occasionally develop when this drug is used to treat opiate overdoses (Henry, 1996). Finally, the patient may have ingested or injected a number of different chemicals, each of which has its own toxicological profile. For these reasons, keep in mind that *known or suspected opiate overdoses are life-threatening emergencies that always require immediate medical support and treatment.*

Is Treatment of Opiate Addiction Worthwhile?

There is a general belief that, once an opiate addict, always an addict, and that treatment for narcotic addiction has a poor prognosis. There seems to be some basis for this pessimism since research has found that 90% of opiate-dependent individuals who are withdrawn successfully from narcotics return to chemical use within 6 months (Schuckit, 1995a). Another pessimistic view of the evolution of narcotics addiction was provided by Hser, Anglin, and Powers (1993). The authors interviewed 581 individuals who were originally identified as addicts by the criminal justice system in the period from 1962 until 1964.

Twenty-four years later, in 1986, the authors found that only 22% of the original sample of 581 narcotics addicts were opiate-free in 1986. Some 7% of the original sample were involved in a methadone maintenance program, and 10% reported engaging in only occasional narcotics use. Almost 28% of the original sample had died, with the main causes of death being homicide, suicide, and accidents, in that order.

After reviewing their data, Hser et al. (1993) concluded that if the narcotics addicts in their sample had not stopped chemical use by their late 30s, they were unlikely to do so; the research team reinterviewed these individuals. They found that a greater percentage of addicts had died than had achieved abstinence by 1986. This is indeed a pessimistic view of the course of narcotics addiction. However, other studies have concluded that more than a third of all opiate addicts ultimately achieve and retain sobriety. For those addicts who survive their addiction, abstinence from opiate use is finally achieved in 6 (T. Smith, 1994) to 9 (Jaffe, 1989; Jenike, 1991) years after the addiction first developed.

Summary

The narcotic family of drugs has been effectively utilized by physicians for several thousand years. After alcohol, the narcotics might be thought of as humans' oldest drug. Members of the narcotic family of drugs have been found to be effective in the control of severe pain, severe cough, and severe diarrhea. The only factor that limits their application in the control of less severe conditions is the addiction potential that this family of drugs represents. The addiction potential of narcotics has been known for hundreds, if not thousands, of years. Opiate addiction was a common complication of military service in the nineteenth century and was called the "Soldier's disease."

It was not until the advent of the chemical revolution, however, when synthetic narcotics were first developed, that new forms of narcotic analgesics became available to drug users. Fentanyl and its chemical cousins are products of the pharmacological revolution that began in the late 1800s and that continues to this very day. This chemical is estimated to be several hundred, to several thousand, times as powerful as morphine, and promises to remain a part of the drug abuse problem for generations to come.

Over-the-Counter Analgesics

Unexpected Agents of Abuse

Medications used in the control of pain can be classified into three different groups. First, there are the *local anesthetics*, medications that interfere with the transmission of pain messages from the site of the injury to the brain. Cocaine is one such agent, and although it has been replaced by newer medications, it was once the local anesthetic of choice for many purposes. Even now, cocaine is still occasionally used by physicians under special circumstances, as it offers a number of advantages over other medications.

The next group of medications are the *global analgesics*. These drugs work within the brain to nonselectively alter the individual's perception of pain. The drugs in the narcotic family are most frequently utilized as global analgesics.

Finally, there are the *nonnarcotic analgesics*, which are thought to interrupt the chemical sequence that results in pain at the site of an injury. This latter class of medications includes aspirin,[1] ibuprofen, naproxen,[2] and acetaminophen, chemicals that are normally considered over-the-counter (or OTC) medications.[3] Cocaine and the narcotic analgesics have been reviewed in earlier chapters. In this chapter, we discuss the most popular OTC analgesics.

A Short History of Pain Management

Until the introduction of aspirin in the late 1800s, physicians were forced to use narcotic-based analgesics in the control of even mild to moderate levels of pain. However, the opiates are addictive and have a depressant effect on the central nervous system. These factors limited the usefulness of the opiates in the control of pain and made physicians hesitate to utilize narcotic-based analgesics except in the case of severe pain (Giacona, Dahl, & Hare, 1987).

Aspirin, or *acetylsalicylic acid*, was developed from silicin, which is found in the bark of certain willow trees. Aspirin was first developed in 1827, but was not commercially marketed until 1898 (Gay, 1990; Mann & Plummer, 1991). Actually, the very term *aspirin* is a historical accident. The Bayer pharmaceuticals company introduced "Aspirin" (with a capital "A") as the brand name for acetylsalicylic acid around the turn of the century. Over time, however, aspirin (with a small "a") has come to mean *any* preparation of acetylsalicylic acid. The manner in which this happened lies beyond the scope of this chapter, but is reviewed in excellent detail by Mann and Plummer (1991).

Shortly after it was isolated, researchers quickly discovered that aspirin is effective in controlling

---

[1] Aspirin belongs to a family of related compounds, many of which have some analgesic, antiinflammatory, antipyretic (or, antifever) action. However, since these other aspirinlike chemical compounds are not as powerful as aspirin, they will not be discussed.

[2] Naproxen was available only by prescription until 1994, when it was approved for use as an over-the-counter sales, in modified dosage levels.

[3] An over-the-counter medication is one that can be legally purchased without a prescription.

mild to moderate levels of pain, while avoiding the danger of addiction found with the narcotic family of analgesics. Further, aspirin was found to have other applications that the narcotic family of analgesics did not, such as the control of inflammation and its ability to reduce fever. Because of its multiple uses, aspirin has become the most frequently used drug in the world (Mann & Plummer, 1991). In 1993, the estimated worldwide consumption was 38,000 tons (76 million pounds) (Castleman, 1994). In the United States alone, 80 million aspirin tablets are consumed each day (Graedon & Ferguson, 1993; Graedon & Graedon, 1996; Stolberg, 1994).

Since the 1950s, four other OTC analgesics have been introduced: ibuprofen, acetaminophen, naproxen, and ketoprofen. Since the time of their introduction, these aspirinlike OTC analgesics have collectively come to take the lion's share of the $2.7 billion spent on OTC analgesics in the United States in 1990 away from aspirin. However, aspirin remains a popular OTC analgesic, and it still accounts for 28% of the OTC analgesic sales in this country ("Take 2 Aspirins," 1994).

Acetaminophen was introduced as an OTC analgesic in this country in the 1950s. The term "acetaminophen" is based on a form of chemical shorthand. The true name of this chemical is N-acetyl-para-aminophenol, from which the term acetaminophen is obtained. The drug was actually first isolated in 1878, and its ability to reduce fever was identified shortly after its discovery. But at the time, it was thought that acetaminophen would share the dangerous side effects found in a close chemical cousin, para-aminophenol. So it was set aside, and chemists did not pay much attention to this chemical for many years (Mann & Plummer, 1991).

In the early 1950s, sufficient evidence had accumulated to show that acetaminophen was much safer than para-aminophenol and that it did not have the same potential for harm found in aspirin. A massive advertising campaign followed the introduction of acetaminophen, playing on the fact that aspirin might irritate the stomach, while acetaminophen does not. By the early 1970s, acetaminophen had carved a small, but respectable, niche for itself in the OTC analgesic market. By 1996, acetaminophen

had become the most popular OTC analgesic in the United States ("Strong Medicine," 1995).

Ibuprofen emerged as a prescription-only drug in the United States in 1974, following an extensive search by pharmaceutical companies for a drug with the effectiveness of aspirin, but without its side effects. In 1984, the Food and Drug Administration approved the sale of ibuprofen without prescription, in modified dosage forms. Since its introduction as an OTC medication, ibuprofen has become the second most popular OTC analgesic in the United States ("Strong Medicine," 1995).

The Food and Drug Administration of the United States Government granted permission for *naproxen* to be classified as an over-the-counter medication in 1994. Prior to this time, naproxen was available only as a prescribed medication. In the OTC form, it is expected that naproxen will be recommended for treating the aches and pains of the common cold, headache, minor dental pain, the discomfort of menstrual cramps, and in reducing fever (Gannon, 1994). Naproxen has not been available as an OTC medication for a long enough period to determine how popular it will be with consumers. However, there is a very good chance that it will become a popular OTC medication and will capture some of the market now held by aspirin and ibuprofen (Gannon, 1994).

While these medications are indeed useful, since the early 1990s physicians have discovered that they are far more toxic to the user, even at normal dosage levels, than had been thought earlier ("Strong Medicine," 1995). Aspirin itself was introduced before the modern rules and regulations that govern medication distribution in this country were developed. The truth is that aspirin is such a potent drug that, were it to be discovered today rather than a century ago, its use would be closely regulated and it would be available only by prescription (Graedon & Ferguson, 1993).

Further, although the OTC analgesics are not recreational drugs in the traditional sense of the word, they all have an abuse potential. Even naproxen, which until recently had only been available by prescription, had a history of occasionally being abused by patients who were taking it under a physician's supervision. Further, each chemical has been found to have potentially harmful side effects, under certain conditions. Thus chemical dependency professionals should have a working knowledge of the OTC analgesics.

Medical Uses of the OTC Analgesics

The Origin of the Term NSAID

Aspirin, ibuprofen, and naproxen all have an antiinflammatory effect. But, if one were to examine the chemical structure of these drugs, it would become clear that they have a different chemical structure than the steroids, another class of antiinflammatory drugs. Because of this, they are often called Non-Steroidal AntiInflammatory Drugs (or, NSAIDs).

Aspirin

Scientists are still discovering new uses for the oldest OTC analgesic in use, aspirin. Aspirin is used in the control of mild to moderate levels of pain (Giacona et al., 1987; Supernaw, 1991). Aspirin has also been found effective in treating common headaches, neuralgia, the pain associated with oral surgery, toothache, and musculosketal pain (Giacona et al.). There is evidence that aspirin might slow the development of cataracts (Payan & Katzung, 1995). Further, just one aspirin tablet every other day has been found to reduce the frequency of migraines by 20% in some patients with this disorder (Gilman, 1992; Graedon & Ferguson, 1993; Graedon & Graedon, 1991).

In addition, there is evidence to suggest that aspirin might be of value in controlling a form of hypertension that occasionally complicates pregnancy (Graedon & Ferguson, 1993; Graedon & Graedon, 1991; Patrono, 1994). Further, aspirin has been found to be helpful in relieving the symptoms of dysmenorrhea, and reducing inflammation; and despite its age, aspirin is still the most effective drug available to reduce fever (Payan & Katzung, 1995).

This latter effect is brought on, in part, by aspirin's ability to cause peripheral vasodilation and sweating in the patient, which helps lower the body temperature (Shannon et al., 1995). Aspirin also is thought to interfere with prostaglandin production in the hypothalamus, a region of the brain that helps

to control temperature (Laurence & Bennett, 1992). This effect, in turn, helps to limit fever (but does not lower the body temperature below normal).

Surprisingly, since it has been in use for more than a century, physicians have only recently discovered that it may be an important adjunct to the treatment of either the initial or subsequent myocardial infarction (a "heart attack") (Shannon et al., 1995; American Society of Hospital Pharmacists, 1994; "Aspirin for Prevention," 1989; "Aspirin Reduces," 1989). There is even evidence that low doses of aspirin may be of value in the treatment of an evolving myocardial infarction in which a blood vessel is blocked by a blood clot (Graedon & Graedon, 1996; Hennekens, Jonas, & Buring, 1994; Patrono, 1994; Stolberg, 1994).

Aspirin's utility in the fight against cardiovascular disease was discovered in a research project involving 22,000 male physicians that began in the 1980s (Ridker, Cushman, Stampfer, Tracy, & Hennekens, 1997). The authors examined the level of a chemical in the blood known as the *C-reactive protein* of 543 physicians who subsequently had a myocardial infarction, stroke, or a blood clot that blocked another vessel (a *venous thrombosis*) against the level of C-reactive protein in 543 male physicians who had not developed such a disorder. The authors found that (a) blood levels of C-reactive protein seem to predict the individual's level of risk for myocardial infarction, and (b) because aspirin lowers the level of C-reactive protein in the blood, it is able to significantly reduce the individual's risk for a heart attack in those men with the highest levels of C-reactive protein. These findings were consistent with those of an earlier study that found that those physicians who took just one 325 mg aspirin tablet every other day suffered 44% fewer heart attacks when compared with the physicians who took a placebo ("Aspirin in the Prevention," 1989). This beneficial effect was noted only for individuals older than 50 years of age and was strongest for those individuals with lower blood cholesterol levels.

Physicians have discovered that aspirin is of value in the treatment of a rare neurological disorder known as *transient ischemic attacks* (TIAs), in which the patient loses his/her memory for a short period. Further, aspirin has been found useful in the control of inflammation caused by rheumatoid arthritis, osteoarthritis, and other forms of arthritis (Giacona et al., 1987; Graedon & Graedon, 1991; McGuire, 1990).

Although this is not technically a recognized medical application of aspirin, researchers have discovered evidence that suggests the regular use of aspirin might inhibit the growth of tumors in the colon (Giovannucci et al., 1994). The authors reported on an ongoing project involving 47,900 male health care professionals who participated to a questionnaire mailed to them in 1986, 1988, and again in 1990. The questionnaire included inquiries about aspirin use and the respondent's health status. Examination of the answers revealed that regular users of aspirin (more often than 2 times a week) had a significantly lower risk for colorectal cancer than did occasional users of aspirin, after factoring out the impact of such variables as diet and parental history of cancer.

The exact mechanism by which aspirin might inhibit the growth of colorectal cancer is still not clear. There is evidence to suggest that aspirin's ability to inhibit prostaglandin synthesis (a process discussed in the next section) might interfere with the cell growth patterns of some types of colorectal tumors (Muscat, Stellman, & Wynder, 1995; Thun, Namboodiri, & Heath, 1991). Some forms of prostaglandin increase the rate of cell growth and division, traits common to cancer (Muscat et al., 1995). Thus, by inhibiting prostaglandin synthesis throughout the body, it is possible that aspirin might slow the rate of growth of some types of colorectal cancers, allowing for the cancer to be more easily detected and treated.

A second theory is that aspirin may stimulate the body's immune response in some unknown manner, allowing the body to fight the invading cancer more effectively. Finally, Thun et al. (1991) suggested that aspirin's side effect of causing gastrointestinal bleeding might increase the tendency for a tumor to bleed, a factor that often results in the discovery of a tumor in the colon. By causing the tissues of the gastrointestinal tract to bleed, aspirin might also contribute to the tendency for the tissue in the tumor to start to bleed when the tumor is still in the earlier stages of growth. This would, in turn, make the tumor vulnerable to detection at an earlier stage than would be the case of a patient who did not use aspirin on a regular basis.

However, the team of Giovannucci et al. (1994) discounted the latter theory on the basis of their research, suggesting that the total number of colorectal cancers detected among aspirin users was significantly lower in their research sample, even after the variable of tumor bleeding was controlled for. The authors called for further research into this topic, to determine the exact mechanism by which aspirin might inhibit the growth of tumors in the colon.

In addition to all of its known uses, some research suggests aspirin might be of value in the prevention of gallstones and cataracts (Graedon & Ferguson, 1993). Some researchers even believe that aspirin might be of value in treating HIV infection (Stolberg, 1994). Preliminary laboratory research suggests that aspirin might prevent the AIDS virus from being able to replicate, in some unknown manner, and researchers are busy exploring this effect to see if it is of value in treating those infected with HIV. Thus, while the primary use of aspirin is as an analgesic, researchers continue to discover new applications for this "old" drug.

Acetaminophen

Because acetaminophen has no significant antiinflammatory effect, it is not usually classified as a NSAID (Supernaw, 1991). Nevertheless, acetaminophen is not without its uses. Acetaminophen has been found to be as effective in the control of fever as aspirin (American Society of Hospital Pharmacists, 1994). Further, as an OTC analgesic, acetaminophen is as potent as aspirin, and may be used for virtually every painful condition that aspirin is used for. Unfortunately, given its popularity as an analgesic, acetaminophen did not seem to affect tumor growth, or to facilitate the detection of colon tumors.

Ibuprofen

This drug was developed as a result of an intensive search by pharmaceutical companies to find a drug with the analgesic, antipyretic, and antiinflammatory actions of aspirin, but that was safer to use. Aspirin is a potentially dangerous chemical that, on occasion, may even cause fatal side effects. Ibuprofen is thought to be about 30 times as effective as aspirin in both combating inflammation and in controlling pain (Mann, 1994). Further, ibuprofen is thought to be about 20 times as effective as aspirin in controlling fever, according to the author.

An exciting research discovery involving ibuprofen was made by Stewart, Kawas, Corrada, and Metter (1997). The authors followed a sample of 1686 individuals enrolled in the Baltimore Longitudinal Study of Aging and examined the relationship between the use of NSAID agents such as aspirin and ibuprofen, and the development of a neurodegenerative disorder known as Alzheimer's disease (AD). The authors found that those older individuals who used ibuprofen for an extended period (2 years or longer) tended to have a lower risk for the development of Alzheimer's disease. Aspirin use was found to have a smaller, statistically nonsignificant impact on the development of AD, while long-term acetaminophen use was found to have no effect whatsoever on the potential development of AD. While the authors' work does not suggest that ibuprofen or similar NSAIDs will entirely prevent the development of AD, it does hint at a possible avenue for the treatment/prevention of AD in older adults.

Another application of ibuprofen's antiinflammatory action has been the control of the tissue inflammation caused by cystic fibrosis (CF). Cystic fibrosis is a genetic disorder that first manifests itself in childhood. As a result of a genetic mutation, the body of the person with CF is unable to eliminate chloride ions effectively, a deficiency that affects a number of different body systems, including the lungs. Patients afflicted with this genetic disorder frequently develop chronic inflammation and infections of the lungs. The team of Konstan, Hoppel, Chai, and Davis (1991) found that, like the anabolic steroids, dosage levels of 300–600 mg of ibuprofen were effective in controlling CF-related lung inflammation. The authors concluded that the dosage levels had to be adjusted to match the child's body size, but that ibuprofen was able to achieve acceptable levels of control over the lung tissue inflammation, without the harsh side effects seen with anabolic steroid use.

In a follow-up study, Konstan, Byard, Hoppel, and Davis (1995) gave either ibuprofen or a placebo to a sample of 85 patients, ages 5–30 years, who suffered from CF, and followed their subjects for four years. At the end of that time, the authors evaluated the patients' lung function, and found that the disease process in those patients with CF who had received high doses of ibuprofen was significantly slowed. While the use of ibuprofen in CF was not a "cure" for the pulmonary problems caused by this disorder, this NSAID did help to significantly slow the progression of the characteristic lung tissue damage of CF.

In another medical application of the OTC analgesics, aspirin, acetaminophen, and ibuprofen have all been found to be effective in helping to control the pain associated with some forms of cancer (Fishman & Carr, 1992). Researchers have also concluded that aspirin and ibuprofen, when used in combination with narcotic analgesics, may lower the patient's postoperative need for narcotic pain killers, at least in some cases (Murphy, 1993).

Naproxen

This is another chemical compound that emerged from the search by pharmaceutical companies for compounds that offered the advantages of aspirin without the dangerous side effects inherent in the use of the older analgesic. Long available in the United States only by prescription, naproxen has been found to be able to control mild to moderate levels of pain. Further, naproxen has an antiinflammatory effect that makes it useful in treating such conditions as rheumatoid arthritis, dysmenorrhea, gout, tendinitis, and bursitis. As an OTC analgesic, naproxen is recommended for the treatment of headaches, the aches of the common cold, backache and muscle aches, arthritis, and the discomfort of menstrual cramps, in addition to the control of fever (Gannon, 1994).

There is strong evidence to suggest that naproxen, in addition to its antiinflammatory effects, may have other uses. For example, physicians have discovered that, when used in combination with the antibiotic ampicillin, naproxen seems to reduce the distress felt by children with respiratory infections. Most certainly, as medical researchers continue to seek new uses for the OTC analgesics, these "old" drugs will prove of value in the treatment of disease well into the 21st century.

Ketoprofen

This medication, like naproxen, is an NSAID that was once only available by prescription. In 1996, the Food and Drug Administration approved ketoprofen as an OTC medication, in modified dosage form. Like the other NSAIDs discussed in this chapter, ketoprofen is thought to work by inhibiting prostaglandin synthesis. It is also an effective antipyretic (antifever), and can be used to control mild to moderate levels of pain secondary to injuries. However, the NSAIDs are about equally as effective in this regard, and the prototype NSAID, aspirin, is much cheaper than more recently developed members of the NSAID family.

Occasionally, somebody will ask why a new NSAID is needed. For reasons that are not well understood, when treating inflammatory diseases such as rheumatoid arthritis, different patients seem to respond more to one NSAID than to others. Thus, like the other NSAIDs, ketoprofen is often used to treat inflammatory diseases. But while ketoprofen, like the other NSAIDs, is effective in controlling inflammation, it must be taken for up to two weeks before it has much effect on inflammation.

Although OTC analgesics have often been thought of as being less powerful than prescription medications, the truth is that OTC analgesics are potent drugs. Ibuprofen, naproxen, and ketoprofen were originally sold as prescription-only medications, which were eventually approved for OTC use in modified dosage forms.

Pharmacology of the OTC Analgesics

Aspirin

Aspirin is usually administered by mouth. In the body, acetylsalicylic acid is transformed into salicylic acid, which is the active agent for aspirin's effects (Peterson, 1997). The drug is rapidly absorbed, and when it is taken on an empty stomach, aspirin begins to reach the bloodstream in as little as one minute (Rose, 1988). However, its primary site of absorption

is the small intestine, so that while it is possible to detect the first atoms of aspirin in the blood in approximately one minute, it usually takes somewhat longer to achieve therapeutic blood levels.

After a single dose, peak blood levels of aspirin are achieved in between 15 minutes (Shannon et al., 1995) and 1 to 2 hours (McGuire, 1990). Aspirin is biotransformed mainly in the liver into water-soluble metabolites, which are then rapidly removed from the blood by the kidneys (Payan & Katzung, 1995). Only about 1% of a single dose of aspirin is excreted unchanged from the body. Aspirin normally has a biological half-life of 2 hours, but when used at high dosage levels for longer than a week, the half-life of aspirin might be extended to between 8 (Kacso & Terezhalmy, 1994) and 15 (Payan & Katzung) hours.

Unlike the narcotic analgesics, which seem to work mainly within the brain, aspirin appears to have a different mechanism of action. First, aspirin does not seem to work within the cortex of the brain (Kacso & Terezhalmy, 1994). Rather, aspirin appears to work both at the site of the injury, in the hypothalamic region of the brain, and within the spinal cord (Fishman & Carr, 1992; Kacso & Terezhalmy, 1994).

To understand how aspirin works at the site of the injury, it is necessary to investigate the body's response to injury. Each cell in the human body contains several chemicals that are released when that cell is damaged, to warn neighboring cells of the damage and to activate the body's repair mechanisms. Some of these chemicals include *histamine*, *bradykinin*, and a group of chemicals collectively known as the *prostaglandins*. The inflammation and pain that results when these chemicals are released serves both to warn the individual that he/she has been injured, and, to activate the body's repair mechanisms.

Aspirin's analgesic effect at the site of the injury can be attributed to its power to inhibit the production of the prostaglandins (American Society of Hospital Pharmacists, 1994; Bushnell & Justins, 1993). Aspirin does this by inhibiting the production of an enzyme known as *cyclooxygenase*. This enzyme, in turn, is involved in the production of the prostaglandins. By blocking the action of cyclooxygenase, aspirin is able to block prostaglandin production, lowering the level of pain and reducing inflammation. Researchers have also found evidence that aspirin reduces pain perception by acting on the spinal cord although the exact mechanism by which this is accomplished is still not clear (Fishman & Carr, 1992; Graedon & Ferguson, 1993).

The ability of aspirin to inhibit the formation of blood clots by the platelets appears to be caused by its ability to indirectly inhibit the synthesis of the protein *thromboxane A$_2$* (Patrono, 1994). This protein is found in blood platelets and is essential to the formation of blood clots. Blood platelets have a normal lifetime of between 8 and 10 days, and once the thromboxane A$_2$ in a given platelet has been destroyed, the body must wait until new platelets have been produced before the clotting mechanism returns to normal. By blocking the process by which the body forms blood clots, aspirin has been found to be quite useful in the treatment of heart attacks, strokes, and other conditions (Patrono. 1994). Eventually, these aspirin-inhibited blood platelets will be replaced with new ones, as part of the normal process of platelet replacement. Thus, it is necessary for the patient to take a new dose of aspirin every day, or every other day, to provide optimal inhibition of blood clot formation.

Acetaminophen

Acetaminophen is usually administered orally, although it may also be administered as a rectal suppository. Oral preparations include tablet, capsule, or liquid forms, and virtually 100% of the medication is absorbed through the gastrointestinal tract (Shannon et al., 1995). The peak effects are seen in ½ to 2 hours after a single dose, and acetaminophen is metabolized in the liver. Virtually 100% of the drug is eliminated in the urine, although some acetaminophen is also found in breast milk of nursing mothers.

In terms of its analgesic and fever-reducing potential, acetaminophen is thought to be as powerful as aspirin (Supernaw, 1991). In terms of its analgesic or antifever effects, acetaminophen might be substituted for aspirin on a milligram-for-milligram basis. As discussed later in this chapter, when used at dosage levels above those recommended by the manufacturer, there is a danger of acetaminophen

toxicity. However, liver toxicity/damage from acetaminophen is quite rare, as long as the user does not ingest more than 4000 mg of acetaminophen per day (Cherny & Foley, 1996) or use the drug for more than 10 days (Peterson, 1997).

The exact manner by which acetaminophen reduces pain or fever remains unknown (Shannon et al., 1995). One theory suggests that, like aspirin, acetaminophen also interferes with prostaglandin synthesis. However, unlike aspirin, acetaminophen-induced inhibition of prostaglandin takes place mainly in the central nervous system, which is why acetaminophen does not possess a significant antiinflammatory potential (Peterson, 1997). Further, unlike aspirin, acetaminophen does not interfere with the normal clotting of the blood (Shannon et al.). Finally, individuals who are allergic to aspirin do not usually suffer from adverse reactions when they take acetaminophen. These features often make acetaminophen an ideal substitute for individuals who are unable to take aspirin due to any of the following conditions: the patient is allergic to it, the patient is prone to bleeding disorders, or aspirin might interfere with another medication being used by the patient.

Ibuprofen

Ibuprofen is usually administered orally, and about 80% of the medication is absorbed from the gastrointestinal tract following a single dose. The medication is metabolized in the liver, with the half-life of ibuprofen being between 2 and 4 hours (Shannon et al., 1995). About 99% of the ibuprofen molecules will become protein-bound following absorption into the general circulation (Olson, 1992). The therapeutic half-life of ibuprofen is between 1.8 and 2.6 hours (American Medical Association, 1994). Peak plasma levels following a single oral dose are achieved in between 30 minutes and 1.5 hours. Ibuprofen and its metabolites are mainly eliminated by the kidneys, although a small amount of ibuprofen is eliminated through the bile.

Like aspirin, ibuprofen has been found to be effective in the control of mild to moderate levels of pain, and in the control of fever (Shannon, Wilson & Stang, 1995). Further, like aspirin, ibuprofen is thought to inhibit the action of the enzyme cyclooxygenase, which, in turn, blocks prostaglandin production. But this does not mean that ibuprofen can automatically be substituted for aspirin to control inflammation. Indeed, there is disagreement as to ibuprofen's effectiveness as an antiinflammatory agent.

Payan and Katzung (1995) stated that when used at a dosage level of 2400 mg/day,[4] ibuprofen is as effective as aspirin in the control of inflammation in the average adult. However, when used at a dosage level lower than 2400 mg/day, ibuprofen is far less effective as an antiinflammatory agent than is aspirin (Payan & Katzung, 1995). Mann (1994), on the other hand, suggested that when used at effective dosage levels, ibuprofen is 30 times as effective in fighting inflammation as aspirin. As is obvious from these reports, researchers still disagree as to the exact antiinflammatory potential of ibuprofen.

There is strong evidence to suggest that, when ibuprofen is taken concurrently with aspirin, each of these two chemicals interferes with the antiinflammatory action of the other (Payan & Katzung, 1995). Thus, ibuprofen should not be used by a patient taking aspirin, except when the attending physician recommends the concurrent use of these two NSAIDs. Further, ibuprofen's antiinflammatory effects are seen only after 2 to 4 weeks of continuous drug use (Fischer, 1989). While this would argue that one would do better to utilize aspirin for the control of inflammation, one must remember that aspirin is irritating to the stomach. Ibuprofen, on the other hand, is about one-fifth to one-half as irritating to the stomach as aspirin (Giacona et al., 1987). Thus, ibuprofen is often utilized if the individual is unable to tolerate the gastrointestinal irritation caused by aspirin. But, while ibuprofen is less irritating to the stomach, it has been estimated that 4% to 14% of those who use ibuprofen still experience some degree of gastrointestinal irritation (Graedon & Graedon, 1996).

Further, just as aspirin can cause gastrointestinal bleeding when used for prolonged periods, researchers estimate that approximately 3 out of every 1000 users will also experience some degree of ibuprofen-induced gastrointestinal bleeding (Carlson et al., 1987). The team of Taha, Dahill, Sturrock,

Lee, and Russell (1994) found that 27% of their sample who had used ibuprofen for an extended period had evidence of ulcer formation in their gastrointestinal tract. However, the number of ibuprofen-using subjects in their sample was quite small, and it was not clear how representative these findings were of the ability of ibuprofen to contribute to gastrointestinal ulcer formation.

Naproxen

The mechanism of action of naproxen is similar to that of aspirin (American Society of Hospital Pharmacists, 1994). In other words, naproxen is thought to interfere with the production of prostaglandins. However, naproxen may be more effective as an antiinflammatory agent than aspirin (American Medical Association, 1994; American Society of Hospital Pharmacists, 1994; Graedon & Graedon, 1991). This makes it of value for the treatment of inflammatory conditions, although at this time it is not clear whether naproxen will be marketed as an antiinflammatory agent in the OTC market.

Like aspirin, naproxen has an antipyretic effect. Researchers are not sure of the exact mechanism through which naproxen reduces fever. However, it is thought that naproxen may suppress the synthesis of prostaglandins in the hypothalamus (American Society of Hospital Pharmacists, 1994). The hypothalamus is a region of the brain that helps to regulate body temperature. Thus, it is logical to assume that naproxen somehow helps to modify the action of the hypothalamus, reducing the individual's fever.

When used as an analgesic, naproxen begins to have an effect in 1 hour, and its effects last for 7 to 8 hours (American Medical Association, 1994). The biological half-life of naproxen in the healthy adult is approximately 10 to 20 hours. About 30% of a given dose of naproxen is metabolized by the liver into the inactive metabolite *6-desmethylnaproxen* (American Society of Hospital Pharmacists, 1994). Only 5% (American Medical Association, 1994) to 10% (American Society of Hospital Pharmacists, 1994) of a standard dose of naproxen is excreted unchanged. The majority of a standard dose of naproxen is excreted in the urine as either metabolized or unmetabolized drug.

---

[4] The 2400 mg is taken in divided doses, not all at once.

As stated earlier, naproxen binds to proteins in the blood plasma, which can absorb only so much of the medication before reaching a saturation point. Research suggests that the concentration of naproxen reaches a plateau if the patient takes 500 mg twice daily for 2 to 3 days (American Society of Hospital Pharmacists, 1994).[5] Thus, the typical dosage level does not exceed 500 mg/bid.

Ketoprofen

The mechanism of action of ketoprofen is similar to that of aspirin. Like aspirin, ketoprofen is thought to inhibit the production of prostaglandins in the body. When used to treat arthritis, improvement usually begins within a couple of weeks of continual use, with maximum benefit appearing after several weeks of continuous use.

When ketoprofen was sold as a prescription drug, patients were advised not to take *more* than 300 mg/day, and it was usually recommended that they take the medication with food to minimize irritation to the gastrointestinal tract. Ketoprofen is well absorbed from the GI tract, with peak blood levels appearing in 30 minutes to 2 hours after a single dose taken on an empty stomach (American Medical Association, 1994). It is more slowly absorbed when taken with food, but, eventually, all the ketoprofen will be absorbed even when taken with a meal. Ketoprofen is extensively bound to plasma proteins, with 99% of the drug molecules being protein-bound. There are no known active metabolites of ketoprofen.

The elimination half-life is, in part, dependent on the efficiency of the individual's liver and kidneys. In young adults, the half-life is 3 hours, while in the elderly, this might be increased to 5 hours, following a single oral dose. Because of this characteristic, it is recommended that older patients, or patients with impaired kidney function, consult with their physician before taking this medication, to determine whether they should use ketoprofen or use a modified dosage.

As noted earlier, all the OTC analgesics can control mild to moderate levels of pain. These medication effects are both an advantage and a danger for the patient. For the control of pain or a fever provides only symptomatic relief. Even after controlling pain and/or fever, the physician must still identify and treat the cause to ensure adequate medical care for the patient (Fishman & Carr, 1992).

Normal Dosage Levels of Over-the-Counter Analgesics

There is conflicting evidence as to whether aspirin's analgesic effects are dose-related (Giacona et al., 1987). But there is mixed evidence suggesting little or no additional analgesic benefits from increasing the dosage levels above 600 mg every 4 hours for an adult. At this dosage level, aspirin or acetaminophen have a significant analgesic potential. McGuire (1990) reported that 650 mg of aspirin or acetaminophen, a standard dose of two regular strength tablets of either medication, provided an analgesic effect equal to that of 50 mg of the narcotic painkiller meperidine (Demerol). Kaplan and Sadock (1990) suggested that 650 mg of aspirin has the same analgesic potential as 32 mg of codeine, or 65 mg of Darvon (propoxyphene), or a 50 mg oral dose of Talwin (pentazocine).

Kacso and Terezhalmy (1994) reported that a single 1300 mg dose of aspirin seemed to provide a greater degree of relief from pain than did a single 600 mg dose. However, dosage levels above 1300 mg in a single dose did not provide a greater degree of analgesia and actually put the user at risk for a toxic reaction from the aspirin, according to the authors. In contrast, Aronoff, Wagner, and Spangler (1986) postulated that there was a "ceiling effect" (p. 769) for aspirin, beyond which higher dosage levels would not provide greater pain relief. The authors reported that this ceiling level was "approximately 1000 mg every 4 hr" (p. 769). A dosage level of aspirin higher than this "only increases the threat of a toxic reaction" (McGuire, 1990, p. 30).

The American Society of Hospital Pharmacists (1994) recommends a normal adult oral dosage level of aspirin is 325 to 650 mg every four hours, as

---

[5] It should be noted that a patient should not take 500 mg of naproxen twice a day, except under a physician's supervision.

needed for the control of pain. Furthermore, this text warns that aspirin should not be continuously used for longer than 10 days by an adult, and longer than 5 days for a child under the age of 12, except under a doctor's orders.[6]

When taken by mouth, aspirin is rapidly and completely absorbed from the gastrointestinal tract and is distributed by the blood to virtually every body tissue and fluid. The actual speed at which aspirin is absorbed by the user depends on the acidity of the stomach contents (Sheridan et al., 1982). When taken on an empty stomach, the rate at which aspirin is absorbed depends on how quickly the tablet crumbles, after reaching the stomach (Rose, 1988). After the tablet crumbles, the individual aspirin molecules pass through the stomach lining into the general circulatory system.

When the individual takes aspirin either with food, or right after eating, it may take 5 to 10 times longer to reach the bloodstream and, thus, longer to have a therapeutic effect on the individual (Pappas, 1990). Ultimately, however, all the aspirin will be absorbed from the gastrointestinal tract. This is useful knowledge, since Rodman (1993) suggested that the patient take aspirin with meals, or at least a snack, to limit aspirin-induced irritation to the stomach lining. However, in some cases, it is desirable to achieve as high a blood level of aspirin as possible. The patient should discuss with his/her physician or pharmacist whether to take aspirin on an empty stomach or with a meal before attempting to use this technique to limit stomach irritation.

Aspirin is sold both alone and in combination with agents designed to reduce the potential irritation to the stomach. In theory, time-released and enteric-coated tablets can reduce this irritation. However, both of these forms of aspirin have been known to bring about erratic absorption rates, making it harder to achieve the desired effect (Shannon

et al., 1995). Some patients take aspirin with antacids, to reduce the irritation to the stomach caused by aspirin. When antacids are mixed with aspirin, the patient's blood level of aspirin will be 30% to 70% lower than when aspirin is used without antacids (Graedon & Graedon, 1996; Rodman, 1993). This is a matter of some concern for individuals who are taking the drug for the control of inflammation or pain, since lower blood levels of aspirin mean that less of the drug is available to help control the pain.

The American Society of Hospital Pharmacists (1994) noted that the usual adult dose of acetaminophen is also 325 to 650 mg every 4 hours, as needed for the control of pain. In many ways, dosage recommendations for aspirin and acetaminophen are similar. Aronoff et al. (1986) observed that acetaminophen's antipyretic and analgesic effects are equal to those of aspirin, and that the ceiling level of acetaminophen is the same for these two drugs.

Peak blood concentrations were achieved in 30 minutes to 2 hours after an oral dose of acetaminophen (Shannon et al., 1995). The half-life of an oral dose of acetaminophen is normally from 1 to 4 hours. However, since this chemical is metabolized in the liver, persons with significant liver damage might experience a longer acetaminophen half-life than is normally the case and should avoid the use of acetaminophen except under the supervision of a physician.

Sands et al. (1993) go even further and recommend that patients with alcohol-related liver damage totally avoid the use of acetaminophen. A small amount (about 4%) of acetaminophen is biotransformed into a toxic metabolite, even in users with normal liver function (Peterson, 1997). Normally, this poses no danger to the user. But, the bodies of individuals with alcohol-induced liver damage often have trouble dealing with this toxic acetaminophen metabolite, even at recommended dosage levels. For this reason, individuals with alcohol-related liver damage should not use acetaminophen (Peterson, 1997; Sands et al., 1993). Finally, because of its toxic effects on the liver, it is recommended that acetaminophen *not* be used for longer than 10 days at any dosage level (Kacso & Terezhalmy, 1994).

---

[6]A physician may, when using aspirin in the treatment of arthritis, for example, elect to have the patient take it at a higher-than-normal dosage levels for extended periods. This represents a special application of aspirin's antiinflammatory effect, and the physician will weigh the advantages of using aspirin at such high dosage levels against the potential for harm to the patient. Since this is a special application of aspirin, however, it is not discussed in this chapter.

Ibuprofen occupies a unique position, in that it is both available over-the-counter and is still utilized as a prescription medication. When used as a non-prescription analgesic, the recommended dose of ibuprofen is 200–400 mg every 4 hours (Dionne & Gordon, 1994). As a prescription medication, individual dosage levels of 400–800 mg are often utilized, depending on the specific condition being treated.

Shannon et al. (1995) recommended that 400–800 mg of ibuprofen be used 3 to 4 times a day by adults who suffer from inflammatory diseases. The authors suggest that 400 mg every 4 to 6 hours be utilized in the control of mild to moderate pain. However, there is some disagreement as to the analgesic potential of ibuprofen. Dionne and Gordon (1994) noted that the greatest degree of relief from pain is achieved with doses of 400–600 mg, and that additional ibuprofen above this level is unlikely to result in greater levels of analgesia. In contrast to this, however, Rosenblum (1992) stated that 800 mg of ibuprofen provided greater control of postoperative pain than did therapeutic doses of the narcotic fentanyl, in a small sample of women who had laparoscopic surgery.

It is necessary to keep in mind that the OTC dosage levels of ibuprofen are limited to 200–400 mg every 4 hours. A physician who prescribes this medication might elect to use a higher dosage level. However, even when it is used as a prescription medication, it is not recommended that the total daily dosage level exceed 3200 mg per day, in divided doses (Dionne & Gordon, 1994; Shannon et al., 1995).

Ibuprofen is rapidly absorbed when used orally, and the drug is rapidly distributed throughout the body. About 80% of a single oral dose is absorbed from the intestinal tract. Following a single oral dose, peak blood plasma levels are achieved in 1 to 2 hours (American Society of Hospital Pharmacists, 1994). The drug's half-life is between 1.8 and 2.6 hours, and the effects of a single dose of ibuprofen last for about 6 to 8 hours following a single oral dose (Shannon et al., 1995).

Naproxen was available only by prescription in the United States for a number of years, but was finally approved for over-the-counter use in 1994. One brand name of OTC naproxen is "Aleve," which is sold in tablet form, each tablet containing 200 mg of naproxen and 20 mg of sodium (Gannon, 1994). According to a package insert, users are advised to take up to 3 tablets, twice a day.

As a prescription medication, ketoprofen was available in 25, 50, and 75 mg capsules. Recommended dosage levels were 50–75 mg every 8 hours, up to a maximum of 300 mg/day. There is no evidence that dosage levels above 300 mg/day are more effective than lower doses, and the manufacturer does not recommend that ketoprofen be used in dosage levels above 300 mg per day (Medical Economics Company, 1995). In the modified OTC analgesic form, it is sold in 25-mg tablets.

Complications Caused by Use of Over-the-Counter Analgesics

The OTC analgesics are hardly "safe" medications. In general, these drugs may ". . . be harmful, even deadly, if used too often, in combination with one another, or by the wrong people at the wrong time" (Morgenroth, 1989, p. 36). Although they are available without a prescription, the OTC analgesics pose a significant potential for harm. Many people tend to forget this fact since these medications are available without a prescription.

Aspirin

Aspirin is the most commonly used drug in this country. The statistics reveal the popularity of aspirin: Americans consume between 20 billion (Rapoport, 1993) and 40 billion (Talley, 1993) tablets of aspirin a year. Steele and Morton (1986) gave another measure of aspirin use in this country, stating that between 30 and 74 million pounds of aspirin are consumed in the United States each year. On a worldwide basis, one hundred million pounds of aspirin are consumed each year (Mann & Plummer, 1991).

Because aspirin is a popular over-the-counter medication, many people underestimate both its usefulness and its potential for causing serious side effects (Jaffe & Martin, 1990). For example, each year in the United States, between 500 and 1,000 people die as a result of aspirin-induced bleeding disorders (Grinspoon & Bakalar, 1993).

Even therapeutic doses of aspirin interfere with the body's ability to control blood loss. After just a single dose of aspirin, virtually every user experiences some degree of gastrointestinal bleeding (Pappas, 1990; Talley, 1993). The aspirin-induced gastrointestinal bleeding that follows a single dose is usually minor, but up to 15% of those individuals who occasionally take aspirin at the recommended dosage levels experience at least one significant, potentially fatal, adverse side effect (Rapoport, 1993). When used on a chronic basis, aspirin causes a significant percentage of individuals to experience adverse side effects. Forty percent of the patients who use aspirin at recommended doses on a chronic basis experience an erosion in their stomach lining, and between 17% (Kitridou, 1993) and 30% (Taha et al., 1994) will actually develop stomach ulcers.

Thus, it should not be surprising to learn that, when used on a regular basis, it may contribute to the formation of a "bleeding" ulcer.[7] Indeed, in more than 20% of all cases of bleeding ulcers, doctors conclude that the patient's use of aspirin was a major contributing factor (Talley, 1993). Wilcox, Shalek, and Cotsonis (1994) gave an even higher estimate of the percentage of the cases of aspirin-related gastrointestinal (GI) hemorrhage. The authors noted that 41% of the patients admitted to the hospital because of a GI hemorrhage had consumed aspirin in the week prior to admission. Even dosage levels as low as 75 mg/day have been found to significantly increase the individual's risk for damage to the lining of the gastrointestinal system (Guslandi, 1997).

In addition to its effects on the stomach lining, the regular use of aspirin can contribute to the formation of potentially life-threatening ulcers in the small intestine (Allison, Howatson, Torrance, Lee, & Russell, 1992). For these reasons, aspirin should not be used in persons with a history of ulcers, bleeding disorders, or other gastrointestinal disorders (American Society of Hospital Pharmacists, 1994). Further, people should not take aspirin with acidic foods such as coffee, fruit juices, or alcohol, which might further irritate the gastrointestinal system (Pappas, 1990).

This is not to say that every patient who uses aspirin for a protracted period will experience a major gastrointestinal hemorrhage or ulcers. But, a significant number of patients who use aspirin for extended periods develop bleeding severe enough to require hospitalization. Further, many of the ulcers that form as a result of aspirin use fail to produce major warning symptoms (Taha et al., 1994). Thus, the potential benefit for the use of aspirin must be weighed against the potential harm that the drug can cause the user.

Aspirin's ability to cause gastric irritation is thought to be a side effect of aspirin's nonselective ability to interfere with the production of prostaglandins (Mortensen & Rennebohm, 1989). Scientists have found several subtypes of prostaglandin in different regions of the body. But since aspirin is a nonselective antiprostaglandin, its use can result in the disruption of the production of the prostaglandins necessary for the proper function of different organ systems, including that of the gastric lining. Thus, while blocking the production of prostaglandins at the site of an injury, aspirin can cause irritation and bleeding in the stomach and gastrointestinal tract. This is why such a large percentage of chronic aspirin users experience gastrointestinal problems.

When used at recommended dosage levels for extended periods, aspirin has also been known to cause breathing problems in up to 33% of the patients (Kitridou, 1993). This side effect seems to be related to aspirin's ability to cause allergic reactions in some users. Approximately 0.2% of the general population is allergic to aspirin. However, of those individuals with a history of *any* kind of allergic disorder, approximately 20% will be allergic to aspirin. Patients who are sensitive to aspirin are likely also to be sensitive to ibuprofen or naproxen, as cross-sensitivity between these drugs is common (Fischer, 1989; Shannon et al., 1995).

[7]This is the formation of a stomach ulcer over a blood vessel in the stomach wall. The blood vessel is gradually exposed to stomach acid as the surrounding tissue is destroyed by the stomach acid and ultimately ruptures. The ulcer is now "bleeding." This is a serious medical emergency that may result in the patient's death.

Symptoms of an allergic reaction to aspirin may include rash and breathing problems (Zuger, 1994). Patients with symptoms of the "aspirin triad" (i.e., a history of nasal polyps, asthma, and sensitivity to aspirin) should not use any NSAID except under the supervision of a physician (Craig, 1996).

Aspirin has been known to trigger fatal asthma attacks in patients with this disorder (Zuger, 1994). All the NSAIDs are capable of causing an exacerbation of the symptoms of asthma as a result of their ability to inhibit prostaglandin production (Craig, 1996; Mackman, 1995). Persons with a history of chronic rhinitis should not use aspirin except under a physician's supervision (Shannon et al., 1995). These conditions are warning signals for individuals at risk for an allergic reaction to aspirin or similar agents. About 5% to 15% of those individuals who suffer from asthma will experience an adverse reaction if they use an NSAID (Craig, 1996; Mackman, 1995). If the asthma patient also has a history of nasal polyps, the possibility of an adverse reaction to a NSAID may be as high as 40%, according to the authors.

Aspirin can cause a number of other side effects, including anorexia (loss of desire to eat), nausea, and vomiting (Sheridan et al., 1982). Because of its ability to cause gastrointestinal bleeding, individuals who use aspirin on a regular basis may actually develop anemia as a result of the constant internal blood loss. Due to the effects on blood clotting, aspirin, naproxen, or ibuprofen should not be utilized by persons with a bleeding disorder such as hemophilia (American Society of Hospital Pharmacists, 1994; Shannon et al., 1995). Even in persons who do not have a bleeding disorder, a single dose of aspirin can prolong bleeding time for between 3 to 7 days after the last use of that drug (Shannon et al.). This is why persons who are undergoing anticoagulant therapy involving such drugs as heparin or warfarin should not use aspirin except when directed by a physician (Rodman, 1993). The combined effects of aspirin and the anticoagulant may result in significant, unintended blood loss for the patient, especially if he/she were to have an accident.

Patients being treated for hyperuricemia (a buildup of uric acid in the blood often found in gout as well as other conditions) should not use aspirin. When used at normal dosage levels, aspirin reduces the body's ability to excrete uric acid, contributing to the problem of uric acid buildup. Further, if the individual is taking the prescription medication probenecid, one of the drugs used to treat hyperuricemia, he/she should not take aspirin. At therapeutic doses, aspirin inhibits the action of probenecid, allowing uric acid levels to build up in the blood. Acetaminophen has been advanced as a suitable substitute for patients who suffer from gout and who need a mild analgesic (Shannon et al., 1995).

Aspirin also should not be used in patients who are receiving medications for the control of their blood pressure, except under a physician's supervision. It has been found that aspirin, or the other NSAIDs, may interfere with the effectiveness of some antihypertensive medications (Fischer, 1989). The exact mechanism by which this happens is unclear; however, it may reflect the impact of aspirin use on prostaglandin production within the kidneys, resulting in fluid retention ("Strong Medicine," 1995).

Patients taking other NSAIDs such as ibuprofen or naproxin should not take aspirin, except under a physician's supervision. The combined effects of these medications can cause significant gastrointestinal tract irritation (Rodman, 1993). Aspirin, naproxen, and ibuprofen may all cause a condition known as "tinnitus" (loss of hearing and a persistent "ringing" in the ears). The patient's hearing will usually return to normal when the offending medication is immediately discontinued. Also, aspirin use may result in a very rare side effect known as *hepatotoxicity.*

In such cases, aspirin prevents the liver from being able to filter the blood effectively (Gay, 1990). This will allow the buildup of certain toxins in the blood, which may appear suddenly. The available literature would suggest that hepatotoxicity caused by the use of aspirin or ibuprofen is extremely rare, but it has been documented (Gay, 1990). Another rare complication from aspirin use is a drug-induced depression (Mortensen & Rennebohm, 1989).

The elderly are especially susceptible to toxicity from aspirin and similar agents. Although the reasons are not entirely clear, this may be because their bodies are unable to metabolize and excrete this family of drugs as effectively as younger adults. Bleidt and Moss (1989) suggested that a contributing factor is that as people grow older, there is a reduction in blood flow to the liver and kidneys. This results in difficulties in metabolizing and excreting many drugs, including aspirin. Another complication of aspirin use in the elderly is the development of drug-induced anxiety states (Sussman, 1988).

Aspirin or related compounds should not be used with children who are suffering from a viral infection, except when directed to do so by a physician. Research strongly suggests that aspirin may increase the possibility of the child developing Reye's syndrome as a complication to the viral infection (American Medical Association, 1994; Sagar, 1991). Reye's syndrome is a serious medical condition that usually develops in children between the ages of 2 to 12. The condition usually follows a viral infection such as influenza or chickenpox, and may have symptoms such as swelling of the brain, seizures, disturbance of consciousness, a fatty degeneration of the liver, and coma, and in about 30% of the cases results in death (Graedon & Graedon, 1996; Sagar, 1991).

Individuals who plan to consume alcohol should not use aspirin immediately prior to, or while they are, actively drinking. The research team of Roine, Gentry, Hernandez-Munoz, Baraona, and Lieber (1990) found that the use of aspirin prior to the ingestion of alcohol will decrease the activity of gastric alcohol dehydrogenase, an enzyme produced by the stomach that starts to metabolize alcohol even before it reaches the bloodstream. This will result in a higher than normal blood alcohol level even in the rare social drinker who had ingested aspirin shortly before drinking alcohol.

Aspirin has been implicated in the failure of intrauterine devices (IUDs) to prevent pregnancy. The antiinflammatory action of aspirin is thought to interfere with the effectiveness of intrauterine devices, which normally act to prevent pregnancy. Aspirin has also been implicated in fertility problems for couples who wish to have children. The use of aspirin at therapeutic dosage levels may reduce the ability of sperm to move (sperm motility)

by up to 50%, a side effect that may reduce the chances of successful conception for at least some couples. While this is not to say that aspirin could serve as a method of birth control, the reduction in sperm motility might interfere with the couple's ability to conceive, when they want to do so.

Ibuprofen

Ibuprofen has been implicated as the cause of blurred vision of patients (Nicastro, 1989). Graedon and Graedon (1996) suggested that persons using ibuprofen who experience some change in their vision discontinue the medication, and consult with their physician immediately. In addition to the 3% to 9% of the patients on ibuprofen who experience skin rashes or hives as a side effect, ibuprofen has been implicated in the formation of cataracts (Graedon & Graedon, 1996) and as the cause of migraine headaches in both men and women (Nicastro, 1989).

When ibuprofen was first introduced as a prescription medication in 1974, it was manufactured by the Upjohn Company, and sold under the brand name *Motrin*. The Upjohn Company warned that ibuprofen has been found to cause a number of side effects including heartburn, nausea, diarrhea, vomiting, nervousness, hearing loss, and congestive heart failure in persons who had marginal cardiac function, changes in vision, and elevation of blood pressure (Medical Economics Company, 1995).

Recent research has also suggested that ibuprofen can cause, or contribute to, kidney failure in persons with high blood pressure, kidney disease, or other health problems (Squires, 1990). This may be a side effect of ibuprofen's ability to block the production of prostaglandin. Research has shown that by blocking the body's production of prostaglandin, ibuprofen also reduces the blood flow throughout the body, especially to the kidneys. If the individual is already suffering from a reduction in blood flow to the kidneys for any reason, including "normal aging, liver or cardiovascular disease or simply dehydration from vomiting, diarrhea and fever accompanying the flu" (Squires, 1990, p. 4E), ibuprofen might either cause, or at least contribute to, acute kidney failure.

Patients who are suffering from systemic lupus erythematosus (often simply called "lupus" or SLE) should not use ibuprofen, except under a physician's supervision. Occasionally, ibuprofen has been the cause of the development of a condition known as *aseptic meningitis,* within hours of the time that a patient with SLE ingested ibuprofen. In extremely rare cases aseptic meningitis is also a complication in a patient who does *not* have SLE (Zuger, 1994). However, there have been less than 40 reported cases of this side effect of ibuprofen in patients who do not have SLE or some other autoimmune disorder.

When used by a client who is also taking lithium, ibuprofen may also increase the blood levels of lithium by 25% to 60% (Jenike, 1991; Rodman, 1993). This effect is most pronounced in the older individual and may contribute to lithium toxicity in some individuals, according to the author. Close monitoring of blood lithium levels would be necessary in patients who use both lithium and ibuprofen concurrently, to avoid the danger of lithium toxicity. Patients who are on lithium should report any use of ibuprofen, even over-the-counter preparations, to the physician who is prescribing the lithium, so that appropriate steps may be taken.

Patients taking the prescription medication methotrexate should not use ibuprofen, since this drug reduces the rate at which methotrexate is excreted from the body (Rodman, 1993). Reduced excretion rates may result in toxic levels of methotrexate building up in the patient, according to the author. If an OTC analgesic should be required, Rodman recommended the use of acetaminophen. Also, ibuprofen should not be used in conjunction with other NSAIDs, including aspirin, except under a physician's supervision (Rodman). The combined effects of NSAIDs may result in excessive irritation to the gastrointestinal tract and, possibly, severe bleeding.

Acetaminophen

Acetaminophen is metabolized by the liver, which, as outlined in Chapter 5, may be damaged by the chronic use of alcohol. It has been observed that the chronic use of alcohol may lower the dosage level necessary for the person to become toxic from acetaminophen (American Medical Association, 1994). A few chronic alcohol users have become toxic on acetaminophen at dosage levels only slightly higher than the normal recommended dose (Mitchell, 1988). For this reason, active or recovering alcoholics should not utilize acetaminophen for any reason, except under a doctor's supervision (Shannon et al., 1995).

A rare, but not unknown, complication of acetaminophen use is the development of anaphylactic reactions on the part of the user. Acetaminophen has also been found to be *nephrotoxic,* which is to say that if used too often, or at too high a dosage level, it may be toxic to the cells of the kidneys. Since the 1950s, a number of research studies have concluded that OTC analgesics may be nephrotoxic. To explore this possibility, Perneger, Whelton, and Klag (1994) examined the drug use pattern of 716 patients with what is known as end stage renal disease (ESRD) and compared this data with the drug use pattern of 361 individuals of the same age, who did not suffer from kidney disease. The authors found that patients who had taken as few as 1000 acetaminophen tablets during the course of their lifetime were twice as likely to develop ESRD as were patients who did not use acetaminophen. Further, the authors found evidence to suggest a dose-related danger of ESRD when the patient consumed either more than 365 acetaminophen tablets in a year's time, or a total of 1000 tablets in a lifetime. In other words, the authors suggest that beyond the cutoff limit, the greater the individual's use of this acetaminophen, the greater the chances of that individual ultimately developing ESRD.

While ESRD is a rare complication of OTC analgesic use, Perneger et al. (1994) estimated that from 8% to 10% of all cases of end state renal disease were caused by acetaminophen use. Their findings suggest that, as with all medications, acetaminophen should be utilized only when the benefits obtained through this OTC analgesic outweigh the potential dangers inherent in its use.

Naproxen

Much of the information available on naproxen and its effects is based on experience obtained with prescription forms of this chemical. Naproxen has been found to be a factor in potentially fatal allergic reactions in some users. Patients with the "aspirin triad" (discussed earlier) should not use naproxen except under a physician's supervision. This medication may also contribute to the formation of peptic ulcers and gastrointestinal bleeding. In rare cases, male users have experienced naproxen-induced problems achieving an erection, and the loss of the ability to ejaculate (Finger et al., 1997).

On occasion, naproxen has contributed to drowsiness, dizziness, feelings of depression, and vertigo. Patients have been known to experience diarrhea, heartburn, constipation, and vomiting while taking naproxen. Between 3% and 9% of the patients who used prescription-strength naproxen experienced such side effects as constipation, heartburn, abdominal pain, and nausea. The team of Taha et al. found that 44% of their sample who had used naproxen for extended periods had evidence of gastrointestinal ulcers. While it was not clear how representative these findings were of naproxen's ability to contribute to the formation of ulcers, it was recommended that naproxen not be utilized by patients with a history of peptic ulcer disease (Dionne & Gordon, 1994).

The study by Perneger et al. (1994) suggested that there is a cumulative dose threshold for NSAIDs, above which the patient runs the risk of developing end stage renal disease. The authors found that patients who had consumed more than 5000 tablets of an over-the-counter NSAID over the course of their lives were significantly more likely to develop ESRD than were patients who had consumed less than 5000 tablets in their lifetime. The authors did not identify the mechanism by which NSAIDs might contribute to the development of ESRD, but they did find that aspirin did not seem to contribute to the development of ESRD.

There have been rare reports of patients who developed side effects such as a skin rash, diarrhea, headache, insomnia, sleep problems, problems with their hearing, and/or tinnitus, after using naproxen. There have also been reports of potentially fatal liver dysfunctions that seem to have been caused by naproxen. Thus, as with all medications, naproxen should be used only when the benefits of this drug outweigh the potential dangers of its use.

Animal research has suggested the possibility of damage to the eyes as a result of naproxen use,

although it is not clear whether this medication may cause damage to the visual system of a human being.

Ketoprofen

The side effects of Ketoprofen are essentially the same as those seen with naproxen, or other NSAID agents.

Overdose of OTC Analgesics

Acetaminophen

In addition to its value as an OTC analgesic, acetaminophen is also the drug most commonly ingested in an overdose attempt (Anker & Smilkstein, 1994; Lipscomb, 1989). In 1993, there were 94,287 cases of acetaminophen overdose in the United States, while in 1994 there were 102,619 cases reported to medical authorities (Cetaruk, Dart, Horowitz & Huribut, 1996; Sporer & Khayam-Bashi, 1996). These figures are misleading in the sense that only 100 people died as a result of an acetaminophen overdose in 1994 (Cetaruk et al., 1996). But this drug is an extremely dangerous chemical to ingest in excess.

Acetaminophen is often ingested by individuals, especially adolescents, who want to make a suicide gesture. While the individual who makes this gesture rarely intends to suicide, the relatively low dose necessary to produce a toxic reaction to acetaminophen makes it a poor choice for an overdose. Because the first evidence of acetaminophen toxicity may not appear until 12 to 24 hours after the drug was ingested, the individual may falsely conclude that he/she is not at risk for adverse effects from the suicide gesture, and not seek medical assistance until several hours, or even days, have elapsed.

This is unfortunate because while an antidote to acetaminophen overdose is available, it must be administered *within 12 hours after taking the overdose* to be fully effective. This antidote is a chemical known as *N-acetylcysteine*. When it is administered within several hours of the initial overdose, N-acetylcysteine is effective in the treatment of acetaminophen poisoning (American Medical Association, 1994). But if, as all too often happens, the individual waits until the symptoms of acetaminophen toxicity develop before seeking help, it may be too late to prevent permanent liver damage, or even death.

When taken in large doses, acetaminophen destroys the liver enzyme *glutathione*. Glutathione is a chemical produced by the liver to protect itself from various toxins (Anker & Smilkstein, 1994). A dose of just 7.5–15 grams of acetaminophen (just 15–30 extra-strength tablets) in a single dose, or 5–8 grains per day (650–975 mg/day or 2–3 regular strength tablets/day) for several weeks, is enough to cause a toxic reaction in the healthy adult (American Medical Association, 1994; Whitcomb & Block, 1994). For children, the toxic level is approximately 140 mg per kilogram of body weight.[8]

A factor that seems to contribute to liver damage in at least some cases is whether the individual ingested the acetaminophen on an empty stomach (Whitcomb & Block, 1994). The authors concluded that taking the medication while abstaining from food (fasting) seemed to contribute to hepatotoxicity, at least for those cases where the patient had taken a "moderate overdose" (p. 1849). Thus, for some patients, food might serve a protective function.

Supernaw (1991) also suggested that individuals who use acetaminophen at high dosage levels for extended periods of time (i.e., 5000 mg/day for 2–3 weeks) were also at risk for drug-induced liver damage. However, Supernaw did not identify factors other than the chronic ingestion of above-normal acetaminophen doses that might contribute to liver damage. The studies suggest, however, that at least for certain individuals, acetaminophen has the potential to cause toxic reactions at dosage levels just above the normal therapeutic dosage range.

Aspirin

Aspirin is commonly ingested in suicide gestures/attempts. To underscore this role of aspirin, one need only consider that there were 19,916 intentional aspirin overdoses treated in health care facilities in 1993 (Sporer & Khayam-Bashi, 1996). Although scientists have learned a great deal about how an aspirin overdose affects the body in the past 40 years (Yip, Dart, & Gabow, 1994), it remains a potentially dangerous chemical. In 1990, aspirin caused approximately as many deaths in the United States as did heroin overdoses ("Forum," 1991).

The average dosage level necessary to produce a toxic reaction to aspirin is about 10 grams for an adult, and about 150 mg of aspirin for every kilogram of body weight for children. A dose of 500 mg of aspirin per kilogram of bodyweight is potentially fatal. Symptoms of aspirin toxicity include headache, dizziness, tinnitus, mental confusion, increased sweating, thirst, dimming of sight, and hearing impairment (Shannon et al., 1995). Other symptoms of aspirin toxicity include restlessness, excitement, apprehension, tremor, delirium, hallucinations, convulsions, stupor, coma, hypotension and, at higher dosage levels, possible death (Sporer & Khayam-Bashi, 1996). While these symptoms are most often seen in the person who has ingested a large dose of aspirin, even small doses can result in toxicity for the aspirin-sensitive individual.

Ibuprofen

Ibuprofen's popularity as an OTC analgesic has resulted in an increasing number of overdose attempts involving this drug (Lipscomb, 1989). Symptoms of overdose include seizures, acute renal failure, abdominal pain, nausea, vomiting, drowsiness, and metabolic acidosis (Lipscomb). There is no specific antidote for a toxic dose of ibuprofen, and medical care is often aimed at supportive treatment only.

Naproxen

The *Physician's Desk Reference* (Medical Economics Company, 1995) reported that the life-threatening dose of naproxen in humans is not known. Animal research involving dogs suggests that a dose of 1000 mg/kg is potentially fatal, although in hamsters the estimated LD_{100} was estimated to be 4100 mg/kg. No specific antidote is known for an overdose of naproxen, and medical care is limited to supportive treatment only.

There are no symptoms specific to a naproxen overdose. Symptoms of a NSAID overdose include lethargy, drowsiness, nausea, vomiting, epigastric

---

[8]*Any* suspected chemical overdose should be evaluated by a physician.

pain, respiratory depression, coma, and convulsions. The NSAIDs are capable of causing G.I. bleeding in overdose situations and may cause either hypotension or hypertension (Medical Economics Company, 1995). An overdose of naproxen is considered a medical emergency, and the overdose victim should be evaluated by a physician.

Ketoprofen

There is limited information about ketoprofen overdoses. The *1995 Physician's Desk Reference* identified 26 overdoses for the prescription form of ketoprofen known as Orudis (Medical Economics Company, 1995). No fatalities were noted. In general, ketoprofen overdoses will cause any or all of the symptoms seen in naproxen overdoses, since both drugs are NSAIDs.

There are no symptoms specific to a ketoprofen overdose. Symptoms of NSAID overdose include lethargy, drowsiness, nausea, vomiting, epigastric pain, respiratory depression, coma, and convulsions. The NSAIDs cause GI bleeding in overdose situations and may cause either hypotension or hypertension (Medical Economics Company, 1995). An overdose of naproxen is considered a medical emergency, and the overdose victim should be evaluated by a physician. The basic treatment procedures involve supportive treatment as well as specific interventions designed to treat the individual's symptoms as they emerge (Medical Economics Company, 1995).

Summary

Over-the-counter analgesics are often discounted by many as not being "real" medications. Despite this fact, aspirin is America's most popular pharmaceutical. Each year, more than 20,000 tons of aspirin are manufactured and consumed in this country alone, and aspirin accounts for only about 28% of the OTC analgesic sales.

Aspirin, acetaminophen, naproxen, and ibuprofen are all quite effective in the control of mild to moderate levels of pain, without exposing the patient to the side effects found with narcotic analgesics. Some of the OTC analgesics have also been found to be useful in controlling the inflammation of autoimmune disorders and in helping to control postsurgical pain. Researchers have discovered that the OTC analgesics are of value in controlling the pain associated with cancer and, in the case of aspirin, may even contribute to the early detection of some forms of cancer. The oldest OTC analgesic, aspirin, was introduced more than a century ago, but medical researchers are still discovering new applications for this potent medication and its chemical cousins.

Although they are available over-the-counter, the OTC analgesics carry significant potential for harm. Acetaminophen has been implicated in toxic reactions in chronic alcoholics at near-normal dosage levels. It also has been implicated as the cause of death in people who have taken acetaminophen overdoses. Aspirin and ibuprofen have been implicated in fatal allergic reactions, especially in those who suffer from asthma. The use of aspirin for children with viral infections is not recommended.

The Hallucinogens

It has been estimated that about 6000 different species of plants can be used for their psychoactive properties (Brophy, 1993). Several species of mushrooms may also be used to produce hallucinations (Rold, 1993). Many of these plants and mushrooms have been used for centuries in religious ceremonies and healing rituals, and for predicting the future (Berger & Dunn, 1982; Kaplan & Sadock, 1990). Sometimes, their effects were used to prepare warriors for battle (Rold, 1993). Even today, certain religious groups use mushrooms with hallucinogenic properties as part of their worship, although in the United States this is illegal (Rold, 1993).

Over the years, researchers have identified approximately 100 different hallucinogenic compounds that might be found in various plants or mushrooms. Many of these compounds have been extensively studied by scientists. Indeed, it was through during a clinical research project that the effects of one hallucinogenic, lysergic acid diethylamide-25 (LSD-25, or simply, LSD) were accidentally discovered, and recorded. LSD is a substance obtained from the rye fungus ergot *Claviceps purpurea* (Lingeman, 1974). The chemical was first isolated in 1938 by chemists who were looking for a cure for headaches (Monroe, 1994). In 1943, a scientist accidentally ingested a small amount of LSD-25 while conducting an experiment. Later that day, he experienced LSD-induced hallucinations for the first time. After he recovered, the scientist correctly concluded that the source of the hallucinations was the specimen of *Claviceps purpurea* on which he had

been working. He again ingested a small amount of the fungus, and experienced hallucinations for the second time, and confirmed his original conclusion.

Following World War II, there was a great deal of scientific interest in the hallucinogenics, especially in light of the similarities between the subjective effects of these chemicals and various mental illnesses. Because the hallucinogenics were so potent, certain agencies of the U.S. government such as the Department of Defense and the Central Intelligence Agency experimented with chemical agents, including LSD, as possible chemical warfare weapons (Budiansky, Goode, & Gest, 1994). At one point, scientists questioned whether LSD might be useful in the treatment of alcoholism (Henderson, 1994a).

The hallucinogens were hardly a well-kept secret, and in the 1960s, these chemicals moved from the laboratory into the streets, where they quickly became popular drugs of abuse (Brown & Braden, 1987). The popularity and widespread abuse of LSD in the 1960s prompted the classification of this chemical as a controlled substance in 1970 (Jaffe, 1990). But the classification of LSD as a controlled substance did not solve the problem of its abuse. Over the years, LSD has waxed and waned in popularity declining in the late 1970s, but now appearing to increase once more (Henderson, 1994a; *Mayo Clinic Health Letter*, 1989).

One hallucinogen, phencyclidine (PCP) deserves special mention. Because of its toxicity, PCP fell into disfavor in the early 1970s (Jaffe, 1989). In the 1980s, however, a form of PCP that could be smoked was introduced, and it again became popular with illicit drug users. Currently, PCP seems to be in less demand although it is still being sold on the illicit drug market, often in the guise of other more desired substances.

Another drug, N, alpha-dimethyl-1,3-benzodioxole-t-ethanamine (or, MDMA), became quite popular as a chemical of abuse in the late 1970s and early 1980s. This drug is frequently sold on the streets under the name of "ecstasy." Both PCP and MDMA are discussed in later sections of this chapter.

Scope of the Problem

It is difficult to estimate the number of casual hallucinogenic users in the United States. Monroe (1994) reported that 2.8 million people in this country use LSD at least once a year. Further, there is evidence to suggest that LSD is gaining in popularity with adolescents (Gold, Schuchard, & Gleaton, 1994; Kaminer, 1994). Indeed, the authors reported that 5.3% of the high school seniors questioned admitted to having used LSD at least once. The team of Johnston, O'Malley, and Bachman (1996) found that 11.7% of the seniors of the class of 1995 admitted to having used LSD at least once, a significant increase over the percentage of seniors from the previous year who admitted to the use of LSD during their lifetime.

These figures suggest also that high school seniors are more likely to accept experimental LSD use than were students from past years. Further, these figures suggest a trend toward increasing acceptance of LSD use by adolescents. In years past, the majority of those who used the hallucinogens such as LSD were those who experimented with the drug, then either totally avoided further hallucinogen use, or went on to only use hallucinogens on an episodic basis (Jaffe, 1989). However, in recent years, LSD has been repackaged and reformulated, so that current preparations contain lower dosage forms than were typical in past years (Gold et al., 1994). Thus, much of what was discovered about the effects of LSD on the user in the 1960s and 1970s may not apply to the current user, since he/she might have ingested a far smaller dose of LSD than was typical 20 years ago.

Pharmacology of the Hallucinogens

The commonly abused hallucinogenics can be divided into two major groups on the basis of their chemical structure (Jaffe, 1989). First, there are the hallucinogens that bear a structural resemblance to the neurotransmitter serotonin. These hallucinogenics include LSD, psilocybin, and the chemical dimethyl-tryptamine (DMT). A second group of hallucinogenics is chemically related to the neurotransmitters dopamine and norepinephrine. The chemical structure of these agents also resembles that of the amphetamine family (Jaffe, 1989). These hallucinogenics include mescaline, MDMA, and DOM (which is also known as STP).

Despite the chemical differences between hallucinogens and differences in potency, illicit drug users tend to adjust their intake of the drug(s) being used to produce similar effects (Schuckit, 1995a). Thus, because of the tendency for the user to modify his/her dose to produce similar drug-induced experiences, the effects of the hallucinogenics tend to be similar. One exception to this rule is DMT. The effects of DMT only last about 20 minutes, and for this reason, DMT is often called a "businessman's high." The drug experience may fit into a typical half-hour lunch break, making it a popular drug of abuse for some of the business community. With this one exception, however, DMT is very similar to the other hallucinogens discussed in this chapter.

It is common for a person under the influence of one of the hallucinogens to believe that he/she has a new insight into reality. But, these drugs do not generate new thoughts so much as alter one's perception of existing sensory stimuli (Snyder, 1986). Despite their chemical differences, these chemicals also produce hallucinations, or hallucinatory-like experiences, which are usually recognized by the user as being drug-induced (Lingeman, 1974). Thus, the terms *hallucinogen* and *hallucinogenic* are usually applied to this class of drugs.

LSD has long been considered the prototypical hallucinogenic. It is also the third most commonly used drug, ranking behind alcohol and marijuana (Schwartz, 1995). Since the effects of other hallucinogens are often compared with those of LSD, the major focus of this chapter is on the hallucinogens

LSD, MDMA, and PCP. Other hallucinogens are only briefly discussed.

The Pharmacology of LSD

In terms of relative potency, LSD is one of the most potent chemicals known to scientists. Researchers have compared LSD with hallucinogenic chemicals naturally found in plants, such as psilocybin and peyote, and found that LSD is between 100 and 1000 times as powerful as these natural hallucinogens (Schwartz, 1995). However, it is also weaker than synthetic chemicals such as the hallucinogenic DOM/STP (Schuckit, 1995a).

For the casual user, LSD might be effective at doses as low as 50 micrograms although the classic LSD "trip" usually requires that the user ingest twice that amount (Schwartz, 1995). LSD is usually administered orally, but it is possible to administer LSD by intraveneous injection (Henderson, 1994a). Despite the claims of some users whose chemical use was detected by urine toxicology testing, it is not possible to absorb LSD through the skin (Henderson, 1994a). Thus, the user must actively ingest the chemical, for it to have an effect.

The LSD molecule is water-soluble. When taken by mouth, LSD is rapidly absorbed from the gastrointestinal tract, and is quickly distributed to all body tissues including the brain (Mirin et al., 1991). Because it is distributed throughout the body, only about 0.01% of the original dose actually reaches the brain (Lingeman, 1974). Thus, if the user were to ingest a 50-microgram dose of LSD, only five-tenths of a microgram would actually reach the brain. The chemical structure of the LSD molecule is similar to that of the neurotransmitter serotonin. In the brain, the LSD molecules seem to bind to one of the many subtypes of serotonin receptor sites (Schwartz, 1995).[1] This would seem to account for the ability of LSD to cause perceptual and mood distortions, since serotonin is a neurotransmitter involved in the process of perception and the modification of mood (Henderson, 1994a).

One theory about how LSD exerts its effect is that the drug inhibits the activity of serotonin in the region of the brain known as the dorsal midbrain raphe (Mirin et al., 1991). This theory was challenged by Jaffe (1989), who suggested that LSD exerted an effect at various sites in the central nervous system, ranging from the cortex of the brain itself down to the spinal cord, including (but not limited to) the midbrain sites identified by Mirin et al.

Another theory is that LSD's psychoactive effects are caused by the drug's actions in the region of the brain known as the temporal lobes (Restak, 1994). The author supported this theory with the observation that individuals who suffer from temperal lobe epilepsy often report similar experiences to that of LSD users. However, this is only a theory, and after more than 50 years of research, the exact mechanism of action for LSD is still not entirely known (Henderson, 1994a; Jaffe, 1989).

Tolerance to the effects of LSD develops quickly, often within 2 to 4 days of continual use (Henderson, 1994a; Mirin et al., 1991; Schwartz, 1995). If the user has become tolerant to the effects of LSD, then increasing the dosage level will have little if any effect (Henderson). However, the individual's tolerance to LSD's effects also abate in just 2 to 4 days of abstinence (Henderson, 1994a; Jaffe, 1989; Lingeman, 1974). Cross-tolerance between the different hallucinogens is also common (Jaffe, 1989; Lingeman, 1974). Thus, most LSD users alternate between periods of active drug use and periods of abstinence.

In terms of direct physical mortality, LSD is perhaps the safest drug known to modern medicine (Brown & Braden, 1987; Weil, 1986). There are only two known reports of death resulting from the use of LSD alone (Schwartz, 1995). In another incident reported by Lingeman (1974) an elephant who received a massive dose of LSD (297,000 micrograms, or 5,940 doses at 50 micrograms each) died.[2] While this suggests that LSD might prove toxic to the user, in reality the approximate lethal

---

[1] In specific terms, LSD seems to bind to the 5-HT$_2$ receptor site in the brain although it may also bind to other receptor sites yet to be discovered.

[2] Lingeman (1974) did not, however, mention how the elephant happened to ingest the LSD in the first place.

dose of LSD in humans is simply not known.[3] Henderson (1994a) stated "The risk of death from an overdose of LSD is virtually nonexistent" (p. 43). But, indirectly, LSD has been implicated as the cause of death in some users, usually as a result of accidents.

The biological half-life of LSD is not known with any certainty. It is known that the drug is rapidly biotransformed by the liver, and thus it is rapidly eliminated from the body. Indeed, so rapid is the process of LSD biotransformation and elimination that traces of the major metabolite of LSD, 2-oxy-LSD, will remain in the user's urine only for 12 to 36 hours after the last use of the drug (Schwartz, 1995). The estimates of the half-life of LSD range from 2 or 3 hours (Jaffe, 1989, 1990; Karch, 1996; Shepherd & Jagoda, 1990; Weiss et al., 1994) to 5 hours (Henderson, 1994a).

Surprisingly, the effects of LSD in humans seem to last about 8 to 12 hours (Kaplan & Sadock, 1990; Monroe, 1994). Researchers have not identified how LSD's effects can last such a long time, given the short half-life of the chemical in the body. Only about 1% of the LSD ingested is excreted unchanged, with the rest being biotransformed by the liver and excreted in the bile (Henderson, 1994a). Thus, LSD continues to challenge researchers, who have yet to understand how—when the person ingests such a small dose and when such a small portion of the total dose ingested actually reaches the brain—LSD can have such a profound impact on the user's state of mind.

Subjective Effects of Hallucinogens

Subjectively, the user will begin to feel the first effects of a dose of LSD in about 5 to 10 minutes. These initial effects include such symptoms as anxiety, gastric distress, and tachycardia (Schwartz, 1995). In addition, the user may also experience increased blood pressure, increased body temperature, pupillary dilation, nausea, and muscle weakness during the period following the ingestion of the drug (Jaffe, 1989). Other side effects of LSD include an

exaggeration of normal reflexes (a condition known as "hyperreflexia"), dizziness, and some degree of muscle tremor (Jaffe). Lingeman (1974) characterized these changes as "relatively minor" (p. 133) although they might cause some anxiety for the inexperienced user.

The hallucinogenic effects of LSD usually begin anywhere between 30 minutes and an hour after the user first ingested the drug (Henderson, 1994a). Scientists are still not sure how LSD causes the user to hallucinate (Ciraulo et al., 1995). However, the effects of a hallucinogen will vary depending on factors such as (a) the individual's personality makeup, (b) expectations for the drug, and (c) the environment in which the drugs are used (Kaplan & Sadock, 1990).

Users often refer to the effects of LSD on the user as a "trip." It appears that the LSD trip moves through several distinct phases (Brophy, 1993). First, within a few minutes of taking LSD, there is a release of inner tension. This stage, which lasts 1 to 2 hours (Brophy) is characterized by either laughing or crying as well as a feeling of euphoria (Jaffe, 1989). The second stage usually begins between 30 and 90 minutes (Brown & Braden, 1987) to 2 or 3 hours (Brophy) after the ingestion of the drug. During this period, the individual experiences the perceptual distortions such as visual illusions and hallucinations that are the hallmark of the hallucinogenic experience.

Mirin et al. (1991) described this phase as being marked by "wavelike perceptual changes" (p. 290) and noted that synthesthesia is often experienced during this phase. Synthesthesia is a phenomenon where information from one sense may "slip over" into another sensory system. A person who is experiencing synthesia may report being able to "taste" colors, or "see" music.

The third phase of the hallucinogenic experience begins 3 to 4 hours after the drug is ingested (Brophy, 1993). During this phase of the LSD trip, the person experiences a distortion of the sense of time. The person may also experience marked mood swings and a feeling of ego disintegration. Feelings of panic are often experienced during this phase as are occasional feelings of depression (Lingeman, 1974). These LSD-related anxiety reactions are discussed in the next section. It is during the third stage of the

---

[3] This margin of safety, however, does not extend to the other hallucinogens, and it is possible to both overdose and to die from some of the other popular hallucinogens.

LSD trip that the individuals may express a belief that they possess quasi-magical powers or are magically in control of events around them (Jaffe, 1989). This loss of contact with reality has resulted in fatalities as individuals have jumped from windows or attempted to drive motor vehicles. For this reason, LSD has been indirectly implicated as the cause of death in a number of cases.

The effects of LSD start to wane 4 to 6 hours after ingestion. As the individual begins to recover, he or she experiences "waves of normalcy" (Mirin et al., 1991, p. 290; Schwartz, 1995) that gradually blend into the normal state of awareness. Within 12 hours, the acute effects of LSD have cleared although he/she may experience a "sense of psychic numbness, [that] may last for days" (Mirin et al., 1991, p. 290).

Hallucinogenics and "Bad Trips"

As noted, it is not uncommon for the individual who has ingested LSD to experience significant levels of anxiety, which can reach the levels of panic reactions. This is known as a "bad trip." The likelihood of a bad trip seems to be determined by three factors: (a) the individual's expectations for the drug (which is known as the "set"), (b) the setting in which the drug is used, and (c) the psychological health of the user (Mirin et al., 1991).

The LSD bad trip seems most likely to occur with inexperienced LSD users (Mirin et al., 1991); the inexperienced user's set seems to contribute to the development of the bad trip. If the person develops a panic reaction to the LSD experience, he/she will often respond to calm, gentle reminders from others that these feelings are caused by the drug and will pass. This is known as "talking down" the LSD user.

In extreme cases, the individual may require pharmacological support to deal with the LSD-induced panic attack. Physicians have several pharmaceuticals that can help lower the individual's anxiety. But there is some disagreement as to which medications offer the greatest potential for relief during an LSD-related panic reaction. Kaplan and Sadock (1990) recommend that the physician utilize diazepam or, in extreme cases, haloperidol.

However, Jenike (1991) warned *against* the use of benzodiazepines such as diazepam in aborting an LSD-related panic reaction. He based his warning on the fact that the benzodiazepines tend to distort the individual's sensory perception. Normally, this distortion is so slight as to be unnoticed by the typical patient. But when combined with the effects of LSD, the benzodiazepine-induced sensory distortion may cause the patient to have even more anxiety than before, according to Jenike. The antipsychotic medication haloperidol was suggested as the drug of choice for use by medical personnel to abort the LSD-related panic attack (Jenike). Schwartz (1995) recommended that 2–4 mg of haloperidol might be administered by intramuscular injection every hour, until the patient's anxiety was under control.

Many samples of hallucinogens sold on the street are adulterated with belladonna, or other anticholinergics (Henderson, 1994a; Kaplan & Sadock, 1990). When mixed with phenothiazines, these substances may bring about coma and death through cardiorespiratory failure. Thus, it is imperative that the physician treating a bad trip know what drug/s have been used and, if possible, obtain a sample of the drug(s) ingested, to determine what medication is best in treating the patient.

The LSD-induced bad trip normally lasts only a few hours and typically will resolve itself as the drug's effects wear off (Henderson, 1994b). However, LSD may also have long-lasting effects on the user. Some researchers believe that in rare cases LSD is capable of activating a latent psychosis (Henderson). But researchers are not sure whether this reflects the activation of a preexisting psychiatric disorder in the patient or the development of a drug-induced psychotic break.

One reason it is so difficult to identify LSD's relationship to the development of psychiatric disorders is that the:

> . . . LSD experience is so exceptional that there is a tendency for observers to attribute *any* later psychiatric illness to the use of LSD. (Henderson, 1994b, p. 65, italics added for emphasis)

As the author points out, psychotic reactions that develop weeks, months, or even years after the last use of LSD have been attributed to the individual's use of this hallucinogen, rather than to nondrug factors. Thus, it has been suggested that LSD is capable of causing long-term complications such as a drug-induced psychosis. However, this theory has also been challenged by other researchers.

An extremely rare complication of LSD use is the overdose (Schuckit, 1995a). Some symptoms of an LSD overdose include convulsions and hyperthermia. Medical care is necessary in any suspected hallucinogenic overdose, to control the drug-induced seizures and monitor the individual's vital signs. In a hospital setting, the physician can take appropriate steps to monitor the patient's cardiac status, and to counter the seizures and elevation in body temperature.

The LSD Flashback

The "flashback" is another long-term consequence of LSD use that is not well understood. The flashback is a "spontaneous recurrence" (Mirin et al., 1991, p. 292) of the drug experience that might take place days, weeks, or in some cases even months after the last time LSD was used.

Schwartz (1995) stated that the "majority" (p. 409) of those who use LSD at least 10 times would experience flashbacks. The flashback experience might be brought on by stress, fatigue, marijuana use, emerging from a dark room, illness, and occasionally by intentional effort on the part of the individual. They usually last a few seconds to a few minutes, although occasionally they last from 24 to 48 hours or even longer (Kaplan & Sadock, 1990). Approximately 50% of those people who develop flashbacks do so in the first 6 months following their last use of LSD. In about 50% of the cases, the individual continues to experience flashbacks for longer than 6 months, possibly for as long as 5 years (Schwartz, 1995; Weiss et al., 1994).

Flashback experiences occasionally are frightening to the individual. Some individuals have been known to become depressed, develop a panic disorder, or become suicidal after having had a LSD-related flashback (Kaplan & Sadock, 1990). On the other hand, some LSD users seem to enjoy the visual hallucinations, flashes of color, halos around objects, the perception that things are growing smaller or larger, and feelings of depersonalization common in a LSD flashback (Mirin, Weiss, & Greenfield,1991). Thus, different individuals will respond to the development of LSD-related "flashbacks" in different ways.

The only treatment usually needed for the patient having an LSD flashback is reassurance that it will end. Occasionally, benzodiazepines are needed to help control the anxiety that may accompany the LSD-related flashback in the patient who is distressed by his/her unexpected drug experience.

Posthallucinogen Perceptual Disorder

This is a rare, poorly understood complication of LSD use/abuse (Hartman, 1995). For reasons that are poorly understood, some chronic users of LSD experience a disturbance in their visual perceptual system that may, or may not, become permanent. Victims of this disorder report seeing afterimages, or distorted "trails" following behind objects in the environment, for extended periods after their last use of LSD (Hartman, 1995). The exact mechanism by which LSD might cause these effects is not known at this time.

Although LSD has been studied by researchers for the past 50 years, there still is a lot that remains to be discovered about this elusive chemical. For example, there is one case report of a patient who developed grand mal seizures after taking LSD while taking the antidepressant fluoxetine (Ciraulo, Creelman, et al., 1995). The reason for this interaction is not known, but underscores that there is still much to learn. Unfortunately, even before scientists were able to learn all that there is to learn about LSD, another popular hallucinogen appeared. This hallucinogen is called PCP.

Phencyclidine (PCP)

The drug *phencyclidine* (PCP) was introduced in 1957 as an experimental intravenously administered surgical anesthetic (Milhorn, 1991). By the mid-1960s, researchers had discovered that 10% to 20% of the patients who had received PCP experienced a drug-induced delirium, and the decision was made to discontinue using the drug with humans (Brown & Braden, 1987; Milhorn, 1991). However, phencyclidine continued to be used in veterinary medicine in the United States until the mid-1970s.

In 1978, all legal production of PCP in this country was discontinued, and the drug was declared a controlled substance under the Comprehensive Drug Abuse Prevention and Control Act of 1970

(Slaby et al., 1981). However, it continues to be used as a veterinary anesthetic in other parts of the world, and is legally manufactured by pharmaceutical companies in other parts of the world (Kaplan et al., 1994). In the United States, PCP production continues in illicit laboratories that are centered mainly in and around Los Angeles (Office of National Drug Control Policy, 1996).

There are two major reasons PCP appears to be a popular drug of abuse. First, despite its harsh effects (to be discussed), PCP is easily manufactured in illicit laboratories (Slaby et al., 1981). Because PCP can be produced in illicit laboratories with minimal training in chemistry, it is often mixed into other street drugs to enhance the effects of chemicals produced in underground laboratories. PCP is also frequently sold under the guise of other chemicals that are more difficult to manufacture (Brophy, 1993; "Consequences of PCP," 1994). For example, it is common for a person who thought that he/she had purchased LSD, or ketamine, to actually have purchased PCP produced in an illicit laboratory. Another example of PCP abuse is the practice of mixing PCP with marijuana before it is sold to unsuspecting users, to make the marijuana seem more potent. Thus, illegal drug producers like PCP because they can substitute it for other, possibly more expensive, recreational chemicals.

The second reason PCP became so popular is that users discovered smoking PCP allowed them to more easily control the symptoms of PCP intoxication. If the symptoms became too harsh and aversive, the user simply stopped smoking the PCP-laced cigarette for a while. This ability to titrate the effects could not be achieved through the other methods of PCP abuse (to be discussed). These two factors contributed to the popularity of PCP in the past two decades.

Methods of PCP Administration

There are many ways to administer PCP: it can be smoked, used intranasally, taken by mouth, injected into the muscle tissue, or injected intravenously (Brown & Braden, 1987; Slaby et al., 1981). The most common method is for the user to smoke a cigarette that contains PCP (Grinspoon & Bakalar, 1990). This allows a great deal of control over the drug's effects, since the user can stop smoking when a desired state of intoxication is reached.

Pharmacology of PCP

Chemically, phencyclidine is a weak base, which is soluble in both water and lipids. Because it is a base, it is absorbed mainly through the small intestine rather than through the stomach lining (Zukin & Zukin, 1992). This slows the absorption of the drug, which must pass through the stomach to reach the small intestine. But the effects of an oral dose of PCP are still generally seen in just 20 to 30 minutes, and last for 3 to 5 hours ("Consequences of PCP," 1994).

When smoked, PCP is rapidly absorbed through the lungs, and symptoms of PCP intoxication appear within about 2 or 3 minutes after smoking the drug (Milhorn, 1991; Shepherd & Jagoda, 1990). However, only about 30% to 50% of the PCP in the cigarette actually is absorbed. Crowley (1995b) said that only about one-third of the PCP in the cigarette is absorbed. Much of the rest of the PCP in the cigarette is converted into the chemical *phenylcyclohexene* by the heat of the cigarette (Shepherd & Jagoda, 1990).

When injected or ingested orally, between 70% and 75% of the available PCP reaches the circulation (Crowley, 1995b). The effects of injected PCP last for about 3 to 5 hours, while the effects of an oral dose usually last 5 to 8 hours ("Consequences of PCP," 1994). PCP is very lipid-soluble, and because of this, it tends to accumulate in fatty tissues and in the tissues of the brain. The level of PCP in the brain might be 31 to 113 times as high as blood plasma levels (Shepherd & Jagoda, 1990). Further, animal research data suggests that PCP remains in the brain for up to 48 hours after it is no longer detectable in the blood (Hartman, 1995). Once in the brain, PCP tends to act at a number of different receptor sites, including blocking those utilized by a neurotransmitter known as N-methyl-D-aspartic acid (NMDA) (Zukin & Zukin, 1992). This seems to be the receptor site most strongly affected at low doses. It has also been suggested that PCP binds to one of the numerous opioid receptor sites (the sigma opioid receptor site) (Daghestani & Schnoll, 1994), although Crowley disputed this theory. Thus, the question of whether PCP binds to any of the opioid receptor sites has yet to be resolved.

In the human body, PCP has some unusual effects. Depending on the dosage level and the route of administration, PCP may function as an anesthetic, a stimulant, a depressant, or a hallucinogenic (Brown & Braden, 1987; Weiss & Mirin, 1988). In part, this happens because PCP affects several different neurotransmitters within the brain, rather than just one (D. Roberts, 1995). Thus "few drugs seem to induce so wide a range of subjective effects" as PCP (Jaffe, 1990, p. 557).

Some of the desired effects include a sense of euphoria, decreased inhibitions, a feeling of immense power, a reduction in the level of pain, and altered perception of time, space, and the user's body image (Milhorn, 1991). However, not all the drug's effects are benign. "Most regular users report unwanted effects" (Mirin et al., 1991, p. 295) caused by PCP. Some of the more common negative effects include feelings of anxiety, restlessness, and disorientation.

In some cases, the user retains no memory of the period of intoxication, a reflection of the anesthetic action of the drug (Ashton, 1992). Other negative effects of PCP include disorientation, mental confusion, assaultiveness, anxiety, irritability, and paranoia (Weiss & Mirin, 1988). So many people have experienced so many different undesired effects from PCP that researchers are at a loss to explain why the drug is so popular (Newell & Cosgrove, 1988).

A PCP-induced depressive state is common among users (Berger & Dunn, 1982). In extreme cases, the individual's level of depression can reach suicidal proportions (Jenike, 1991; Weiss & Mirin, 1988). This is consistent with the observations of Berger and Dunn (1982), who, in drawing on the wave of PCP abuse that took place in the 1970s reported that the drug would bring the user either to "the heights, or the depths" (p. 100) of emotional experience.

PCP is biotransformed by the liver into a number of inactive metabolites, which are then excreted mainly by the kidneys (Zukin & Zukin, 1992). Following a single dose of PCP, only about 10% (Shepherd & Jagoda, 1990) to 20% (Crowley, 1995b) of the drug will be excreted unchanged. One characteristic of PCP is that it takes the body an extended period to biotransform/excrete the drug. The half-life of PCP following an overdose may be as long as 20 (Kaplan et al., 1994) to 72 hours (Jaffe, 1989), up to a period of weeks (Grinspoon & Bakalar, 1990).

One reason for the extended half-life of PCP is that it tends to accumulate in the body's adipose (fat) tissues. In chronic users, PCP molecules can remain in the user's fat cells for days, or even weeks, following the last dose of the drug. There have even been cases where a chronic PCP user has lost weight, either as a result of dieting, or because of trauma, and unmetabolized PCP still in the person's adipose tissue has been released back into the general circulation, causing the user to have flashback experiences long after his/her last use of the drug (Zukin & Zukin, 1992).

Some physicians believe that it is possible to reduce the half-life of PCP in the body by making the urine more acidic. This is done by having the patient ingest large amounts of ascorbic acid or cranberry juice (Kaplan & Sadock, 1990; Grinspoon & Bakalar, 1990). However, a potentially dangerous complication of this technique is the possible development of a condition known as myoglobinuria, which may cause the kidneys to fail (Brust, 1993). Because of this potential complication, many physicians do not recommend the acidification of the patient's urine.

Although it is possible for the user to become tolerant to the effects of PCP, only a limited degree of tolerance is thought to develop to the effects of this drug (Crowley, 1995b). There is no evidence of physical dependence to PCP (Newell & Cosgrove, 1988; Weiss et al., 1994).

Symptoms of Mild Levels of PCP Intoxication

Small doses of PCP, usually less than 1 mg, do not seem to have an effect on the user (Crowley, 1995b). At dosage levels of about 5 mg, the individual experiences a state resembling that seen in alcohol intoxication (Crowley, 1995b; Mirin et al., 1991). The individual experiences muscle incoordination, staggering gait, slurred speech, and numbness of the extremities (Jaffe, 1989). Other effects of mild doses of PCP include agitation, some feelings of anxiety, flushing of the skin, visual hallucinations, irritability, possible sudden outbursts of rage, and feelings of euphoria, nystagmus, changes in the body image, and depression (Beebe & Walley, 1991; Crowley, 1995b; Milhorn, 1991).

The acute effects of a small dose of about 5 mg of PCP last between 4 and 6 hours. Following the period of acute effects is a post-PCP recovery period that can last 24 to 48 hours (Beebe & Walley, 1991; Milhorn, 1991). During the post-PCP recovery period, the user gradually "comes down," or returns to normal.

Symptoms of Moderate Level of PCP Intoxication

As the dosage level increases to the 5–10 mg range, many users experience a range of symptoms, including a disturbance of body image, where different parts of their bodies no longer seem "real" (Brophy, 1993). The user may also experience slurred speech, nystagmus, dizziness, ataxia, tachycardia, and an increase in muscle tone (Brophy, 1993; Weiss & Mirin, 1988). Other symptoms of moderate levels of PCP intoxication might include paranoia, severe anxiety, belligerence, and assaultiveness (Grinspoon & Bakalar, 1990) as well as unusual feats of strength (Brophy, 1993; Jaffe, 1989) and extreme salivation (Brendel, West, & Hyman, 1996). Some people have experienced drug-induced fever, an excess of salivation, drug-induced psychosis, and violence.

Symptoms of Severe Levels of PCP Intoxication

As the dosage level reaches the 10–25 mg level, or higher, the individual's life is in extreme danger. At this dosage level, PCP may cause vomiting, seizures, and—if the user is still conscious—serious impairment of reaction time. The user who ingests in excess of 10 mg of PCP may experience hypertension and severe psychotic reactions similar to schizophrenia (Grinspoon & Bakalar, 1990; Kaplan & Sadock, 1990; Weiss & Mirin, 1988). The coma brought on by an extreme dose of PCP may last up to 10 days (Mirin et al., 1991).

In addition to the possibility of a coma, the individual who has ingested 10–20 mg of PCP may develop cardiac arrythmias, encopresis, visual and tactile hallucinations, and a drug-induced paranoid state. PCP overdoses have caused death from respiratory arrest, convulsions, and hypertension (Brophy, 1993).

Complications of PCP Abuse

As noted earlier, PCP has been implicated as causing a drug-induced psychosis that may last for days, weeks (Jaffe, 1989; Jenike, 1991; Weiss & Mirin, 1988), or months (Ashton, 1992) following the last use of the drug. This PCP psychosis seems to be most likely in those persons who either have suffered a previous schizophrenic episode (Mirin et al., 1991), or who are vulnerable for such an episode (Jaffe).

There is no way to predict who might develop a PCP-induced psychosis. Grinspoon and Bakalar, (1990) reported that 6 out of 10 patients who had developed a PCP psychosis went on to develop chronic schizophrenia. This suggests a predisposition for schizophrenia in at least some of those who experience a PCP psychosis. Ashton (1992), on the other hand, suggested an alternative theory: the apparent PCP-induced psychosis might result from organic brain damage induced by chronic PCP use. Thus, there is no clear understanding of the mechanism through which PCP induces a psychotic reaction.

The PCP psychosis usually progresses through three stages, each of which lasts approximately five days (Mirin et al., 1991; Weiss & Mirin, 1988). The first stage of the PCP psychosis is usually the most severe, and is characterized by paranoid delusions, anorexia, insomnia, and unpredictable assaultiveness. During this phase, the individual is extremely sensitive to external stimuli (Jaffe, 1989; Mirin et al., 1991), and the talking-down techniques that might work with an LSD bad trip will not usually work with a person experiencing a PCP-induced psychosis (Brust, 1993; Jaffe, 1990).

The middle phase is marked by continued paranoia and restlessness, but the individual is usually calmer, and in intermittent control of his/her behavior (Mirin et al., 1991; Weiss & Mirin, 1988). This phase also usually lasts 5 days and gradually blends into the final phase of the PCP psychosis recovery process. This final phase is marked by a gradual recovery over 7 to 14 days; however, in some patients the PCP psychosis may last for months (Mirin et al., 1991; Slaby et al., 1981; Weiss & Mirin, 1988). Social withdrawal and severe depression are also common following chronic use of PCP (Jaffe, 1990).

There appear to be some minor withdrawal symptoms following prolonged periods of hallucinogen use. Chronic PCP users have reported memory problems, which seem to clear when they stop using the drug (Jaffe, 1990; Newell & Cosgrove, 1988). Recent evidence suggests that chronic PCP users demonstrate the same pattern of neuropsychological deficits found in other forms of chronic drug use; thus PCP may cause chronic brain damage (Grinspoon & Bakalar, 1990; Newell & Cosgrove, 1988).

Research has also revealed that at high dosage levels, PCP can cause hypertensive episodes (Lange et al., 1992). These periods of unusually high blood pressure may then cause the individual to experience a cerebral vascular accident (CVA, or "stroke") (Brust, 1993; Daghestani & Schnoll, 1994). Although research into this area is lacking, the possibility exists that this is the mechanism through which PCP causes brain damage.

The majority of PCP users who die do so because of traumatic injuries that they suffer while under the drug's effects ("Consequences of PCP," 1994). Because of the assaultiveness frequently induced by PCP, many users end up either as the victim of homicide or as the perpetrator of a homicide while under the drug's effects (Ashton, 1992). Given its effects on the user, researchers are mystified as to why anybody would want to use PCP.

Ecstasy: Latest in a Long Line of "Better" Hallucinogens?

In the past two decades, substance abuse professionals have been dealing with a "new" hallucinogenic, the chemical formula for which is N, alpha-dimethyl-1,3 benzodioxole-t-ethanamine. On the streets, this drug is called by such names as "ecstasy," "XTC," "M&M," "Adam" (Beebe & Walley, 1991), or "rave," or simply by the letter "E" (Henry, Jeffreys, & Dawling, 1992), Clinicians and chemists simply refer to the drug by the initials "MDMA."

Although classified by some as a new "designer" drug, MDMA actually was first synthesized by scientists in 1914.[4] But a medical use for MDMA was

never identified, and the chemical remained little more than a curiosity until the 1970s (Climko, Roehrich, Sweeney, & Al-Razi, 1987; Cook, 1995; Mirin et al., 1991; Sternbach & Varon, 1992). One exception to this was the U.S. Army, which briefly considered MDMA as a possible chemical warfare agent in the 1950s before moving on to other compounds (Abbott & Concar, 1992). Because nobody really seemed interested in MDMA, it was not classified as a controlled substance when the drug classification system currently in use was set up in the early 1970s. The British government banned MDMA in 1977 (Abbott & Concar, 1992), while in this country the Drug Enforcement Administration did not classify MDMA as a controlled substance until 1985 (Climko et al., 1987).

MDMA is a chemical cousin of the amphetamines and has a similar chemical structure. For this reason, MDMA is occasionally referred to as a "psychedelic amphetamine" (Cook, 1995). The chemical structure of MDMA is also similar to that of another hallucinogen, MDA (Creighton, Black & Hyde, 1991; Kirsch, 1986). MDMA briefly surfaced as a drug of abuse during the 1960s. But, because LSD was more potent and did not cause the nausea or vomiting often experienced by MDMA users, LSD became the more popular hallucinogenic.

MDMA was all but forgotten by drug users until the mid-1970s. Then illicit drug manufacturers "decided to resurrect, christen, package, market, distribute, and advertise" (Kirsch, 1986, p. 76) MDMA. An apparent reason for this decision was that MDMA was not then classified as a controlled substance in the United States. In the mid-1970s, manufacturers could legally produce MDMA in this country without having to fear the harsh penalties for the manufacture of such controlled substances as LSD or amphetamines.

Within the drug underworld, marketing plans and possible product names were discussed (Kirsch, 1986). The possible name of "empathy" was considered; however, "ecstasy" was finally selected. In effect, this brought the techniques of big business to the drug world. The unknown drug manufacturers first created a demand for a "product," which was then conveniently met by the very people who had first manipulated the public into clamoring for

---

[4]Cook (1995) says that MDMA was patented in 1913, not 1914.

MDMA. The original samples of ecstasy included a "package insert" (Kirsch, 1986, p. 81) that "included unverified scientific research and an abundance of 1960s mumbo-jumbo" (p. 81). However, these same package inserts warned the user not to mix ecstasy with other chemicals (including alcohol), to only occasionally use the drug, and to take care to ensure a proper set for using it.

By the late 1970s, MDMA was a popular drug of abuse both in the United States and in Europe. The official response in the United States was swift: the Drug Enforcement Administration (DEA) classified MDMA as a controlled substance effective July 1, 1985 (Climko et al., 1987). As of that date, "trafficking in MDMA (was made) punishable by fifteen years in prison and a $125,000 fine" (Kirsch, 1986, p. 84). Immediately after this, several "labs" known to be involved in the production of MDMA were shut down by the DEA. By the time that the drug was classified as a controlled substance, it had become a popular drug of abuse, and the demand for MDMA was being met by street "chemists" who were more than happy to supply the drug . . . for a price. This practice has continued until the present day.

Scope of the Problem of MDMA Abuse

Since its reintroduction in the 1970s, MDMA has remained a popular drug of abuse for many people. Within the "rave" subculture, its use is considered socially acceptable. The rave subculture centers around parties that are frighteningly similar to the LSD parties of the 1960s and early 1970s. At these parties, MDMA is supplied to all participants (Randell, 1992). Such parties have been common in the United Kingdom and have been reported here in the United States as well. Further, the drug is viewed by many as a "dance making drug," because users feel the urge to dance for extended periods ("The Agony," 1994).

To understand the popularity of MDMA, consider the following: In 1976 one illicit drug lab manufactured and distributed an estimated 10,000 doses of MDMA per month (Kirsch 1986). By the year 1984, this same lab was manufacturing and distributing approximately 30,000 doses of the drug per month. In 1985, the year that the manufacture of

MDMA was finally declared illegal, this same lab was thought to be turning out some 500,000 doses per month, according to Kirsch. This illicit drug laboratory has since been closed by the authorities, but the demand for MDMA is still there, and underground laboratories are busy producing the drug.

Early demand for MDMA in the United States was fueled by news stories in the popular press about ecstasy's supposed value in psychotherapy ("Drug Problems," 1990). In the United States, 3% of college students surveyed in 1995 admitted to having used MDMA at least once (Johnston et al., 1996). Despite being illegal in England, an estimated 750,000 doses of MDMA are consumed in that country each weekend (Cook, 1995).

MDMA users tend to have different drug-use patterns than is the case for the other chemicals of abuse. During the mid-1980s, it was found that the *median* number of MDMA doses ingested by students who had used this drug was 4.0 (Peroutka, 1989). The author found that the *average* number of doses reported being 5.4 per student. The dosage levels being reported were 60–250 mg. Further, the author observed that recreational users of MDMA tend to use the drug only once every 2 or 3 weeks, if not less frequently than this. This rather unusual drug use pattern reflects that MDMA users become tolerant to the drug's effects rather quickly, and the desired effects become weaker as tolerance develops.

As the individual becomes tolerant to MDMA, he/she is more likely to experience the negative side effects associated with its use. Surprisingly, taking a double dose does not increase the desired effects of MDMA, but rather makes it more likely that the individual will experience unpleasant side effects (Peroutka, 1989), and increases the chances of MDMA-induced brain damage (McGuire & Fahy, 1991). However, the high cost of the chemical ($20–$25 per dose) has caused some users to turn to amphetamines as an alternative ("The Agony," 1994).

Subjective and Objective Effects of MDMA Abuse

Much of what is known about the MDMA's effects are based on observations of illicit drug users. Although it has been a popular drug of abuse for more than a decade, there has been little objective research into the pharmacological or toxicological effects of MDMA (Karch, 1996). Researchers believe that MDMA works by inhibiting the reabsorption of the neurotransmitter serotonin after it has been released by neurons in the brain.

The effects of one dose of MDMA usually begin in about 20 minutes, and peak within an hour (Cook, 1995). The drug's effects last 4–6 hours and the half-life of MDMA is estimated to be approximately 8 hours (Karch, 1996). Research using animals suggests that the LD_{50} following a single intravenous dose of MDMA is approximately 8–23 mg/kg in dogs, and 17–28 mg/kg in Rhesus monkeys (Karch). One study, which used a single volunteer subject, found that almost three-fourths of the MDMA ingested was excreted unchanged in the urine, within 72 hours of the time that the drug was first used.

At dosage levels of 75–100 mg, the individual experiences a sense of euphoria, and improved self-esteem (Beebe & Walley, 1991). At this dosage level, the user might also possibly experience mild visual hallucinations (Evanko, 1991). Following the period of acute drug intoxication, some users experience some degree of confusion, anxiety, and depression following their use of MDMA (Weiss et al., 1994). These feelings reportedly lasted for several hours, to several days following the individual's use of MDMA.

At one point, some psychiatrists advocated the use of MDMA as an aid to psychotherapy (Price et al., 1989, 1990). Climko et al. (1987) reported that one "uncontrolled study" (p. 365) found that MDMA brought about a positive change in mood. But the authors also pointed out that MDMA has also been reported to cause:

> . . . tachycardia, an occasional "wired" feeling, jaw clenching, nystagmus, a nervous desire to be in motion, transient anorexia, panic attacks, nausea and vomiting, ataxia, urinary urgency . . . insomnia, tremors, inhibition of ejaculation, and rarely, transient hallucinations. (p. 365)

Some of the other effects of a typical dose of MDMA include an increase in heart rate, muscle tremor, tightness in jaw muscles, bruxism (grinding of teeth), nausea, insomnia, headache, and sweating. People who are sensitive to the effects of MDMA may experience numbness and tingling in extremities of the body, vomiting, increased sensitivity to cold, visual hallucinations, ataxia, crying, blurred vision, nystagmus, and the experience of having the floor appear to shake. MDMA has been implicated as the cause of decreased sexual desire, as well as inhibition of the ejaculatory reflex and erectile problems in men (Finger et al., 1997).

Complications of MDMA Use

There have been a number of reports involving fatal reactions to MDMA, usually as a result of cardiac arrhythmias (Beebe & Walley, 1991). It is thought that MDMA has the same ability to alter cardiac function as its chemical cousins, the amphetamines (Karch, 1996). There have also been reports of intracranial hemorrhage in some victims (Sternbach & Varon, 1992), and one case report of a young woman who developed a condition known as cerebral venous sinus thrombosis after ingesting MDMA at a rave party (Rothwell & Grant, 1993). The authors speculated that dehydration may have been a factor in the development of the cerebral venous sinus thrombosis in this case and warned of the need to maintain adequate fluid intake while under the influence of MDMA.

Some MDMA users have developed an extreme elevation of the body temperature, a condition known as hyperthermia, which may be fatal without proper treatment. At one point, it was thought that this temperature elevation was most common in those who engaged in heavy exercise (such as prolonged, vigorous dancing) after taking the drug (Ames, Wirshing, & Friedman, 1993; Beebe & Walley, 1991; Cook, 1995; Randall, 1992). But researchers have been unable to isolate the factor(s) that bring about hyperthermia in MDMA users (Bodenham & Mallick, 1996).

There are also isolated reports of liver toxicity in persons who had ingested MDMA, although it is not clear whether the observed toxic reactions were the result of the drug itself or from one or more contaminants in the dose consumed by the user (Cook, 1995; Henry et al., 1992; Jones et al., 1994). It has been suggested that the MDMA user may experience flashbacks similar to those seen with LSD use

(Creighton et al., 1991). These MDMA flashbacks usually develop in the first few days following the use of the drug (Cook).

In another interesting drug effect seen at normal dosage levels, the user will occasionally "relive" past memories. The experienced memories are often ones that were suppressed because of the pain associated with those events (Hayner & McKinney, 1986). Thus, the individual might find him/herself reliving an experience that he/she did not want to remember. This effect, which many psychotherapists thought might prove beneficial in the therapeutic relationship, may be so frightening to the user as to be "detrimental to the individual's mental health" (p. 343). Long-time use has contributed to episodes of violence, and also to suicide, according to the journal *Medical Update* ("The Agony," 1994).

The therapeutic index of MDMA is small, with a significant overlap existing between the usual dose of the drug, and the amount necessary to cause a toxic reaction (Karch, 1996). Symptoms of an MDMA overdose include restlessness, agitation, sweating, tachycardia, hypertension, hypotension, heart palpitations, renal failure, muscle rigidity, and visual hallucinations (Jaffe, 1995a). Seizures may be induced by extreme elevations in body temperature (Henry, 1996). MDMA use may prove fatal, although fatalities are relatively rare. The *Economist* ("Better than Well," 1996) estimated that MDMA causes one death for each 3 million doses. Evidence suggests, however, that MDMA "can potentially kill at doses that were previously tolerated in susceptible individuals" (Hayner & McKinney, 1986, p. 342). Some potential treatments available to physicians for toxic reactions to MDMA are methysergide maleate or beta-blockers (Ames et al., 1993).

In addition to the acute toxic effects of MDMA, it may also cause residual effects, such as anxiety attacks, persistent insomnia, rage reactions, and a drug-induced psychosis (Hayner & McKinney, 1986; Karch, 1996; McGuire & Fahy, 1991). The MDMA-induced psychosis is thought to be most commonly seen in chronic users of MDMA, and resembles paranoid schizophrenia (Cook, 1995; Sternbach & Varon, 1992). Researchers are still not sure of the exact mechanism by which MDMA causes a drug-induced psychosis. It is thought that, like the amphetamines, MDMA is able to activate a psychotic reaction because of a suspected biological predisposition on the part of the user (McGuire & Fahy).

Animal research suggests that once MDMA reaches the brain, it functions as a selective neurotoxin,[5] causing damage to those neurons that use serotonin as a neurotransmitter (Fischer, Hatzidimitriou, Wlos, Klatz, & Ricaurte, 1995; Jaffe, 1995a; Sternbach & Varon, 1992). The mechanism through which MDMA functions as a neurontoxin remains unknown. But to put the danger of MDMA as a toxin into perspective, a rat in a laboratory might receive 10,000 times the normal human dose of LSD in an experiment and not demonstrate any signs of neurotoxicity. However, rats, guinea pigs, and monkeys that receive only two or three times the normal dose of MDMA have been found to show symptoms of neurotoxicity (McGuire & Fahy, 1991; M. Roberts, 1986). Thus, there is strong evidence that MDMA is neurotoxic in animals and possibly in humans as well.

Many of the studies that suggest MDMA might be neurotoxic in humans have been challenged, however, on the grounds that the experimental animals were forced to ingest high doses of MDMA twice a day, for several days in a row ("MDMA May Not," 1996). As stated earlier, most human MDMA users ingest the drug only rarely, and for the most part use fewer than 10 doses. The animal research thus does not follow a dosage pattern similar to that found in human MDMA users, raising questions as to its applicability in humans.

But there is still significant evidence suggesting that MDMA is neurotoxic in human users. Even limited MDMA use has been found to cause a 35% reduction in 5-HT metabolism (an indirect measure of serotonin activity in the brain) for men, and almost a 50% reduction in 5-HT metabolism in women (Hartman, 1995). Thus, there is evidence that MDMA may be neurotoxic to human users although there is no information on whether this brain damage is permanent ("Drug Problems," 1990; Grob, Bravo, & Walsh, 1990; Karch, 1996; Mann, 1994).

---

[5] A neurotoxin is a chemical that destroys nerve cells, which are known as neurons.

Peroutka (1989) argued that, while there is no evidence to suggest that MDMA is addictive, there is evidence to suggest "a long-term, and poentially irreversible, effect of MDMA on the human brain" (p. 191). Price et al. (1989, 1990) found indirect evidence suggesting that MDMA indeed causes neurotoxicity in humans. It was found that MDMA users responded differently to a test designed to measure serotonin levels in the body. Admittedly, the measured differences between MDMA users and normal control subjects were not statistically significant in the study conducted by Price et al. (1989). However, the authors still concluded that the results were suggestive of neurotoxicity caused by ecstasy use.

These findings are especially frightening because of those college students who admitted to using MDMA, the average dose was 60–250 mg, a dosage level found to cause neurotoxicity in animals (Peroutka, 1989). Some research evidence suggests that MDMA is toxic to certain brain cells in animals and possibly in humans. Thus, the latest drug to emerge from the nation's illicit laboratories may very well cause organic brain damage in the user, a sharp contrast to its reputation on the streets as a warm, relaxing, loving drug.

Summary

Weil (1986) suggested that people initially use chemicals to alter the normal state of consciousness.

Hallucinogen use in this country, at least in the past generation, has followed a series of waves, as first one drug and then another becomes the current drug of choice for achieving this altered state. In the 1960s, LSD was the major hallucinogen, and in the 1970s and early 1980s, it was PCP. Now, MDMA seems to be gaining in popularity as the hallucinogen of choice although research suggests that MDMA may cause permanent brain damage, especially to those portions of the brain that utilize serotonin as a primary neurotransmitter.

If we accept Weil's (1986) hypothesis as correct, then it is logical to expect that other hallucinogens will emerge over the years, as people look for a more effective way to alter their state of consciousness. It is likely that these drugs will, in turn, slowly fade as they are replaced by newer hallucinogenics. Just as cocaine faded from the drug scene in the 1930s and was replaced for a while by the amphetamines, so wave after wave of hallucinogen abuse can be expected, as new drugs become available. Thus, chemical dependency counselors will have to maintain a working knowledge of an ever-growing range of hallucinogens in the years to come.

CHAPTER FOURTEEN

Inhalants and Aerosols

The inhalants are unlike the other chemicals of abuse. They are a group of toxic substances that include cleaning agents, herbicides, pesticides, gasoline, kerosene, various forms of glue, laquer thinner, and felt-tipped pens, to name a few chemicals that may potentially be abused as inhalants. These agents are not primarily intended to function as recreational substances. But, many of the chemicals in these compounds will, when inhaled, alter the manner in which the brain functions. In part because of this characteristic, and in part because they are so easily accessible to children and adolescents, inhalant abuse has become the most rapidly growing form of chemical abuse in the United States (Heath, 1994).

Subjectively, at low doses, inhalants may cause the user to experience a sense of euphoria. Further, it is often possible for adolescents, or even children, to purchase many agents that have the potential to be abused by inhalation. For these reasons, children, adolescents, or even the rare adult will occasionally abuse chemical fumes. Because these chemicals are inhaled, they are often called *inhalants* although Esmail, Meyer, Pottier, and Wright (1993) made a case for calling this class of chemicals "volatile substances." In this text, we use the term "inhalants."

The History of Inhalant Abuse

The first recent historical episodes of inhalant abuse involve the practice of anesthetic abuse, dating back to the last century. The earliest documented use of the anesthetic gasses appears to have been for recreation, and historical records from the 1800s document the use of such agents as nitrous oxide for "parties." The use of gasoline fumes to get high is thought to have started prior to World War II (Morton, 1987), with the first documentation of this practice being found in the early 1950s (Blum, 1984).

By the mid-1950s and early 1960s, attention was being paid to the practice of "glue sniffing" in the popular press (D. Anderson, 1989a; Morton, 1987; Westermeyer, 1987). In this practice, the individual uses model airplane glue as an inhalant. The active agent of model glue in the 1950s was often toluene. Nobody knows how the practice of glue sniffing first started, but there is evidence that it began in California, when teenagers accidentally discovered the intoxicating powers of toluene-containing model glue (Berger & Dunn 1982).

The first known reference to this practice was in 1959, in the magazine section of a Denver newspaper (Brecher, 1972). Local newspapers soon began to carry stories on the dangers of inhalant abuse, in the process giving explicit details of how to use airplane glue to become intoxicated and what effects to expect. Within a short period, a "nationwide drug menace" (Brecher, 1972, p. 321) emerged in the United States. Inhalant abuse is thought to be a worldwide problem (Brust, 1993), and is especially common in Japan and Europe (Karch, 1996).

Brecher (1972) suggested that an inhalant abuse "problem" was essentially manufactured through distorted media reports. The author went on to point out that in response to media reports of deaths due to glue sniffing, one newspaper tracked down several stories and found only nine deaths that could be attributed to glue sniffing. Of this number, six deaths were due to asphyxiation: each victim had used an airtight plastic bag and had suffocated.

In one case, there was evidence that asphyxiation was also the cause of death, while in the eighth case there was no evidence that the victim had been using inhalants. Finally, in the ninth case, the individual was found to have been using gasoline as an inhalant but was reported to be in poor health prior to this incident. Furthermore, Brecher (1972) notes that "among tens of thousands of glue-sniffers prior to 1964, no death due unequivocally to glue vapor had as yet been reported. The lifesaving advice children needed was not to sniff glue with their heads in plastic bags" (p. 331).

In reading Brecher's (1972) work, one is left with the question of how serious the glue-sniffing problem was before the news media in this country began to publish reports about it. Without doubt, the media contributed to and enlarged the problem. However, subsequent research has found that inhalants may introduce potentially toxic chemicals into the user's body (Brunswick, 1989; Jaffe, 1989). Some of the consequences of inhalant abuse include cardiac arrhythmias, anoxia, damage to the visual perceptual system, and neuropathies (Hansen & Rose, 1995). Thus, while the media might have played a role in the development of this crisis back in the late 1950s and early 1960s, by the 1990s it has become a legitimate health concern.

The Pharmacology of the Inhalants

As discussed in Chapter 3, many chemical agents reach the brain more rapidly and efficiently when inhaled than when ingested by mouth or injected. When a chemical is inhaled, it is able to enter the bloodstream without its chemical structure being altered in any way by the liver. Once in the blood, one factor that influences how fast that chemical reaches the brain is whether the molecules are able to form chemical bonds with the lipids in the blood. As a general rule, inhalants are quite lipid-soluble

(Henretig, 1996). This feature allows them to reach the brain in an extremely short period, usually within seconds (Blum, 1984; Hartman, 1995; Heath, 1994; Watson, 1984).

Cone (1993) grouped all the inhalants into two broad classifications: (a) anesthetic gasses, and (b) volatile hydrocarbons. In contrast, Monroe (1995) suggested three classes of chemicals that might be inhaled:

1. *Solvents.* Glues, paint, paint thinner, gasoline, kerosene, lighter fluid, fingernail polish, fingernail polish remover, correction fluids for office use, felt tip markers, and so on.
2. *Gasses.* Butane cigarette lighters, propane gas, propellant in whipping cream cans, cooking sprays, and so on.
3. *Nitrites.* Butyl nitrite, amyl nitrite, and so on.

However, D. Anderson (1989a)[1] suggested four classes:

1. *Volatile organic solvents* such as those found in paint and fuel.[2]
2. *Aerosols*, such as hair sprays, spray paints, and deodorants.
3. *Volatile nitrites* (such as amyl nitrite or its close chemical cousin, butyl nitrite).
4. *General anesthetic agents* such as nitrous oxide.

As these classification systems suggest, there are many chemicals, with a multitude of uses, that can be used to produce fumes that will alter the user's sense of reality. Of the different classes of inhalants commonly abused, children and adolescents most often abuse the first two classes of chemicals. Children or adolescents have limited access to the third category

---

[1] Children and adolescents have only limited access to volatile nitrites. In some states, butyl nitrite is sold without a prescription. Thus potentially, children or adolescents have access to the volatile nitrites in some parts of the country. Except in rare cases, the abuse of surgical anesthetics usually involves a small percentage of health care workers, since access to anesthetic gasses is limited to that group.

[2] Technically, alcohol might be classified as a solvent. However, since the most common method of alcohol use/abuse is through oral ingestion, ethyl alcohol is not discussed in this chapter.

of inhalants, and extremely limited access to general anesthetics, the final class of inhalants.

The chemistry of inhalants is quite complex, making it difficult to talk about the "pharmacology" of inhalants. First, there are so many different agents that can be used as an inhalant, each of which has a unique chemical structure. Also, many of the chemicals used as inhalants are designed for industrial or for household use, not human consumption. Thus, there is little research into the specific effects of many inhalants on the human body, since this s not the purpose for which these chemicals were developed.

Also, multiple chemical agents are often combined to achieve the purpose for which these materials are designed, which is to say to meet the needs of industry. The exact combination of chemicals included in any mixture often is dependent on the purpose for which that solvent is to be used, and the conditions under which it is to be used. Again, there is little research into the effects of these chemical compounds on the body, since they were never developed for human inhalation.

Finally, even when the user wants the effects of just one compound, such as cleaning fluid, *all* the chemicals in that compound are introduced into the body when the individual inhales the fumes. In such a case, so many different chemicals are contained in the mixture being inhaled that it is difficult to identify the agent or agents that might cause euphoria, or the chemicals that might cause physical damage (D. Anderson, 1989a; Jaffe, 1989; Morton, 1987).

Once in the brain, the inhalants are thought to alter the normal function of the membranes of the neurons. The exact mechanism by which each inhalant is able to achieve this effect is not known (Henretig, 1996). There is no standard formula for estimating the biological half-life of an inhalant, since so many different chemicals are abused. However, the half-life of most solvents tends to be longer in obese users than in those individuals who lack a significant amount of body fat (Hartman, 1995). As a general rule, the half-life of the compounds commonly abused through inhalation might range from hours to days, depending on the exact chemicals being abused (Brooks, Leung, & Shannon, 1996). The process of removing the inhalants from the body

usually involves a combination of pulmonary exhalation, excretion of the inhalant and/or metabolites in the urine, and biotransformation of the chemicals inhaled by the user's liver (Brooks et al., 1996).

Either directly or indirectly, the compounds inhaled for recreational purposes are all toxic to the human body to one degree or another (Blum, 1984; Fornazzazri, 1988; Morton, 1987). But, there is little research into the effects of industrial chemical compounds at the concentrations used by inhalant abusers. For example, the maximum permitted exposure to toluene fumes in the workplace is 100 parts per million (ppm) (Crowley, 1995a). But, when used as an inhalant, it is not uncommon for the individual to willingly expose him/herself to levels 100 times as high as the maximum permitted industrial exposure level. There has been little research into the effects of most chemicals at this level of exposure (Blum, 1984; Fornazzazri, 1988; Morton, 1987). Further, most of what is known about these chemicals is based on the short-term impact on the individual. There is very little research into the effects of chronic exposure to many of the compounds abused by inhalant users.

Thus, it is difficult to talk about the pharmacology of the inhalants.[3] Ultimately, the material devoted to this topic would fill many tens of thousands of pages, since there are literally thousands of compounds that might be abused by inhalation. But, behavioral observations of animals who have been exposed to inhalants suggest that many inhalants act like alcohol or barbiturates, on the brain. Indeed, alcohol and the benzodiazepines have been found to potentiate the effects of many inhalants such as toluene. However, ultimately, the pharmacology of a given inhalant will depend on the chemicals in the specific compound being abused. Such compounds often contain dozens or, in some cases, scores of different chemicals.

Scope of the Problem

It has been suggested (Newcomb & Bentler, 1989), that these agents are usually the first consciousness-

[3] Hartman (1995) provides an excellent technical summary of the neuropsychological effects of chronic exposure to some of the more common industrial solvents.

altering agents utilized by children. The inhalants tend to be most popular among boys in their early teens, especially in poor or rural areas where more expensive drugs of abuse are not easily available (Henretig, 1996; Jaffe, 1989). In a sense, inhalant abuse is a sporadic fad among teenagers that usually lasts for about year or two (Crowley, 1995a; Henretig, 1996).

As a general rule, inhalant abuse peaks between 11 and 13 years of age, after which it declines in popularity (Brooks et al., 1996). But there is at least one case report of children as young as five years old abusing inhalants (Beauvais & Oetting, 1988), and regular use has been reported in children as young as seven or eight years of age (Henretig, 1996). Further, there is evidence that inhalant abuse is becoming more popular with younger age groups than was true in the past (Hansen & Rose, 1995). The current evidence suggests that inhalant abuse begins somewhere in middle to late childhood, and continues through middle adolescence. For example, Johnston et al. (1996) found that 22% of the students in eighth grade who were asked admitted to the use of an inhalant at least once. Brooks et al. (1996) also found that approximately 1 in 5 students in the eighth grade admitted to the use of an inhalant at least once. Hansen and Rose (1995) found that 12.8% of their sample of 10,198 high school students from Forsyth County, North Carolina, admitted to having ever used an inhalant, with 4.6% having done so in the 30 days preceding the survey. This suggests that older adolescents continue to abuse inhalants in significant numbers.

While these figures are frightening, there is a positive note: Morton (1987) found that of those adolescents who abuse inhalants, 30% to 40% do so only on a few occasions. Another 40% to 50% abuse inhalants over a period of a few weeks to a few months and then discontinue the use of inhalants, according to the author. Only about 10% of those who try inhalants are thought to become "habitual abusers" (Morton, 1987, p. 454). But some of those who do continue to abuse inhalants, many do so for as long as 15 years or more (Schuckit, 1995a; Westermeyer, 1987).

The actual percentage of those persons who are using solvents remains unknown (Miller & Gold, 1991a). However, it has been suggested that for children and adolescents, inhalants are the most commonly abused substance after alcohol and tobacco (Wilson-Tucker & Dash, 1995). The practice of abusing inhalants appears to involve boys more often than girls by a ratio of 3:1 (Crowley, 1995a). Inhalant users are usually between 10 and 15 years of age (Miller & Gold, 1991a). In England, 3% to 10% of the adolescents asked admitted to the use of inhalants at least once, and about 1% were thought to be current users (Esmail et al., 1993).

For a minority of those who abuse them, the inhalants appear to function as a gateway chemical that opens the way to further drug use in later years (D. Anderson, 1989a). Research suggests that approximately one-third of the children who abuse inhalants go on to abuse one or more of the traditional drugs of abuse within 4 years (Brunswick, 1989). Crowley (1995a) reported, for example, that persons who admitted to the use of inhalants were 45 times as likely to have used self-injected drugs, while those individuals who admitted to both the use of inhalants and marijuana were 89 times as likely to have injected drugs as the general population.

Inhalant abuse may thus be the first warning sign of a later substance use problem. Crowley (1995a) suggested that a warning sign also might be found in the personality of the children abusing inhalants. Those children with an oppositional-defiant disorder who abused inhalants seemed more likely to progress to the use of other chemicals, according to the author. However, there has been little research into the relationship between childhood personality patterns and subsequent drug use patterns.

S. Cohen (1977) identified several reasons for the inhalants' popularity as chemicals of abuse. First, these chemicals have a rapid onset of action, usually on the order of a few seconds. Second, inhalant users report pleasurable effects, including a sense of euphoria, when they use these chemicals. Third, and perhaps most important, the inhalants are relatively inexpensive and are easily available to teenagers. They are so easily obtained by adolescents that they have been called a "household drug" (Wisneiwski, 1994, p. 8Ex).

Virtually all the commonly used inhalants may be easily purchased without legal restrictions on their sale to teenagers. An additional advantage for the user is that these inhalants are usually available in small, easily hidden packages. Brunswick (1989) identified some of the more popular inhalants as being:

> ... accessible and cheap. They are found at the corner drug store, in the garage, or under the kitchen sink. They take the form of magic markers, glue, and fingernail polish. They produce a short but intense high that some have likened to the rush from rock cocaine, or "crack." (p. 6A)

As discussed in the next section, many of the inhalants can harm the user, if not actually causing death. The inhalant abuser thus runs a serious risk whenever he/she begins to "huff."[4]

Method of Administration

McHugh (1987) noted that inhalant abuse is "a group activity" (p. 334), as opposed to a solitary habit. There are a number of ways that inhalants can be abused, depending on the specific chemical involved. Glue and adhesives may be poured into a plastic bag, or a milk carton, which is then placed over the mouth and nose (Esmail et al., 1993). The individual then inhales the fumes from the bag. Liquids such as cleaning fluids may be dripped onto a cloth, or into a small container (such as an empty plastic bottle), and the fumes inhaled from the container or cloth. Fumes from aerosol cans may be directly inhaled, or sprayed directly into the mouth, according to the authors.

To inhale the fumes of glue, the user sometimes squirts the glue into a paper bag. Then, the individual covers his or her face with the bag, and inhales (Mirin et al., 1991). Another technique that children often use is to simply squirt the chemical into a rag, and inhale the fumes from the rag (Brunswick, 1989). There are a multitude of other ways for inhaling fumes from household chemicals, far too many to list in this text. However, a common feature of every method is that the user is able to inhale concentrated fumes from a chemical not normally meant to be admitted into the body.

Subjective Effects of Inhalants

The initial effects of the fumes on the individual might include a feeling of hazy euphoria, somewhat like the feeling of intoxication caused by alcohol (Blum, 1984; Crowley, 1995a; Henretig, 1996). Other reported effects include a floating sensation, decreased inhibitions, and possible amnesia, slurred speech, excitement, double vision, ringing in the ears, and hallucinations (Blum, 1984; Kaminski, 1992; Morton, 1987; Schuckit, 1995a). Occasionally, the individual feels omnipotent, and episodes of violence have been reported (Morton). In most cases, the effects of a single exposure may last up to 45 minutes (Mirin et al., 1991).

One of the initial experiences of inhalant abuse is a feeling of euphoria although nausea and vomiting may also occur (McHugh, 1987). The inhalant-induced euphoria lasts less than 30 minutes in most cases. After the initial euphoria, depression of the central nervous system (CNS) develops. The individual may become confused, anxious, disoriented, develop a headache, and experience a loss of inhibitions (Hartman, 1995; Kaminski, 1992; McHugh, 1987). If the individual continues to inhale the fumes beyond this stage, stupor, seizures, and cardiorespiratory arrest may develop (McHugh).

Where the individual has used a solvent only once or twice, the effects usually disappear "fairly quickly, and, with the exception of headache, serious hangovers are usually not seen" (Schuckit, 1995a, p. 217). If there is some degree of inhalant hangover, this usually clears "in minutes to a few hours" (Westermeyer, 1987, p. 903). In some cases, however, the user experiences a residual sense of drowsiness, and/or stupor that lasts for several hours after the last use of inhalants (Kaplan et al., 1994; Miller & Gold, 1991a). Further, there have been reports where an inhalant-induced headache has lasted for several days after the last use of the inhalant (Heath, 1994).

Complications from Inhalant Abuse

When the practice of abusing the inhalants first surfaced, most health care professionals did not think many serious complications could result from this

---

[4] "Huff" is a street term for inhaling the fumes of an inhalant.

practice. However, in the past 25 years, researchers have found that inhalant abuse is a causal factor in a wide range of physical problems. Depending on the concentration of the solvent being abused, even a single episode of use might result in the user developing symptoms of solvent toxicity (Hartman, 1995).

A partial list of the possible consequences of inhalant abuse includes (D. Anderson, 1989a; Brunswick, 1989; Hansen & Rose, 1995; Hartman, 1995; Henretig, 1996; Karch, 1996; Monroe, 1995; Morton, 1987):

Cardiac arrhythmias (irregularities in the heartbeat that may be fatal if not corrected).

Liver damage.

Kidney damage/failure, which may be permanent.

Transient changes in lung function.

Respiratory depression, possibly to the point of respiratory arrest.

Reduction in blood cell production, possibly to the point of aplastic anemia.

Possible permanent organic brain damage (including dementia).

Permanent muscle damage secondary to the development of rhabdomyolysis.

Vomiting, with the possibility of the user aspirating some of the material being vomited, resulting in his/her death.

In addition, inhalant abuse may also cause damage to the bone marrow of the user, sinusitis (irritation of the sinus membranes), erosion of the nasal mucosal tissues, and laryngitis (Henretig, 1996; Westermeyer, 1987). These complications "usually resolve after some weeks of abstinence" (Westermeyer, 1987, p. 903).

The impact of the inhalants on the CNS are perhaps the most profound, if only because inhalant abusers are usually so young. Many of the inhalants have been shown to cause damage to the central nervous system, causing such problems as cerebellar ataxia,[5] tremor, peripheral neuropathies, and

deafness (Brooks et al., 1996; Fornazzazri, 1988; Maas, Ashe, Spiegel, Zee, & Leigh, 1991). Inhalant abuse also can cause such problems as coma, convulsions, cirrhosis, or even death (Henretig, 1996; McHugh, 1987; Mirin et al., 1991). Inhalant-related death is "one of the leading causes of death in those under 18" (Esmail et al., 1993, p. 359). Each year, between 100 and 1000 deaths in the United States are directly attributable to inhalant abuse (Hartman, 1995; Wisneiwski, 1994).

Depending on the compound being used, the individual using an inhalant(s) may be exposed to toxic levels of heavy metals such as copper or lead (Crowley, 1995a). For example, gasoline sniffing by children is a major cause of lead poisoning (Henretig, 1996; Monroe, 1995; Parras, Patier, & Ezpeleta, 1988). Exposure to lead is a serious condition that may have long-term consequences for the child's physical and emotional growth.

Although in the 1970s it was not thought that inhalant abuse could result in physical damage to the body, it is now known that this is not true. There is significant evidence that inhalant abuse may cause permanent damage to the central nervous system. For example, chronic exposure to solvents has been found to be a cause of organic brain damage in European workers (Hartman, 1995). Further, although the standard neurological examination is often unable to detect signs of solvent-induced organic brain damage until it is quite advanced, sensitive neuropsychological tests often find signs of significant neurological dysfunction in workers who are exposed to solvent fumes on a regular basis (Hartman).

Toluene is found in many forms of glue, and is the solvent that is most commonly abused (Hartman, 1995). Researchers have found that chronic toluene exposure might result in intellectual impairment, deafness, and a loss of the sense of smell (Maas et al., 1991; N. Rosenberg, 1989). The chronic exposure to toluene might result in such extensive injury to the brain that it is visible on the magnetic resonance imaging (MRI) procedures utilized by physicians to identify the physical structure of the brain.

Finally, researchers have identified what appears to be a withdrawal syndrome that develops following extended periods of inhalant abuse (Blum, 1984; Mirin et al., 1991). This syndrome appears similar to

---

[5]A loss of coordination caused by physical damage to the region of the brain that is responsible for coordinating muscle movements.

that of alcohol-induced "delirium tremens" (DTs), according to the authors. The exact withdrawal syndrome that develops after episodes of inhalant abuse depends on the specific chemicals being abused, the duration of inhalant abuse, and the dosage levels being administered (Miller & Gold, 1991a). Some of the symptoms seen when a chronic inhalant user stops include muscle tremors, irritability, anxiety, insomnia, muscle cramps, hallucinations, sweating, nausea, and possible seizures (Crowley, 1995a). Thus, the inhalants may be physically addictive when used on a chronic basis.

Anesthetic Misuse

Berger and Dunn (1982) reported that nitrous oxide and ether, the first two anesthetic gasses, were introduced as recreational drugs prior to their introduction as surgical anesthetics. These gases were routinely used as intoxicants for quite some time before they were utilized by medicine. Horace Wells, who introduced the medical profession to nitrous oxide, noted the painkilling properties of this gas when he observed a person under its influence trip and gash his leg, without any apparent pain (Brecher, 1972).

As medical historians know, the first planned demonstration of nitrous oxide as an anesthetic was something less than a success. The patient returned to consciousness in the middle of the operation, and started to scream in pain. However, despite this rather frightening beginning, physicians began to understand how to properly use nitrous oxide to bring about surgical anesthesia, and it is now an important anesthetic agent (Brecher, 1972).

Julien (1992) noted that the pharmacological effects observed with the general anesthetics are the same as those observed with the barbiturates. There is a dose-related range of effects from the anesthetic ranging from an initial period of sedation and relief from anxiety on through sleep and analgesia. At extremely high dosage levels, the anesthetic gasses can cause death.

Nitrous oxide presents a special danger in that precautions must be observed to maintain a proper oxygen supply to the individual's brain. For this reason, Lingeman (1974) reported that nitrous oxide is rarely used as an anesthetic unless it is combined with other agents. Julien (1992) warned that ordinary room air will not provide sufficient oxygen to the brain when nitrous oxide is used. Thus, unless the patient receives a special mixture of oxygen and nitrous oxide, he/she may develop hypoxia (a decreased oxygen level in the blood that can result in permanent brain damage if not corrected immediately). In surgery, the anesthesiologist must ensure that the patient has an adequate oxygen supply.

However, a person using nitrous oxide for recreational purposes lacks the support resources available to the surgical team and runs the risk of serious injury, or even death. It is possible to achieve a state of hypoxia from virtually any of the inhalants, including nitrous oxide (McHugh, 1987). Despite this danger, nitrous oxide is a popular drug of abuse in some circles (Schwartz, 1989). Recreational users report that the gas brings about a feeling of euphoria, giddiness, hallucinations, and a loss of inhibitions (Lingeman, 1974). Dental students, dentists, medical school students, and anesthesiologists, all of whom have access to this gas through their professions occasionally abuse surgical anesthetics such as nitrous oxide, ether, chloroform, trichlorothylene, and halothane. Also, because nitrous oxide is also used as a propellant in certain whipping cream cans, such as "Reddi Whip," children and adolescents occasionally abuse this chemical by finding ways to release the gas from the container. On rare occasions, the user attempts to make his/her own nitrous oxide risking possible death from impurities in the compound (Brooks et al., 1996).

The volatile anesthetics are not metabolized by the body to any significant degree, but enter and leave the body essentially unchanged (Glowa, 1986). Once the source of the gas is removed, the concentration of the gas in the brain begins to drop and normal circulation brings the brain to a normal state of consciousness within moments. While the person is under the influence of the anesthetic gas, however, the ability of the brain cells to react to painful stimuli seems to be reduced.

The use of nitrous oxide, chlorform, and ether is confined, for the most part, to dental or general surgery. Very rarely, however, one encounters a person who has used, or is currently using, these agents.

There is little information available concerning the dangers of this practice, nor is there much information as to the side effects of prolonged use.

Abuse of Nitrites

Two different forms of nitrites commonly abused: *amyl nitrite* and, its close chemical cousin *butyl nitrite*. When inhaled, amyl nitrite functions as a coronary vasodilator, which is to say that it will cause the coronary arteries to dilate, allowing more blood to flow to the heart. Because of this, amyl nitrite was once commonly used in the control of angina pectoris. The drug was administered in small glass containers, embedded in cloth layers. The user would "snap" or "pop" the container and inhale the fumes to control the chest pain of angina pectoris.[6]

With the introduction of nitroglycerine preparations, which are equally effective as amyl nitrite and lack many of its disadvantages, few people now use amyl nitrite for medical purposes (Schwartz, 1989). It continues to have a small role in diagnostic medicine and for the emergency treatment of cyanide poisoning. For the most part, however, the medical uses of amyl nitrite are limited (Schwartz).

While amyl nitrite is available only by prescription, butyl nitrite is often sold legally by mail-order houses, or in specialty stores, depending on specific state regulations. In many areas, butyl nitrite is sold as a "room deordorizer," and is packaged in small bottles that may be purchased for under 10 dollars. Both chemicals are thought to cause the user to experience a prolonged, more intense orgasm, when they are inhaled just before the individual reaches orgasm. However, amyl nitrite is also known to be a cause of delayed orgasm and ejaculation in the male user (Finger et al., 1997). Aftereffects include an intense, sudden headache, increased pressure of the fluid in the eyes (a danger for those with glaucoma),

possible weakness, nausea, and possible cerebral hemorrhage (Schwartz, 1989).

When abused, both amyl nitrite and butyl nitrite cause a brief (90-second) rush that includes dizziness, giddiness, and the rapid dilation of blood vessels in the head (Schwartz, 1989), which in turn causes an increase in intracranial pressure ("Research on," 1989). It is this increase that may, on occasion, contribute to the rupture of unsuspected aneurysms, causing the individual to experience a cerebral hemorrhage (a "stroke").

The use of nitrites is common among male homosexuals and may contribute to the spread of the virus that causes AIDS ("Research on," 1989; Schwartz, 1989). It has been suggested that by causing the dilation of blood vessels in the body, including the anus, the use of either amyl or butyl nitrite during anal intercourse (a common practice for male homosexuals) may actually aid the transmission of the HIV from the active to the passive member of the sexual unit ("Research on," 1989). Given the multitude of adverse effects, one may ask why it is popular during sexual intercourse.

Summary

For many, the inhalants are the first chemicals abused for recreational purposes. For the most part, inhalant abuse seems to be a phase that mainly involves teenagers, although occasionally young children will abuse an inhalant. During this phase, teenagers tend to engage in the abuse of inhalants on an episodic basis.

Individuals who use inhalants do not usually do so for more than one or two years. But a few individuals continue to inhale the fumes of gasoline, solvents, certain forms of glue, and so on, for many years. The effects of these chemicals on the individual seem to be rather short-lived. There is evidence, however, that prolonged use of certain agents can result in permanent damage to the kidneys, brain, and liver. Death, either through hypoxia or through prolonged exposure to inhalants, is possible. Very little is known about the effects of prolonged use of this class of chemicals.

---

[6]It is from the distinctive sound of the glass breaking within the cloth ampule that both amyl nitrite and butyl nitrite have come to be known as "poppers" or "snappers" by those who abuse these chemicals.

Anabolic Steroids

Unlike alcohol, marijuana, or virtually every other drug of abuse, the anabolic steroids (or, simply, steroids) are not primarily abused for their ability to bring about a sense of euphoria. Rather, the anabolic steroids are abused because of persistent rumors that these chemicals enhance athletic performance. So common has the use of steroids become in certain athletic training programs that some athletes look on these drugs as a "nutritional supplement" (Breo, 1990, p. 1697), rather than as potent chemical agents.

Very little is actually known about the problem of anabolic steroid abuse (Bower, 1991). This is unfortunate, because despite their considerable potential to harm the user, many teenagers and young adults are abusing one or more steroids. The growing recognition of the problem of anabolic steroid abuse demands that mental health and chemical dependency professionals have a working knowledge of the effects of this class of medications.

An Overview of the Anabolic Steroids

The term *anabolic* refers to the action of this family of drugs to increase the speed of growth of body tissues, while *steroids* refers to their chemical structure (Redman, 1990). These drugs are chemically similar to testosterone, the male sex hormone and because of this have a masculinizing (androgenic) effect on the user (Hough & Kovan, 1990; Landry & Primos, 1990). At times, this class of chemicals is referred to as the *anabolic-androgenic steroid* family of drugs.

It has been suggested that, when abused, these drugs may cause the user to experience a feeling of euphoria (M. Johnson, 1990; Kashkin, 1992; Lipkin, 1989; Schrof, 1992). However, this is not the primary reason most people abuse them. Rather, steroids are mainly abused either to stimulate the growth of muscle tissue or simply to slow the process of muscle tissue breakdown. Repeated, heavy, physical exercise can actually damage muscle tissues. The anabolic steroids have been found to stimulate protein synthesis, a process that indirectly may help muscle tissue development, increase muscle strength and, it is thought by users, limit the damage to muscle tissues through heavy physical exercise (Gottesman, 1992; Hough & Kovan, 1990; Pettine, 1991; Pope & Katz, 1990).

In addition to athletes who abuse steroids, many nonathletic users believe that steroid use will help them look more physically attractive (Bahrke, 1990; Brower, 1993; Corrigan, 1996; M. Johnson, 1990; Pettine, 1991; Pope, Katz, & Champoux, 1986; Schrof, 1992). Between 25% (Fultz, 1991) and 40% (Whitehead, Chillag, & Elliott, 1992) of adolescent steroid abusers take the drug out of a belief that it will give them a better looking appearance. In addition, there is a subgroup of people, especially some law enforcement officers and security officers, who abuse steroids because of the belief that these drugs will increase their strength and aggressiveness (Corrigan, 1996; Schrof, 1992).

Medical Uses of Anabolic Steroids

Although the anabolic steroids have been in use since the mid-1950s, there still is no clear consensus on how they work (Wadler, 1994). It is thought that the steroids force the body to increase protein synthesis and inhibit the action of chemicals known as the glucocorticoids, which cause tissue breakdown. In a medical setting, the anabolic steroids are used by physicians to promote tissue growth and help damaged tissue recover from injury (Shannon et al., 1995).

Physicians may also use one of the steroid family of drugs to treat certain forms of anemia, help patients regain weight after a severe illness, treat endometriosis, and as an adjunct to the treatment of certain forms of breast cancer in women (Bagatell & Bremner, 1996; United States Pharmacopeial Convention, 1990b). The steroids may also promote the growth of bone tissue following injuries to the bone in certain cases. The Council on Scientific Affairs of the American Medical Association (1990b) suggested that steroids might be useful in the treatment of osteoporosis.

The anabolic steroids can be broken down into two classes: (a) those that are active when used orally, and (b) those that are active only when injected into muscle tissue. Anabolic steroids intended for oral use tend have a shorter half-life, but are also more toxic to the liver than parenteral forms of steroids (Bagatell & Bremner, 1996; Tanner, 1995).

The Legal Status of Anabolic Steroids

In 1990, Congress outlawed the use of anabolic steroids, except for medical purposes. Thus, the steroids, like narcotic analgesics, are considered to be a "controlled substance." As of 1990, the anabolic steroids were listed under the Controlled Substances Act of 1970 as a Schedule III controlled substance. These medications are available, with a doctor's prescription, for certain medical purposes. However, the sale of any of 28 different forms of anabolic steroids for nonmedical purposes or by individuals who are not licensed to sell medications is a

crime that may be punishable by a prison term of up to 5 years (10 years if the steroids are sold to minors) (Fultz, 1991).

Scope of the Problem of Steroid Abuse

There has been little research into the scope of the problem of steroid abuse in the United States (Brower, 1993; Kashkin, 1992). Estimates of the scope of steroid abuse in the United States range from a low estimate of 300,000 current and 1 million former anabolic steroid abusers (Bagatell & Bremner, 1996; Franklin, 1994; Karch, 1996), to a middle estimate of 1 million people currently abusing steroids (Middleman & DuRant, 1996; Porterfield, 1991; Schrof, 1992) to a high estimate of 3 million current, and at least 1 million former steroid abusers (Corrigan, 1996).

Adolescents of high school age, although known to abuse anabolic steroids, do not seem to make up the majority of steroid abusers. Compared with the approximately 20% of college athletes who are thought to have used steroids on at least one occasion (Hough & Kovan, 1990), only 2.3% of the high school seniors of the class of 1995 admitted to the use of steroids (Johnston et al., 1996). In terms of actual numbers, it is thought that between 250,000 (DuRant, Rickert, Ashworth, Newman, & Slavens, 1993) and 500,000 (Schrof, 1992; Wadler, 1994) high school students are either current or former users of anabolic steroids. For this reason, the majority of those college athletes who abuse steroids are thought to have started to do while in college (Brower, 1993).

Sources and Methods of Steroid Abuse

Anabolic steroids are widely available through illicit sources including drugs smuggled into the United States or legitimate pharmaceuticals that are diverted to the black market. Another common source of steroids are veterinary products, which are then sold on the street for use by humans. Whatever the source, steroids tend to be available through an informal distribution network found in health clubs or gyms (M. Johnson, 1990; Schrof, 1992).

Frequently, the steroid abuser's physician confronts him/her with the evidence of steroid abuse and the patient confesses to using anabolic steroids for personal reasons. All too often, the physician then offers to prescribe anabolic steroids to the user, on the condition that he/she *only* take the steroids prescribed by the doctor (Breo, 1990). This offer is made by the physician in the hope of being able to monitor and control the individual's use of these drugs. However, athletes rarely will limit themselves to the prescribed medications and obtain steroids from other sources to increase their daily dosage. Thus, the physician should not attempt to control the user's daily dose of steroids by prescribing it, according to Breo (1990).

Many users obtain their steroids by diverting prescribed medications, or by obtaining multiple prescriptions for steroids from different physicians. "Diverting" refers to a process by which prescribed medications are used by individuals for whom these medications were never prescribed. Sometimes, the medications are stolen from drugstores, or medicine cabinets, while on other occasions an individual with a legitimate need for steroids will (for a fee) visit several different doctors, obtain a prescription for medications from each physician, and then sell the excess medication to others.

Between 80% (Bahrke, 1990) and 90% (Tanner, 1995) of the steroids used by athletes comes from the black market.[1] Many of the steroids smuggled into this country originate in Mexico or Europe (M. Johnson, 1990). Estimates of the scope of the illicit steroid market in the United States range from $100 million (DuRant et al., 1993; Middleman & DuRant, 1996) to $300–$500 million (Council on Scientific Affairs, 1990b; Fultz, 1991; Wadler, 1994) to $1 billion a year (Hoberman & Yesalis, 1995).

Anabolic steroids may be injected into muscle tissue, taken orally, or both intramuscular and oral doses of the medication may be used at once. This latter practice is known as "stacking" steroids (Brower, 1993). Injectable steroids are known as "injectables," while oral forms of these drugs are known as "orals" (Bahrke, 1990) or "juice" (Fultz, 1991). Fully 61% of steroid-abusing weight lifters were found to have engaged in stacking steroids (Brower, Blow, Young, & Hill, 1991). Another way in which the steroids are abused is through the practice of "pyramiding." The abuser using this method starts a cycle of steroid abuse by initially taking the smallest dose and gradually increasing the daily dosage level so that by the midcycle the user is taking a massive amount of steroids. Then, the daily dosage level is gradually tapered, until by the last week in the cycle the abuser is again taking a relatively small daily dose.

Episodes of pyramiding are alternated with periods of abstinence from anabolic steroid use that may last several weeks or months (Landry & Primos, 1990), or perhaps even as long as a year (Kashkin, 1992). During the periods of abstinence, much of the muscle mass gained by the use of steroids will be lost, sometimes quite rapidly. When this happens, anabolic steroid abusers often become frightened into prematurely starting another cycle of steroid abuse, to recapture the muscle mass that has disappeared (Corrigan, 1996; Schrof, 1992; Tanner, 1995).

Problems Associated with Anabolic Steroid Abuse

Much of what is known about the anabolic steroids is based on clinical experience from patients who are taking steroids under a physician's care, using specific recommended dosage levels to achieve a specific goal (Medical Economics Company, 1989). Adverse effects have been documented at relatively low doses in cases where these medications are used to treat medical conditions (Hough & Kovan, 1990). The consequences of long-term steroid abuse at the dosage levels usually utilized by abusers are simply not known (Kashkin, 1992; Schrof, 1992; Wadler, 1994).

What little is known about the consequences of anabolic steroid abuse is usually based on clinical data from male steroid abusers. In large part, this reflects the tendency for steroid abusers to be male. Karch (1996) observed that 7% of high school boys,

---

[1]As used here, the term "black market" applies to any steroid obtained from illicit sources and then sold for human consumption.

but only 1% of high school girls surveyed admitted to the use of anabolic steroids. As a result of this male bias, virtually nothing is known about the long-term effects of anabolic steroid abuse on women (Gottesman, 1992).

The adverse effects of anabolic steroids depends on the (a) route of administration, (b) the specific drugs taken, (c) the dose utilized, (d) the frequency of use, (e) the health of the individual, and (f) the age of the individual (M. Johnson, 1990). However, even at recommended dosage levels, steroids are capable of causing sore throat or fever, vomiting (with or without blood being mixed into the vomit), dark colored urine, bone pain, nausea, unusual weight gain or headache, and a range of other side effects (United States Pharmacopeial Convention, 1990b).

Many adolescents and young adults who abuse steroids do so at dosage levels that are often 10 (Hough & Kovan, 1990), 40 (M. Johnson, 1990), 100 (Brower, Catlin, Blow, Eliopulos, & Beresford, 1991), or even 1000 times the maximum recommended dosage level (Council on Scientific Affairs, 1990b; Wadler, 1994). The research team of Brower, Blow, et al. (1991), for example, found that the dosage range of steroids being used by their sample of weight lifters was 2 to 26 times the recommended dosage level for these agents.

Another study found that the *lowest* dose of anabolic steroids being used by a group of weight lifters was still 350% above the usual therapeutic dose (Landry & Primos, 1990). There is very little information available on the effects of the anabolic steroids on the user at these dosage levels (M. Johnson, 1990; Kashkin, 1992). It is known that the effects of the anabolic steroids on muscle tissue last for several weeks after the drugs are discontinued (Pope & Katz, 1991). Thus, muscle builders who abuse steroids may discontinue the drugs shortly before competition, to avoid having their steroid use detected by urine toxicological screens.

Other illicit steroid users abuse specific forms of anabolic steroids that are hard to detect or that are thought to be undetectable by current laboratory tests. Thus, a clean urine sample does not rule out steroid use in modern sporting events or rule out the possibility that the individual is at risk for any of a wide range of complications.

Complications of Steroid Abuse

Reproductive System

Males who utilize steroids at the recommended dosage levels may experience enlargement of breasts (to the point where breast formation similar to that seen in adolescent girls takes place). The male steroid abuser may also experience increased frequency of erections or continual erections (a condition known as priapism, which is a medical emergency), unnatural hair growth/hair loss, and a frequent urge to urinate.

Steroid abuse in males may also bring about degeneration of the testicles, enlargement of the prostate gland, impotence, and sterility (Council on Scientific Affairs, 1990b; Hough & Kovan, 1990; Kashkin, 1992; Pope & Katz, 1994). On rare occasions, steroid abuse has resulted in carcinoma (cancer) of the prostate (M. Johnson, 1990; Landry & Primos, 1990; Tanner, 1995), and urinary obstruction (Council on Scientific Affairs, 1990b).

Women who use steroids at recommended dosage levels may experience an abnormal enlargement of the clitoris, irregular menstrual periods, unnatural hair growth and/or unusual hair loss, a deepening of the voice, and a possible reduction in the size of the breasts (Hough & Kovan, 1990; Pope & Katz, 1988; Redman, 1990; Tanner, 1995). The menstrual irregularities caused by steroid use often disappear after the steroids are discontinued (M. Johnson, 1990). The Council for Scientific Affairs (1990b) suggested that women who use steroids may experience beard growth, which is an example of the unnatural hair growth pattern caused by these drugs. Another possible outcome for women is the development of "male pattern" baldness. Often, steroid-induced baldness in the woman is irreversible (Tanner, 1995).

Liver, Kidneys, and Digestive Systems

Steroid abusers may experience altered liver function, which may be detected through the blood tests such as the serum glautamic-oxaloacetic transaminase (SGOT), and the serum glautamic-pyruvic transaminase (SGPT) (M. Johnson, 1990). As noted, oral forms of anabolic steroids may be more likely to result in liver problems than injected forms

(Tanner, 1995). Anabolic steroid abuse has been implicated as a cause of hepatoxicity (liver failure). In addition, there is evidence to suggest that, when used for an extended period at excessive doses, steroids might contribute to the formation of both cancerous and benign liver tumors (Council for Scientific Affairs, 1990b; Karch, 1996; Tanner, 1995).

Cardiovascular System

Anabolic steroid abuse may result in the user developing high blood pressure, cardiomyopathy, and heart disease as a result of a steroid-induced reduction in high-density lipoprotein levels and an increase in the low-density lipoprotein levels (Council for Scientific Affairs, 1990b; Fultz, 1991; M. Johnson, 1990; Tanner, 1995). In effect, the anabolic steroids may contribute to accelerated atherosclerosis of the heart and its surrounding blood vessels.

Anabolic steroid abuse might also result in the user experiencing a thrombotic stroke, which is to say a stroke caused by a blood clot in the brain (Karch, 1996; Tanner, 1995). Such strokes are a side effect of high doses of the anabolic steroids, which cause blood platelets to clump together, forming clots. Researchers have also found evidence that suggests steroids have a direct, dose-related, cardiotoxic effect (Slovut, 1992). There is evidence of physical changes in the structure of the heart of some steroid users although the mechanism by which steroids cause this effect is not known (Milddleman & DuRant, 1996).

Central Nervous System

The anabolic steroid family of drugs has been suspected as being capable of causing behavioral changes in the user. To explore this belief, the research team of Wolkowitz et al. (1990) administered 80 mg of a pharmaceutical steroid known as prednisone daily for 5 days, to a sample of healthy volunteers. The authors found that "prednisone administration was associated with decreases in . . . levels of several biologically and behaviorally active neuropeptides or neurotransmitters" (p. 966). In other words, the authors found measurable changes in the levels of neuropeptides or neurotransmitters in their sample, after only 5 days. However,

despite these measured changes in biochemical levels, the authors found "no significant prednisone-associated changes . . . in group mean behavioral ratings" (p. 967).

Although the team of Wolkowitz et al. (1990) utilized only a 5-day period to explore whether prednisone might cause behavioral changes, abusers of steroids often do so for far longer than 5 days, and at dosage levels far above 80 mg of prednisone each day. As noted, individuals who abuse steroids often do so at dosage levels between 40 (M. Johnson, 1990) to 1000 times the maximum recommended dosage level (Medical Economics Company, 1995). It requires several weeks of constantly increasing dosage levels to achieve this level of steroid abuse.

At these grossly inflated dosage levels, anabolic steroids are suspected of being able to cause psychotic symptoms in the chronic user (M. Johnson, 1990; Kashkin, 1992; Pope & Katz, 1994; Pope et al., 1986). At the very least, the unpleasant side effects of anabolic steroids may be an incentive for the person to use recreational drugs to self-medicate their discomfort or control side effects (Schrof, 1992). Kashkin (1992) reported that about 50% of steroid abusers abuse other substances to control the side effects of the anabolic steroids. Some of the drugs that the author noted might be abused included diuretics (to counteract steroid-induced "bloating") and antibiotics (to control steroid induced acne).

The team of Pope and Katz (1987) examined 31 weight lifters who had admitted to the use of steroids, and found that 22% of their sample experienced some symptoms of psychosis, apparently as a side effect to their steroid use. In a later study, Pope and Katz (1988) examined 41 athletes who had used steroids, and found that 9 subjects (22%) had experienced either a manic or a depressive reaction while using steroids, while another 5 subjects (12%) had experienced an apparent drug-induced psychotic reaction.

In 1990, the authors reported that, in their opinion, steroid abuse had contributed to the violent behavior of three individuals, to the point where homicide or attempted homicide, was the end result in all three cases. This drug-induced reaction is often known as a " 'roid rage" by illicit steroid users

(Fultz, 1991; Redman, 1990). Up to 90% of those who abuse steroids may experience an increase in aggressive or violent behaviors (M. Johnson, 1990).

The team of Pope and Katz (1994) investigated the psychiatric side effects of anabolic steroid abuse. Their research sample was made up of 88 steroid-abusing athletes, and 68 individuals who were not abusing steroids. Twenty-three percent of the steroid-abusing athletes were found to have experienced a major mood disturbance such as mania, or depression, which was attributed to their steroid use. They also became more physically aggressive. One member of the sample of steroid abusers examined by Pope and Katz started to smash three different automobiles out of frustration over a traffic delay. Another individual was implicated in a murder plot, while yet a third beat his dog to death. Still another individual in the research sample rammed his head through a wooden door, and several others were expelled from their homes because of their threatening behavior (*The Back Letter*, 1994). Other psychiatric effects of anabolic steroid abuse include loss of inhibition, lack of judgment, irritability, a "strange edgy feeling" (Corrigan, 1996, p. 222), impulsiveness, and antisocial behavior (Corrigan).

An interesting possible explanation for this increased level of violence while under the influence of anabolic steroids was offered by Yesalis, Kennedy, Kopstein, and Bahrke (1993). The authors examined earlier studies that suggested a relationship between violent behavior and anabolic steroid use, but failed to find a causal relationship. Two different theories were suggested Yesalis et al. (1993) to account for this misperception. First, the authors suggested that for some unknown reason, anabolic steroid abusers might have exaggerated their self-report of violent behavior noted in earlier studies. A second possibility, according to the authors, was that violent individuals are prone to abuse steroids for some unknown reason, giving the illusion of a causal relationship. In either case, there is a need for further research to further explore the relationship between anabolic steroid use and violence, according to the authors of this study.

Steroids may cause depression in both men and women even when used at recommended dosage levels. As Pope and Katz (1994) found, depression was a common side effect encountered by steroid abusers. These drugs may also produce a toxic reaction if the individual is using too high a dose for his/her body chemistry. Symptoms of a toxic reaction to steroids include a drug-induced psychotic reaction, manic episodes, delirium, dementia, or a drug-induced depressive reaction that may reach suicidal proportions (Lederberg & Holland, 1989).

Other Complications

Patients with medical conditions such as certain forms of breast cancer, diabetes mellitus, diseases of the blood vessels, kidney, liver, or heart disease, or males who suffer from prostate problems should not utilize steroids unless the physician is aware that the patient has these problems (United States Pharmacopeial Convention, 1990). The anabolic steroids are thought to be possible carcinogens (M. Johnson, 1990), and their use is not recommended for patients with either active tumors or a history of tumors, except under a physician's supervision.

Other side effects caused by steroid use include severe acne (especially across the back) and possibly a foul odor on the breath (Redman, 1990). There has been an isolated case of unnatural bone degeneration attributed to the long-term use of steroids by a weight lifter (Pettine, 1991). Also, animal research suggests that anabolic steroids may contribute to the degeneration of tendons, a finding that is consistent with clinical case reports of athletes who are using anabolic steroids having tendons rupture under stress (Karch, 1996).

Although anabolic steroids are often abused to improve athletic performance, the evidence to support the theory that steroids actually do improve the user's athletic abilities is mixed (Tanner, 1995). One factor that complicates research into athletic performance is the individual's belief that these drugs will improve his/her abilities. The authors suggested that the athlete's expectation of improved performance could contribute, at least in part, to the observed performance on the part of the user.

Growth Patterns in the Adolescent

Adolescents who use steroids run the risk of stunted growth, as these drugs may permanently stop bone growth (Council on Scientific Affairs, 1990b;

M. Johnson, 1990; Schrof, 1992). A further complication of steroid abuse by adolescents is that the tendons do not grow at the same accelerated rate as the bone tissues, resulting in increased strain on the tendons and a higher risk of injury to these tissues (Hough & Kovan, 1990; M. Johnson, 1990).

Anabolic Steroid Abuse and Blood Infections

In addition to the complications of steroid abuse itself, individuals who abuse steroids through intramuscular or intraveneous injection often share needles. These individuals run the same risk of infections being transmitted by contaminated needles seen in heroin or cocaine addicts. There have been cases of athletes contracting AIDS from a needle that had been used by an infected athlete (Kashkin, 1992; Scott & Scott, 1989).

Drug Interactions between Steroids and Other Chemicals

The anabolic steroids interact with a wide range of medications, including several drugs of abuse. Potentially serious drug interactions have been noted in cases where the individual has utilized acetaminophen in high doses, while on steroids. The combination of these two drugs—steroids and acetaminophen—should be avoided except when the individual is being supervised by a physician. Patients who utilize Antabuse (disulfiram) should not take steroids, nor should individuals who are taking Trexan (naltrexone) anticonvulsant medications such as Dilantin (phenytoin), Depakene (valproic acid), or any of the phenothiazines (United States Pharmacopeial Convention, 1990).

Are Anabolic Steroids Addictive?

Surprisingly, when used for extended periods at high dosage levels, the anabolic steroids have an addictive potential. Some users have reported preoccupation with the use of these chemicals and craving when they were not using steroids (Middleman & DuRant, 1996). Further, anabolic steroids have been known to bring about a sense of euphoria both when used for medical purposes and when abused (Fultz, 1991; Middleman & DuRant, 1996).

This may explain why steroid use is so attractive to at least some of those who abuse this family of drugs.

There also is evidence to suggest that the user may become either physically, or psychologically, dependent on the anabolic steroids (M. Johnson, 1990). Bower (1991), for example, found that up to 57% of weight lifters who used steroids ultimately became addicted to these drugs. Dreyfuss (1990) concluded that fully one-quarter of the current users of steroids at the time of his study were either physically or psychologically dependent on these drugs.

Remember that one hallmark of physical dependence on a chemical is a characteristic withdrawal syndrome. In the case of anabolic steroid addiction, the withdrawal syndrome seems to be similar to that seen with cocaine withdrawal. Symptoms of withdrawal from steroids include depressive reactions, possibly to the point of suicide attempts (Hough & Kovan, 1990; Kashkin, 1992; Kashkin & Kleber, 1989). Other symptoms often reported during or after withdrawal from steroids include sleep and appetite disturbances, which seem to be part of the poststeroid depressive syndrome (Bower, 1991), fatigue, restlessness, anorexia, insomnia, and decreased libido (Brower, Blow, et al., 1991).

Like their drug-using counterparts, many steroid abusers require gradual detoxification from the drugs over time as well as intensive psychiatric support, both to limit the impact of withdrawal on the individual's life and to forestall a return to steroid use (Bower, 1991; Hough & Kovan, 1990; Kashkin & Kleber, 1989). Robert Dimeff, Donald Malone, and John Lombardo (cited in Bower, 1991) listed several symptoms of steroid addiction:

1. The use of higher doses than originally intended.
2. A loss of control over the amount of steroids used.
3. A preoccupation with further steroid use.
4. The continued use of steroids despite awareness of the problems caused by their use.
5. The development of tolerance to steroids in the dosages originally used, and the need for larger doses to achieve the same effects.
6. The disruption of normal daily activities by steroid use.
7. The continued use of steroids to control or avoid withdrawal symptoms.

The authors suggested that individuals with three or more of these symptoms are probably dependent on steroids. Kashkin (1992) suggested that those individuals who have gone through 5 or more cycles of steroid use are very likely to be "heavy" steroid users.

The Treatment of Anabolic Steroid Abuse

The first step in the treatment of the steroid abuser is identification of those individuals who are indeed abusing anabolic steroids. The physician, on the basis of clinical history, blood, and/or urine tests, may be the first person to suspect that a patient is abusing steroids and is in the best position to confront the user. The addictions counselor is not thought to have a significant role to play in the treatment of the anabolic steroid user, at least in the earliest stages.

Once the steroid abuser has been identified, close medical supervision of the patient to identify and treat potential complications of steroid abuse is necessary. The attending physician may need to consider the need for a gradual detoxification program for the steroid abuser. Most medical complications caused by steroid abuse will usually clear up after the individual stops the use of steroids (Hough & Kovan, 1990); however, some of the complications caused by steroid abuse (i.e., heart tissue damage) may be permanent. Surgical intervention may be possible to correct some of the side effects of steroid use (Hough & Kovan); however, this is not always feasible.

Following detoxification from anabolic steroids, staff members should work with the patient to identify why he/she started using steroids. Self-concept issues should be identified, and the proper therapy initiated to help the person learn to accept him/herself without leaning on an artificial crutch such as anabolic steroids. Proper nutritional counseling may be necessary to help the athlete learn how to enhance body strength without using potentially harmful substances such as anabolic steroids, and individual support programs should be started to help the individual learn how to substitute social support for the chemical support that he/she once used.

Summary

Within the past decade, a surprising new group of drugs, the anabolic steroids, have emerged as drugs of abuse in many circles. However, steroids are not the "typical" drug of abuse. Adolescents and young adults abuse steroids because they believe these substances will increase aggressiveness, athletic ability, and improve personal appearance. Little is known about the effects of these drugs at the dosage levels utilized by abusers of steroids. The identification and treatment of steroid abusers is primarily a medical issue, but substance abuse counselors should have a working knowledge of the effects and complications of steroid abuse.

Tobacco and Nicotine

Historians believe that the natives of the New World had used tobacco for many hundreds, if not thousands, of years before the arrival of the first European explorers. Tobacco was used both in religious ceremonies and for recreational purposes. Following the discovery of the American continents, the art of smoking was carried back across the Atlantic to Europe by early explorers, many of whom had themselves adopted the habit of smoking tobacco during their time in the Americas.

In Europe, the use of tobacco for smoking was received with some skepticism, if not outright hostility. In Germany, public smoking was once punishable by death, while in Russia, castration was the sentence for the same crime (Berger & Dunn, 1982). In Asia, the early Chinese rulers made the use or distribution of tobacco a crime punishable by death, while smokers were executed as infidels in Turkey. Despite these harsh measures, smoking became popular, and within a few decades, the use of tobacco spread across Europe and into Asia (Schuckit, 1995a).

The practice soon became at least moderately acceptable in European society. Initially, tobacco was thought to be a medicine by European physicians. Later, especially during the past two centuries, its use was interpreted as a mark of sophistication both in Europe and North America. Only in the last generation or two has tobacco use been widely associated with public criticism.

When one reviews the face of tobacco use over the years, it is important to keep in mind that today's tobacco differs greatly from the tobacco grown centuries ago. The tobacco in the New World when the first European explorers arrived was possibly "more potent and may have contained high concentrations of psychoactive substances" (Schuckit, 1995a, p. 259) when compared with the tobacco of today. But European tobacco growers soon learned to substitute milder, more acceptable *Nicotiana tabacum* for the more potent *Nicotina rustica* used by the Native Americans for their religious ceremonies (Hilts, 1996).

Starting in the mid-19th century, several different forces combined to change the shape of tobacco use. First, new varieties of tobacco were planted, allowing for a greater yield than in previous years. Second, new methods of curing the leaf of the tobacco plant were found, speeding up the process of preparing the leaf for use. Third, the manner in which tobacco was used changed. The advent of the industrial age brought with it machinery capable of manufacturing the cigarette, a smaller, cheaper, neater way to smoke than cigars, which were manufactured by hand—a slow, expensive process. James A. Bonsack invented a machine that could produce 120,000 cigarettes a day. The development of such machines greatly accelerated production, and the increased supply reduced the price, making it possible for less affluent groups to afford tobacco products.

Finally, changes in the tax laws also lowered the price of the cigarettes, which soon became a favorite of the poor (Tate, 1989). By the year 1890, the price of domestic cigarettes had fallen to the price of a nickel for a pack of 20 (Tate, 1989), making them affordable to all but the poorest smoker. But this rapid acceptance of cigarettes was not always automatic. By 1909, no less than ten different states had laws that prohibited the use of cigarettes.

Prior to the introduction of the cigarette, the major method of tobacco use had been chewing. The practice of chewing tobacco, then spitting into the ever present cuspidor, contributed to the spread of tuberculosis and other diseases (Brecher, 1972). Because of this, public health officials, after the year 1910, began to campaign against chewing tobacco. The new cigarette, manufactured in large numbers by the latest machines, provided a more sanitary and relatively inexpensive alternative to chewing tobacco.

Cigarette smokers soon discovered that, unlike cigars or pipes, the smoke of the new cigarette was also so mild that it could be inhaled (Burns, 1991). The smoke from pipes or cigars is much more bitter, making it unlikely that the smoker will inhale deeply. For many, cigarette smoking became the preferred method for servicing their nicotine addiction. The world has never been the same since.

Scope of the Problem

In the United States, the use of cigarettes grew in popularity following World War I, and peaked in the mid-1960s (Schuckit, 1995a). The social climate was one of "total social acceptance" (Jaffe, 1989, p. 680) of tobacco use. "Until quite recently, tobacco use was so common and socially acceptable . . . (that) . . . almost everyone tried smoking" (p. 680). By the mid-1960s, when cigarette smoking was most popular in this country, approximately 52% of adult American males and 32% of adult American females were cigarette smokers (Schuckit, 1995a).

Then, in 1964, the Surgeon General of the United States released a report stating that cigarette smoking was dangerous to the smoker's health and outlined the problems that were thought to be caused by smoking. In doing so, the Surgeon General has joined a battle against smoking that has been going on since the late 1800s (Tate, 1989). Gradually, since that 1964 report, the number of adults who continue to smoke in this country has declined (see Figure

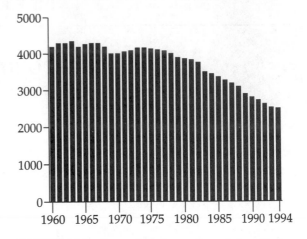

FIGURE 16.1   Per capita consumption of cigarettes in the United States by year.

16.1). However, there is evidence that the number of smokers in this country has leveled off and after declining for many years might even be gradually increasing (Calabresi, Fowler, Scala, Thompson, & Willwerth, 1994).

In the year 1960, approximately 4171 cigarettes were smoked for every man, woman, and child over the age of 18 (Massachusetts Medical Society, 1994). In the year 1964 when the Surgeon General released his famous report, this number had increased to 4194 cigarettes for every man, woman, and child over the age of 18. Per capita consumption peaked in 1966, when 4287 cigarettes were smoked for every person over the age of 18 in this country. Since then, this figure has gradually been dropping. In 1994, the per capita consumption of cigarettes dropped to 2493 cigarettes for every person over the age of 18 (Massachusetts Medical Society).

Researchers suggest that 78% of the men between the ages of 15 and 54, and 73% of the women between 15 and 54, have smoked at least one cigarette (Anthony et al., 1995). It is not too much to assume that the majority of those who smoke one cigarette do so out of curiosity. However, these authors also suggest that one in every three individuals who smoke that first cigarette will continue to smoke until becoming addicted. For these individuals, the interval between experimental cigarette use and daily smoking is 2 to 3 years (Schwartz, 1996).

Of the estimated 265 million people in the United States, approximately 46 million are thought to smoke cigarettes. Of this number, approximately 24 million are male, and, 22 million are female. Although the purchase of cigarettes by adolescents is illegal, 3.1 million of those who smoke are teenagers (Roberts & Watson, 1994).

While only a small minority of cigarette smokers abuse other chemicals, substance abusers often are also heavy smokers (Bobo, Slade, & Hoffman, 1995). Estimates of the prevalence of cigarette use suggest that cigarette smoking is 2 to 3 times higher in substance-abusing populations than in the general population, according to the authors. An estimated 74% of alcohol-dependent individuals, 77% of cocaine-dependent persons, and 85% of those who are dependent on heroin are also cigarette smokers, according to Bobo et al.

In addition to the changes in smoking patterns in the United States, there is evidence suggesting that cigarette smoking is on the increase in many parts of the world, especially the so-called developing countries (Phillips, Savigny, & Law, 1995). There are an estimated 300 million cigarette smokers in China alone, a number that is thought to be about 25% of the total number of smokers in the world.

At the time of the 1964 report, smoking appeared to be a relatively simple phenomenon: either you smoked, or you did not. Now, more than 40 years later, we know that cigarette smoking is a complex behavior that spans the individual's life. Many individuals begin to smoke at an extremely early age. By the age of 12, fully one-half of the schoolchildren in Canada have already experimented with tobacco (J. Walker, 1993), and the average age of smoking initiation is estimated to be 15 years (Cohen et al., 1996). But the individual's attitudes toward smoking are established before using that first cigarette. Research suggests that prosmoking attitudes are formed in childhood or, at the latest, by early adolescence. This is true even if the individual does not *begin* to smoke until late adolescence or early adulthood.

Thus, the first stages of nicotine addiction are established early in life. Almost 90% of tobacco smokers are addicted to nicotine before the age of 20 (J. Walker, 1993). In a real sense, smoking is a lifelong problem with its deepest roots in childhood

and adolescence, and the final fruits of this addictive process often developing in the individual's adult years.

Pharmacology of Cigarette Smoking

In the United States, the primary method of tobacco consumption is the smoking of cigarettes (Schuckit, 1995a) although, in recent years, tobacco chewing and cigar smoking have again become popular. For this reason, the terms *cigarette* and *tobacco* are used interchangeably in this chapter, except when other forms of tobacco (i.e., tobacco prepared for chewing, or for smoking in cigars) are discussed.

The pharmacology of tobacco smoking is complicated because several variables influence the composition of tobacco smoke. According to Jaffe (1990), these variables include (a) the exact composition of the tobacco being used, (b) how densely the tobacco is packed in the cigarette, (c) the length of the column of tobacco (for cigarette or cigar smokers), (d) the characteristics of the filter being used (if any), (e) the paper being used (for cigarette smokers), and (f) the temperature at which the tobacco is burned. To further complicate matters, the cigarette of today is far different from the cigarette of 1900, or even the cigarette of 1950. According to Hilts (1996), up to 40% of today's typical cigarette is composed of "leftover stems, scraps, and dust" (p. 44). Where, in 1955, it took 2.6 pounds of tobacco leaves to produce a thousand cigarettes, the use of these fillers has reduced the amount of tobacco needed to produce a thousand cigarettes to 1.7 pounds (Hilts).

Cigarette tobacco smoke contains some 4000 different compounds, of which some 2550 come from the unprocessed tobacco itself (Burns, 1991). According to the author, the other 1450 compounds found in cigarette smoke come from additives, pesticides, and organic or metallic compounds that either intentionally or unintentionally find their way into cigarettes. A partial list of the compounds found in tobacco smoke includes:

> carbon monoxide, carbon dioxide, nitrogen oxides, ammonia, volatile nitrosamines, hydrogen cyanide, volatile sulfur-containing compounds, nitrites and other nitrogen-containing compounds, volatile hydrocarbons, alcohols, and aldehydes and keytone

(e.g., acetaldehyde, formaldehyde and acrolein). (Jaffe, 1990, p. 545)

In addition to all these compounds, perfumes are added to the tobacco leaves to give the cigarette its distinctive aroma (Hilts, 1996). Other compounds found in cigarettes or the paper wrapper include various forms of sugar, humectants (to give the tobacco a characteristic aroma), insecticides, herbicides, fungicides, rodenticides, pesticides, and manufacturing machine lubricants that come into contact with the tobacco leaves/paper as these products move through these machines in the manufacture of cigarettes (Glantz, Slade, Bereo, Hanauer, & Barnes, 1996). There has been virtually no research into the effects on the human body when these chemicals are smoked.

The concentrations of many chemicals found in cigarette smoke, such as carbon monoxide, are such that "uninterrupted exposure" (Burns, 1991, p. 633) would result in death. The author noted that the concentration of carbon monoxide found in cigarettes is "similar to that found in automobile exhaust" (p. 633), a known source of potentially dangerous concentrations of this chemical.

Researchers have found that cigarette smoke also contains radioactive compounds, such as polonium 210 (Evans, 1993; Jaffe, 1990), and lead 210 (Brownson, Novotny, & Perry, 1993). These compounds for the most part are found in the soil in which tobacco is grown and are incorporated into the tobacco plant. When the individual smokes, these radioactive compounds are carried into the lungs along with the smoke. Over a 1-year period, the cumulative radiation exposure for a two-pack/day smoker is equal to what a person would receive if he/she had 250–300 chest X rays (Evans).

Further, cigarette smoke is known to contain a small amount of arsenic (Banerjee, 1990). All of these—and a multitude of other—chemicals are inhaled when a person smokes. Some of the chemicals found in tobacco smoke, like benzene, are documented carcinogens. A carcinogen is a chemical that is known or strongly suspected to cause cancer in humans. At least 43 known, or suspected, carcinogens are found in cigarette smoke (Burns, 1991; Hilts, 1996). Thus, cigarette smoking introduces a wide range of known or suspected carcinogenic chemicals directly into the body.

Nicotine

As a result of legal action against tobacco companies within the past decade, it has come to light that these companies have long known that nicotine is the major psychoactive agent inn cigarettes. Indeed, there is evidence that suggests that tobacco companies have long viewed cigarettes as little more than a single dose container of nicotine that will quickly administer the chemical to the user since the 1960s (Benowitz & Henningfield, 1994; Glantz, Barnes, Bero, Hanauer, & Slade, 1995; Glantz et al., 1996; Hilts, 1996). Further, there is strong evidence that suggests that at least one tobacco company has selectively grown strains of tobacco plants with high nicotine[1] levels in the leaves, for use in producing cigarettes for smoking (*60 Minutes*, 1996b).

Although nicotine is well absorbed through the gastrointestinal tract, much of the nicotine that is absorbed when the drug is ingested orally is biotransformed by the liver by the "first-pass metabolism" effect (see Chapter 3). Thus, in order to achieve a high blood level of nicotine, another means of use other than oral ingestion must be utilized. The preferred method of nicotine administration, according to tobacco industry memos that have become available to the public, is through smoking.

In the brain, the psychoactive effects of nicotine are very similar to those of other drugs of abuse. When nicotine reaches the brain, the user experiences a "high," a sense of release from stress, or possibly a sense of euphoria, when they smoke (Fiore, Jorenby, Baker, & Kenford, 1992). As will be discussed in a later section of this chapter, nicotine shares another characteristic with the other drugs of

---

[1] Despite these internal memos, however, the Chief Executive Officer (CEO) of the Philip Morris Tobacco Company characterized tobacco as being about as addictive as "Gummy Bears" (a form of candy), in one televised interview. Dr. Alexander Spears, who runs the company that makes Kent cigarettes defended his definition of tobacco as being nonaddicting on the grounds that it did not cause intoxication and compared it to caffeine (*60 Minutes*, 1997b).

abuse besides the ability to cause euphoria: it can also cause the individual to become physically addicted to it.

In the average healthy adult, a lethal dose of nicotine is estimated to be a single dose of about 60 milligrams (mg) (Ashton, 1992). The "typical" cigarette contains between 6–11 mg of nicotine (Henningfield, 1995). But the bioavailability of nicotine from one cigarette is only 3% to 40% (Benowitz & Henningfield, 1994). Because nicotine is not able to cross over from the alveoli of the lungs to the blood very easily, the typical smoker only absorbs 1–3 mg of nicotine from each cigarette (Henningfield, 1995). Thus, the typical smoker receives between 1/60 and 1/24 of the estimated lethal dose of nicotine, each time he/she smokes a cigarette. But this figure is for a single cigarette. Over the course of the typical day, the average smoker absorbs a cumulative dose of 20–40 mg of nicotine (Henningfield).

Once in the body, nicotine is rapidly distributed to virtually every blood-rich tissue in the body, including the brain (Henningfield & Nemeth-Coslett, 1988). Nicotine is both water-soluble and lipid-soluble, and thus is able to cross over the blood-brain barrier quickly to reach the brain. Indeed, the brain is one of the organs where the highest levels of nicotine accumulate. Measured levels of nicotine in the brain can be twice as high as the level of nicotine found in the blood (Fiore et al., 1992). Between 0.05 and 2.5 mg of the nicotine from each cigarette reaches the brain (Ashton, 1992; Lee & D'Alonzo, 1993). High concentrations of nicotine also are found in the lungs and the spleen of cigarette smokers.

In the brain, nicotine is known to have "properties similar to those of cocaine and amphetamine" (Rustin, 1988, p. 18). As discussed in earlier chapters, these are chemicals with strong reinforcing effects on the user. However, researchers disagree as to the relative potency of nicotine. Jaffe (1989) suggested that as a reinforcer, nicotine is less powerful than cocaine or the amphetamines. Weil (1986), on the other hand, stated that nicotine is a more powerful reinforcer than the amphetamines. In terms of relative potency, the reward potential of intravenous nicotine is thought to be five to ten times more potent than that of intravenous cocaine (Henningfield & Nemeth-Coslett, 1988).

Researchers also disagree about the speed with which smoking cigarettes allows nicotine to reach the brain. Estimates of the speed which nicotine reaches the brain after the first "puff" of a cigarette range from 7 seconds (Fiore et al., 1992), to 8 (Hilts, 1996; Jaffe, 1990) seconds, up to 19 seconds (Benowitz, 1992). However, while different researchers might differ as to their opinion of how quickly nicotine might reach the brain, they all agree that it reaches the brain very quickly after the smoker starts to smoke a cigarette.

Within the brain, nicotine is thought to facilitate the release of the neurotransmitter dopamine within the region of the limbic system known as the nucleus accumbens (Miller & Gold, 1993), and the neurotransmitter acetylcholine in the peripheral regions of the body. Another region of the brain where nicotine exerts a major effect is the medulla. This is the region of the brain responsible for such functions as swallowing, vomiting, respiration, and the control of blood pressure (Restak, 1984). This is also why many first-time smokers experience both nausea and vomiting (Jaffe, 1990). However, with repeated exposure to the nicotine in tobacco, the smoker becomes tolerant to the nausea that smoking can cause. Thus, it is necessary for the beginning cigarette smoker to force him/herself through the nausea and vomiting that nicotine causes, until he/she can become tolerant to this effect of the chemical.[2]

The smoker's heart rate is also modified by nerve impulses from the medulla, which accounts at least in part for nicotine's immediate effects on the cardiovascular system. These effects include an increase in heart rate, an increase in blood pressure, and an increase in the strength of heart contractions. While the heart rate is increased, the peripheral blood flow in the body is reduced as nicotine causes the blood vessels in the outer regions of the body to constrict (Schuckit, 1995a). This process contributes to the tendency for nicotine to increase blood pressure levels.

---

[2] Hilts (1996) suggested that chewing tobacco made of tobacco leaves with a low nicotine content was introduced to help the smoker-to-be become tolerant to the nausea experienced by first-time smokers. Later, when the individual was no longer able to absorb enough nicotine by chewing to avoid withdrawal he/she would be tempted to switch to cigarette smoking, to achieve a higher blood level of nicotine and avoid going into withdrawal.

In addition to its effects on the brain, nicotine causes a decrease in the strength of stomach contractions (Schuckit, 1995a), and cigarette smoke itself can cause irritation of the tissues of the lungs and pulmonary system. Cigarette smoking deposits potentially harmful chemicals in the lungs and causes a decrease in the motion of the cilia (small hairlike projections that help to clean the lungs). These features of cigarette smoking are thought to contribute to the development of pulmonary problems in long-term smokers.

The peak concentrations of nicotine are reached in the first minutes after the cigarette is smoked, and then the level of nicotine in the blood starts to drop. The biological half-life of nicotine is between 100 minutes (Rustin, 1992) and 2 hours, (Fiore et al., 1992). Since only 50% of the nicotine from one cigarette is metabolized in the half-life period, and the typical smoker uses more than one cigarette every 8–10 hours, over the course of a day, a reservoir of unmetabolized nicotine is established in the smoker's body. Some degree of tolerance to the effects of nicotine develops in a matter of hours, but this acquired tolerance is lost just as rapidly during the night hours, when the typical smoker abstains from cigarette use (Bhandari, Sylvester, & Rigotti, 1996). This is why many smokers find that the first cigarette of the day has such a strong effect.

Only 5% to 10% of the nicotine that enters the body is excreted unchanged. The rest is biotransformed by the liver. About 90% of the biotransformed nicotine is turned into *cotinine*, a metabolite of nicotine that has no known psychoactive properties. The other 10% of the nicotine is biotransformed into *nicotine-n-oxide*. These chemicals are then excreted from the body in the urine.

At one point, it was thought that cigarette smokers might be able to biotransform nicotine more quickly than nonsmokers. This assumption was based on the observation that the nicotine in the smoker's blood would cause the body to biotransform some medications more quickly than in the nonsmoker, and it was assumed that this was one reason new smokers gradually increased the frequency with which they smoked cigarettes in the first few years. However, Benowitz and Jacob (1993) tested this hypothesis, and found that smokers and nonsmokers biotransform nicotine more or less at the same rate. The authors concluded that their data did not support the theory that, as smokers became more adept at the biotransformation of nicotine, they would gradually smoke more frequently. Thus, the question of why beginning smokers gradually smoke more and more often over time remains to be answered.

Acetaldehyde

Nicotine is not the only psychoactive chemical in tobacco. In addition, tobacco smoke includes a small amount of acetaldehyde. It is interesting to note that acetaldehyde is the first metabolite produced by the liver when the body biotransforms alcohol. Acetaldehyde is thought to be more potent than alcohol in terms of psychoactive potential. Also, like alcohol, acetaldehyde has a sedative effect on the user (Rustin, 1988). Thus, while nicotine may have the strongest effect on the user, other compounds in tobacco smoke also have some impact on the smoker's state of mind.

Does Cigarette Smoking Protect against Alzheimer's Disease?

In 1993, the team of Brenner et al. suggested that there was a "negative association" (p. 293) between cigarette smoking and the later development of Alzheimer's disease. Based on their research, the authors suggested that those individuals who had smoked cigarettes at one point in their lives were less likely to develop Alzheimer's disease, which is commonly a disease of old age. The authors hypothesized that low doses of nicotine might alter the sensitivity of certain neurons in the brain to acetylcholine in such a way as to make these neurons more sensitive to this neurotransmitter. This, in turn, could make it possible for those same neurons to function effectively even with reduced levels of acetylcholine.

Another mechanism that might account for the apparent protective influence of cigarette smoking on Alzheimer's disease was suggested by Riggs (1996). The author noted that as people in any given age cohort die as a result of accident and/or disease, their genes are removed from the gene pool for that age group. The genetic heritage of the surviving members of that age cohort is thus altered with each death. The author offered by way of illustration that the original genetic heritage of the age cohort born in 1926 is far different now, when a significant percentage of its members have died, than it was in 1927, when virtually all its members were still present.

To understand the logic behind this argument, consider these points: (a) neurodegenerative disorders such as Alzheimer's disease seem to have a genetic component, (b) neurodegenerative disorders such as Alzheimer's disease usually do not manifest themselves until the individual reaches age 65 or later, and (c) cigarette smokers are prone to premature death as a result of cigarette-induced illness. As a result of factor (c), a significant percentage of cigarette smokers will have died from smoking-related illness before they have a chance to develop a neurodegenerative disorder of late life such as Alzheimer's disease, according to Riggs. Thus, it is not clear at this time whether cigarette smoking offers *any* protection against Alzheimer's disease.

Drug Interactions between Nicotine and Other Chemicals

Drug interactions between nicotine and various other therapeutic agents are well documented. Cigarette smokers, for example, require more morphine for the control of pain (Bond, 1989; Jaffe, 1990). Tobacco smokers may experience less sedation from benzodiazepines than do nonsmokers (Barnhill et al., 1995). Thus, the physician treating the patient who smokes might need to adjust the individual's daily benzodiazepine dose to achieve the desired level of sedation.

Nicotine also seems to counteract some of the sedation seen with alcohol use, which might be why many drinkers smoke.[3] Tobacco also interacts with many anticoagulants, as well as the beta-blocker propranol and caffeine (Bond, 1989). Women who use oral contraceptives and who smoke are more likely to experience strokes, myocardial infarction, and thromboembolism than their nonsmoking counterparts, according to the author.

After cigarette smokers who use the medication theophylline stop smoking, they will experience a 36% rise in theophylline blood levels over the first week of abstinence. This seems to be caused by the effects of such chemicals as benzopyrene, which are found in the tobacco smoke (Henningfield, 1995). Also, the concentration of caffeine in the blood may increase by as much as 250 percent following smoking cessation. Since one of the effects of this high concentration of caffeine is to cause anxietylike symptoms, cigarette smokers often associate the sensation of anxiety with the practice of smoking another cigarette. The result is that former smokers who experience caffeine-related anxiety symptoms may interpret this as a sign that they should have a cigarette.

Nicotine use has been found to decrease the blood levels of clozapine and haloperidol by as much as 30% (American Psychiatric Association, 1996). It has been found to increase the blood levels of medications such as clomipramine, and antidepressant medications such as desipramine, dozepin, and nortriptyline, according to the American Psychiatric Association. While the list of potential interactions between nicotine and various pharmaceuticals reviewed in the preceding paragraphs does not list every chemical that might interact with nicotine, it highlights that nicotine has a strong effect on how other chemicals work in the human body.[4]

Subjective Effects of Nicotine Use

The exact mechanism by which nicotine affects the central nervous system is unknown. However, nicotine is thought to bring about a dose-dependent, biphasic response at the level of the individual neurons of the brain, especially those that utilize the neurotransmitter acetylcholine (Ashton, 1992; Benowitz, 1992; Restak, 1991). Initially, nicotine stimulates these neurons, possibly contributing to the feeling of increased alertness on the part of the smoker. However, over longer periods the nicotine blocks the

---

[3] The author of this text has met many alcohol abusers who report, for example, that they *only* smoke while they are drinking, and that they avoid cigarette use at other times.

[4] To avoid potentially dangerous interaction effects between a pharmaceutical and a compound found in cigarettes, you should ask a physician or a pharmacist if there is any danger in taking that medicine while smoking.

effects of acetylcholine, reducing the rate at which those neurons "fire."

This theory would seem to account for the observed effects of cigarette smoking. Smokers are known to experience stimulation of the brain (Schuckit, 1995a), as well as decreased muscle tone (Jaffe, 1990). This is one reason many smokers find that cigarette smoking helps them to relax when they are under pressure. About 90% of cigarette smokers report a sense of pleasure when they smoke (Ashton, 1992). This may, as animal research suggests, reflect the ability of nicotine to stimulate the release of the neurotransmitters norepinephrine and dopamine (Jaffe), chemicals known to be used by the brain's pleasure system.

Initially, the first-time smoker will report a sense of nausea and may possibly even vomit (Restak, 1991). However, if the individual persists in attempts to smoke, the stimulation of the neurotransmitter systems will eventually result in an association between smoking and the nicotine-induced pleasurable sensations. Thus, with repeated episodes of nicotine use over time, the individual comes to associate smoking with pleasurable sensations, as the neurotransmitters norepinephrine and dopamine are released within the brain.

Nicotine Addiction

There is evidence, in the form of internal memos and research studies, that at least one major tobacco company understood that nicotine is addictive as early as 1963 (Slade, Bero, Hanauer, Barnes, & Glantz, 1995). However, these memos and research studies were apparently suppressed by the tobacco company until copies were "leaked" to researchers more than 30 years later. According to one such memo from 1963, cited by Slade et al. (1995) researchers openly stated in their internal memo that their company was "in the business of selling nicotine, an addictive drug" (p. 228) to smokers. However, it was not until 1997 that a major tobacco company in the United States, the Liggett Group, admitted in court that tobacco is addictive (Solomon, Rogers, Katel, & Lach, 1997).

The average layperson tends to underestimate the addictive potential of nicotine. Cocaine, for example,

has the reputation of being extremely addictive. However, only 3% to 20% of those who try cocaine once go on to become addicted to it (Musto, 1991). In contrast, between one-third and one-half of those individuals who experiment with smoking go on to become addicted (Henningfield, 1995; Pomerleau, Collins, Shiffman, & Pomerleau, 1993). Further, like the other drugs of abuse, the more that the individual experiments with the practice of smoking, the more likely that he/she will become addicted to it. Jaffe (1989) concluded that "a very high percentage" (p. 680) of those who smoke 100 cigarettes go on to become daily smokers. J. Walker (1993) gave an even lower figure, noting that children who smoke just 4 or more cigarettes stand a 94% chance of continuing to smoke.

Thus, nicotine appears to be significantly more likely to bring about physical addiction than cocaine, despite the latter's reputation. But not everybody who begins to smoke goes on to become addicted to nicotine (Henningfield & Nemeth-Coslett, 1988). Despite nicotine's addictive potential, a small minority (perhaps 5–10%) of those who smoke are not addicted to nicotine (Jarvik & Schneider, 1992; Shiffman et al., 1990). These individuals, who demonstrate an episodic pattern of nicotine use, are classified as cigarette "chippers."

As a group, chippers do not appear to smoke in response to social pressures, and they do not seem to smoke to avoid the symptoms of withdrawal (Shiffman et al., 1990). One of the defining characteristics of tobacco chippers is that they do not experience withdrawal symptoms from nicotine when they stop smoking. This suggests that the chipper is not addicted to nicotine, according to the authors. Very little beyond this is known about the phenomenon of tobacco chipping, and there is much to learn about this phenomenon.

Remember, however, that only 5% to 10% of those who smoke cigarettes are thought not to be addicted to nicotine. This means that the other 90% to 95% of those who smoke are indeed addicted. These individuals demonstrate all the necessary characteristics typically seen in drug addiction: (a) tolerance, (b) withdrawal symptoms, and (c) drug-seeking behaviors (Rustin, 1988, 1992). In addition, tobacco users develop highly individual drug-using rituals.

These smoking rituals seem to provide the individual with a sense of security in an insecure world, and contribute to the individual's tendency to engage in smoking behaviors when anxious.

Chemical addiction to nicotine is a very real problem. To place the strength of nicotine addiction in perspective, consider that only 2% to 3% of those individuals who try to quit cigarette smoking each year are able to do so (Henningfield, 1995). Kozlowski et al. (1989) asked some 1000 individuals in treatment for a drug addiction to rate the relative difficulty of quitting smoking, compared with their drug of choice. Surprisingly, 74% rated the task of quitting cigarette use at least as difficult as giving up their drug of choice, a finding that underscores the addiction potential of tobacco.

Some researchers believe that chronic smokers tend to smoke in such a way as to regulate the nicotine level in the blood. Smokers will increase or decrease their cigarette use to achieve, and then maintain, an individually specific blood level of nicotine (Benowitz, 1992; Pomerleau et al., 1993; Sherman, 1994; Shiffman et al., 1990). This would explain why, when given cigarettes of a high nicotine content, smokers will use fewer cigarettes, while the reverse is true when a smoker is given low-nicotine cigarettes (Benowitz, 1992; Jaffe, 1990).

Henningfield and Nemeth-Coslett (1988) challenged this conclusion, however, noting that research has suggested that cigarette smokers are "remarkably insensitive" (p. 45s) to changes in nicotine levels in the blood. The authors noted that the hypothesis that cigarette smokers will regulate their use to maintain a constant blood plasma level of nicotine has "never been convincingly demonstrated" (p. 46s). The authors, in reviewing the rapid changes in blood plasma nicotine levels across the span of a single day, concluded that the research data does not support the constant-level hypothesis. However, the final answer to this question has not, as yet, been determined.

Nicotine Withdrawal

Withdrawal symptoms usually begin within 2 hours of the last use of tobacco, peak within 24 hours (Kaplan & Sadock, 1990), then gradually decline over the next 10 days to several weeks (Hughes, 1992; Jaffe, 1989). The exact nature of the withdrawal symptoms varies from person to person. Surprisingly, in light of the horror stories often heard about the agony of giving up cigarette smoking, research has found that approximately one-quarter of those who quit cigarettes report no significant withdrawal symptoms at all (Benowitz, 1992).

The exact reason for this is not clear, although it has been suggested that a higher daily intake of nicotine may be associated with stronger withdrawal symptoms (Jaffe, 1990). The reverse is also thought to be true: those individuals who report little or no withdrawal from nicotine may be smokers who are smoking fewer cigarettes to begin with. But this is only a theory, and the exact relationship between the number of cigarettes an individual smokes and the severity of his/her withdrawal from nicotine is still unclear.

Some symptoms of nicotine withdrawal include anxiety, sleep disturbance, irritability, impatience, difficulties in concentration, restlessness, a craving for tobacco, hunger, gastrointestinal upset, headache, and drowsiness (Fiore et al., 1992; Hughes, 1992). Other possible symptoms of nicotine withdrawal include depression, hostility, fatigue, lightheadedness, headaches, a tingling sensation in the limbs, constipation, and increased coughing (Jarvik & Schneider, 1992).

Most of those people who try to quit smoking will return to the active use of cigarettes in the first week, when their withdrawal symptoms are at their peak (Henningfield, 1995). For the most part, the withdrawal symptoms from cigarettes will gradually decrease in frequency and intensity after the first week or two following abstinence. But there are exceptions to this rule. The research team of Hughes, Gust, Skoog, Keenan, and Fenwick (1991) concluded that up to a quarter of their sample continued to experience withdrawal symptoms from nicotine a full month after they had stopped smoking. Even 6 months after they had stopped smoking, up to three-quarters of those who were abstinent experienced at least occasional craving for nicotine, according to the authors.

Very soon after the individual stops smoking cigarettes, heart rate and blood pressure decrease, and peripheral blood flow patterns improve. Jarvik and Schneider (1992) suggested that the heart rate drops after about 10 days of abstinence. Hughes (1992) however, reported that the heart rate begins to decline as soon as the second day of abstinence from nicotine, with further decreases being noted on the 7th and 14th day following the last cigarette. Thus, it is not clear at this time how cigarette cessation affects the heart rate although researchers agree that, ultimately, cardiac function improves if the individual stops smoking.

The possibility that the withdrawal process might exacerbate preexisting depressive disorders in some people has been suggested (Breslau, Kilbey, & Andreski, 1993; Jaffe, 1990). Research has revealed that 60% of those smokers who try to quit have histories of major depression. However, this does not mean that the cigarette withdrawal process caused the individual to become depressed. Rather, researchers now believe that cigarette smoking and depression are separate conditions that seem to be influenced by the same genetic factors (Breslau et al., 1993; Glassman, 1993). However, this is only a theory, and the exact nature of the relationship between smoking and depression remains to be identified.

What *is* known is that cigarette smokers tend to use nicotine to cope with negative emotional states, of which depression is a good example (Sherman, 1994). Other negative emotional states include anxiety, boredom, or sadness, according to the author. Nicotine quickly becomes an easily administered, quick method for coping with these feelings, and the smoker soon learns that he/she can control negative emotional states through the use of cigarettes.

Cigarette Cessation and Weight Gain

Smokers who stop smoking often report a distressing increase in weight during the first few weeks of abstinence. Although researchers have attempted to understand the relationship between cigarette smoking and low body weight, the exact mechanism by which weight gain comes about following cigarette cessation remains unknown (Eisen, Lyons, Goldberg, & True, 1993).

One theory holds that cigarette smoking helps to suppress the individual's appetite (Jaffe, 1990). It would thus seem logical to assume that this smoking-related loss of appetite is reversed when the person stops smoking. A smoker also tends to retain less fluid compared with a nonsmoker, and some of the

weight gain noted after a person stops smoking might reflect fluid weight gain.

While many smokers attempt to avoid this weight gain, researchers have come to view the exsmoker's weight gain in a more positive light within the past few years. The research team of Hughes et al. (1991) concluded that those individuals who gained weight were more likely to remain abstinent following the decision to stop smoking. Further, the authors concluded that weight levels "returned to precessation levels at 6 months" (p. 57), suggesting that weight gain may be a time-limited phenomenon for those individuals who experience this side effect of abstinence.

The team of Williamson et al. (1991) explored the problem of weight gain in exsmokers, using a sample of 748 male and 1137 female smokers, compared with 409 men and 359 women who had abstained from the use of tobacco for one year. It was found that the average male smoker gained 2.8 kilograms[5] (6.1 pounds), and the average female smoker gained 3.8 kilograms (8.4 pounds) after they stopped smoking. For a minority of exsmokers, some 10% of the men and 13% of the women who stopped smoking, however, the authors found a larger weight gain of 13 kilograms (28.6 pounds).

The team of Williamson et al. (1991) uncovered an interesting twist to the problem of weight gain following the individual's decision to quit smoking, however. The authors of this study found that the average smoker in their sample actually weighed less than individuals who had never smoked. Further, by "the end of the study . . . the mean body weight of those who had quit had increased only to that of those who had never smoked" (p. 743). The implication of this study, as the authors concluded, is that tobacco use interferes with weight gain, through some unknown mechanism. The weight gain following the decision to quit tobacco use may reflect the body's readjustment to the same level as those individuals who never smoked to begin with, according to Williamson et al. (1991).

Increased weight is a known risk factor for cardiovascular disease. However, even if the former cigarette smoker does gain weight following smoking

---

[5] There are 2.2046 pounds per kilogram.

cessation, the health benefits obtained by giving up cigarette use far outweigh the potential risks associated with postcigarette weight gain (Eisen et al., 1993). A former smoker would have to gain 50 to 100 pounds after giving up cigarettes before the health risks of the extra weight came close to the health risks inherent in cigarette smoking (Brunton, Henningfield, & Solberg, 1994). Most former smokers gain far less weight than this. As we have seen, most former smokers gain only a modest amount of weight when they give up cigarette smoking.

Complications of the Chronic Use of Tobacco

Although nicotine is not without its dangers, most of the tobacco-related disorders discussed in this section appear to be caused by compounds other than nicotine found in tobacco smoke (American Psychiatric Association, 1996). To further complicate matters, the impact of smoking on any given individual is quite difficult to determine. For example, consider the manner in which the exact amount of nicotine, tar, and carbon monoxide obtained from a specific brand of cigarette is determined: the cigarette is "smoked" by a test machine, and the composition of the smoke is then analyzed (Hilts, 1994).

Because this is a mechanical process, the test data obtained through this method has little relationship to the amount of tar and nicotine the average smoker will inhale.[6] This is because the machine will smoke a cigarette in a predictable manner, while the smoking methods utilized by different individuals cause significant variability in both the specific chemical combinations generated by each cigarette and the chemicals that are absorbed into the smoker's body. For example, some smokers inhale the cigarette smoke more deeply into their lungs than other smokers. Other smokers hold their cigarette in such a way as to block the air holes in filters (thus altering the content of the smoke). These smoker-specific behaviors make it difficult to determine exactly what chemicals, and in what concentrations, have been introduced into the body of any given individual when he/she smokes a cigarette.

But while there is considerable controversy as to the exact chemicals that are absorbed into the body of a cigarette smoker, in the time since the 1964 Report of the Surgeon General on the effects of cigarette smoking, an impressive body of medical literature has emerged, suggesting that the practice of smoking is a cause of illness and death. For a long time, cigarette smoking had been thought to be harmless. This is because it takes time for most of the adverse effects of cigarette smoking to manifest themselves.

To put the problem of cigarette-related illness into historical perspective, remember that cigarette smoking did not become popular until around the turn of the century. At that time, carcinoma (cancer) of the lung was a relatively rare disorder (Bloodworth, 1987). Hard as it is to believe, many physicians of a century ago could go through an entire medical career without ever seeing a case of lung cancer. Even as recently as the year 1921, the association between tobacco use and cancer was not recognized (Foa, 1989). It was not until the year 1923 that lung cancer was included in the *International Classification of Diseases* (*Smithsonian*, 1989). But by 1940, researchers at the Mayo Clinic had suggested that there was a relationship between smoking and coronary artery disease (Bartecchi, MacKenzie, & Schrier, 1994). In the next half century, thousands of research studies identified a relationship between cigarette smoking and other forms of illness.

As we near the year 2000, the association between tobacco use and a wide range of diseases is well known. Nationally, it is estimated that 450,000 (American Medical Association, 1993b; Hilts, 1996) cigarette smokers die each year from smoking-related illness. A smaller number of nonsmokers also die from what is known as "passive," "environmental," or "secondhand" smoke (to be discussed).

It is difficult to put the problem of the risks associated with cigarette smoking into strong enough terms. Statistically, approximately half of all smokers will die a premature death from tobacco-related disease (Benowitz & Henningfield, 1994; Henningfield, 1995). The team of Phillips, Wannamethee, Thomson, and Smith (1996) examined the data from the ongoing British Regional Heart Study,

---

[6]The Federal Trade Commission is aware of this fact, but continues to rely on data provided by the tobacco industry itself to determine the content of cigarette smoke, according to Hilts (1994) and Cotton (1993).

which has followed a sample of 7735 men since the start of the study in 1980. The authors found that 44% of lifelong smokers survived to age 73, while 78% of the nonsmokers in this study reached that same age.

There is a known association between cigarette smoking and the development of cancer. Smokers are estimated to have between 1100 and 2400% greater chance of developing some form of cancer, when compared with nonsmokers of the same age (Pappas, 1995). Fully 30% of all cancer deaths are caused by smoking (Bartecchi et al., 1994; Fiore, Epps, & Manley, 1994). Cigarette smoking is also thought to cause more than 75% of all cases of esophageal cancer, 30% to 40% of all bladder cancers, and 30% of the cases of cancer of the pancreas (Sherman 1991).

When one considers the number of people who die from cigarette-related cancer, and the number of people who die from other forms of cigarette-induced illness, it becomes clear that smoking is the single largest cause of preventable death in this country (Bartecchi et al., 1994). Each year in this country, the use of tobacco products is thought to cause the following deaths (Bartecchi et al.):

- 179,000 deaths from cardiovascular disease.
- 119,920 deaths as a result of lung cancer.
- 31,402 deaths as a result of cancer other than lung cancer.
- 84,475 deaths from respiratory disease other than lung cancer.

From time to time, cigarette smokers defend their addiction on the grounds that it is a "harmless" addiction, that it is inexpensive, or that it is legal. It is neither harmless nor is it inexpensive. The estimated total financial impact of smoking, in terms of lost productivity and health care costs for tobacco-related disease is in excess of $100 billion/year in the United States alone (MacKenzie, Bartecchi, & Schrier, 1994b). Each pack of cigarettes has been estimated to cost society $2.59 in direct and indirect problems (Bhandari et al., 1996). The use of cigarettes often results in hidden financial damages beyond those involved in treating smoking-related health problems. For example, there are an estimated 187,000 smoking-related fires in this country each

year, resulting in an additional loss of $550 million in property damage, according to the authors. Smoking-related fires are the number one cause of property fires in the United States (Bhandari et al.).

Although cigarette smoking is legal if the smoker is an adult, there is hardly a body system that is not affected by cigarette smoking. Tobacco products are the only products sold in this country that are "unequivocally carcinogenic when used as directed" (MacKenzie et al., 1994b, p. 977). What follows is just a short list of the conditions known, or strongly suspected, to be a result of cigarette smoking.

The Mouth, Throat, and Pulmonary System

Chronic cigarette smokers are known to suffer increased rates of respiratory problems during sleep, compared with nonsmokers (Wetter, Young, Bidwell, Badr, & Palta, 1994). The authors examined data from 811 adults who were examined at the sleep disorders program at the University of Wisconsin-Madison medical center, and found that current smokers were at greater risk for such sleep breathing disorders as snoring and sleep apnea than were nonsmokers. The relationship between smoking and sleep disorders is so strong that Wetter et al. recommended that smoking cessation be considered one of the treatment interventions for a patient with a sleep-related breathing disorder.

Phillips and Danner (1995) administered health status questionnaires to 484 individuals, aged 14–84 years. The authors found that for each age group, cigarette smokers were significantly more likely than nonsmokers to report such problems as trouble initiating sleep, insomnia, and daytime sleepiness. A complicating factor, according to the authors, was that the cigarette smokers identified in their research study were also more likely to consume caffeine, which might account for at least some of their findings. However, the relationship between smoking and sleep disorders is so strong that Wetter et al. (1994) recommended that smoking cessation be considered one of the treatment interventions for a patient with a sleep-related breathing disorder.

As discussed earlier in this section, chronic smokers are more likely to develop cancer of the lung, the mouth, the pharynx, the larynx, and the esophagus than nonsmokers. In addition to this increased risk for cancer, cigarette smokers have higher rates for chronic bronchitis, pneumonia, and Chronic Obstructive Pulmonary Disease (COPD) such as emphysema, than nonsmokers. It has been estimated that 81% of all deaths from COPD might be traced to cigarette smoking (Sherman, 1991). Finally, although nonsmokers also develop respiratory disease, research has shown that smokers are more likely to die from a lung disorder, when one develops, than are nonsmokers (Burns, 1991; Jaffe, 1990; Lee & D'Alonzo, 1993; Schuckit, 1995a).

The Digestive Tract

Alcohol and cigarette smoking are both associated with an increased risk of cancer in the upper digestive and respiratory tracts (Garro, Espina, & Lieber, 1992). Research suggests that alcoholics have almost a sixfold greater chance of developing cancer in the mouth and pharynx compared with nondrinkers. Smokers have been found to have a sevenfold increased risk of mouth or pharynx cancer compared with nonsmokers. However, alcoholics who *also* smoke have a 38-fold greater risk for cancer of the mouth or pharynx than do nonsmoking nondrinkers, according to the authors.

There is even evidence to suggest that cigarette smoking is a risk factor for the development of diabetes. The team of Rimm, Chan, Stampfer, Colditz, and Willett (1995) identified a sample of 41,810 men who were free of cancer, cardiovascular disease, or diabetes in 1986, and followed the members of this sample group for a period of 6 years. Questionnaires were administered to identify the incidence of non-insulin-dependent diabetes mellitus at the end of the 6-year period. The authors found that, after controlling for known risk factors, cigarette smoking was still identified as a possible causal factor in the development of non-insulin-dependent diabetes.

The Heart and Cardiovascular System

Smoking is a known risk factor for the development of coronary heart disease, as well as hypertension, the formation of aortic aneurysms, and atherosclerotic peripheral vascular disease. Cigarette smoking is the "single most important preventable risk factor for cardiovascular disease" (Tresch & Aronow, 1996,

p. 24). Fully 30% of all coronary heart disease deaths in the United States can be traced to cigarette smoking, according to the authors.

Cigarette smoking is also a known risk factor for the development of either a cerebral infarction or a cerebral hemorrhage (stroke, or CVA) (Robbins, Manson, Lee, Satterfield, & Hennekens, 1994; Sherman, 1991). Sacco (1995) estimated that cigarette smoking causes 60,000 strokes in the United States each year. Further, cigarette smokers are at increased risk for the development of adult-onset leukemia (Brownson et al., 1993). Although this is not traditionally viewed as a consequence of cigarette smoking, the authors estimated that approximately 14% of all cases of adult onset leukemia in the United States might be traced to cigarette smoking.

Another way that cigarette smoking impacts on the cardiovascular system is by causing the coronary arteries to briefly constrict. The team of Moliterno et al. (1994) measured the diameters of the coronary arteries of 42 cigarette smokers who were being evaluated for complaints of chest pain. The authors found a *7% decrease* in coronary artery diameter for those individuals without coronary artery disease who had smoked a cigarette.

The coronary arteries are the primary source of blood for the muscle tissues of the heart. Anything that causes a reduction in the amount of blood that can flow through the coronary arteries, even if for a short period, holds the potential to damage the heart itself. Thus, the short-term reduction in coronary artery diameter brought on by cigarette smoking may, ultimately, contribute to cardiovascular problems for the smoker.

Another way that cigarette smoking can affect the cardiovascular system is through the introduction of carbon monoxide into the circulation. The blood of a cigarette smoker may lose as much as 15% of its oxygen-carrying capacity as the carbon monoxide binds to the hemoglobin in the blood and blocks the transportation of oxygen to the body's cells (Tresch & Aronow, 1996).

The Visual System

In addition to cigarette-induced cancer, smokers may experience other nonfatal forms of illness. A pair of recent studies revealed that smoking was associated with a higher risk of cataract formation in both men (Christensen et al., 1992) and women (Hankinson et al., 1992). Although the exact mechanism for cataract formation was not clear, current male smokers who used 20 or more cigarettes a day were twice as likely to form cataracts as were nonsmokers (Christensen et al., 1992).

Research also revealed that women who had quit cigarette smoking, even if they had done so a decade earlier, were still at risk for cataract formation (Hankinson et al., 1992). These findings indicate that cigarette-induced disease is far more involved than had previously been thought and suggest that at least some of the physical damage caused by cigarette smoking does not reverse itself if the smoker quits.

Other Complications Caused by Cigarette Smoking

The use of tobacco products is thought to contribute to the formation of peptic ulcers (Jarvik & Schneider, 1992; Lee & D'Alonzo, 1993). Further, cigarette smoking is thought to be a risk factor for the development of psoriasis, although researchers do not know why this might be the case (Baughman, 1993). Although researchers are not sure why, cigarette smokers are also known to suffer from higher rates of cancer of the kidneys than do nonsmokers. Further, researchers have uncovered a relationship between cigarette smoking and a thyroid condition known as *Graves' disease*.

While the exact relationship between cigarette smoking and Graves' disease is not clear, researchers suspect that cigarette smoking "might be one of these environmental stimuli capable of inducing Graves' disease in genetically predisposed individuals" (Prummel & Wiersinga, 1993, p. 479).

Research into how cigarette smoking contributes to the development of Graves' disease in at least some individuals is currently in progress. It appears, however, that cigarette smoking is one of the risk factors for this thyroid dysfunction, in at least some individuals.

As a group, it was found that older women who smoke were physically weaker and had less coordination than did nonsmoking women of the same age (Nelson, Nevitt, Scott, Stone, & Cummings, 1994). The authors examined 9704 women who were at least 65 years of age, who were living independently,

with a battery of physical and neuromuscular function tests. The authors found that their results suggested:

> Women who are current smokers, and to a lesser extent former smokers, are weaker, have poorer balance, and have impaired neuromuscular performance compared with those who have never smoked. (p. 1829)

However, the authors did not identify a mechanism by which cigarette smoking might have interfered with the women's neuromuscular performance. Further, the authors admitted, their study was limited to volunteers who were able to come in to the research center, and thus these women might, in some manner, have been different than those women who were unable to participate in the research study because of ill health, lack of transportation, and so on.

Finally, there is evidence to suggest that smoking can cause changes in brain function, which may persist for many years after the individual stops (Sherman, 1994). There is a measurable decline in mental abilities that begins about 4 hours after the last cigarette. It is not known how long former smokers will need to return to their normal level of intellectual function. However, some former smokers report that they have never felt "right" for as long as *nine years* after their last cigarette. While there has been no research into the long-term effects of cigarette abstinence on cognitive function (Sherman), these reports are quite suggestive.

Smoking and Gender

At least 126,000 of those who die of smoking-related illness in this country each year are women (University of California, Berkeley, 1990c). The annual death toll among women is expected to increase to about 240,000 premature deaths in women by the mid-1990s, as the number of women smokers increases (Peto, Lopez, Boreham, Thun, & Heath, 1992). Women who smoke are at risk for: "invasive cervical cancer, miscarriages, early menopause, and osteoporosis, among other disorders" (University of California, Berkeley, 1990c, p. 7).

Cigarette smoking was estimated to be the cause of 20% to 25% (Simons, Phillips, & Coleman, 1993) and 30% (Bartecchi et al., 1994) of all cases of cervical cancer. The team of Simons et al. (1993) examined a number of women, and found damage to the DNA in the cells of the cervical epithelium to be significantly more common in women who smoked compared with women who have never smoked. This damage is thought to be a factor associated with the ultimate development of cervical cancer and suggests the mechanism through which cigarette smoking contributes to the development of cervical cancer.

The team of Szarewski et al. (1996) examined the size of cervical lesions in 82 volunteer women. Of this sample, all of whom were cigarette smokers, 17 were able to stop smoking, while 11 others reduced the frequency of their cigarette smoking by at least 75%. The authors compared the size of the cervical lesions of these women with those of the remaining smokers, and found that 23 of the 28 women who stopped/reduced their use of cigarettes had a *reduction* in the size of the cervical cancer lesions of at least 20%. Only 13 of the 47 nonquitters had a reduction in the size of the cancerous lesions. The authors interpreted this data to suggest that (a) cigarette smoking is indeed associated with increased rates of cervical cancer, and (b) that quitting cigarette smoking in the early stages of cervical cancer seems to have a beneficial effect on the growth of cancer cells in the cervix.

Approximately 56,000 women die each year as a result of lung cancer, compared with 46,000 women who die each year as a result of cancer of the breast (Bartecchi et al., 1994). Thus, lung cancer has surpassed cancer of the breast to become the leading cause of cancer-related deaths in women in the United States. There is also significant evidence to suggest that cigarette smoking is associated with accelerated calcium loss in women, following menopause. Hopper and Seeman (1994) measured bone density in pairs of female identical twins, only one of whom smoked cigarettes. The authors found that the twin who smoked cigarettes tended to have a greater degree of bone loss following menopause. The authors did not identify a mechanism through which the smoking twin lost more bone mass following menopause, but they suggested that cigarette smoking would contribute to a tendency toward greater levels of reabsorption

of bone minerals. If this theory is correct, then the authors have identified both another negative consequence of cigarette smoking for women and the mechanism through which smoking is able to contribute to increased bone loss in older female smokers.

The Degrees of Risk

There is a dose-related risk of premature death caused by cigarette smoking. Robbins et al. (1994) found that male physicians who smoked less than a pack of cigarettes a day still had a significantly higher risk of both ischemic and hemorrhagic stroke than did nonsmokers. The authors found that male physicians who smoked more than a pack of cigarettes a day had an even higher risk of stroke, and concluded that *any* cigarette use significantly increased the individual's risk of stroke.

Many smokers believe that if they limit their cigarette use they will reduce their risk of cancer. However, research has shown that smokers who use only 1–9 cigarettes a day are still *five times as likely* to develop lung cancer as are nonsmokers (The Wellness Letter, 1990). For those who smoke 10–19 cigarettes a day, the risk increases to nine times as likely to develop lung cancer. As these figures make clear, "No amount of smoking is free of risk" (The Wellness Letter).

The Passive Smoker

Nor is the danger of smoking-related death limited to the smoker. Researchers have found that a significant percentage of the population of the United States is exposed to tobacco smoke either at home or the workplace, although they do not themselves smoke. The team of Pirkle et al. (1996) examined blood samples of 10,642 individuals selected to reflect the population characteristics of the entire United States, in order to determine what percentage of nonsmokers had cotinine (a metabolite of nicotine) in their blood. The authors determined that 87.9% of nonsmokers had cotinine in their blood, suggesting that the majority of individuals in the United States are routinely exposed to cigarette smoke even though they do not themselves smoke.

This "passive smoking" (i.e., being around smokers so that you inhale cigarette smoke even if you do not smoke, also known as "secondhand" smoke) is thought to cause the death of between 50,000 (American Medical Association, 1993; Glantz & Parmley, 1995) and 62,000 (Tresch & Aronow, 1996) nonsmokers in the United States each year. Of this number, approximately 35,000 to 40,000 die as a result of heart disease caused by environmental tobacco smoke, and 3000 Americans die as a result of lung cancer caused by secondhand smoke (Fontham et al., 1994; Pappas, 1995). Other researchers give even higher estimates of the number of lives lost to the effects of secondhand cigarette smoke.

The Environmental Protection Agency (EPA) estimated that what it termed "environmental tobacco smoke" causes some 300,000 cases of various forms of respiratory disease yearly (Bartecchi et al., 1994). Pappas (1995) went even further, stating that secondhand smoke causes between 150,000 and 300,000 respiratory infections just in the 5.5 million children in this country who are under the age of 18 months. Further, secondhand smoke is thought to cause 150,000 heart attacks yearly (Associated Press, 1994b). Environmental tobacco smoke has been identified as the third most common preventable cause of death by Glantz and Parmley (1995). Only active smoking and alcohol use result in a greater number of preventable deaths in this country each year.

The EPA has now classified secondhand tobacco smoke as a major carcinogen. Evidence in support of the EPA's recommendation that secondhand tobacco smoke be classified as a carcinogen is found in the study by a team of Greek researchers (Trichopoulos et al., 1992). The authors examined lung tissue samples from 400 recently deceased individuals from the Athens, Greece, region. They found that nonsmokers living with cigarette smokers had "possibly precancerous" (p. 1697) changes in the lung tissue samples of the same type found in lung tissue samples from recently deceased cigarette smokers.

In addition to this study, the team of Fontham et al. (1994) also found evidence supporting the theory that secondhand smoke is dangerous to nonsmokers. The authors examined the risk factors associated with the development of lung cancer in 653 nonsmoking women with that disease and compared the

data with data from 1253 control subjects who were not commonly exposed to tobacco smoke. The authors concluded that, overall, nonsmoking women who were exposed to secondhand smoke had a 30% greater chance of developing lung cancer than did nonsmoking women who were not routinely exposed to tobacco smoke. The authors of both studies concluded that their research had uncovered significant evidence to link environmental tobacco smoke and lung cancer. Further, the results of these studies raise serious questions as to the impact that cigarette smoking might have on others in the smoker's environment.

Nor does secondhand smoke limit its effects to the lungs. The team of Morabia, Bernstein, Heritier, and Khatchatrian (1996) examined the effects of active smoking, a history of having smoked cigarettes before quitting, and passive smoking, on the development of breast cancer in women. They found that while former smokers had a reduced risk of breast cancer compared with current smokers, both groups had a significantly higher risk of breast cancer than did women who had never smoked cigarettes. The authors noted that many of the carcinogenic chemicals found in tobacco smoke are filtered from the breast tissue only slowly, allowing those substances to continue to cause damage to the tissues of the breast long after the individual has stopped smoking. These chemicals are absorbed by women who are exposed to environmental tobacco smoke, as well as by women who actively smoke cigarettes, and thus those women who had never been exposed to tobacco smoke had the lowest risk of breast cancer of the three groups of women.

The team of Klonoff-Cohen et al. (1995) examined the smoking patterns of adults in 200 households where an infant had died of sudden infant death syndrome (SIDS), and compared this data with the smoking pattern in 200 households with healthy children (Chapter 20). The authors found a statistical relationship between the child's exposure to secondhand smoke and SIDS. Thus, those children raised in homes where there were no cigarette smokers had the lowest risk of death from SIDS. Further, the authors found that the greater the degree of exposure of the infant to environmental smoke, the greater that child's chances of death by SIDS.

In other words, those infants raised in a home where smoking around the baby was banned had a lower risk of death from SIDS than those infants who were raised in a home where the parents smoked near the child. Further, the more that the parents smoked at home, the greater the child's chances of death by SIDS, according to the authors' findings. While this study did not reveal a specific mechanism by which parental smoking might increase the infants' chance of SIDS, the statistical relationship was such that the authors recommended that physicians warn their patients of this potential danger.

The most common cause of death for those who are exposed to environmental tobacco smoke is coronary artery disease (Kritz, Schmid, & Sinzinger, 1995). Each year, fully 70% of those people in the United States who die from secondhand smoke, or an estimated 62,000 individuals, will do so from coronary heart disease caused by their passive smoking, according to Tresch and Aronow (1996).

One reason passive cigarette smoke is so dangerous to those who are near the smoker is that the passive smoker is being exposed to many of the same toxins that cause damage to the smoker's cardiovascular system (Glantz & Parmley, 1995). Further, the passive smoker is being exposed to these toxins in sufficient concentrations that his/her cardiovascular system is being damaged by the same chemicals that cause so much damage to the cardiovascular system of cigarette smokers. Finally, the authors suggested that secondhand tobacco smoke causes between 30,000 and 60,000 fatal heart attacks and three times this number of nonfatal heart attacks each year in nonsmokers.

As these studies suggest, the dangers of cigarette smoking are not limited to the smoker alone.

Complications Caused by Chewing Tobacco

There are three types of smokeless tobacco: moist snuff, dry snuff, and chewing tobacco (Westman, 1995). It is thought that 5.6% of men, and 0.6% of the adult women in the United States use smokeless tobacco (Spangler & Salisbury, 1995). Of these three forms of smokeless tobacco, chewing tobacco is the most common.

Although many of those who use chewing tobacco believe that the use of oral tobacco is safer

than cigarette smoking, the practice is actually dangerous. A person who uses chewing tobacco achieves blood nicotine levels that approximate those achieved by smoking one cigarette (Gottlieb, Pope, Rickert, & Hardin, 1993). At least three compounds in smokeless tobacco are capable of causing hypertension: nicotine, sodium, and licorice (Westman, 1995). Further, there are 28 different chemical compounds capable of causing the growth of tumors in smokeless tobacco (Bartecchi et al., 1994).

Thus, it would be natural to expect that individuals who use oral forms of tobacco would be at increased risk for cancer of the mouth and throat. This assumption has been proven correct. In one study cited by Spangler and Salisbury (1995) 93% of the patients with oral cancer reported using snuff and 6% admitted to the use of chewing tobacco. Other possible consequences that seem to be caused by the use of smokeless tobacco include damage to the tissues of the gums, staining of the teeth, and damage to the teeth (Spangler & Salisbury).

While it is not clear whether tobacco chewers have the same degree of risk for coronary artery disease as do cigarette smokers, they have a greater incidence of coronary artery disease than do individuals who neither chew nor smoke tobacco. Further, smokeless tobacco can contribute to problems with the control of the individual's blood pressure (Westman, 1995). Thus, while smokeless tobacco is often viewed as "the lesser of two evils," it is certainly not without risk.

The Cost of Cigarette Smoking around the World

The problem of cigarette-induced disease is not limited to this country. It has been estimated that tobacco use around the world is responsible for 3 million premature deaths each year (Phillips et al., 1995). Further, if present trends continue, it is estimated that by the year 2020 cigarette smoking will cause 10 million premature deaths around the world each year, or 27,300 deaths each day from cigarette-related illness (Sagan, 1995). Seventy percent of these premature deaths will take place in the developing countries of the so-called Third World, according to Phillips et al. (1995). It has been estimated by the World Health Organization that, by the year 2020, 1 in every 10 deaths around the world will be caused by tobacco-related illness (*Wisconsin State Journal*, 1996). As these figures suggest, cigarette smoking would seem to be a most dangerous pastime.

Recovery from Risk

Over time, the smoker who learns to abstain from the use of tobacco enjoys a reduced risk for many of the complications caused by cigarette smoking. The risk of lung cancer gradually decreases, until by 10 to 15 years after the last use of cigarettes former smokers have about the same risk for developing lung cancer as nonsmokers (Lee & D'Alonzo, 1993). Former smokers enjoy a reduced risk of coronary artery disease, with the rate of coronary artery disease for former smokers reaching the same levels as nonsmokers in 2 to 3 years for women and 5 years for men, according to the authors.

The team of Wannamethee, Shaper, Whincup, and Walker (1995) conducted a prospective study of cardiovascular disease in 7735 men who were between the ages of 40 and 59. The names of these men were drawn at random from the health records of a number of towns in England. Smokers were found to have a fourfold greater risk of stroke than nonsmokers. When the authors examined the effects of giving up tobacco smoking (including pipes and cigars), they found that there was a reduction in the individual's risk of smoking over the first 5 years following the last use of tobacco. However, it was found, heavy smokers who stopped still had a twofold greater risk of stroke compared with nonsmokers. Thus, for the heavier smoker, giving up the use of tobacco products will reduce the risk of stroke, but not reduce it to the level of a nonsmoker.

Other improvements in the exsmoker's health status include a slowing of peripheral vascular disease and improved sense of taste and smell, according to Lee and D'Alonzo (1993). In addition, the team of Grover, Gray-Donald, Joseph, Abrahamowicz, and Coupal (1994) found that former cigarette smokers as a group added between 2.5 and 4.5 years to their life expectancy when they stopped smoking. The authors found that cessation of cigarette use was several times as powerful a force in prolonging life as was changing one's dietary habits. Finally, as a

group, former smokers show less cardiac impairment and lower rates of reinfarction than do smokers who continue to smoke after having a heart attack. As these findings suggest, there are very real benefits to giving up cigarette smoking.

The Treatment of Nicotine Addiction

When one asks a cigarette smoker why he/she continues to smoke, despite the dangers of this habit, the response is often "I can't help myself. I'm addicted." Indeed, it is believed that the addictive power of nicotine is why 90% to 98% of those who attempt to quit smoking in any given year will ultimately fail (Benowitz & Henningfield, 1994; Henningfield, 1995; Sherman, 1994).

Although health care workers have tried for many years to identify the factors that contribute to a person's successful attempt to quit smoking, they have met with little success (Kenford et al., 1994). Thus, cigarette cessation programs are something of a hit-or-miss affair, in which neither the leaders nor the participants have much knowledge of what *really* works. Smoking cessation training programs usually help between 70% to 80% of the participants to stop smoking on a short-term basis. But, of those who attempt to stop smoking, two-thirds may stop for a very few days, but only 2% to 3% will be tobacco-free a year later (Henningfield, 1995). The research team of Hughes et al. (1991) found that 65% of their experimental sample relapsed within the first month of quitting, suggesting that the first month is especially difficult for the recent exsmoker.

The reason for this may be that in the first 3 to 4 weeks following cessation of cigarette smoking, the individual is especially vulnerable to smoking cues, such as being around other smokers (Bliss, Garvey, Heinold, & Hitchcock, 1989). At such times, the individual is less likely to effectively cope with the urge to smoke and is in danger of a relapse into active cigarette smoking.

Lichtenstein and Glasgow (1992) presented a model for smoking cessation in which recovery is viewed as a multistage process (see Table 16-1). Their model follows the same stages as those for recovery from other forms of drug abuse/addiction (discussed in Chapter 35). This similarity underscores that nicotine affects the same nerve pathways in the brain's pleasure center that are stimulated by the other drugs of abuse, and thus there is little distinction between nicotine and the other recreational drugs discussed in this text.

According to Lichtenstein and Glasgow (1992), the first stage of recovery from nicotine dependence is that of *precontemplation*. This is the stage of tobacco use prior to the individual's decision to try to quit smoking. During this phase, the individual is still smoking but has occasional, vague, thoughts about quitting "one of these days."

Once the smoker makes a conscious decision to think about giving up tobacco use within the next 6 months, he/she is viewed as having moved into the *contemplation* phase. When the smoker embarks on an effort to give up tobacco and actually begins the cigarette cessation program, he/she has entered the *action* phase of smoking cessation. Finally, after the individual has been smoke-free for 6 months, he/she enters the *maintenance* phase. During the maintenance phase, the individual works on remaining smoke-free. This is often a difficult task for the former smoker, and this period is associated with a high relapse rate.

As noted earlier in this chapter, there appears to be an association between the frequency of cigarette smoking and the difficulty associated with giving up tobacco use. The research team of Cohen et al. (1989) reviewed data from ten different research projects that involved a total of 5000 subjects who were attempting to stop smoking cigarettes.

The authors found that light smokers (defined as those who smoked less than 20 cigarettes each day) were significantly more likely to be able to stop smoking on their own than were heavy smokers.

Cohen et al. (1989) also found that the number of previous attempts to quit smoking was not an indication of hopelessness. Rather, the authors found that the number of unsuccessful previous attempts was unrelated to whether the smoker would be able to quit this time. They concluded that "most people who fail a single attempt (to quit smoking) will try again and again and eventually quit" (p. 1361).

Another factor that seems to be associated with the difficulty smokers experience when attempting to quit is their *expectancies* for the nicotine withdrawal process. The team of Tate et al. (1994) formed 4 subgroups from their research sample of 62 cigarette smokers. Those former smokers who were led to believe that they would not experience any significant distress during the nicotine withdrawal process reported significantly fewer physical or emotional complaints than did the other research groups. It appeared to the authors that the individual's expectations for the nicotine withdrawal process might play a role in how the individual interprets and responds to the symptoms experienced during early abstinence. The team of Kviz, Clark, Crittenden, Wearnecke, and Freels (1995) found that for smokers over the age of 50, the perceived degree of difficulty in quitting was negatively associated with the individual's actual attempts to quit smoking. That is, especially for smokers over the age of 50, the harder the individual expected the task of quitting to be, the less likely that person was to do so. Thus, the individual's expectations for quitting were found to play a significant role in whether the individual quit smoking cigarettes.

Researchers now believe that smokers who want to quit require an average of 3 to 4 attempts (Prochaska, DiClemente, & Norcross, 1992), to perhaps as many as 5 to 7 "serious attempts" (Brunton et al., 1994, p. 105; Sherman, 1994) before being able to

TABLE 16-1 The Stages of Smoking Cessation

Precontemplation phase	*Contemplation phase*	*Action phase*	*Maintenance phase*
Smoker is not considering an attempt to stop smoking. Smoker is still actively smoking.	Smoker is now seriously thinking about trying to give up smoking in the next 6 months.	Day to stop smoking is selected. The individual initiates his/her program to stop smoking.	Having been smoke-free for 6 months, ex-smoker works to remain smoke-free.

stop smoking. But the reader should keep in mind that these figures reflect the *average* number of attempts smokers must make before being able to quit. Some people are able to quit on the first or second attempt, while other people may require nine or ten attempts, before they succeed.

Individuals who want to give up smoking should be warned that cigarette cessation is a "Dynamic Process" (Cohen et al., 1989, p. 1361), in which periods of abstinence are intermixed with periods of relapse:

> The return to smoking . . . occurs so frequently that it should be thought of as a part of the process of quitting and not as a failure in quitting. (Lee & D'Alonzo, 1993, p. 39)

Thus, the smoker who wants to quit should be warned that the struggle against cigarette smoking is a lifelong one. Further, former smokers should be warned that they will be vulnerable to relapsing back to cigarette smoking for the rest of his/her life.

Although there has been a great deal of emphasis on formal cigarette cessation treatment programs, perhaps as many as 90% (Brunton et al., 1994; Fiore et al., 1990) to 95% (Hughes, 1992; Kozlowski et al., 1989; Peele, 1989) of cigarette smokers who quit do so without participating in a formal treatment program. Of those smokers who do quit, it would seem that the individual's motivation to quit smoking is most "critical" (Jaffe, 1989, p. 682) to the success of their efforts. These conclusions raise serious questions as to whether extensive treatment programs are necessary for tobacco dependence. But formal treatment programs may be of value to heavy smokers or those who are at risk for tobacco-related illness.

Summary

Tobacco use, once limited to the New World, was introduced to Europe by Columbus's men. The practice of smoking or chewing tobacco spread rapidly in Europe. Following the introduction of the cigarette around the turn of the century, smoking became more common, rapidly replacing tobacco chewing as the accepted method of tobacco use.

The active psychoactive agent of tobacco, nicotine, has been found to have an addiction potential similar to that of cocaine or narcotics. A significant percentage of those who are currently addicted to nicotine will attempt to stop smoking cigarettes, but will initially be unsuccessful in doing so. Current treatment methods have been unable to achieve a significant cessation rate, and more comprehensive treatment programs have been suggested for nicotine addiction. These comprehensive programs are patterned after alcohol addiction treatment programs, but have not demonstrated a significantly improved cure rate for cigarette smoking. It has been suggested that such formal treatment programs may be of value for those individuals whose tobacco use has placed them at risk for tobacco-related illness.

CHAPTER SEVENTEEN

The Medical Model of Chemical Addiction

In Chapters 1 through 16, the major drugs of abuse were discussed. This is important information for the chemical dependency or human services professional. However, knowledge of what each drug of abuse might do to the user does not answer a simple, and yet, very difficult, set of questions: (a) Why do people begin to use these chemicals, (b) why do they continue to use recreational chemicals, and (c) why do people become addicted to them? In this chapter, the answers to these questions are examined from the perspective of what has come to be known as the "medical" or "disease" model of addiction.

Why Do People Use Chemicals?[1]

At first, this question may seem simplistic. People use drugs because they choose to do so. The drugs of abuse are part of the environment. Every day, perhaps several times a day, each one of us has to make a decision to use/not use recreational chemicals. Admittedly, for most of us, this choice is relatively simple. Usually the decision not to use chemicals does not even require conscious thought. But, whether we acknowledge them or not, we are faced with opportunities each and every day to use one or more recreational chemicals. Each day, we must decide either consciously or unconsciously whether to engage in recreational chemical use.

[1] This question is a reference not to those people who are addicted to chemicals, but to those people who use chemicals for recreational purposes.

Although some people may challenge the issue of personal choice, there is a grim logic to the statement in the preceding paragraph. Stop for an instant, and think: Where is the nearest liquor store? If you wanted to do so, where could you buy some marijuana? If you are above the age of about 15, the odds are very good that you could either answer both of these questions or find somebody who could answer them. But, why didn't you go out and buy any of these chemicals on your way in to work, or to school, this morning? Why didn't you buy a recreational drug or two on your way home last night?

If you did not, the reason is that you made a choice not to do so. Your decision not to use chemicals might have been so automatic that you made it without any conscious thought. But, on some level, you chose either to stop and buy alcohol or some other form of recreational drug, or you chose not to do so. So, in one sense, the answer to the question of why people use the drugs of abuse is because they choose to do so. But other factors are involved in making the decision to use or not to use recreational chemicals.

Factors That Influence Recreational Drug Use

The Physical Reward Potential

Actually, the question of why a person might use alcohol or another drug of abuse is complex. The novice chemical user may decide to try one or more drugs in response to peer pressure or because the person anticipates that the drug will have pleasurable effects. Researchers call this the "pharmacological potential," or the "reward potential" of the chemical (Meyer, 1989a). Not surprisingly, virtually all the drugs of abuse have a high reward potential (Crowley, 1988). Stated very simply, the drugs of abuse make the user feel good. To illustrate this point, consider that cocaine's effects have been likened to that of sexual orgasm by some users and that the rush from intravenously administered narcotics or cocaine has been described in similar terms. Indeed, so powerful is cocaine for some users that they prefer the drug to a human lover! On a similar note, it is not unusual for AA members to speak of alcohol as their "best friend" (Knapp, 1996, p. 96).

One of the basic laws of behavioral psychology is that if something (a) increases the individual's sense of pleasure, or (b) decreases his/her discomfort, then the person is likely to repeat that behavior. If a certain behavior (c) increases the individual's sense of discomfort, or (d) reduces the person's sense of pleasure, he/she is unlikely to repeat that behavior. Any immediate consequence (either reward or punishment) has a stronger impact on behavior than delayed consequence.

When one applies these rules of behavior to the problem of substance abuse, it becomes evident that the immediate consequences of chemical use (i.e., the immediate pleasure) has a stronger impact on behavior than the delayed consequences (i.e., possible addiction or disease at an unspecified later date). Within this context, it should not be surprising to learn that, since many people find the effects of the drugs of abuse[2] to be pleasurable, they are tempted to use them again and again.

The Social Learning Component of Drug Use

Many people do not initially find that the drugs of abuse cause them to feel pleasure. Sometimes, the user must be taught to (a) recognize the drug's effects and (b) interpret them as pleasurable. For

example, first-time marijuana users must be taught by their drug-using peers: (a) how to smoke it, (b) how to recognize the effects of the drug, and, (c) why marijuana intoxication is so pleasurable (Kandel & Raveis, 1989; Peele, 1985). In much the same way, first-time heroin users are taught by more experienced users what drug-induced effects to look for and why these drug-induced feelings are so desirable (Lingeman, 1974).

A similar learning process takes place with alcohol. It is not uncommon for the first-time drinker to become so ill after a night's drinking that he/she will swear never to drink again. However, more experienced drinkers will help the novice learn such things as how to drink, what effects to look for, and why these alcohol-induced physical sensations are so pleasurable. This feedback is often informal, and comes through sources such as a "drinking buddy," newspaper articles, advertisements, television programs, conversations with friends and co-workers, and casual observations of others who are drinking. The outcome of this social learning process is that the novice drinker is taught how to drink and how to enjoy the alcohol consumed.

Individual Expectations as a Component of Drug Use

The individual's expectations for a drug have been found to be a strong influence on how that person interprets its effects. This has been found to be true for nicotine-containing gum (Gottlieb, Killen, Marlatt, & Taylor, 1987), and for certain effects thought to be produced by alcohol (Gordis, 1996a). In the former case, researchers have found that it is the individual's expectation of receiving nicotine-containing gum, rather than whether he/she actually receives gum containing nicotine, that moderates the individual's cigarette withdrawal symptoms. In the case of alcohol, the individual's expectations seem to shape his/her response to a beverage that he/she thinks contains alcohol. The team of Brown, Goldman, Inn, and Anderson, (1980) found that—among other things—their subjects expected that low to moderate doses of alcohol would positively enhance life experiences, magnify physical and social pleasure, and increase sexual performance. Further, the authors found that their subjects fully expected that moderate alcohol use would increase

---

[2] Obviously, the OTC analgesics are exceptions to this rule, since they do not cause the user to experience "pleasure." However, they are included in this text because of their significant potential to cause harm.

social aggressiveness, make them more assertive, and reduce tension.

The individual's expectations for alcohol or drugs are formed well before he/she first begins to experiment with chemicals (G. Smith, 1994). It would appear that these expectations are formed in childhood or the early years of adolescence. Once established, the individual's expectations then play a powerful role in shaping the individual's later drinking behavior. Werner, Walker, and Greene (1995) measured the expectations for alcohol for a sample of 260 students at the start of their freshman year of college, and again at the end of their junior year. The authors found that those individuals who became "high-risk drinkers" (p. 737) by the end of their junior year of college had significantly stronger expectations that alcohol use would be a positive experience for them than did nondrinkers or those classified as "low risk" by the authors (p. 737).

The individual's expectations for alcohol/drugs are not fixed, but may be modified on the basis of both personal experience and social feedback. For example, if the adolescent finds alcohol's effects to be pleasurable, this then sets the stage for increased alcohol use as adolescence progresses (G. Smith, 1994). The individual's expectations for a recreational chemical's effects are thought to contribute to the likelihood that an LSD user will have a "bad trip." Novice LSD users tend to anticipate unpleasant consequences from the drug, and this anxiety seems to help start the negative drug experience (bad trip).

Thus, establishing expectations about recreational chemical use is a complex process. Individual expectations about a drug's effects are often learned from several sources, including more experienced chemical users. Over time, the individual is exposed to information about (a) how to use a drug of abuse, (b) what effects to expect from that drug, and (c) why these effects are so desirable. Based on all this information, the individual then evaluates the anticipated outcome of the possibility of recreational chemical use, to determine whether the use of a chemical(s) at this time is likely to be a rewarding experience.

If a person's expectations about a specific drug are extremely negative, he/she will not even experiment with that chemical. An example of this might be seen in the reaction that people have when you

suggest that they experiment with a well-known poison, such as cyanide. Their usual response is something along the lines of "Are you crazy, or something?" But those individuals who contemplate the possibility of using one or more recreational chemicals in a more positive light create a psychological predisposition to actually experiment with that chemical(s). Further, the individual's preconceptions will influence how he/she interprets the effects of the chemical, possibly encouraging future repetitions of use. This may be why Werner et al. (1995) found that those college students who engaged in problem drinking at the end of their junior year were more likely to have had positive expectations for alcohol several years earlier, when they entered college.

Society as the Model for Chemical Use

The individual's decision to use, or not use, one or more chemicals is made within a cultural context. Within each culture, certain attitudes and feelings evolve that govern the use of mood-altering chemicals (Westermeyer, 1995). These cultural attitudes and beliefs then form the framework within which the individual's decision about personal recreational chemical use is made. The cultural attitudes and beliefs also provide a standard by which the individual's chemical use is measured. Thus, for each individual, cultural influences serve as significant determinants of drug use patterns (Peele, 1985). Cultural influences may encourage, or inhibit, the actual development of addiction:

> In cultures where use of a substance is comfortable, familiar, and socially regulated both as to style of use and appropriate time and place for such use, addiction is less likely and may be practically unknown. (Peele, 1985, p. 106)

Thus, according to Peele (1985), it is only if a given society *fails to regulate* (a) the style of chemical use, (b) the time that the chemical may be used, or, (c) the place in which that chemical may be used, that chemical abuse becomes a problem. Developing rules to govern the use of a new recreational substance may take a culture generations, or centuries (Westermeyer, 1995) because cultural standards of behavior result from the slow process of social evolution, while new drug use patterns and new recreational chemicals have been emerging on a year-to-year basis. Thus, the problem of substance abuse can be viewed as a failure of this society to regulate substance use in an acceptable way, rather than to eliminate all drug use by the members of this society (Peele).

An excellent example of the power of social rules to govern chemical use might be found in the observation that, for both the Jewish and Italian American cultures, drinking was limited mainly to religious or family celebrations. In these cultures, excessive drinking was strongly discouraged, and "proper" (i.e., socially acceptable) drinking behavior was modeled by the adults during religious or family activities. It is no coincidence that these two subgroups have relatively low rates of alcoholism.

A comparison of the role that alcohol plays in two subcultures in the United States also helps to illustrate the manner in which social rules control recreational chemical use. In the Chinese American subculture, adults model proper drinking behavior to their children, and alcohol is neither viewed as a rite of passage into adulthood, nor is its use associated with social power (Peele, 1985). In contrast, however, the Irish American culture has viewed alcohol use far more liberally, as a rite of passage, and peer groups have encouraged the use of alcohol. For these reasons, Peele (1984, 1985) concluded that the Irish American subculture subsequently has demonstrated higher rates of alcoholism than the Chinese Americans.

Kunitz and Levy (1974) explored the different drinking patterns of the Navajo and Hopi Indian tribes. This study is significant in that these cultures coexist in the same part of the country and share similar genetic histories. However, Navajo tribal customs hold that public group drinking is acceptable, while solitary drinking is a mark of deviance. For the Hopi, however, drinking is more likely to be a solitary experience, for alcohol use is not tolerated within the tribe, and those who drink are shunned. These two groups, who live in close geographic proximity to each other, demonstrate how different social groups develop different guidelines for members' alcohol use.

In some subcultures, the individual's use of chemicals is seen as a sign of maturity, with the specific drugs being abused serving as a signpost of the individual's "growth." For example, in the United States, adolescents often look upon drinking as a sign of their entry into adulthood, almost as a "rite of passage" (Leigh, 1985). Within this context, it should not be surprising to learn that the adolescent peer subculture frequently encourages repeated episodes of chemical abuse (Swaim, Oetting, Edwards, & Beauvais, 1989).

For the most part, the discussion has been limited to the use of alcohol in this section. This is because alcohol is the most common recreational drug used in the United States. However, this is not always true for other cultural groups. For example, the American Indians of the Southwest frequently ingest mushrooms with hallucinogenic potential, as part of their religious ceremonies. In the Mideast, alcohol is prohibited, but hashish is an accepted recreational drug. In both cultures, strict social rules dictate when these substances may be used, the conditions under which they may be used, and the penalties for unacceptable substance use.

The point to remember is that cultural rules provide the individual with guidance about what is acceptable or unacceptable substance use. But within each culture, there are various social subgroups which accept the rules of the parent culture to a greater or lesser degree. For example, in one social group, alcohol use might be strictly prohibited, while another social group might accept alcohol use only on religious holidays and a third social group might advocate the free use of alcohol within certain limits. Thus, different social groups might have quite different standards for alcohol use behavior, despite the fact that they are all part of the same culture. The relationship between different social groups and the parent culture is demonstrated in Figure 17.1.

Social Feedback Mechanisms and Drug Use

There is a subtle, often overlooked feedback mechanism between the individual and his/her social group. While the group shapes the individual's behavior at least in part, the individual, by choosing to associate with that group, also helps to shape its behavioral expectations. For example, alcoholics (and other drug users) tend to drift toward social groups where the use of their chemical use is at least tolerated, if not

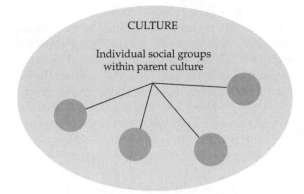

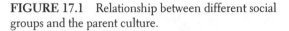

FIGURE 17.1 Relationship between different social groups and the parent culture.

actively encouraged. At the same time, the person addicted to chemicals tends to avoid social groups where drug use is discouraged.

Kandel and Raveis (1989) found that one important predictor of whether a person would use cocaine was whether he/she had friends who also used cocaine. The authors found that a given individual's cocaine use pattern was extremely similar to that of his/her friends. Those individuals who used cocaine tended to associate more with others who also used cocaine, and those who avoided cocaine use tended to associate with those who also did not use this drug. In a similar study, Simpson, Crandall, Savage, and Pava-Krueger (1981) noted that, prior to their participation in a substance abuse treatment program, 60% of their sample of narcotics addicts spent "a lot" (p. 38) of time engaged in "street" leisure activities. Such recreational activities center on behaviors involving other addicted individuals. After the completion of treatment, only 13% of their sample continued to associate with active narcotics addicts.

Within each culture, guidelines evolve that specify (a) which chemicals may—or may not—be used, (b) the frequency of use that is permitted within that culture, and (c) the sanctions that apply if these rules are violated. For example, crack cocaine is found mainly in the inner cities, while powdered cocaine is found more often in the suburbs. If as is often the case, there are social sanctions against the use of that chemical, then the individual must (a) try to find a way to reconcile further use of that drug while remaining in the

same social group, (b) decide how important the use of that drug is compared with membership in a given social group, or, (c) try to find a social group that permits continued drug use.

Admittedly, most people do not think in these exact terms. However, their thinking would parallel these themes. There are many people who, if questioned, would admit to being "closet" drug users. Such people go to great trouble to hide their use of alcohol or other recreational chemicals from neighbors and friends. Caroline Knapp (1996) described how she (and other alcoholics that she knew) would go to a different liquor store each day, so that the clerk would not know the full extent of her drinking. The housewife, or husband, who sneaks around the neighborhood hiding empty alcohol bottles in the neighbors' trash cans is another example of how a person may attempt to reconcile personal use of alcohol with social expectations. The discovery of too many empty alcohol bottles might lead to unpleasant questions by friends and co-workers about personal alcohol use. To counter this threat, many closet drinkers try to hide the evidence of excessive alcohol use.

There are also those who would, if closely questioned, admit to having experimented with one or more of the drugs of abuse. But, these same individuals would also admit that, while the drug's effects were pleasurable, they stopped using it because further use was not compatible with their social status. For example, if one were to question large numbers of those who used marijuana and hallucinogenics during the "hippie" era (late 1960s to the mid-1970s), most of these former drug users would say something to the effect that the drug use was simply a "phase that I was going through."

There are, however, those who find that the chemical's effects are desirable enough to encourage further abuse. These individuals continue to use the drug despite social sanctions against its use. Further, in the service of their use of their drug of choice, they drift toward social groups where the use of that drug is encouraged and supported.

The Effect of Individual Life Goals on Chemical Use

Another factor that influences the individual's decision to either begin, or continue, the use of chemicals is whether the use of a specific drug or drugs is consistent with that person's long-term goals, or values. This is rarely a problem with socially approved drugs, such as alcohol and, to a smaller degree, tobacco. But, consider the example of a junior executive who has just won a much hoped for promotion, only to find that the new position is with a division of the company with a strong "no smoking" policy.

This executive might find that giving up the habit of smoking is not as serious a problem as he once thought, if it is part of the price he has to pay for the promotion. The executive in question has evaluated the degree to which further use of that drug (tobacco) is consistent with his life goal of a major administrative position with a large company. However, the individual in question might also have elected to search for a new position rather than to accept the restriction on cigarette use. In such a case, the individual would have considered the promotion and weighed the cost of giving up cigarettes against the benefits of not making a major lifestyle change.

All these factors have been found by researchers to play a role in a given individual's decision to begin to use alcohol or other drugs. A flowchart of the decision-making process might look something like Figure 17.2.

Note, however, that we are discussing the individual's decision to use alcohol or drugs on a recreational basis. The factors that *initiate* chemical use are not the same factors that *maintain* chemical use (Zucker & Gomberg, 1986). For example, a person may begin to use narcotic analgesics because these chemicals make it easier to deal with painful memories. However, after that individual has become physically addicted to the narcotics, usage may continue because of fear of withdrawal.

What Do We Mean When We Say That Someone Is Addicted to Chemicals?

The truth is, there is no single definition of addiction to alcohol/drugs. Rather, there are a number of competing definitions. But, although many of these theories appear to have some validity in certain situations, a comprehensive theory of addiction has yet

to be developed. It is known that many people experiment with recreational chemical use, and that a percentage of these people become either physically or psychologically dependent on alcohol or recreational drugs. In this text, addiction is defined by the criteria outlined in the American Psychiatric Association's (1994) *Diagnostic and Statistical Manual of Mental Disorders* (4th edition) *(DSM-IV)*. According to the *DSM-IV*, the signs of alcohol/drug addiction include:

1. *Preoccupation* with use of the chemical between periods of use.
2. *Using more of the chemical* than had been anticipated.
3. *Development of tolerance* to the chemical in question.
4. A *characteristic withdrawal syndrome* from the chemical.
5. *Use of the chemical to avoid or control withdrawal symptoms.*
6. *Repeated efforts to cut back or stop* the drug use.
7. *Intoxication at inappropriate times* (e.g., at work), or when *withdrawal interferes with daily functioning* (e.g., hangover makes person too sick to go to work).
8. A *reduction in social, occupational, or recreational activities* in favor of further substance use.
9. *Chemical use* that continues despite the individual having suffered social, emotional, or physical problems related to drug use.

Four or more of these signs, in any combination, identify the individual who is said to suffer from the "disease" of addiction. The "disease model" of substance abuse, or the "medical model" as it is also known, holds that: (a) addiction is a medical disorder, as much as cardiovascular disease or a hernia might be, (b) there is a biological predisposition toward addiction, and (c) the disease of addiction is progressive. An unspoken assumption on which the disease model of drug addiction rests is the concept that some people have a biological vulnerability to the effects of chemicals that is expressed in the form of a loss of control over the use of that substance (Foulks & Pena, 1995).

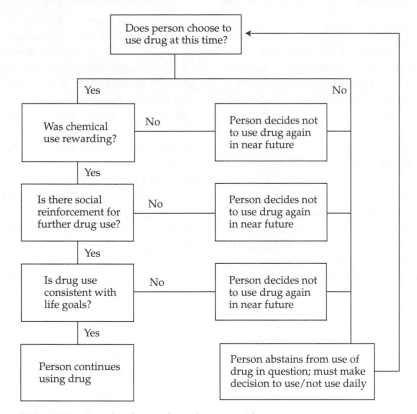

FIGURE 17.2   The chemical use decision-making process.

The Medical Model of Drug Addiction

The medical model of addiction is, perhaps, the most difficult aspect of drug abuse to write about. There are several reasons for this. First of all, although substance abuse professionals often speak of the disease model of addiction, in reality there is no single, universally accepted "disease model." Instead, a group of loosely related theories state that alcohol/drug abuse/addiction is the outcome of a biomedical or psychobiological process. Depending on which theory one is reading, virtually every one of the factors that influences recreational chemical use reviewed in this chapter has been suggested as "the" cause of drug abuse.

Essentially, the core feature of the disease model of the addictions is that, because of the theoretical biological basis of chemical dependency, it should be classified as a disease. But the disease model of chemical dependency has not met with universal acceptance. There are those who argue with equal fervor that alcohol and drug addiction meet the criteria for a disease about as well as the proverbial square peg in the round hole. It has even been suggested that the issue of whether addiction is a true disease is nothing more than a turf battle between the mental health and medical professions (Goodwin & Warnock, 1991, p. 485).

In the United States, however, the treatment of chemical addiction is considered to fall within the realm of medicine. In this section, the disease model of addiction is discussed, along with some of the research that, according to proponents of this treatment model, supports their belief that the compulsive use of chemicals is a true disease.

Jellinek's Work

The work of E. M. Jellinek (1952, 1960) has had a profound impact on the evolution of the medical model of addiction. Jellinek concentrated on the prototypical addiction: alcoholism. Prior to the American Medical Association's decision to classify alcoholism as a formal disease in 1956, it was viewed as a moral disorder. Alcoholics were viewed as being immoral individuals both by society in general and by the majority of physicians.

As others before him had argued, Jellinek (1952, 1960) believed that alcoholism was a disease, like cancer or pneumonia. Certain characteristics of the disease, according to Jellinek, included: (a) the individual's loss of control over his/her drinking, (b) a specific progression of symptoms, and (c) the fact that if it was left untreated, alcoholism would result in the individual's death.

In an early work on alcoholism, Jellinek (1952) suggested that the addiction to alcohol progressed through four stages. The first of these stages, which he called the *prealcoholic* phase, is marked by the individual's use of alcohol for the relief from social tensions encountered during the day. In the prealcoholic stage, one sees the roots of the individual's loss of control over his/her drinking, in that the individual is no longer drinking on a social basis, but has started to drink for relief from stress and anxiety.

As the individual continues to engage in "relief drinking" for an extended period, he/she enters the second phase of alcoholism: the *prodromal* stage (Jellinek, 1952). This second stage is marked by the development of memory blackouts, secret drinking (also known as hidden drinking), a preoccupation with alcohol use, and feelings of guilt over one's behavior while intoxicated.

With the continued use of alcohol, the individual eventually becomes physically dependent on alcohol, a hallmark of what Jellinek (1952) called the *crucial* phase. Other symptoms of this third stage of drinking are a loss of self-esteem, a loss of control over one's drinking, social withdrawal in favor of alcohol use, self-pity, and, a neglect of proper nutrition while drinking. During this phase, the individual attempts to reassert his/her control over the alcohol by entering into periods of abstinence, only to return to the use of alcohol after short periods.

Finally, with continued alcohol use, Jellinek (1952) thought that the alcoholic enters the *chronic* phase. The symptoms of the chronic phase include a deterioration in one's morals, drinking with social inferiors, the development of motor tremors, an obsession with drinking, and, for some, the use of substitutes when alcohol is not available (e.g., drinking rubbing alcohol). Figure 17.3 is a graphic representation of these four stages of alcoholism.

In 1960, Jellinek presented a theoretical model of alcoholism that was both an extension and a revision of his earlier work. According to Jellinek, the alcoholic was unable to consistently predict in advance how much he/she would drink at any given time. Alcoholism, like other diseases, was viewed by Jellinek as having specific symptoms, which included the physical, social, vocational and emotional complications often experienced by the compulsive drinker. Further, Jellinek continued to view alcoholism as having a progressive course which, if not arrested, would ultimately result in the individual's death.

However, in his 1960 book, Jellinek went further than he had previously, by attempting to classify different patterns of addictive drinking. Like Dr. William Carpenter in 1850, Jellinek came to view alcoholism as being a disease that might be expressed in several forms, or styles, of drinking (Lender, 1981). Unlike Dr. Carpenter, who thought that there were three types of alcoholics, Jellinek identified five subforms of alcoholism. Jellinek used the first five letters of the Greek alphabet to identify the most common forms of alcoholism found in the United States, although he also admitted that other subtypes might exist in different parts of the world. Thus, Jellinek's model was a culture-specific model that recognized the possibility that there were other forms of alcohol use than those found in the United States.

The first of Jellinek's (1960) subtypes of alcoholics was the *Alpha* pattern of alcoholism. Jellinek suggested that the Alpha alcoholic was psychologically dependent on alcohol, but did not suffer from any of the physical complications caused by chronic

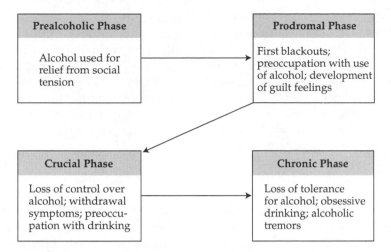

FIGURE 17.3   Jellinek's four stages of alcoholism.

alcohol use. Further, Jellinek believed that this individual could abstain from alcohol use for short periods if necessary. An example of the Alpha drinker might be the businessman, who "needs" a martini or two before dinner, to unwind from the day's troubles.

As noted, Jellinek (1960) did not view the Alpha pattern of drinking as reflecting a physical dependency on alcohol. Further, Jellinek did not believe that the Alpha pattern of drinking was automatically progressive. This drinking pattern was thought to be stable for an extended period, as seen in the case of a businessman who has had two (and only two!) martinis after work every day for 15 years. According to Jellinek, if the Alpha alcoholic were to progress to a more serious form of drinking, it would be to the *Gamma* form of alcoholism. The Gamma pattern is discussed in more detail, later. The point to remember here is that Jellinek viewed the *Alpha* form of alcoholism as a relatively stable pattern that only rarely progressed to more severe forms of alcohol use.

Jellinek (1960) also classified some drinkers as *Beta* alcoholics. The Beta drinking pattern was very similar to the Alpha pattern, but in addition to psychological dependency, the Beta drinker had also developed physical complications from alcohol use. Thus, the Beta alcoholic might demonstrate medical symptoms of chronic alcohol use, such as alcoholic gastritis and cirrhosis of the liver, both of which develop only after extended periods of alcohol use. If the Beta alcoholic progressed, it was also to the *Gamma* form of drinking, according to Jellinek.

The third pattern of drinking was classified as *Delta* by Jellinek. The alcoholic whose drinking fell into the Delta pattern was thought to demonstrate physical dependence on alcohol, including the development of tolerance to alcohol, craving when he/she could not drink, a loss of control over alcohol but few or no physical complications that might be traced to use of alcohol. In contrast, the *Gamma* alcoholic was seen by Jellinek (1960) as demonstrating physical withdrawal symptoms, craving, physical dependence on alcohol, and various medical complications caused by alcohol use. The Gamma alcoholic also demonstrated a progressive loss of control over alcohol use, according to Jellinek. As noted, the Alpha and, less frequently, Beta alcohol use patterns might progress to the Gamma pattern of alcohol use over time.

Finally, the *Epsilon* alcoholic might best be classified as the "binge" drinker. This form of alcoholism was least frequently encountered in the United States according to Jellinek (1960), where the Alpha and the Gamma drinking patterns were most common. Jellinek noted that there were other culturally related patterns of drinking (i.e., "fiesta drinking") that were worthy of study but that were possibly not true forms of alcoholism.

Advanced in an era when the majority of physicians viewed alcohol dependence as being caused by a moral weakness, Jellinek's (1960) model of alcoholism offered them a new paradigm. First, it provided a diagnostic framework within which physicians could classify different patterns of drinking, as opposed to the restrictive dichotomous view in which the patient was either alcoholic or not, that had previously prevailed. Second, Jellinek's model of alcoholism as a physical disease made it worthy of study, and suggested that the person with this disorder was worthy of "unprejudiced access" (Vaillant, 1990, p. 5) to medical treatment. Finally, the Jellinek model attributed the individual's use of alcohol to a medical disorder, *not* to a failure of personal willpower (Brown, 1995).

Since the time that Jellinek (1960) proposed his model of alcoholism, several research studies have been carried out in an attempt to determine whether this model is valid. Schuckit et al. (1993) examined the drinking patterns of 636 male inpatients, hospitalized because of alcoholism. The authors found that while there was remarkable variation in the specific problems encountered by the subjects in their study, there was clear evidence of a progression in the severity of problems encountered by their subjects as a result of their alcohol use.

Further, by their late 20s, just under three-quarters of the sample studied by the authors had started to engage in the morning use of alcohol and had started to experience alcohol-related job problems. According to the authors, many of the men in their study started to experience alcohol-related health problems by their mid-30s, characteristic of the progressive nature of alcohol dependence according to the Jellinek (1960) model. However, they admitted that the specific symptoms encountered by their subjects were different from those reported by Jellinek. Thus, it appears that there is evidence supporting Jellinek's theory that alcoholism is a progressive disorder, that results in more serious consequences for the individual over time, unless he/she stops drinking.

Although Jellinek (1952, 1960) introduced his theory only as a theoretical model of alcoholism, it has become the standard model for alcohol addiction in this country. Further, Jellinek's model has been used, without significant modification, since it was introduced. Surprisingly, although Jellinek's model was developed as a theory for alcoholism, it has also been applied to virtually every other pattern of drug abuse/addiction. Yet, as discussed in Chapter 18, there are serious flaws in the Jellinek model.

The Genetic Inheritance Theories

In the past two decades, scientists have accumulated an impressive body of research that suggests there is a strong genetic component to alcohol addiction. As we near the start of the 21st century, the majority of scientists have come to believe that alcoholism is mediated by the individual's genetic heritage (Hill, 1995). The question that seems to face scientists now is the degree to which genetic factors and environmental factors influence the development of alcohol dependence for both men and women.

In a series of studies that have spanned two decades, teams of researchers under the direction of Robert Cloninger have examined the adoption records from Sweden, where some of the best records of parental history and adoption are available for study. In 1981, Cloninger, Gohman, and Sigvardsson, announced that after reviewing the records of 3000 individuals who were adopted, they had discovered that the children of alcoholic parents were likely to grow up to be alcoholic themselves, even in cases where the children were reared by nonalcoholic adoptive parents almost from birth (see Table 17-1).

TABLE 17-1   Relationship between Biological Parents' and Adopted Children's Alcoholism

Did biological parent abuse alcohol?		*Percentage of children adopted into other families who abused alcohol*	
Father	*Mother*	*Boys*	*Girls*
No	No	14.7	2.8
Yes	No	22.4	3.5
No	Yes	26.0	10.3
Yes	Yes	33.3	9.1

Source: Based on Cloninger, Sigvardsson, and Bohman (1996).

The authors also found that the children who grew up to be alcoholic essentially fell into two groups. The first subgroup was made up of three-fourths of the children whose parents were alcoholic and who themselves went on to develop alcohol-use disorders. During young adulthood, these individuals drank only in moderation. It was only later in life that their drinking progressed to the point where they could be classified as alcoholic. Even so, Cloninger et al. (1981) found that these individuals tended to function within society, and were only rarely involved in antisocial behaviors. The authors classified these individuals as "Type I" alcoholics (Goodwin & Warnock, 1991).

In their study, Cloninger et al. (1981) found that there was a strong environmental impact on the possibility that the adopted child would be alcoholic. For example, the authors found that children of alcoholic parents, if adopted by a middle-class family in infancy, actually had only a 50–50 chance of being alcoholic in adulthood. While this is still markedly higher than what one would expect based on the knowledge that only 3% of the general population is alcohol dependent, it is still lower than the outcome found for children of alcoholic parents who were adopted and raised by poor parents. In this latter case, the chances were greater that this child would grow up to be an alcoholic. The authors interpreted these findings as evidence of a strong environmental influence on the evolution of alcohol use, despite the individual's genetic inheritance.

The second, smaller, group of alcoholics found by the research team of Cloninger et al. (1981) were male, more violent, alcoholics who were more likely to be involved in criminal activity. These individuals were classified as having "Type II" (or "male-limited") alcoholism (Goodwin & Warnock, 1991). A male child born to a "violent" alcoholic ran almost a 20% chance of himself becoming alcoholic, no matter what social status the child's adoptive parents were. Because a male child whose father was a violent alcoholic stood a significantly greater chance of himself becoming alcoholic than what one would expect on the basis of chance alone, the authors concluded that there was a strong genetic influence for this subgroup of alcoholics.

In 1996, the team of Sigvardsson, Bohman, and Cloninger (1996) successfully replicated this earlier study on the inheritability of alcoholism. The authors examined the adoption records of 557 men and 600 women who were born in Gothenburg, Sweden, and who were adopted at an early age by nonrelatives. The authors found that the earlier identification of two distinct subtypes of alcoholism for men was confirmed in this new study. Further, the authors found that the Type I and Type II subtypes appear to be independent, but possibly related, forms of alcoholism. Where one would expect 2% to 3% of their sample to have alcohol use problems on the basis of population statistics, the authors found that 11.4% of their male sample fit the criteria for Type I alcoholism, while 10.3% of the men in their study fit the criteria for Type II alcoholism. But, in contrast to the original studies, which suggested that Type II alcoholism was limited to males, there is now evidence that a small percentage of alcohol-dependent women might also be classified as Type II alcoholics (Cloninger et al., 1996; Del Boca & Hesselbrock, 1996).

The distinction between Type I and Type II alcoholics has lent itself to a series of research studies designed to identify possible personality traits unique to each group of alcohol dependence. Researchers have found that, as a group, Type I alcoholics tend to engage in harm-avoidance activities, whereas Type II alcoholics tend to be high in the novelty-seeking trait (Cloninger et al., 1996). Other researchers have found differences in brain wave activity between the Type I and Type II alcoholics on the electroencephalograph (EEG). Further, as a group, Type I alcoholics tend to have higher levels of the enzyme monoamine oxidase (MAO) than Type II alcoholics do. It was hypothesized that this lower MAO level in Type II alcoholics might account for their tendency to be more violent than Type I alcoholics (Cloninger et al., 1996). Thus, the Type I–Type II typology seems to have some validity for classifying different patterns of alcohol use/abuse.

The Biological Differences Theories

Over the past 50 years, a number of researchers have suggested that those who are alcohol-dependent are somehow different from those who are not alcohol-dependent. The range of this research is far too extensive to discuss in this chapter, but the general theme is that alcohol-dependent individuals seem to metabolize alcohol differently than nondependent drinkers, that the site/mechanism of alcohol biotransformation is different in the alcoholic when compared with the nonalcoholic, or that the alcoholic seems to react differently than nonalcoholics to the effects of that chemical.

The general thrust of these research articles is that there is a biological difference between the alcoholic and nonalcoholic. This has resulted in a number of studies being conducted by researchers who have attempted to identify the exact difference that might exist between alcoholic and nonalcoholic individuals. One example is the study conducted by the team of Ciraulo et al. (1996). The authors selected a sample of 12 women who were adult daughters of alcoholic parents, and 11 women whose parents were not alcohol-dependent, and then administered either a 1-mg dose of alprazolam or a placebo to their subjects. The authors found that the women who had alcoholic parents who received the alprazolam found it to be more enjoyable than did those women whose parents were not alcohol-dependent. This finding, along with an earlier study using male subjects conducted by the same team, was interpreted as evidence that children of alcoholic parents were also at risk for benzodiazepine abuse/dependence in addition to their higher risk for alcohol use disorders.

In 1990, the team of Blum et al. explored the possibility that a specific gene, known as the *dopamine D_2 receptor gene,* was involved in the predisposition toward alcoholism. Dopamine is one of the neurotransmitters affected by alcohol, and researchers have identified two subtypes of receptors in the brain that respond to dopamine, which they have called the "D_1" and "D_2" receptors. The authors utilized samples of brain tissue from 70 cadavers for their research. Half of the brain tissue samples were from known alcoholics, whereas the other half were not. The authors found that 77% of the alcoholics, but only 28% of the nonalcoholics, possessed the dopamine D_2 receptor gene. This discovery was interpreted as suggesting that there was a genetic basis for alcohol use.

In an extension of the original research, Noble, Blum, Ritchie, Montgomery, and Sheridan (1991)

utilized tissue samples from the brains of 33 known alcoholics and a matched group of 33 nonalcoholic controls. The authors concluded, on the basis of their "blind" study of the genetic makeup of the tissue samples[3] that there was strong evidence of a genetic foundation for severe alcoholism involving the D_2 dopamine receptor. As discussed in Chapter 18, however, these studies have been challenged by other researchers.

Marc Schuckit (1994) utilized a different approach to try to identify biological predictors to alcoholism. In the early 1980s, the author tested 227 men who were the sons of alcoholics and found that 40% of the sons of alcoholics but only 10% of the men who did not have an alcoholic parent were "low responders" to a standard dose of alcohol. The author found that the low responders did not seem to have been as strongly affected by the alcohol that they had received as were the individuals in the control group. Ten years later, the author again was able to contact 223 of the original sample of men who were raised by alcoholic parents. It was found that, of the men who had an abnormally low response to the alcohol challenge test, 56% had become alcoholic. Of the men raised by alcoholic parents who did not demonstrate an abnormally low physiological response to a standard dose of alcohol when originally tested, only 14% had become alcoholic in the intervening decade (Schuckit, 1994; Schuckit & Smith, 1996).

This data was interpreted to suggest that low responders were somewhat insensitive to the effects of alcohol. It was suggested that this insensitivity could, in turn, contribute to a tendency for the individual to drink more often and to consume more alcohol per session, than individuals who were not low responders (Schuckit, 1994). As discussed in Chapter 18, however, although this study seems to suggest some significant differences between those who do, and do not, become alcoholic, it still does not provide a final answer to the question of what

---

[3]A "blind" research study is one where the data is examined, without the researcher knowing if any given piece of data is from the research sample or the control sample. In this case, the tissue samples were examined by a researcher who did not know whether the tissue sample came from an alcoholic or nonalcoholic person.

biochemical factors predict the later development of alcoholism.

Thus, the controversy over whether there are measurable biochemical or biophysical differences between alcoholics and nonalcoholics remains unanswered. Clinical research hints that such a difference does exist. But, to date, no *unequivocal* biochemical or biophysical difference has been identified by researchers. The discovery of such a unique difference would provide a basis for the identification of the biological foundation of alcoholism and, by extension, the other forms of drug addiction. The research findings have been suggestive of biological differences between those who are/are not alcohol-dependent. But, there is a need for further research into the exact nature of the physical differences between those who do/do not abuse alcohol or drugs.

The Personality Predisposition Theories of Substance Abuse

Many researchers believe that substance abuse can be traced back to the individual's personality structure. This perspective is known as the *characterological model* (Miller & Hester, 1995). Murphy and Khantzian (1995) suggested that the ego structures of some individuals "predispose them to depend on substances" (p. 1689), thus creating a psychological predisposition toward addictive behaviors. From this perspective, substance abuse and the physical addiction to chemicals are the end product of a process where the individual comes to use drug-induced effects as a way of coping with emotional states that are overwhelming, confusing, or simply too painful to face (Murphy & Khantzian, 1995; Shaffer & Robbins, 1995).

An early proponent of this model was Karen Horney (1964), who spoke of alcohol as being a way to "narcotize" (p. 45) anxiety. As shown in Table 17-2, the modern psychoanalyst views substance abuse as a way to counter a wide range of emotional states.

Although recreational chemicals may offer a short-term means of coping with these painful emotional states, they do so at the expense of the individual's long-term adjustment (Murphy & Khantzian, 1995). Thus, the promise of relief from these painful feeling states initially offered by the drugs of abuse is not fulfilled in the longer term.

There is significant evidence to suggest that individuals who abuse chemicals have suffered significant psychological trauma in their lives. For example, ongoing research suggests a relationship between the individual's having been either physically and/or sexually abused during childhood or adolescence and his/her later development of a substance use disorder (Miller & Downs, 1995). The emotional aftermath of such victimization is thought to contribute to the development of lifelong patterns of emotional distress, which the individual then attempts to self-medicate through the use of alcohol and/or chemicals (Kaufman, 1989).

Even if the child is not abused by his/her primary caregivers, the child's family of origin may still be so dysfunctional that it virtually prevents normal development for its members. In such cases, the individual often finds that recreational chemical use provides a means to escape, if only for a short time, the shame that he/she experiences as a result of the emotional distress in the family (Bradshaw, 1988a). But if the individual begins compulsively to use the same method to cope with emotional pain time after time, the seeds of addiction take root. For it is when the person compulsively uses one, and only one, method of escaping from the emotional distress, that he/she is in danger of becoming addicted to that system of control.

TABLE 17-2   Drug of Choice and Emotional State

Class of chemical being abused	*Affective state that chemical of abuse is thought to control*
Alcohol and CNS depressants (barbiturates, benzodiazepines, etc.)	Loneliness, emptiness, isolation
Opiates (heroin, morphine, etc.)	Rage and aggression
CNS stimulants (cocaine, amphetamines, etc.)	Depression, a sense of depletion, anergia (sense of no energy), low self-esteem

Source: Chart based on Murphy and Khantzian (1995).

The control of psychological pain through any form of compulsive behavior is effective only for a short time. Although "compulsive behaviors may help us temporarily avoid feelings or problems, they don't really stop the pain" (Beattie, 1989, p. 14). Further, the individual's repeated exposure to the drugs of abuse results in the development of physical tolerance to the effects of those chemicals. Eventually, the individual will be faced with the problem of how to cope with the same emotional pain, with a drug that is no longer effective in the dose previously used.

Franklin (1987) suggested that there is a psychological predisposition toward narcotics abuse. Perhaps, the author suggested, the addict suffered from an ongoing depressive disorder that predisposed him/her to use narcotics. Further, it was suggested that before the individual began to use narcotics, he/she saw the feelings of depression as a normal emotional state. After being introduced to drugs, however, the individual would come to learn that the distress was not "normal," and that there is at least a chemical escape from continuous emotional pain. The narcotics then would provide the individual with at least the illusion of control over his/her depression. However, ultimately, the illusion of "control" comes to dominate the user's life, as the person becomes addicted to narcotics.

According to psychodynamic theory, alcohol might also be utilized by the individual to self-medicate depression. However, as discussed in Chapter 5, the chronic use of alcohol can cause depressive reactions that are very similar to clinical depression. Further, as discussed in Chapter 21, the role of depression in the individual's personality pattern is dependent on a number of factors, including the drinker's sex. Thus, it is not possible to make a general statement to the effect that the chronic drinker who is depressed is automatically using alcohol to self-medicate his/her depression.

A number of researchers have suggested that certain personality characteristics that predispose the individual toward alcoholism, or other forms of chemical abuse. Some of these theories have been quite suggestive. There appear to be certain personality traits that are associated with substance use disorders. However, it is difficult to identify whether these personality traits precede the development of the drug dependency or are a result of the frequent use of illicit chemicals. To date, no clearly identified causal factor has been found, and research continues into possible personality factors might predispose one toward alcohol or substance abuse.

Summary

This chapter has explored some of the leading theories that attempt to explain why people use recreational chemicals and why they might become addicted to these drugs. Several factors that help to modify the individual's substance use pattern were explored, including the physical reinforcement value of the drugs being abused, the social reinforcement value, cultural rules that govern recreational chemical use, and the individual's life goals.

The medical or disease model of addiction has come to play an important role in the treatment of substance abuse in this country. Based on the work of E. M. Jellinek, the disease model of alcoholism has come to be applied to virtually every other form of substance abuse besides alcohol. Jellinek viewed alcoholism as a progressive disorder that advanced through specific stages. In a time when the image of the alcoholic was that of a social failure who resorted to the bottle, Jellinek suggested that the individual suffered from a disease that would, if not treated, result in death. In time, the field of medicine came to accept this new viewpoint, and alcoholism came to be seen as a medical disorder.

Since the early work of Jellinek, other researchers have attempted to identify the biophysical dysfunction that forms the basis for the addictive disorders. Most recently, drawing on medicine's growing understanding of human genetics, scientists have attempted to identify the genetic basis for alcoholism and the other forms of drug addiction. To date, however, the exact biochemical or genetic factors that predispose one to become addicted have not been identified.

Are People Predestined to Become Addicted to Chemicals?

The disease model of substance addiction, which was discussed in Chapter 17, has not met with universal acceptance. There are many health care professionals and scientists who maintain that there are no biological or personality traits that automatically predispose the individual to abuse chemicals. Some researchers even question the possibility that alcohol/drug addiction is a true disease. Others concede that while there is evidence of biological or psychosocial predispositions toward substance abuse, certain environmental forces are needed to activate the biopsychosocial predisposition toward addiction. In this chapter, some of these reactions against the disease model of substance abuse are examined.

Reaction against the Disease Model of Addiction

It is tempting to speak of the disease model of alcohol/drug abuse as if there were a single, universally accepted definition of substance use problems. But, in reality, there are often subtle and, on occasion, not so subtle, philosophical differences in how physicians view the same disease. For example, treatment protocols for a condition such as a myocardial infarction might vary from one hospital to another, because of the differing treatment philosophies for that disorder at the different health care facilities.

Many experts in the field of substance abuse rehabilitation question whether alcoholism or drug addiction can be classified as a "disease." One component

of a disease, as the term is used in the United States, is the existence of a biophysical dysfunction of some kind that interferes with the normal function of the body. In infectious diseases, this is the bacteria, virus, or fungus that invades the host organism. Another class of diseases are those that are caused by a genetic disorder, which results in abnormal growth or functioning of an organism. A third class of diseases are those where the optimum function of the organism is disrupted by acquired trauma. In each case, however, the optimal functioning of an organism is disrupted by the disease process in one way or another.

As noted in previous chapters, the general consensus is that there is a genetic loading for alcoholism, although the exact nature of predisposition has not been clearly identified (Goodwin & Warnock, 1991). It is argued that, if such a genetic predisposition exists for alcoholism, then one must exist for all forms of substance addiction, since alcohol is just one of a variety of recreational chemicals. If there is a genetic predisposition for addictive behaviors, then chemical dependency is very much like the other physical disorders where there is a genetic predisposition. In this sense, substance abuse might be said to be a "disease," which is what E. M. Jellinek proposed in 1960.

Reaction to the Jellinek Model

As discussed in the previous chapter, the "Jellinek" model has become *the* model of the addictions. However, in the 40 years since Jellinek advanced his theoretical model, a number of flaws have come to light. First, he based his work on surveys that were mailed to members of Alcoholics Anonymous (AA). But, of the many hundreds of surveys mailed out, only 98 were returned.

It was on the data generated from these 98 responses that Jellinek based his model of alcoholism. Yet, in using this data, Jellinek violated one of the basic assumptions of research, for it is assumed that those individuals who volunteer to participate in a research study are *not* automatically representative of the population as a whole. For example, some people agreed to participate in the study while the majority of those contacted did not. If there is one major difference between groups, there may very well be other significant differences.

In the case of Jellinek's work, he violated this rule of research by assuming that those individuals who volunteered to return his questionnaire were the same as those AA members who either received the survey but did not take the time to fill it out, or, those AA members who never received his questionnaire. He then went on to generalize from the data obtained from those who did return his survey forms, to suggest a general theory of alcoholism that he applied to both AA members and nonmembers. But, as discussed in Chapter 34, there is little evidence that members of AA are the same as nonmembers. Thus, researchers have started to question both Jellinek's methods and, his conclusions.

One of the cornerstones of the Jellinek (1960) theory is that alcoholism is a progressive disorder. Yet, researchers have found mixed evidence that alcoholism is automatically progressive (Skog & Duckert, 1993). At best, the progression of alcohol-related symptoms suggested by Jellinek is actually found only in a minority (25–30%) of the cases (Toneatto et al., 1991). The Joint Committee of the National Council on Alcoholism and Drug Dependence as much as admitted this in its current definition of alcoholism by stating that alcoholism is "often [but not automatically] progressive" (Morse & Flavin, 1992, p. 1013). Schuckit et al. (1993) found that alcoholics tend to alternate between periods of abusive and nonabusive drinking, a finding that challenges Jellinek's conclusion that alcohol dependence is a progressive disorder.

Further, Jellinek's theory assumes that alcoholics have lost control over their drinking. But research has failed to suggest that alcoholics experience a loss of control (Skog & Duckert, 1993). There is significant evidence that drinking patterns often change over time, a finding that is inconsistent with the loss-of-control hypothesis (Vaillant, 1983). Scientists now believe that alcohol-dependent individuals tend to regulate their drinking to achieve a desired emotional state (Peele, 1989). At best, alcoholics might be said to demonstrate *inconsistent* control over their drinking, consuming different amounts of alcohol at different points in their lives (Toneatto et al., 1991; Vaillant, 1990). But, there is no evidence supporting the concept of loss of control over one's alcohol use, as suggested by the Jellinek model.

Thus, the Jellinek model rests on a foundation of flawed assumptions. Despite this, the Jellinek model has been used as the basis for planning treatment programs for untold thousands of alcoholics who have entered treatment in the years since he first advanced his theory.

To be fair, Jellinek (1960) presented his model as being a *preliminary* theory of what he viewed as an unrecognized disease, not the perfect theory of alcoholism. Nevertheless, and despite its many flaws, the Jellinek model has become "virtually gospel in the field of alcohol studies" (Lender, 1981, p. 25) and in the treatment of other forms of drug addiction.

The Genetic Inheritance Theories

In the past 30 years, a growing body of research has suggested a possible biological predisposition toward alcohol/drug dependence. This biological predisposition is assumed to reflect the individual's genetic inheritance. However, continued research has yet to identify the nature of this genetic loading or its impact on the individual. Further, a number of researchers still question whether there even is a genetic basis for alcoholism (Hill, 1995).

In the previous chapter, the research of Cloninger et al. (1981) was briefly discussed. Their work is often used by proponents of the medical model to support the contention that there is a biological predisposition for alcoholism. Yet the methodology utilized by Cloninger et al. (1981) was seriously flawed

(Hall & Sannibale, 1996). The authors based their classification of the parental alcohol abuse not on interviews they conducted, but on the records on file at the social service agencies that placed the children for adoption and accepted the word of others (the social service agency employees) as to whether the biological parents did/did not have an alcohol use problem. This raises serious questions as to whether the social service agency employees used the same criteria to define alcohol use problems.

Then, researchers have questioned whether Cloninger et al. (1981) might not have selected inappropriate statistical models to test their data (Hall & Sannibale, 1996). Because of these methodological flaws, their data must be viewed as tentative, at best. For example, although Cloninger et al. claimed that the alcohol-dependent males in their study fell into two different subgroups (the Type I/Type II typology discussed in Chapter 17), Hall and Sannibale suggested that fully 90% of the alcohol-dependent individuals who are admitted to treatment actually have characteristics of both Type I and Type II alcoholics. If true, the Type I–Type II alcoholism typology suggested by Cloninger et al. reflects a flawed classification system that does little to further our understanding of alcohol use disorders.

It should also be noted that although the original intent of the study by Cloninger et al. (1981) was to explore the genetics of alcoholism, the authors uncovered strong evidence suggesting that environmental forces also help to shape alcohol use disorders. Cloninger et al. found that even where the child's genetic inheritance seemed to predispose that child to alcoholism, if he/she had been adopted by a middle-class family in infancy, the chances of actually being alcoholic in adulthood were no greater than chance alone.

For the child adopted into a poor family, however, the chances were greater that this child would grow up to be an alcoholic. These findings suggest a strong environmental influence on the evolution of Type I alcoholism, despite the individual's genetic inheritance. Because of this environmental influence, Type I alcoholism is also called "milieu-limited alcoholism" by some researchers. In contrast to the Type I alcoholics identified by Cloninger et al. (1981) were the Type II alcoholics. This subgroup is often

called "male-limited" alcoholism. These individuals tend to be both alcoholic and involved in criminal behaviors. The adopted male offspring of a "violent" alcoholic ran almost a 20% chance of himself becoming alcohol dependent regardless of the social status of the child's adoptive parents. However, here again the statistics are misleading. For, while almost 20% of the male children born to a violent alcoholic might themselves become alcoholic, this means that more than 80% of the male children born to these fathers do *not* follow this pattern. This suggests that additional factors, such as environmental forces may play a role in the evolution of alcoholism for Type II alcoholics.

The research team of Pickens et al. (1991) attempted to isolate the impact of genetic inheritance on the development of alcohol dependence in pairs of both male and female twins. The authors concluded that "the influence of genetic factors appears to be somewhat weaker than the influence of shared environmental factors, especially for female subjects" (p. 25).

This conclusion was contradicted by the results of a study conducted by Kender, Heath, Neale, Kessler, and Eves (1992). The authors of this study examined the drinking patterns of over 1000 pairs of female twins and reached several conclusions. First, the authors concluded that environmental influences were a significant factor in the development of alcoholism in women and that these environmental factors accounted for 40% to 50% of the inheritability of alcoholism. However, equally important, the authors concluded that 50% to 60% of the liability for the development of alcoholism in the women studied was the result of the woman's genetic inheritance. The authors thus concluded that genetic inheritance was a major factor in the development of alcoholism.

Hill (1995) pointed out that there are significant variations in the ratio between males and females who are dependent on alcohol in different cultures around the world. For example, the ratio of men in the United States who develop an alcohol abuse/addiction problem at some point in their lives compared with the ratio of women who develop an alcohol use problem at some point in their lives was 5.4 : 1. Yet this same ratio was approximately 14 : 1 in Israel, 9.8 : 1 in Puerto Rico, 29 : 1 in Taiwan, 20 : 1 in

South Korea, and 115 : 1 in the Yanbian region of China. These differing ratios between the extent of alcohol use problems at some point in their lives for men and women from these different countries suggests that there are strong environmental/cultural influences on the evolution of alcohol use patterns.

Thus, the research suggests that both a biological predisposition toward alcohol addiction and strong environmental forces help to shape the individual's alcohol use pattern. However, researchers have yet to determine the exact role that either genetic inheritance or environmental influences play in the evolution of addictive alcohol abuse or addiction for either sex. One reason for this uncertainty is that up to 60% of known alcoholics come from families where there is no prior evidence of alcohol dependence (Cattarello et al., 1995).

Do Genetics Rule?

Admittedly, there appears to be a genetic predisposition, or a "loading," for alcohol/drug dependence. But the genetic "loading" for a certain condition does not guarantee that it will develop (Kahn, 1996; Restak, 1995). The individual's degree of genetic loading should be viewed only as a rough measure of his/her degree of risk, not the individual's predestination (Gordis, 1996). Scientists now believe that social, environmental, historical, and cultural forces all play a role in determining whether a given genetic potential will/will not be activated. The individual's genetic inheritance is but one of many factors that determine his/her behavior (Cattarello et al., 1995). For example, Schuckit (1987) suggested that such environmental factors as coming from an unstable home environment in the early years, a relatively low-status occupation for the father, and an extended neonatal hospital stay for the infant, all seemed to identify the individual at risk to later grow up to become an alcoholic. Thus, while there is evidence to suggest a genetic component to alcoholism, there is also strong evidence suggesting that cultural, social, and environmental forces play an equally strong role in the evolution of this substance use disorder.

The Dopamine D_2 Connection

In Chapter 17, the theory that a specific gene controlling the development of the dopamine D_2 receptor within the brain was discussed as a possible cause of alcoholism (Blum et al., 1990; Noble et al., 1991). This line of research, while suggestive of a possible biological foundation for alcoholism, has not been supported by subsequent research (Bolos et al., 1991; Parsian & Cloninger, 1991).

Bolos et al. (1991) used a different, more extensive methodology than did Blum et al. (1990), subtyping their subjects according to the age of onset of alcoholism, severity of alcoholism, whether the subject qualified for a diagnosis of antisocial personality disorder, and family history. The authors concluded that there was no evidence for a "widespread association between the D_2 receptor gene and alcoholism" (p. 3160).

Parsian et al. (1991) also explored the genetics of alcoholism and concluded that no "specific gene influencing the risk or expression of alcoholism has been identified" (p. 655) although the authors admitted that several possible biological factors had been uncovered by research. The authors concluded, after an extensive research project that is far too complicated to discuss in detail in this text, that their results "cast doubt on the D_2 receptor locus having a major and direct causative role in most cases of alcoholism" (p. 662). In other words, their results did not suggest that the dopamine D_2 receptor gene was the biological foundation for alcoholism.

The research team of Uhl, Persico, and Smith (1992) reviewed the current literature on the dopamine D_2 receptor gene and its possible association with alcoholism. The authors concluded that while this line of research seemed to identify at least one genetic factor for alcoholism, the existing research had failed to utilize a random sample of alcohol users and control subjects. Thus, it was possible that differences in the genetic makeup of various ethnic groups, or some other, undiscovered, variable, might have resulted in the apparent association between the dopamine D_2 receptor gene and alcoholism.

Even if the dopamine D_2 connection does play a major role in the biochemistry of addiction:

> Knowing that drug dependence has a neurochemical basis does not tell us why some people but not others use drugs regularly and heavily, why they use them in some circumstances and not others, and why different people prefer different drugs. ("Addiction–Part I," 1992a, p. 2)

Further the theory that the D_2 receptor gene plays a role in the development of alcoholism has been challenged by Gelernter, Goldman, and Risch (1993), who concluded:

> Based on all we know about the genetics of alcoholism, it would seem that a single gene is unlikely to be in itself responsible for a large proportion of illness. (p. 1673)

But that is exactly what proponents of the dopamine D_2 theory were looking for: a single gene that could account for alcoholism.

In the previous chapter, a study by Marc Schuckit (1994) was presented as evidence of a biological predisposition toward alcohol abuse/dependence on the part of certain men. In this study, the author reexamined 223 men who had, when tested a decade earlier, demonstrated an abnormally low physical response to a standard dose of an alcoholic beverage. At the time of his earlier study, Schuckit had found that fully 40% of the men who had been raised by alcoholic parents, but only 10% of his control group, demonstrated this unusual response when given a standard dose of alcohol.

A decade later, in 1993, the author found that 56% of the men who had the abnormally low physiological response to alcohol had progressed to the point of alcoholism. The author interpreted this finding as evidence that the abnormally low physical response to a standard dose of an alcoholic beverage might identify a biological marker for alcoholism. But, only a minority of the men who had been raised by an alcoholic parent demonstrated this abnormally low physiological response to the alcohol challenge test. Only 91 men of the experimental group of 227 men had this abnormal response. Further, a full decade later, only 56% of these 91 men (or, just 62 men of the original sample) appeared to have become dependent on alcohol. Thus, while Schuckit's (1994) study suggests possible biochemical mechanisms for the development of alcoholism, this study also illustrates that biological predisposition does not predestine the individual to develop an alcohol use disorder.

Other Challenges to the Disease Model of Addiction

No matter how you look at it, addiction remains a most curious "disease." Even Vaillant (1983), who has long been a champion of the disease model of alcoholism, had to concede that, to make alcoholism fit into the disease model, it had to be "shoehorned" (p. 4). Further, even if alcoholism is a disease, "both its etiology and its treatment are largely social" (Vaillant, 1983, p. 4). This trait suggests that alcohol dependence is an unusual disease.

The possibility has been suggested that what we call "addictions" are actually a misapplication of existing neurobiological reward systems (Rodgers, 1994). According to this view, evolution allowed for the development of a reward system in animals to reinforce behaviors that contributed to survival, such as eating, reproduction, and drinking water. This makes evolutionary sense: those organisms that could reward themselves for doing something that enhanced survival would seem more likely to survive than animals who lacked this ability.

This reward system, however, can be fooled by such chemicals as alcohol, opiates, and cocaine into operating when survival-enhancing activities are not in progress. Sometimes, by coincidence, a chemical happens to be able to trigger the reward system found in human brains, even if the person is not involved in a critical activity. Thus:

> The inescapable fact is that nature gave us the ability to become hooked because the brain has clearly evolved a reward system, just as it has a pain system. (S. Childers, as quoted in Rodgers, 1994, p. 34)

Therefore, we all hold the potential to become addicted because we are all biologically "wired" with a "reward system." However, it is not known why some people are more easily trapped than others by the ability of chemicals to activate the reward system.

A decade ago, Dreger (1986) commented on this fact, for while alcoholism is classified as a disease, it is an unusual disease. Unlike other forms of illness, alcohol (the agent responsible for alcohol abuse/dependence) is "promoted by every Madison Avenue technique and by every type of peer pressure one can imagine. No other disease is thus promoted" (p. 322).

The beer, wine, and liquor manufacturers in the United States spend a combined $1 billion a year on advertising (Knapp, 1996). If alcohol abuse/dependence is indeed a disease, then why is the use of the offending agent, in this case alcohol, promoted through commercial means? The answer to this question raises some interesting questions about the role of alcohol within this society.

The Medical Model and Individual Responsibility

Modern medicine "always gives the credit to the disease rather than the person" (B. Siegel, 1989, p. 12), and this is certainly true for the addictive disorders (Peele, 1989; Tavris, 1990). Pratt (1990) suggested, "Activation of the disease of addiction, once an individual is exposed to activating agents, is genetically predetermined" (p. 18). From this perspective, once the individual has been exposed to the "activating agents," he/she ceases to exist except as a genetically preprogrammed disease process!

This is another, rather extreme, example of the medical model's tendency to "give credit to the disease rather than the person" (B. Siegel, 1989, p. 12). Yet the same process might be seen in the concept behind methadone maintenance. The proponents of the methadone maintenance concept suggested that even a single dose of narcotics would forever change the brain structure of the narcotics addict, making him/her crave further narcotics use (Dole, 1988; Dole & Nyswander, 1965).

Now, if narcotics were so incredibly powerful, then one must account for the phenomenon where thousands of patients receive doses of narcotics for the control of pain, for extended periods, without developing a craving for narcotics after their treatment is ended. Further, even patients who receive massive doses of narcotic analgesics only rarely report a sense of euphoria, or feel the urge to continue their use of opioids (Rodgers, 1994). This seems to cast some doubt on Dole and Nyswander's (1965) theory that exposure to narcotic analgesics causes changes in the brain of the individual that predispose him/her to want to use these chemicals again. In addition, Dole and Nyswander's theory flies in the face of fact, in that many individuals "chip" (occasionally use) narcotics for years, without becoming addicted to these drugs. The whole concept on which methadone maintenance is based is the belief that narcotics are so powerful that just a single dose takes away all the individual's power of self-determination.

Another example of the manner in which the medical model takes away from the individual's power and makes the disease all-powerful is Blum and Payne's (1991) contention that alcohol causes an "Irresistible craving" (p. 237). Yet, when one speaks with alcoholics, they readily agree that they can resist the craving for alcohol, if the reward for doing so is high enough. Many alcoholics successfully resist the desire to drink for weeks, months, years, or decades, casting doubt on the concept of an irresistible craving for alcohol or, by extension, the other drugs of abuse.

A central feature of the medical model of illness is that, once a person has been diagnosed as having a certain disease, he/she is expected to take certain steps toward recovery. According to the medical model, the "proper way to do this is through following the advice of experts (e.g., doctors) in solving the problem" (Maisto & Connors, 1988, p. 425). As was discussed in Chapter 1, however, physicians are not required to be trained in either the identification or the treatment of the addictions. The medical model of addiction thus lacks internal consistency, in the sense that while medicine claims that addiction is a disease, it does not routinely train its practitioners in how to treat this ailment.

Then What Exactly *Are* the Addictive Disorders?

Proponents of the disease model often point out that Dr. Benjamin Rush first suggested that alcoholism was a disease 200 years ago. What they do not point out, however, is that the very definition of disease has changed since the time of Dr. Rush. In his day, a disease was anything classified as being able to cause an imbalance in the nervous system (Meyer, 1996). Most certainly, alcohol appears capable of causing such an imbalance, or disruption in the normal function of the CNS. Thus, by the standards used by Benjamin Rush in the 1700s, alcoholism was indeed a disease.

However, by the criteria used by physicians on the brink of the 21st century, the issue is not so clear. In fact, there still is no standard definition of what constitutes an addiction. There are those who wonder if the addictive use of a chemical is actually a reflection of disease. The most common form of chemical dependency, alcoholism, has been called simply a "bad habit" by Thomas Szasz (1972, p. 84). The addictive use of chemicals has been described simply as "a bad habit that is especially difficult to change" ("Addiction–Part II," 1992b, p. 2). Admittedly, it is up to the individual to try to overcome bad habits, but this does not make it a disease (Szasz, 1972). The author went on to warn, "If we choose to call bad habits 'diseases,' there is no limit to what we may define as a disease" (p. 84).

Twenty years later, Leo (1990) confirmed that society has indeed reached the point where there are no apparent limits as to what is called a disease. The addictions "have been converted into diseases (alcoholism), bad habits have been upgraded and transformed into addictions (yesterday's hard-to-break smoking habit is today's nicotine addiction)" (p. 16).

According to Leo (1990), the outcome of this transformation has been the birth of a multitude of "pseudo ailments" (p. 16), through which people have been able to avoid responsibility for socially unacceptable behaviors. So pervasive has this process become that Leo called the current era the "golden age of exoneration" (p. 16), where virtually every socially deviant behavior is excused on the grounds that the individual has a "disease."

Further, as Ehrenreich (1992) observed, one of the benefits of modern medicine is that while we might not "have a cure for every disease, alas, but there's no reason we can't have a disease for every cure" (p. 88). In other words, now that the treatment industry has established itself, why not discover other "diseases" for which the twelve-step model might be applied? Not surprisingly, this is just what has happened. The twelve-step model pioneered by AA has now been applied to more than 100 different conditions that at least some people believe are a form of addiction ("Addiction–Part II," 1992b). But this does not mean that all these different forms of socially inappropriate behavior are actually diseases. There are those who still believe that alcohol/drug use disorders are themselves a "mythical disease" (Kaiser, 1996; Szasz, 1988, p. 319).

What is often overlooked is that *neither alcohol nor drugs are the enemy.* By itself, a drug has no inherent value (Szasz, 1988, 1996, 1997). It does not matter whether the specific drug in question is a natural agent, such as morphine, or is the product of human ingenuity, such as fentanyl. By themselves, drugs are neither good nor bad. It is the way in which the drugs are used by the individual that determines whether they are helpful or harmful.

To further complicate matters, society has made an arbitrary decision to classify some drugs as "dangerous" and others as being acceptable for social use. For example, the antidepressant medication Prozac (fluoxetine) and the hallucinogen MDMA both cause select neurons in the brain to release the neurotransmitter serotonin, and then block its reabsorption. A small but significant percentage of those patients receiving fluoxetine are doing so not because they require an antidepressant, but because they desire its mood-enhancing effects ("Better than Well," 1996). If a pharmaceutical is being used by a patient because he/she enjoys its effects, where is the line between legitimate need for that medication, and the recreational use of that same chemical? The basis for making this distinction is often not based on scientific studies, but "religious or political (ritual, social) considerations" (Szasz, 1988, p. 316). Since it is more than apparent that people *desire* the recreational drugs for their effects, it appears that the current "war" on drugs is really a "war on human desire" (Szasz, 1988, p. 322). The problem is not so much that people use chemicals, according to Szasz, but that people desire to use them for personal pleasure.

Indirect evidence supporting Szasz's position is found in the observation that an estimated 125,000 die, and an estimated 1.3 million people are injured each year in the United States as a result of "drug mistakes" (Graedon & Graedon, 1996, p. 5). These needless injuries and deaths are the result of mistakes made in the prescription of legitimate pharmaceuticals by health care professionals. The annual toll caused by such mistakes is estimated to be four times the annual number of deaths in the United States caused by recreational drug use, yet there is hardly a whisper heard from Washington about the former while thousands of speeches have been made about the latter.

The Unique Nature of Addictive Disorders

Despite all that has been written about the problem of alcohol/drug use/abuse over the years, researchers continue to overlook an important fact. Unlike the other diseases, *the substance use disorders require the active participation of the "victim" to exist.* The capacity for addiction rests with the individual, not (as so many would have us believe) with the drug itself (Savage, 1993). The addictive disorders do not force themselves on the individual, in the same sense that an infection might. Alcohol or drugs do not magically appear in the individual's body. Rather, the victim of this disorder must go through several steps to introduce the chemical into his/her body.

Consider the case of heroin addiction: the addict must obtain the money necessary to buy the drug. Then, he/she must find somebody who is selling heroin, and actually buy some for use. Next, the user must prepare the heroin for injection by mixing the powder with water, heating the mixture, and pouring it into a syringe, and then must find a vein to inject the drug into and then insert the needle into the vein. Finally, after all these steps, the individual must then actively inject the heroin into his/her own body. This is a complicated chain of events, each step of which involves the active participation of the individual, who is then said to be a victim of a disease process. If it took as much time and energy to catch a cold, pneumonia, or cancer, it is doubtful that any of us would ever be sick a day in our lives.

The team of O'Brien and McLellan (1996) offered a modified challenge to the disease model of the addictions as it now stands. The authors accepted that drug/alcohol addiction is a form of chronic disease. But the authors went on to state that while the addictive disorders were chronic diseases like adult-onset diabetes or hypertension, behavioral factors also helped to shape the evolution of these disorders. Thus, according to the authors:

> Although a diabetic, hypertensive or asthmatic patient may have been genetically predisposed and may have been raised in a high-risk environment, it is also true that behavioral choices . . . also play a part in the onset and severity of their disorder. (p. 237)

Thus, the individual's behavior and decisions help to shape the evolution of the addictive disorders. Ultimately, the individual retains responsibility for

personal behavior, even for a disease such as addiction (Vaillant, 1983, 1990).

In the past 60 years, proponents of the medical model of alcoholism have attempted to identify the biological foundation for abusive drinking. Over the years, a large number of research studies have been published, many of which have suggested that alcoholics (a) seem to metabolize alcohol differently than nonalcoholics, or (b) seem to be relatively insensitive (or, depending on the research study, more sensitive) to the effects of alcohol, when compared with nonalcoholics. Proponents of the medical model of addiction often point to these studies as evidence of a biological predisposition toward alcoholism.

However, the truth is that despite a significant amount of research, no *consistent* difference has been found in the rate of metabolism, the route by which addicted and nonaddicted individuals biotransform chemicals, or, the susceptibility of addicted/nonaddicted individuals to the effects of recreational chemicals. Although substance abuse rehabilitation professionals talk about the "genetic predisposition" toward alcohol/drug use disorders as if this were a proven fact, the truth is that scientists still have virtually no idea how individual genes, or groups of genes, affect the individual's behavior (Siebert, 1996). In the words of David Kaiser (1996):

> Modern psychiatry has yet to convincingly prove the genetic/biologic cause of any single mental illness. However, this does not stop psychiatry from making essentially unproven claims that . . . alcoholism . . . [is] in fact primarily biologic and probably genetic in origin, and that it is only a matter of time until . . . this is proven. (p. 41)

Thus, it does not appear that the disease model of addiction as it now stands provides the answer to why people become addicted to drugs of abuse.

The Disease Model as Theory

Since it was first introduced, the disease model of drug addiction has experienced a remarkable change: although it was first introduced as a theoretical model of alcoholism, it has become the standard model for the treatment of virtually all forms of drug addiction. Further, although the medical model of addiction is but one of several competing theoretical models, proponents do not speak of it as a *theoretical* model, but as an established fact.

The disease model might provide "a useful metaphor or reframe for many clients" (Treadway, 1990, p. 42) to help them understand their compulsion. But he warned that mental health professionals become "uncomfortable when it is presented as scientific fact." The biogenetic foundation of alcoholism (and, by extension, the other forms of drug addiction) has become dogma. Because dogmatists tend to rarely, if ever, question their basic assumptions (Kaiser, 1996), proponents of the disease model seem determined to defend it from all criticism. The proponents of the medical model have adopted a cultlike stance, in that they seem to view those who disagree with the disease model as unenlightened savages.

This process is not uncommon. History has demonstrated time and time again that once a certain theoretical viewpoint has become established, proponents of that position work to protect that theory from both internal and external criticism (Astrachan & Tischler, 1984). This process is apparent in the disease model of addiction. The current atmosphere is one in which legitimate debate over strengths and weaknesses of the different models of addiction is discouraged. There is only one "true" path to enlightenment, according to proponents of the disease model, and you should not question its wisdom.

This tendency for proponents of the disease model to turn a deaf ear to other viewpoints is exacerbated in this country because the disease model has become "big politics and big business" (Fingarette, 1988, p. 64). The disease model has formed the basis of a massive treatment industry, into which many billions of dollars, and thousands of human work-years, have been invested. The biogenetic model has taken on a life of its own.

What is surprising is not that the disease model exists, but that it has become so politically successful. For example, the treatment methods currently in use are those advocated by the proponents of the disease model. Yet these treatment methods have not changed significantly in 40 years (Rodgers, 1994). Imagine, the uproar that would result if a physician were to be found using the technology of 40 years ago

to treat a disorder such as cancer, or cardiovascular disease. Yet, in the field of substance abuse rehabilitation, treatment methods have remained essentially static for the past two generations.

Many current treatment methods in use in the field of substance abuse rehabilitation are based not on clinical research, but on somebody's belief that those treatment methods should work (Gordis, 1996a). Thus, it should not be surprising that there is strong evidence showing that current treatment methods for the addictions are possibly less effective than doing *nothing* for the individual (Peele, 1989). Even such a strong proponent of the medical model as the psychiatrist George Vaillant (1983) concluded that there is no significant difference in recovery rates between those who are treated for alcoholism and those who are not. A number of other studies have reached similar conclusions.

But the disease model has become an industry. Proponents of the medical model are hardly likely to go to insurance companies, or the public, after 50-odd years of claiming that the addictions are diseases, to admit that treatment does not work. Rather, as Peele (1989) pointed out, when the "treatment" of an addictive disorder is unsuccessful, the blame is usually put on the patient. He/she "did not want to quit," or he/she "was still in denial" of having an addictive disorder, or any of a thousand other excuses. But, the blame is never placed on the disease model although an extensive body of evidence suggests it has not been successful in the treatment of the addictive disorders.

Reaction to the Disease Model of Addiction

A welcome breath of fresh air was offered by the chief of the Molecular Neurobiology Laboratory of the National Institute on Drug Abuse, Dr. George Uhl (1992), who suggested that addiction rests on a foundation of 30% genetic predisposition and 70% environmental factors. He suggested that, even if the genetic predisposition is present, if the environment does not support drug use, "They won't become addicted" (p. 4C).

Although the available data seems to point to a biological factor to substance abuse, research has not been able to identify the specific environmental factor, nutritional deficit, or genetic pattern that predisposes the individual to the addictive use of chemicals. Indeed, in their summary of the current state of the research attempting to identify a biological predisposition toward addictive behavior, Goodwin and Warnock (1991), stated that, while alcoholism is known to run in certain families, "We do not believe that alcoholism definitely has been shown to be genetic" (p. 485).

Despite significant efforts to identify a personality or biological predisposition toward addiction, "There's no proof that anyone is chemically, genetically or psychologically doomed" ("Is There an Addictive Personality," 1990, p. 2). Increasingly, researchers in the field of behavioral genetics are viewing alcohol dependence as being "polygenic," which is to say a behavior that reflects the input of a number of different genes (Gordis, 1996). Each of these genes then adds a degree of risk to the individual's total potential for developing an addiction to alcohol. However, environmental influences are also thought to play a significant role in the development of alcohol dependence.

Thus, although the disease model of chemical dependency has dominated the treatment of substance abuse in this country, it is not without its critics. Not surprisingly, in light of this criticism, the medical model of addiction has not found wide acceptance outside this country and, to a lesser degree, Canada.

The Personality Predisposition Theories of Substance Abuse

Personality factors have long been suspected to play a role in the development of addiction (Butcher, 1988; Jenike, 1991). There are a number of variations on this "predisposing personality" theme. Although there are some differences between specific predisposing personality theories, they all are strongly deterministic in the sense that the individual is viewed as being powerless to avoid the development of an addictive disorder if exposed to certain conditions, because of his/her personality predisposition.

A number of studies suggested that dependent individuals were more impulsive, anxious, depressed, or prone to risk taking. These personality traits were then traced to disturbances in the dopamine utilization system in the brains of alcohol abusers/addicts. To test this hypothesis, the team of Heinz et al. (1996) examined the clinical progress of 64 alcohol-dependent individuals and attempted to assess their sensitivity to dopamine through biochemical tests. Despite the expected association between depression, anxiety, disturbances in dopamine utilization, and alcohol use problems, the authors found little evidence to support the popular beliefs that alcoholism is associated with depression, high novelty seeking, or anxiety.

The researcher C. R. Cloninger proposed a "unified biosocial" model of personality, in which certain individuals who were predisposed to exhibit a given personality characteristic (such as risk taking) could have that trait reinforced by social/environmental factors. Cloninger attempted to identify the interaction between genes and environment (Howard, Kivlahan, & Walker, 1997) and then applied his theory of personality to the evolution of alcohol use disorders. He reasoned that individuals who were high on the traits of Harm Avoidance (HA), Novelty Seeking (NS), and Reward Dependence (RD) would be at risk for alcohol use disorders.

The team of Howard et al. (1997) examined a series of research studies that attempted to relate Cloninger's theory of personality to the development of alcohol abuse/addiction. The authors found that even when a test specifically designed to test Cloninger's theory of personality was used, the results did not clearly support the theory that individuals high on the traits of HA and RD were significantly more likely to have an alcohol use disorder. Thus to date, the personality predisposition theoretical models do not allow for more than a general statement that some personality characteristics may increase the long-term risk that a person will become addicted to chemicals. However, it is still unclear which personality characteristics could predispose the individual to become addicted to alcohol and/or drugs. Despite a spirited search for the so-called alcoholic personality that has gone on for the past 50 years, such a personality pattern remains elusive at best (Miller & Kurtz, 1994; Schuckit, Klein, Twitchell, & Smith, 1994).

Although researchers have been unable to identify personality characteristics that consistently identify the person who is at risk for the development of an addictive disorder, certain clinical myths have developed within the field of substance abuse rehabilitation. For example, even though there is limited evidence to support these beliefs, clinicians continue to operate on the assumption that alcoholics are (a) developmentally immature, (b) that the experience of growing up in a disturbed family helps to shape the personality growth of the future alcoholic, and (c) that alcohol-dependent individuals tend to overuse ego defense mechanisms such as denial.

Thus, much of what is called "treatment" in the United States rests on assumptions about the nature of the personality of addicted people that have not been supported in the clinical research. Despite a search that has lasted for more than half a century, researchers have been unable to identify the characteristics of the so-called addictive personality (Brown, 1995; W. Miller, 1995; Woody et al., 1995). Traits identified in one research study as being central to the personality of addicted people are found to be of peripheral importance in subsequent studies, raising a question as to whether there is such a thing as an "addictive personality."

In the face of this evidence, then, one must ask how the myth of the alcoholic personality evolved. Nathan (1988) postulated that the characteristics of the so-called addictive personality found by earlier researchers actually might reflect a misdiagnosis. The author suggested that previous research confused the antisocial personality disorder with a prealcoholic personality pattern. There is a distinct tendency for those who might be diagnosed as having an antisocial personality disorder (APD) to utilize chemicals (Schuckit et al., 1994; Woody et al., 1995). It has even been suggested that substance abuse may be an unrecognized aspect of APD (Peele, 1989).

This is not to suggest that the antisocial personality disorder *caused* the substance use. Rather, the antisocial personality disorder and the addiction to chemicals are two separate disorders that may coexist in the same individual (Schuckit et al., 1994). An alternate theory about how people began to believe there was an addictive personality was suggested by Bean-Bayog (1988). After considering the available evidence, Bean-Bayog postulated that the so-called alcoholic personality emerged as a consequence of

chronic alcohol use on the individual's personality pattern, not the other way around. Which is to say that Bean-Bayog suggested that the personality characteristics often noted in the alcoholic were a result of the disease process, not a factor that aided in the initial development of the addiction.

According to Bean-Bayog (1988), earlier researchers have been blinded by the fact that the personality patterns when the addicted person is admitted to treatment did not precede the addiction. Rather, this personality pattern is viewed as an artifact of the individual's addiction. If this theory is true, then all the research conducted to date on identified addicts has been based on the mistaken assumption that certain personality characteristics precede addiction when actually they are part of the addictive process. It would be as if researchers had thought for years that the pain of a broken leg caused the injury to the bone, rather than that the pain was a signal of a broken limb.

There is little conclusive evidence that there are personality characteristics predisposing the individual toward alcoholism (Schuckit, 1996b). However, the study of the whole area of personality growth and development, not to mention the study of those forces that initially shape and later maintain addiction, is still so poorly defined that it is premature to answer the question of whether there are personality patterns that may precede the development of substance use disorders.

The Abuses of the Medical Model

Since its introduction, the disease model of alcoholism has been misused, or perhaps "misapplied" might be a better term, to the point where:

> Judges, legislators, and bureaucrats . . . can now with clear consciences get the intractable social problems caused by heavy drinkers off their agenda by compelling or persuading these unmanageable people to go elsewhere—that is, to get "treatment." (Fingarette, 1988, p. 66)

Thus, the guardians of social order, the courts and the lawyers, have assumed the power to define who has the disease of addiction and how it is to be treated. As a result of this transformation of the medical model, it has been suggested that the War on

Drugs that began in the early 1980s evolved as a politically inspired program to control those individuals who were defined by conservative Republicans as social deviants (Humphreys & Rappaport, 1993). According to the authors, the War on Drugs essentially served the Reagan administration as a "way to redefine American social control policies in order to further political aims" (p. 896). By shifting the emphasis of social control away from the community mental health center movement to the War on Drugs, the authors suggested, justification was also found for a rapid and possibly radical expansion of the government's police powers, and the "de facto repeal of the Bill of Rights" (Duke, 1996, p. 47).

The charge has been made that the community mental health movement itself has been subverted by government rules and regulations until it has become little more than "an arm of government enforcement" (Cornell, 1996, p. 12). These rather disturbing articles raise serious questions as to whether the social problem of chemical abuse and the medical model of addiction were used as an excuse to extend the government's police powers. Most certainly, drivers who operate motor vehicles while intoxicated present a very real problem of social deviance. However, one must question the wisdom of sending the chronic offender to treatment time and time again, when his/her acts warrant incarceration. As Peele (1989) has argued, incarceration may help bring about a greater behavior change in these people than would repeated exposure to short-term treatment programs.

In an ideal world, one question that would be considered is: At what point should treatment be offered as an alternative to incarceration, and when should incarceration be imposed on the chronic offender? All too often, the courts fail to consider this issue before sending the offender to "treatment" once more.

The Final Common Pathway Theory of Addiction

As should be evident by now, there have been strong challenges to the medical model of substance abuse. In their review of the genetics of alcoholism, Crabbe and Goldman (1993) concluded, "There are many factors associated with whether a person becomes an alcoholic, one of which is genetics" (p. 297, italics in original deleted). At the same time, the psychosocial models of drug use also have been challenged as being too narrow in scope and as not being able to account for the phenomenon of drug/alcohol addiction.

But there is another viewpoint to consider, called the *final common pathway* (FCP) theory of chemical dependency. In a sense, FCP is a nontheory: it is not supported by any single group or profession. Rather, FCP theory holds that there is an element of truth in *each* of the other theories of drug addiction reviewed earlier in this text. But, the final common pathway theory holds that none of these theories about drug abuse is able to account for the phenomenon of drug abuse/addiction by itself.

From the final common pathway perspective, substance use/abuse is viewed not as the starting point, but, as the *end point* of a unique pattern of growth. There is no single cause of drug dependency. Rather, addiction is dependent on the individual. According to this model, a multitude of different factors may influence an individual to become addicted to a chemical(s). These include social forces, psychological conditioning, an attempt on the part of the individual to come to terms with internal pain, a spiritual shortcoming, or some combination of other factors. The proponents of this position admit that there might be a genetic predisposition toward substance abuse. But, they are also willing to accept that a person who lacks the genetic predisposition for drug dependency may become addicted to chemicals, if he/she has the proper life experiences.

The latest neurobiological research findings provide strong support for the final common pathway model of addiction. Researchers have found that, despite the differences between different classes of drugs, by one route or another, the various drugs of abuse all seem to eventually reach and then activate, the so-called pleasure centers of the brain (Restak, 1994). In the past decade, scientists have confirmed what they long suspected: that the pleasure center of the brain involves the *limbic system*. As psychopharmacologists have come to understand the effects of recreational chemicals on the brain, they have discovered that recreational chemicals seem to cause their pleasurable effects by altering the normal pattern of chemical activity within the limbic system (Hyman, 1996; Miller & Gold, 1993).

There is still a lot that researchers have to discover about how the different drugs of abuse alter the function of the limbic system. There is even some question as to whether the drugs of abuse achieve their reinforcing effects by their action on a single part of the limbic system, or whether various drugs affect different subunits of the limbic system. But, for the first time, researchers believe that they have identified the region of the brain where the recreational chemicals all seem to cause the user to experience a sense of pleasure.

Some researchers believe that the various drugs of abuse alter the normal function of the *nucleus accubens,* which is a subunit of the region of the brain known as the basal ganglia (Fischbach, 1992; Fleming, Potter, & Kettyle, 1996; Hyman, 1996; Restak, 1994). Other researchers believe that the drugs of abuse cause the user to feel pleasure by altering the function of the mesolimbic dopamine system of the brain (Beitner-Johnson & Nestler, 1992; Nestler, Fitzgerald, & Self, 1995). This also seems to be the region of the brain most involved in the individual's subjective experience of craving for his/her drug of choice (Anthony et al., 1995). Finally, it is a region of the brain that seems to be involved in the process of drug-seeking behavior (Anthony et al.).

Still other researchers note that all the current drugs of abuse alter the function of the region of the brain known as the *locus ceruleus.* The locus ceruleus appears to be the region of the brain that coordinates the body's response to both novel external stimuli and internal stimuli that signal a danger to the individual (Gourlay & Benowitz, 1995). Thus, the locus ceruleus will respond to such internal stimuli as blood loss, hypoxia, and pain. The locus ceruleus is also involved in the "fight-or-flight" response of fear and anxiety. This makes clinical sense, since in ages past, novel stimuli might have proved to be dangerous to the individual (e.g., a mountain lion running down a path). It also is not surprising that this region of the brain is involved in the body's response to the drugs of abuse.

Nutt (1996) presented the most comprehensive theory of how the drugs of abuse stimulate the user's brain to feel pleasure. According to the author, the primary circuit through which the pleasure center is activated "seems to be the dopamine pathway that runs from the ventral tegmental area (VTA) through the nucleus accumbens to the prefrontal cortex" (p. 35). By activating the neurons along this pathway, the drugs of abuse are able to produce a sense of euphoria and relief from tension, according to Nutt.

Although different researchers have suggested that different regions of the brain are involved in the addictive process, it is important to remember that they have all identified the *limbic system* as being involved in the pleasure response induced by the drugs of abuse. Now they are attempting to identify the sequence of brain regions activated by the drugs of abuse; however, the consensus is that the limbic system seems to be one region of the brain where the recreational chemicals induce a feeling of pleasure.

In the final analysis, the final common pathway model of addiction views alcohol and/or drug addiction as common end points. While there may be different routes, eventually the chemical results in the same end: the activation of the brain's pleasure center. Each different class of recreational chemical may also impact other regions of the brain, but they all induce a state of pleasure by altering the function of at least part of the limbic system. This is not to say that the individual is just a helpless victim of his/her genetic vulnerability to the reinforcing properties of the drugs of abuse. Rather, *both* a genetic predisposition *and* environmental factors interact to bring about a state of vulnerability for drug abuse (Fitzgerald & Self, 1995). If either element were missing, the individual would be unlikely to become addicted to recreational chemicals.

This, then, is the core element of addiction according to the Final Common Pathway theory of addiction: addiction is the common end point for each individual who suffers from the compulsion to use chemicals. To treat the addiction, the chemical dependency counselor must identify the forces that both brought about and support this individual's addiction to chemicals. On the basis of this understanding, the chemical dependency counselor can establish a treatment program that will help the individual abstain from further chemical use.

Summary

Although the medical model of drug dependency has dominated the treatment industry in the United States, this model is not without its critics. For each study that proports to identify a biophysical basis for alcoholism or other forms of addiction, other studies fail to document such a difference. For each study that claims to have isolated personality characteristics that seem to predispose one toward addiction, other studies fail to find that these characteristics have predictive value, or find that the personality characteristic in question is brought about by the addiction, not one that predates it.

It was suggested that the medical model of addiction is a metaphor through which people can better understand their problem behavior. However, the medical model of addiction is a theoretical model that has not been proven and that does not easily fit into the concept of disease, as medicine in this country understands the term. It was suggested that drugs themselves are neither good nor bad, and that it is the use to which people put the chemicals that creates the problem, not the drugs themselves.

CHAPTER NINETEEN

Addiction as a Disease of the Human Spirit

To some, addiction is best understood as a disease of the spirit. For example, the concept of alcoholism as a spiritual disorder forms the basis of the Alcoholics Anonymous program (Miller & Hester, 1995; Miller & Kurtz, 1994). From this perspective, to understand the reality of addiction is, ultimately, to understand something of human nature. Modern society, especially Western medicine, tends to disparage matters of the spirit (Sims, 1994). When the subject is brought up, the "enlightened" person turns away, as if embarrassed by the need to discuss "spiritual" matters. To such a person, the spirit, like spears or clothing made of animal skins, is viewed as a remnant of human's primitive past.

The word "spirit" is derived from the Latin word *spiritus*, which means the divine, living force within each of us. In humans, life, spiritus, has become aware of itself as being apart from nature, and from each other (Fromm, 1956). This awareness is known as "self-awareness." But, with the awareness of self comes the painful understanding that each of us is forever isolated from our fellows. Fromm termed this awareness of one's basic isolation as being an "unbearable prison" (1956, p. 7), in which are found the roots of anxiety and shame. "The awareness of human separation," wrote Fromm, "without reunion by love—is the source of shame. It is at the same time the source of guilt and anxiety" (p. 8).

A flower, bird, or tree cannot help but to be what its nature ordains: a flower, bird, or a tree. A bird does not think about being a bird or what kind of a bird it might become. The tree does not think about "being" a tree. Each behaves according to its gifts, to become a specific kind of bird or tree. But, humans possess the twin gifts of self-awareness and self-determination. They may, within certain limits, be self-aware and decide their own fate. These gifts, however, carry a price. Fromm (1956, 1968) viewed the individual's awareness of fundamental aloneness as being the price paid for the power of self-determination.

Humans have come to know that they are different from the animal world, by their self-awareness. With the awareness of self comes the power of self-determination. But, in becoming self-aware, humans also came to feel isolated from the rest of the universe. Humankind became aware of "self," and in so doing came to know loneliness. It is only through the giving of self to another through love that Fromm (1956, 1968) envisioned the individual as transcending his/her isolation, to become part of a greater whole.

Merton (1978) came to take a similar view of the nature of human existence. Yet Merton clearly understood that one could not seek happiness through the compulsive use of chemicals. He discovered, "There can never be happiness in compulsion" (1978, p. 3). Rather, happiness may be achieved through the love that is shared openly and honestly with others. Martin Buber (1970) took an even more extreme view, holding that it is only through our relationships that our life has definition. Each human stands "in relation" to another. The degree of relation, the relationship, is defined by how much of the self one offers to another and how much is received in return.

The relevance of this material to a text on chemical dependency is found in the observation that the early members of Alcoholics Anonymous came to view alcoholism (and, by extension, the other forms of addiction) as a unique disease. For, in their wisdom, the early members of Alcoholics Anonymous came to recognize alcoholism not only as a disease of the body, but also of the spirit. In so doing, they transformed themselves from helpless victims of alcoholism, into active participants in the healing process of sobriety.

Out of this struggle, the early members of Alcoholics Anonymous came to share an intimate knowledge of the nature of addiction. They came to view addiction not as a phenomenon to be dispassionately studied, but as an elusive enemy that held each member's life in its hands. The early members of Alcoholics Anonymous struggled not to find the smallest common element that might "cause" addiction, but to understand and share in the healing process of sobriety. In this way, the pioneers of AA came to understand that recovery was a process through which the individual regained the spiritual unity that he/she could not find through chemicals.

Self-help groups such as Alcoholics Anonymous and Narcotics Anonymous[1] do not postulate any specific theory of how chemical addiction comes about (E. Herman, 1988). Rather, it is simply assumed that any person whose chemical use interferes with his/her life has an addiction problem. The need to attend AA was, to its founders, self-evident to the individual, in that either you were addicted to alcohol, or you were not.

Addiction itself was viewed as resting on a spiritual flaw within the individual. The drugs do not bring about addiction, but rather the individual comes to abuse or be addicted to drugs because of what he or she believes and holds to be important (Peele, 1989). Such spiritual flaws are not uncommon, and usually

pass unnoticed in the average person. But, the addict's spiritual foundation is such that chemical use is deemed acceptable, appropriate, and desirable.

The expression of this spiritual flaw might be found in Peele's (1989) observation that people tend to try and escape responsibility for their lives. Personal suffering is, in a sense, a way of owning responsibility for one's life, and suffering is an inescapable fact of life. We are thus granted endless opportunities to take personal responsibility for our lives.

Although we often like to think otherwise, the truth is that if we are alive, we will encounter problems and suffering. But some people are unwilling to accept this fact. Indeed, they will:

> go to quite extraordinary lengths to avoid . . . problems and the suffering they cause, proceeding far afield from all that is clearly good and sensible in order to find an easy way out, building the most elaborate fantasies in which to live, sometimes to the total exclusion of reality. (Peck, 1978, p. 17)

In this, the addict is not unique, for it is often difficult to accept the pain and suffering that life offers us. We all must come to terms with personal responsibility, and with the pain of our existence. But the addict chooses a different path from the average person. Addiction can be viewed as an outcome of a process through which the individual comes to use chemicals to avoid recognition and acceptance of life's problems. The chemicals come to lead the individual away from what he/she believes is good and acceptable, in return for the promise of comfort and relief.

Diseases of the Mind—Diseases of the Spirit: The Mind-Body Question

As B. Siegel (1986) and many others have observed, modern medicine has come to enforce an artificial dichotomy between the individual's "mind" and the same individual's "body." As a result, modern medicine has become rather mechanical, with the physician treating symptoms, or diseases, rather than the patient as a whole (Cousins, 1989; B. S. Siegel, 1989).

In a sense, the modern physician might be said to be a very highly skilled technician, who often fails to

---

[1] Although there are many similarities between AA and NA, these are separate programs. On occasion, they might cooperate on certain matters, but each is independent of the other.

appreciate the unique person who is now in the role of a patient. Diseases of the body are viewed as falling in the realm of physical medicine, while diseases of the mind fall into the orbit of the psychological sciences. Diseases of the human spirit, according to this view, are the specialty of clergy (Reiser, 1984). The problem is that the patient is not a "spiritual being" or a "psychosocial being" or a "physical being," but a unified whole. Thus, when a person abuses chemicals, the drug use will affect that person "physically, emotionally, socially, and spiritually" (Adams, 1988, p. 20). Society has difficulty accepting that a disease of the spirit—such as addiction—is just as real as a disease of the physical body.

But, humans are indeed spiritual beings, and self-help programs such as Alcoholics Anonymous and Narcotics Anonymous view addiction to chemicals as being a spiritual illness. Their success in helping people to achieve and maintain sobriety would argue that there is some validity to this claim. However, society struggles to adhere to the artificial mind-body dichotomy and in the process tries to come to terms with the disease of addiction, which is neither totally a physical illness nor exclusively one of the mind.

The Growth of Addiction: The Circle Narrows

Brown (1985), in speaking of the role of alcohol in the alcoholic's life, noted that as the disease of alcoholism progresses, the alcoholic comes to center his/her life around the use of the chemical. Alcohol can be thought of as the axis (Brown, 1985, p. 79) around which the alcoholic's life revolves. Alcohol comes to assume a role of "central importance" (p. 78) both for the alcoholic, and the alcoholic's family. Peele (1989) argued that one reason why alcohol or drugs can assume a central role in the individual's life is that the person's values system tolerates chemical use as being an acceptable behavior.

Those who have never been addicted to chemicals have difficulty understanding the importance that addicts attach to their drug of choice. The addicted person is preoccupied with chemical use and the protection of his/her source of chemicals. It is

not uncommon for cocaine addicts to admit that, if it came down to a choice, they would choose cocaine over friends, lovers, or even family.

The grim truth is that the active addict is, in a sense, insane. One reflection of this moral insanity is that the drug has gained central importance in the addict's life. Other people, other commitments are of secondary importance. Addicts "never seem to outgrow the self-centeredness of the child" (*Triangle of Self-Obsession*, 1983, p. 1).

In exploring this point, the book *Narcotics Anonymous* (1982) noted:

> Before coming to the fellowship of NA, we could not manage our own lives. We could not live and enjoy life as other people do. We had to have something different and we thought we found it in drugs. We placed their use ahead of the welfare of our families, our wives, husbands, and our children. We had to have drugs at all costs [italics in original deleted]. (p. 11)

Kaufmann, in his elegant introduction to Buber's (1970) text, spoke of those whose all-consuming interest is themselves. They care of nothing outside that little portion of the universe known as "self." In this sense, chemical addiction can be viewed as a form of self-love, or perhaps as a perversion of self-love. It is through the use of chemicals that the individual seeks to cheat his/her self of the experience of reality, replacing it with the distorted desires of the self.

It is difficult, however, for the nonaddicted person to understand the importance that the addicted person attaches to further drug use. To say that the addict demonstrates an ongoing preoccupation with chemical use is something of an understatement. The addicted person may also demonstrate an exaggerated concern about maintaining a supply of the drug and may avoid those who might prevent further drug use. For example, an alcoholic with six or seven cases of beer in storage in the basement may go out to buy six more cases "just in case." This behavior demonstrates the individual's preoccupation with maintaining an "adequate" supply.

Other people (when their existence is recognized at all) are viewed by the addict either as being helpful in the further use of chemicals or as being impediments to drug use. But to the extent possible, nothing is allowed to come between the individual and his/her drug. It is for this reason that recovering addicts speak of their still addicted counterparts as being morally insane.

The Circle of Addiction: Addicted Priorities

The authors of the book *Narcotics Anonymous* concluded that addiction was a disease composed of three elements: (a) a compulsive use of chemicals, (b) an obsession with further chemical use, and (c) a spiritual disease expressed through total self-centeredness. It is this self-centeredness, the spiritual illness which causes the person to demand "what I want when I want it!" that makes the individual vulnerable to addiction.

As the disease of addiction progresses, the individual comes to center his/her life around continued use of the chemical. This reflects the obsession with drug use, and chemical dependency professionals often speak of the addict's preoccupation with drug use. But, for the addict to admit to this would be to accept the reality of personal addiction. So, persons who are addicted to chemicals begin to use the defense mechanisms of denial, rationalization, projection, and/or minimization to justify their increasingly narrow range of interests both to themselves and to significant others.

To support the addiction, the individual must renounce more and more of his/her self in favor of new beliefs and behaviors that make it possible to continue to use chemicals. This is the spiritual illness that is found in addiction, for the individual comes to believe that "nothing should come between me and my drug use!" No price is too high, nor is any behavior unthinkable, if it allows for further drug use. This is, as Peele (1989) pointed out, a value judgment made by the individual.

As the economic, personal, and social cost of continued drug use mount, the individual often begins to lie, cheat, and steal to maintain his/her addiction. Addicted persons have been known to sell prized possessions, steal money from trust accounts, misdirect medications prescribed for patients, deny any significant feelings for a spouse or family members, and engage in theft, all to maintain the addiction.

While many an addict has examined the cost demanded of drug use, and turned away from chemicals with or without formal treatment, there are those who accept this cost willingly. These individuals go through great pains to hide the evidence of their drug addiction. More than one "hidden" alcoholic has confessed to how he/she would "take the dog for a walk" at night in order to hide empty bottles in neighbors' trash cans. Addicts have been known to hide drug supplies under certain rocks in the countryside, behind books in the living room, under the sink in the kitchen, behind the headboard of the bed, and in a multitude of other places. They have done so to maintain the illusion that they are not using chemicals.

Even the addict is confused as to what brought about this change in personality. The book *Alcoholics Anonymous* (1976) noted that, when you ask the alcoholic why he/she uses alcohol, you are unlikely to learn the real reason. At the same time, the addict is likely to envy and be mystified by the average person's ability to say "no" to chemical use. Addicts simply do not know why they started, or why they continue to use the drugs. They are, in a real sense, spiritually blind.

As the addiction comes to control more and more of life, addicts must expend greater and greater effort to maintain the illusion that they are living a normal life. Gallagher (1986) related how one physician, addicted to a synthetic narcotic known as fentanyl, ultimately would buy drugs from the street because it was no longer possible to divert enough drugs from hospital sources to maintain his drug habit. When the telltale scars from repeated injections of street drugs began to form, this same physician intentionally burned himself on the arm with a spoon to hide the scars.

The addict also finds, as the drug comes to control more and more of his/her life, that significant effort must be invested in the maintenance of the addiction itself. More than one cocaine or heroin addict has had to engage in prostitution (homosexual or heterosexual) to earn enough money to buy more chemicals. Everything is sacrificed to obtain and maintain what the addict perceives as an adequate supply of the chemicals.

To combat the deception inherent in addiction, both Alcoholics Anonymous and Narcotics

Anonymous place a heavy emphasis on the issue of honesty in their respective self-help programs. This is because, as Knapp (1996) noted about alcoholism, one of the core features of the physical addiction to a chemical is "a fundamental inability to be honest . . . with the *self*" (p. 83, italics in original). Drug/alcohol dependency hides behind a wall of deception. Honesty is the way to break through this deception, to bring the person face to face with the reality of the addiction.

Some Games of Addiction

Individuals who are addicted to drugs often seek out sources of legitimate pharmaceuticals, either to supplement their drug supply or to serve as their primary source of chemicals. There are many reasons for this. First, as Goldman (1991) observed, pharmaceuticals may be legally purchased if there is a medical need for the medication. The drug user does not need to fear arrest with a legitimate prescription for the medication.

Second, for the drug addict who can obtain pharmaceuticals, the medication is of a known product, at a known potency level. The drug user does not have to worry about low potency street drugs, impurities that may be part of the drug(s) purchased on the street (e.g., as when PCP is mixed with low-potency marijuana), or misrepresentation (e.g., as when PCP is sold as LSD).

Third, the pharmaceuticals are much less expensive than street drugs. For example, the pharmaceutical analgesic hydromophone costs about $1 per tablet at a pharmacy. On the street, each tablet might sell for as much as $45 to $100 (Goldman, 1991). Thus, there is a demand for pharmaceutical medications, which are obtained by addicts who misdirect the medications onto the street market. To manipulate physicians into prescribing desired medications, addicts are likely to "use ploys such as outrage, tears, accusations of abandonment, abject pleading, promises of cooperation, and seduction" (Jenike, 1991, p. 7).

A favorite manipulative scam is for the addict (or, accomplice) to visit a hospital emergency room (Klass, 1989) or the physician's office to seek medication. The addict then either simulates an illness or uses a real physical illness to obtain desired medications. Sometimes, the presenting complaint is "kidney stones," or a story about how other emergency rooms have not been able to help the patient, who now faces a weekend without relief from some painful condition. In addition to the urinary tract, addicts may complain of bleeding from the alimentary or respiratory tracts (Cunnien, 1988).

When asked for a urine sample, which would show traces of blood if the person suffered from a real kidney stone, addicts have been found secretly pricking their finger with needles to squeeze a few drops of blood into the urine. Another common practice is for the addict to insert foreign objects into the urethra, such as darning needles, to irritate the lining of the urethra. This will cause a small amount of blood to be released by the injured tissues, thus providing a sample of bloody urine. Other manipulative tricks include taking a small wad of cotton, squeezing a couple of drops of blood into it, then inserting the wad of cotton into the urethra just before giving a urine sample. To the casual observer, the addict would seem to have passed a blood clot along with the urine, evidence of a kidney stone to most physicians. Only a close laboratory inspection would reveal that the "clot" was actually cotton. But, the addict knows, most laboratories will not waste the time on a close inspection of the "clot" material, and even if they did, the addict would have long since moved on to a different facility.

The object of this "game" is to obtain a prescription for narcotics from a sympathetic doctor. Addicts have been known to go to an emergency room with a broken bone, have the bone "set," and go home with a prescription for a narcotic analgesic (which was provided to help the patient deal with the pain of a broken bone). Once at home, the addict (or, the accomplice) then removes the cast and appears at yet another hospital emergency room to have yet another cast applied to the injured limb, and to receive yet another prescription for a narcotic analgesic. In a large city, this process might be repeated ten times or more (Goldman, 1991).

Some addicts have even been known to keep detailed records on computer, outlining physicians consulted, pharmacies used to have prescriptions filled, and the dates of the last visit to hospital clinics and emergency rooms so they do not visit the same facility too often. This would raise suspicions that they are actually manipulating medical practitioners to get drugs (Goldman, 1991).

It is also not unusual for addicts to study medical textbooks, to learn what symptoms to fake and how to provide a convincing presentation of these symptoms to health care professionals. The object of this game, again, is to convince the physician to prescribe the desired drug. Salloway, Southwick, and Sadowsky (1990) summarized a case of a 39-year-old narcotics addict who simulated the symptoms of a posttraumatic stress disorder in a Vietnam War veteran, allegedly brought on by an industrial accident. Ultimately, it was discovered that the patient's presenting story was simply an elaborate manipulation designed to obtain narcotics and shelter from the attending physicians of an inpatient psychiatric unit.

Addicts have been known to have "conned" their psychiatrist into keeping a supply of cocaine for him/her. In each case, the addict manipulated the therapist into thinking that he/she was actually interested in therapy. However, the real purpose of this game was in using the therapist to provide a safe "stash" for the cocaine. This allowed the individual to avoid the fear of being caught with cocaine by the police, or having it stolen by other addicts.

The only price that the addict had to pay for this deception was to show up three, four, or perhaps even seven days a week, confess the latest transgression of having purchased more cocaine, then reluctantly allow the therapist to take possession of all but the immediate day's supply of the drug, as an incentive to come back. The addict was then safe from police searches or from other addicts looking for drugs. The therapist in each case apparently thought that, by keeping most of the cocaine, he/she could outmanipulate the addict into staying in therapy.

What the therapist perhaps did not realize was that if the police were to search the office, the therapist (and not the addict), would be in possession of a controlled substance. The addict would not be responsible, since the cocaine was not in his/her immediate possession. The addict could even deny any and all knowledge of the cocaine being there in the first place, since it was the addict's word against that of the therapist. The therapist could then quite possibly face criminal charges, while the addict would look for another place to "stash" (i.e., hide) drugs.

A Thought on Playing the Games of Addiction

A friend who worked in a maximum security penitentiary for men was warned by older, more experienced corrections workers not to try to "out-con a con." Which is to say that a person should not try to outmanipulate the individual whose entire life centers on the ability to manipulate others: "You should remember that, while you are home, watching the evening news, or going out to see a movie, these people have been working on perfecting their 'game.' It is their game, their rules, and in a sense their whole life."

This is also a good rule to keep in mind at all times when working with the addicted person. Addiction is a lifestyle that involves to a large degree the manipulation of others into supporting the addiction. This is not to say that the addict cannot, if necessary, "change his spots," at least for a short time. This is especially true early in the addiction process, or during the early stages of treatment.

Often, addicts go "on the wagon" for a few days, or perhaps even a few weeks, to prove both to themselves and to others that they can "still control it." Addicts who do this overlook the fact that by attempting to "prove" their control, they actually demonstrate their lack of control over the chemicals. They may, as Stuart (1980) observed, be able to give up the drug for a while, if the reward is large enough. However, as the addiction progresses, it takes more and more to motivate addicts to give up their drug, even for a short time. Then, even "a short time" may become too long.

There is no limit to the manipulations that the addicted person may use to support an addiction. Vernon Johnson (1980) spoke at length of how the addict may even use compliance as a defense against treatment. Overt compliance may be, and often is, utilized as a defense against acceptance of one's own spiritual, emotional, and physical deficits. In Johnson's (1980) essay on the subject, compliance is marked by a subtle defiance. It almost appears as if the client is "only going through the motions" to avoid further confrontation. In the struggle to avoid facing the reality of his/her addiction, the client uses a small piece of the truth as a defense against having to accept the whole truth.

Honesty as a Part of the Recovery Process

The authors of the book *Narcotics Anonymous* (1982) warned that the progression toward the understanding that one was addicted was not easy. Self-deception was part of the price that the addict paid for addiction, according to the NA "big book": "Only in desperation did we ask ourselves, 'Could it be the drugs?'" (pp. 1–2).

Addicts will often speak with pride about how they have been more or less "drug-free" for various periods. The list of "reasons" the individual is drug-free is virtually endless. This person is drug-free because his/her spouse otherwise threatened divorce. (But, he or she secretly longs to return to chemical use, and will if he or she can find a way to do so.) Another person is drug-free because his/her probation officer has a reputation for sending people to prison if their urine sample (drawn under strict supervision) is positive for chemicals. (But, he or she is counting the days until probation has ended, and possibly will even sneak an occasional drink, or episode of drug use, if it seems possible to get away with it.)

In each instance, the person is drug-free only because of an external threat. In virtually every case, as soon as the external threat is removed, the individual usually drifts back to chemicals. It is simply impossible for one person to provide the motivation for another person to remain drug-free, forever. (However, as Peele, 1989, pointed out, the individual must choose to avoid further drug use to achieve or maintain sobriety. Personal choice, or commitment to sobriety, is a necessary ingredient to recovery.)

Many an addict in treatment has admitted, often only after repeated and strong confrontation, that they had simply switched addictions to give the appearance of being drug-free. It is not uncommon for an opiate addict in a methadone maintenance program to use alcohol, marijuana, or cocaine. The methadone does not block the euphoric effects of these drugs as it does the euphoria of narcotics. Thus, the addict can maintain the appearance of complete cooperation, appearing each day to take his/her methadone without protest, while still using cocaine, marijuana, or alcohol at will.

In a sense, the addicted person has lost touch with reality. Over time, those who are addicted to chemicals come to share many personality traits. There is some question whether this personality type, the so-called "addicted personality," predates addiction or evolves as a result of the addiction (Bean-Bayog, 1988; Nathan, 1988). However, this chicken-or-the-egg question does not alter that, for addicts, their addiction always comes first.

Many an addicted person has admitted to going without food for days on end, but very few would willingly go without using chemicals for even a short period. Cocaine addicts have spoken about how they would avoid sexual relations with their spouse, or significant other, in order to continue using cocaine. Just as the alcoholic often sleeps with an "eye-opener" (i.e., an alcoholic drink) already mixed by the side of the bed, addicts have spoken about how they had a "rig" (i.e., a hypodermic needle) loaded and ready for use, so that they could inject the drug even before they got out of bed for the day.

Many physicians have boasted of how the patients that they worked with had no reason to lie to them. One physician went so far as to boast that he knew that a certain patient did not have prescriptions from other doctors because the patient ". . . told me so!" The chemical dependency professional needs to keep in mind at all times the twin realities that (a) for the person who is addicted, the chemical comes first, and (b) the addicted person centers his/her life around the chemical. To lose sight of this reality is to run the danger of being trapped in the addict's web of lies, half truths, manipulations, or outright fabrications.

Recovering addicts speak of how manipulative they were and often admit that they were their own worst enemy. For, as they move along the road to recovery, addicts come to recognize that they also were deceiving themselves, as part of the addiction process. One inmate said, "Before I can run a game on somebody else, I have to believe it myself." As the addiction progresses, addicts do not question their perception, but come to believe what they need to believe, to maintain the addiction.

For this reason, the self-help groups of Alcoholics Anonymous and Narcotics Anonymous place heavy emphasis on honesty. They recognize that honesty is their own defense against the self-deception that they used in the past to support their addiction.

False Pride: The Disease of the Spirit

Every addiction is, in the final analysis, a disease of the spirit. Edmeades (1987) related a story of how, in the year 1931, Carl Jung was treating an American, Rowland H. for alcoholism. Immediately after treatment, Rowland H. relapsed, but was not accepted back into analysis by Jung. His only hope of recovery, according to Jung, lay in a spiritual awakening, which he later found through a religious group in America.

Carl Jung identified alcoholism (and by implication all forms of addiction) as diseases of the spirit (Peluso & Peluso, 1988). The *Twelve Steps and Twelve Traditions of Alcoholics Anonymous* (1981) speaks of addiction as being a sickness of the soul. In support of this perspective, Kandel and Raveis (1989) found that a "lack of religiosity" (p. 113) was a significant predictor of continued use of cocaine and/or marijuana for young adults with previous experience with these drugs. The reverse of this is also true: Peluso and Peluso reported that for each of the addicted persons in their book who had achieved sobriety, a spiritual awakening appeared to have been an essential element of recovery.

In speaking with addicts, one is impressed by how often the addict has suffered in his/her lifetime. It is almost as if one could trace a path from the emotional trauma to the addiction. Yet the addict's spirit is not crushed at birth, nor does the trauma that precedes addiction come about overnight. The individual's spirit comes to be diseased over time, as the addict-to-be comes to lose his/her way in life.

Fromm (1968) observed that "we all start out with hope, faith and fortitude" (p. 20). However, the assorted insults of life often join forces to bring about disappointment and a loss of faith. The individual comes to feel an empty void within. Graham (1988) noted that it is at this point that if something is not found to fill the addict's "empty heart, he will fill his stomach with artificial stimulants and seda-

tives" (p. 14). An excellent example of this process is seen in Poland, where many of that country's young adult "no future" generation, whose future has been throttled by years of economic hardship and the martial law of the 1980s, have turned to heroin to ease their pain (Ross, 1991).

Few of us escape this moment of ultimate disappointment, or ultimate awareness (Fromm, 1968). It is at this moment that individuals are faced with a choice. They may come to "reduce their demands to what they can get and do not dream of that which seems to be out of their reach" (Fromm, 1968, p. 21). The Narcotics Anonymous pamphlet *The Triangle of Self-Obsession* (1983) observed that this process is, for most, a natural part of growing up. But the person who is in danger of addiction refuses to reduce those demands. Rather, the addicted person comes to demand "What I want when I want it!" The same NA pamphlet notes that addicts tend to:

> refuse to accept that we will not be given everything. We become self-obsessed; our wants and needs become demands. We reach a point where contentment and fulfillment are impossible. (p. 1)

Despair exists when people view themselves as being powerless. Existentialists speak of the realization of ultimate powerlessness, as awareness of one's nonexistence. In this sense, the individual comes to feel the utter futility of existence. When the person comes to face the ultimate experience of powerlessness, the individual is faced with a choice. He/she may either come to accept his/her true place in the universe or may continue to distort his/her perceptions and thoughts to maintain the illusion of being more than this.

It is only when individuals accept their true place in the universe, and the pain and suffering that life might offer, that they are capable of any degree of spiritual growth (Peck, 1978). When they reach the point of ultimate disappointment, where they realize their true place in the universe, they are faced with a choice: either to accept reality, or, to turn away from it. Many choose to turn away from reality, for it does not offer them what they think they are entitled to. In so doing, these people become somewhat grandiose, and exhibit the characteristic false pride so frequently encountered in addiction.

One cannot accomplish the illusion of being more than what one is without an increasingly large investment of time, energy, and emotional resources. This lack of humility, the denial of what one *is* to give an illusion of being better than this, plants the seeds of despair (Merton, 1961). Humility implies an honest, realistic view of "self" worth. Despair rests on a foundation of a distorted view of one's place in the universe. This despair grows with each passing day, as reality threatens time and again to force on the individual an awareness of the ultimate measure of his/her existence.

In time, external supports are necessary to maintain this false pride. Brown (1985) identified one characteristic of alcohol as being its ability to offer the individual an illusion of control over his/her feelings. This is a common characteristic of every drug of abuse. If life does not provide the pleasure that one feels entitled to, at least comfort and pleasure can be found in a drug, or combination of drugs, that free one from life's pain and misery . . . at least for awhile.

When faced with this unwanted awareness of one's true place in the universe, the addicted person must increasingly distort his/her perception to maintain the illusion of superiority. Into this fight to avoid the painful reality of what is, the chemical injects the ability to seemingly choose one's feelings at will. The chemical, in effect, provides an illusion of control over the emotions, a kingly power to select the feeling one wants to experience.

What the individual does not realize, often not until after the seeds of addiction have been planted, is that the chemical offers an illusion only. There is no substance to the self-selected feelings brought about by the chemical, only a mockery of peace. The deeper feelings made possible through the acceptance of one's lot in life (which is humility) seem to be a mystery to the addicted person. "How can you be happy?" they ask. "You are nothing like me! You don't use!"

Humility, as noted, is the honest acceptance of one's place in the universe (Merton, 1961). Included in this is the honest and open acceptance of one's strengths and one's weaknesses. At the moment when the individual becomes aware of the reality of his/her existence, the individual may come to accept his/her lot in life, or one might choose to struggle against existence itself.

In the struggle against this acceptance, one, in effect, places one's self above all else, to say, "Not as it is, but as I want it!" It is a cry against the ultimate knowledge of being lost that Fromm (1968) spoke of, the knowledge that one is lost. This despair is often so all-inclusive that, ultimately, the self seems unable to withstand its attack. Addicts have described this despair as an empty, black void within. Then, as B. Graham (1988) noted, they have attempted to fill this void with the chemicals that they find around them.

The *Twelve Steps and Twelve Traditions* (1981) view false pride as a sickness of the soul. In this light, chemical use might be viewed as a reaction against the ultimate despair of encountering one's lot in life. It is the false sense of being that says "Not as it is, but as I want it!" in response to one's discovery of personal powerlessness.

Various authors have come to view the substance-abusing person as essentially seeking to join with a higher power. But, in place of the spiritual struggle that Peck (1978, 1993, 1997b) spoke of as being necessary to achieve inner peace, the addict seems to take a shortcut through the use of chemicals. Thus, May (1988) viewed addiction as sidetracking "our deepest, truest desire for love and goodness" (p. 14). In taking the shortcut through chemical abuse, the drugs come to dominate the individual's life. The individual centers his/her life more and more around further chemical use, until at last the person believes that he/she cannot live without it. Further spiritual growth is impossible when the individual views chemical use as being his/her first priority.

In the process of sidetracking the drive for truth and spiritual growth, the addict comes to develop a sense of false pride. This false pride expresses itself almost as a form of narcissism. The clinical phenomenon of narcissism is, itself, a reaction against perceived worthlessness, loss of control, and an emotional pain so intense that it almost seems physical (Millon, 1981). In speaking of the narcissistic personality, Millon observed that such persons view their own self-worth in such a way that ". . . they rarely question whether it is valid" (p. 167). Further,

the narcissistic personality tends to "place few restraints on either their fantasies or rationalizations,
and their imagination is left to run free."

While addicts are not usually narcissistic person-
alities in the pure sense of the word, there are
significant narcissistic traits present in addiction.
Narcissism, or false pride, is based on the lack of
humility, a point Merton (1961) explored at length.
The individual comes to distort not only their perceptions of self, but also of other, in the service of
their pride and their chemical use.

Merton (1961), in speaking of the normal division that takes place within the person's soul, noted
that there are people whose entire life centers on
themselves. Such people:

> . . . imagine that they can only find themselves by
> asserting their own desires and ambitions and ap-
> petites in a struggle with the rest of the world.
> (p. 47)

In this quote are found hints of the seeds of addiction. For, the individual's chemical of choice allows the individual to assert his/her own desires and
ambitions on to the rest of the world. Brown (1985)
speaks at length of the illusion of control over one's
feelings that alcohol gives to the individual. May
(1988) also speaks of how chemical addiction reflects a misguided attempt to achieve complete control over one's life. The drugs of abuse also give an
illusion of control to the user, a dangerous illusion
that allows the individual to believe that he/she is asserting his/her own appetite onto the external world,
while in reality losing his/her will to the chemical.

One often finds addicts speaking with pride of
the horrors that they have suffered in the service of
their addiction. This is known as "euphoric recall," a
process where the addict selectively recalls mainly
the pleasant aspects of drug use, while selectively
forgetting the pain and suffering they experienced
as a consequence (Gorski, 1993). More than one addict, for example, has spoken at length of the quasi-
sexual thrill experienced through cocaine or heroin.
In the process, the addict would dismiss the fact that
this same drug cost him/her a spouse, family, and
several tens of thousand dollars.

There is a name for the distorted view of one's
self and one's world that comes about with chronic
chemical use. It is called the insanity of addiction.

Denial, Rationalization, Projection, and Minimization: The Four Musketeers of Addiction

The traditional view of addiction is that all human
behavior, including the addictive use of chemicals,
rests on a foundation of characteristic psychological
defenses. In the case of chemical dependency, the
defense mechanisms that are thought to be involved
are the triad of denial, rationalization, and projection. These defense mechanisms, like all psychological defenses, are thought to operate unconsciously,
in both the intrapersonal and interpersonal spheres.
They exist to protect the individual from the conscious awareness of anxiety.

Often without knowing it, addicts will utilize
these defense mechanisms to avoid recognizing the
reality of their addiction. For, once the reality of one's
addiction is recognized, there is an implicit social expectation that the person must deal with it. Thus, to
understand addiction, one must also understand
each of these characteristic defense mechanisms.

The traditional view of chemical dependency is
that *denial* is a characteristic defense of the addicted individual. Indeed, the individual's denial of
growing dependence on alcohol is thought to be
the most common reason the individual fails to
seek help for alcoholism (Wing, 1995). Essentially,
denial is "a disregard for a disturbing reality" (Kaplan & Sadock, 1990, p. 20). In this sense, denial
functions as a form of Catch-22 for the addicted
person. It prevents the person from being aware of
the danger signs of the growing addiction to avoid
the awareness of anxiety. But, while avoiding the
experience of anxiety, the individual is also blind to
the growing evidence of his/her addiction to chemicals as well. It is a form of self-deception, used to
help the individual avoid anxiety and emotional
distress (Shader, 1994).

When a person uses denial, it almost seems as if
the individual has selective perception. The Alcoholics Anonymous step program (discussed in more
detail in Chapter 35) calls this selective perception
"tunnel vision." Further, Perry and Cooper (1989)
identified denial as being a rather immature defense
mechanism that is usually found in the person who
is experiencing significant internal and interpersonal distress.

The second of the psychological defense mechanisms commonly found in cases of alcohol/drug addiction is that of *projection*. This defense mechanism is defined by Kaplan and Sadock (1990) as the process through which "what is emotionally unacceptable in oneself is unconsciously rejected and attributed to others" (p. 20). V. Johnson (1980) defined projection differently, noting that the projection is the act of "unloading self-hatred onto others" (p. 31, italics in original deleted).

At times, the defense mechanism of projection expresses itself through the behaviors of misinterpreting the motives or intentions of others (Kaplan & Sadock, 1990). Young children often cry out "See what you made me do?!" when they have misbehaved. This is an expression of projection. Addicts often do this as well, blaming their addiction or unacceptable aspects of their behavior on to others.

Another common defense mechanism utilized in support of continued substance use is the defense mechanism of *rationalization*.This defense mechanism is the process through which "an individual attempts to justify feelings, motives, or behavior that otherwise would be unreasonable, illogical or intolerable" (Kaplan & Sadock, 1990, p. 20). In a later work, the authors also noted that rationalization may express itself through the individual's "invention of a convincing fallacy" (p. 184) through which they seemingly justify their behavior. Some of the examples of rationalization used by addicts include blaming their spouse or family ("if you were married to_____, you would drink, too!") or medical problems (a 72-year-old alcoholic blames his drinking on a bout of pneumonia he had when he was 12).

Anybody who has ever worked with an addicted person can recognize on the basis of personal experience how rationalization is one of the most important of defensive devices utilized by the alcohol/drug-addicted individual. The defense mechanism of *minimization* operates in a different manner than the three preceding defensive operations. In a sense, minimization operates like the defense mechanism of rationalization, but it is more specific. The addicted individual who uses minimization as a defense actively reduces the amount of chemicals that he or she admits to using by a variety of mechanisms.

The alcohol-dependent individual, for example, may pour his/her drinks into an oversized container, perhaps the size of three or four regular glasses, and then claim to having "only three drinks a night!" (overlooking that each drink is equal to three regular-sized drinks). The addict might claim to "only use once a day," and hope that the interviewer does not think to ask whether a "day" means a full, 24-hour day, or just when it is daylight outside. Another trick is for addicts to claim time when they were in treatment, in jail, or hospitalized, as "straight time" (i.e., time when they were not using chemicals), overlooking that they were unable to get alcohol/drugs because they were incarcerated.

These defense mechanisms operate automatically and quite unconsciously, to protect these individuals from a full realization of their addiction. The conscious awareness of one's addiction would be a painful awareness, and thus is something to be avoided. For example, there is the rationalization, offered to this author by a number of different addicts, that marijuana use does not constitute addiction, since marijuana is "a herb," and thus is a natural substance.

A common rationalization is that an individual can only become addicted to artificial chemicals, such as alcohol, amphetamines, or heroin. Obviously, since marijuana grows naturally, it is not possible to become addicted to it, according to this rationalization. Another popular rationalization is that it is "better to be an alcoholic than a needle freak . . . after all, alcohol is legal!" More than one alcohol-dependent individual has denied his/her addiction, despite compelling evidence to the contrary, through the use of one or more of these common defense mechanisms.

Reactions to the Spiritual Disorder Theory of Addiction

Although the traditional view of substance abuse in the United States has been that the defense mechanisms of denial, rationalization, minimization, and projection are traditionally found in cases of chemical dependency, this view is not universally accepted. A small, increasingly vocal, minority has offered alternative frameworks within which substance abuse professionals might view the defense mechanisms that they encounter in their work with addicted individuals.

Stanton Peele, as noted earlier, has been a vocal critic of the medical model of chemical dependency. In his (1989) work on the subject, he discusses at length how treatment centers often utilize the individual's refusal to admit to his/her addiction as confirmation that the individual is addicted. The individual is automatically assumed to be in denial of his/her chemical abuse problem. However, a second possibility, all too often overlooked by treatment center staff, according to Peele, is that the individual might not be addicted to chemicals to begin with!

The automatic assumption that the client is "in denial" may blind treatment center staff to the possibility that the individual's refusal to admit to being addicted to chemicals may reflect reality, and not express denial. This possibility underscores the need for an accurate assessment of the client's substance use patterns, to determine whether there is a need for active intervention or treatment.

Miller and Rollnick (1991) offered a theory that radically departs from the belief that addicts typically utilize denial as a major defense against the admission of being sick. The authors suggest that alcoholics, as a group, do not utilize denial more frequently than any other average group. Rather, the authors suggest that two factors have made it appear that addicts frequently utilize defense mechanisms such as denial, rationalization, and projection in the service of their dependency. First, the authors suggest that the process of selective perception on the part of treatment center staff makes it seem that addicts frequently use the defense mechanisms discussed earlier.

The authors point to the phenomenon known as the "illusion of correlation" to support this theory. According to the illusion of correlation, human beings tend to remember information that confirms their preconceptions and to forget or overlook information that fails to meet their conceptual model. Substance abuse professionals are more likely to remember those clients who use the defense mechanisms of denial, rationalization, projection, or minimization, according to the authors, because that is what they were trained to expect.

Second, Miller and Rollnick (1991) suggest that when substance abuse rehabilitation professionals utilize the wrong treatment approach for the client's unique stage of growth, the resulting conflict is interpreted as evidence of denial, projection, minimization, or rationalization. On the basis of their work with addicted individuals, Berg and Miller (1992) also suggest that denial is found when the therapist utilizes the wrong treatment approach with a client. Thus, both teams of clinicians have concluded that defense mechanisms such as denial are not a reflection of a pathological condition on the part of the client, but the result of the wrong intervention being utilized by the professional working with the individual.

These theories offer challenging alternatives to the traditional model of the addicted person having characteristic defense mechanisms, as discussed in this chapter.

Summary

Many human service professionals who have had limited contact with drug addiction tend to have a distorted view of its nature. Having heard the term "disease" applied to chemical dependency, the inexperienced human service worker may think in terms of more traditional illnesses, and may be rudely surprised at the deception inherent in drug addiction.

While chemical dependency is a disease, it is a disease like no other. It is, as noted in an earlier chapter, a disease that requires the active participation of the "victim." Further, self-help groups such as Alcoholics Anonymous or Narcotics Anonymous view addiction as a disease of the spirit, and offer a spiritual program to help members achieve and maintain their recovery.

Addiction is, in a sense, a form of insanity. The insanity of addiction rests on a foundation of psychological defense mechanisms such as rationalization, minimization, denial, and projection. These defense mechanisms, plus self-deception, keep the person from becoming aware of the reality of his/her addiction until the disease process has progressed quite far. To combat self-deception, Alcoholics Anonymous places emphasis on honesty, openness, and a willingness to try to live without alcohol. Honesty, both with self and with others, is the central feature of the AA program, which offers a program designed to foster spiritual growth to help the individual overcome his/her spiritual weaknesses.

Chemicals and the Neonate

The Consequences of Drug Use during Pregnancy

The problem of maternal drug use during pregnancy is actually part of a more inclusive danger: that of maternal exposure to *any* potentially toxic chemical during pregnancy. Physicians have long been aware that a multitude of chemical compounds are able to cross over the placenta into the fetal circulatory system. Many of these chemicals can severely damage the developing fetus, which is highly vulnerable to maternal drug use for two main reasons. First, the fetus lacks the fully developed liver and excretory systems of the mother and thus will experience the effects of chemical exposure to a far greater extent than will the mother (Chasnoff, 1988). Second, fetal organ systems develop at a rapid rate, and anything that disrupts this process may have lifelong consequences for the child.

Virtually every drug of abuse is able to cross the placenta and enter the fetal circulation (Behnke & Eyler, 1993). While medical science has long been aware of this fact, it has failed to devote much attention to the implications of maternal drug abuse on fetal growth and development (Chasnoff & Schnoll, 1987). Even today, more than a generation after the latest war on drugs began, little is known about either the short-term or the long-term consequences of maternal drug abuse on the fetus (Chasnoff, 1991b; Zuckerman & Bresnahan, 1991).

The possible impact of maternal chemical use on fetal development would not be significant, if it was a rare phenomenon, but this is not the case. Nationally, it is estimated that 19% of all pregnant women use alcohol, 20% smoke cigarettes, and 5.5% use an illicit drug at least once during their pregnancy (Mathias, 1995; Raut, Stephen, & Kosopsky, 1996). Because the rapidly growing fetus is uniquely vulnerable to environmental influences, the danger of maternal chemical use during pregnancy is readily apparent.

Caution. It is most difficult to identify the effects of a given chemical on fetal growth and development. A thousand different factors influence both fetal growth and maternal health. The possibility of maternal illness during pregnancy, polychemical exposure, genetic predisposition toward various medical problems, and the woman's state of health prior to pregnancy are but a few of the factors that the health care professional must consider when studying the effects of chemical use on fetal growth and development.

For example, suppose that a cigarette-smoking woman suffered from a kidney disease before she became pregnant and also failed to receive adequate prenatal care during pregnancy because of her limited financial resources. Should her child's small size at birth be attributed to her cigarette smoking, the mother's poor health, the lack of prenatal care, a poor diet (a common consequence of poverty) or, possibly, to a familial tendency to give birth to smaller children? All these factors must be weighed by the professional who attempts to identify the effects of maternal drug use on the fetus.

The researcher also must consider the extent to which society's attitudes toward drug/alcohol use during pregnancy might interfere with access to prenatal medical care (Irwin, 1995). According to the author, the negative stereotypes that some substance-abusing pregnant women encounter, not to mention their fears that county or state authorities will intervene to take their infant should their substance use problems become known, make them hesitate to seek prenatal care. Social attitudes that condemn substance-abusing pregnant women thus serve to block access to medical care that could reduce fetal risk.

Statement of the Problem

There is significant evidence to suggest that recreational drug use during pregnancy is associated with such complications as preterm labor, early separation of the placenta, fetal growth retardation, and numerous congenital abnormalities. At its most extreme, if the mother is addicted at the time of delivery, the child will share in the mother's addiction. Nationally, more than 1000 children a day are born to mothers who are addicted to chemicals (Byrne, 1989a). These children are addicted to the same chemical(s) at birth.

But, even if the child is not born addicted, maternal drug use may interfere with the normal development of fetal organ systems. The team of Dominguez, Vila-Coro, Aguirre, Slipis, and Bohan (1991) concluded that fetal exposure to recreational drugs during pregnancy was one cause of brain and vision abnormalities later in life.

The medical care of children exposed to recreational drugs is an expensive affair. Chasnoff (1991b) estimated that the median cost of care for children born to mothers who had used illicit chemicals during pregnancy was between $1100 and $4100 higher than for children whose mothers who did not use illicit chemicals while pregnant. Since 350,000 to 739,000 children are exposed to illicit chemicals before birth (Chasnoff), this figure translates into a potential expenditure of between $385 million and $3 billion in medical costs each year for treatment of drug-related neonatal health problems.

When these children reach school age, they may very well require further specialized services that are an additional expense for society. Barden (1991) noted that whereas the average educational cost for a child is approximately $3,000 a year, the cost of the special education classes often required

by children born addicted to drugs can be as high as $15,000 a year per child.

For all these reasons, it is essential that the substance abuse professional have a working knowledge of the impact of the various drugs of abuse on fetal growth and development.

The Fetal Alcohol Syndrome

It is only in the past 25 years that researchers have discovered that women who drink on a regular basis while pregnant run the risk of causing alcohol-induced birth defects in their children, a condition known as the *fetal alcohol syndrome* (FAS). Nobody knows how much, or how often, a pregnant woman must drink before there is a risk of FAS developing. But, FAS is considered the third most common cause of birth defects in the United States (North, 1996). It is also the only cause of birth defects in the United States which is totally preventable (Beasley, 1987).

Researchers believe that 757,000 of the 4 million women who give birth each year consumed alcohol at least once during pregnancy (Mathias, 1995). When an expectant mother drinks, the alcohol quickly crosses the placenta into the fetal bloodstream. Research has shown that when a pregnant woman drinks, the blood alcohol level of the fetus reaches *the same level as the mother's* in only 15 minutes (Rose, 1988). Thus, the fetus is an unwilling participant in the mother's alcohol use. Indeed, if the mother has been drinking shortly prior to childbirth, the smell of alcohol may be detected on the breath of the infant following birth (Rose).

The full prevalence of alcohol-related birth defects is not known (Cordero, 1990). Youngstrom (1992) reported that one child in 700 to 750 suffers from FAS, while Spohr, Willms, and Steinhausen (1993) estimated that 1 to 2 cases of FAS occurred for every 1000 children. Bell and Lau (1995) gave a higher estimate of 2.2 cases for every 1000 live births in this country. But these statistics only reflect the proportion of children with FAS to the total number of live births. Among alcoholic mothers, perhaps between 2.5% (M. Gottlieb, 1994) and 6% (Charness et al., 1989) of the children will be born with FAS. In some communities where maternal alcohol use is common, this figure may be as high as 19% (Hartman, 1995).

Fetal alcohol syndrome is the severe end of a continuum of disabilities brought on by maternal alcohol use during pregnancy (Streissguth et al., 1991). Some infants demonstrate only some of the symptoms of FAS, a condition known as *fetal alcohol effects* (FAE) (Charness et al., 1989; Streissguth et al., 1991). It is thought that perhaps 3 to 5 of every 1000 children suffer from FAE (Spohr et al., 1993).

Researchers now believe that maternal alcohol use during pregnancy affects fetal brain development because alcohol inhibits the production (biosynthesis) of chemicals known as *gangliosides* (A. Rosenberg, 1996). These chemicals play a role in the formation of the brain in the earliest stages of development. Further, two factors seem to play a role in determining whether the child will develop FAS (Charness et al., 1989). These are (a) whether the mother drinks heavily during all, or only part, of her pregnancy, and (b) the genetic vulnerability of the fetus to maternal alcohol use. If the mother drinks heavily throughout pregnancy, and the fetus is especially vulnerable to the effects of the alcohol in the mother's system, then there is a grave danger that the child will be born with fetal alcohol syndrome.

Characteristics of Fetal Alcohol Syndrome Children

Infants who suffer from the full fetal alcohol syndrome usually have a lower than normal birth weight, a characteristic pattern of facial abnormalities, and often a smaller brain size at birth. Noninvasive neurodiagnostic imaging examination of the brains of children who were exposed to alcohol prior to birth reveals damage to such structures of the infant's brain as the cerebral cortex, cerebellum, basal ganglia, hippocampus, and the corpus callosum (Mattson & Riley, 1995). In later life, children with FAS often demonstrate behavioral problems such as hyperactivity, a short attention span, impulsiveness, poor coordination, and numerous other developmental delays (Charness et al., 1989; Committee on Substance Abuse and Committee on Children with Disabilities, 1993; Gilbertson & Weinberg, 1992). Children with FAS also exhibit slower growth patterns following birth and are more likely to be retarded. Maternal alcohol use during pregnancy is thought to be the leading cause of mental retardation

in the United States (Bell & Lau, 1995; Charness et al., 1989; Streissguth et al., 1991).

As a group, children with FAS usually fall in the mild to moderately retarded range following birth, with an average IQ of 68[1] (Chasnoff, 1988). However, some 40% of children with FAS will have measured IQs above 70, a score that is often used to determine which children qualify for special services due to cognitive disabilities (Streissguth et al., 1991). This is not to say that these children have not suffered from the mother's use of alcohol during pregnancy. Rather, these children do not qualify for special support services, because their measured IQ happens to be higher than the cutoff score of 70 typically utilized by most school districts to determine who qualifies for remedial services.

At this point in time, research would suggest that there is no "safe" dose of alcohol during pregnancy (Committee on Substance Abuse and Committee on Children with Disabilities, 1993). Although few heavy drinkers would consider 4 to 6 drinks/day a significant amount of alcohol, research has shown that 4 to 6 drinks/day for the typical woman during pregnancy will result in 33% of the children having FAS, and 33% having FAE (Raut, Stephen, & Kosopsky 1995). The first trimester is a time of hightened vulnerability for the fetus (Pirozzolo & Bonnefil 1996). This is the period of development when the gangliosides that shape neuronal growth are thought to be most active, and alcohol's effects can be especially disruptive on fetal neurological growth during this phase. However alcohol use at *any* point in pregnancy should be avoided (M. Gottlieb, 1994).

Even when children who suffer from FAS are identified at birth, there is evidence that despite the best possible intervention program, they might never achieve normal growth or intelligence, (Mirin et al., 1991; Spohr et al., 1993). For example, Aase (1994) stated that children with "classic" (p. 5) FAS grow at only 60% of the normal rate for height, and 33% of the normal rate for weight gain.

Thus, once the damage has been done during pregnancy, the child appears to be unlikely to recover

---

[1]An IQ of 68 falls in the mildly retarded range of intellectual function. The average IQ is 100, with a standard deviation of 15 points. An IQ of 68 is thus more than 2 standard deviations below the mean.

even if special efforts are made to help the child following birth. In terms of academic performance, one study found that only 6% of those students with FAS could function in regular school classes, without special help (Streissguth et al., 1991). These researchers found that the average reading level for these adolescent and adult FAS victims was fourth grade, while the average arithmetic skill level for their sample was second grade. Such scores highlight the lifelong consequences of maternal alcohol use on the child's subsequent growth and development.

It has been found that "major psychosocial problems and lifelong adjustment problems were characteristic of most of these patients" (Streissguth et al., 1991, pp. 1965–1966). Surprisingly, the low birth weight characteristic of FAS seemed to at least partially resolve itself by adolescence, according to the authors. Nevertheless, "none of these (adolescent or young adult) patients were known to be independent in terms of both housing and income" (p. 1966) at the time of the study. These findings again underscore the lifelong impact of maternal alcohol use during pregnancy on the child.

Breast-Feeding and Alcohol Use

Animal research would suggest that, even if the mother does not drink during pregnancy, if she drinks during the period she is breast-feeding, the infant may still absorb alcohol through the mother's milk (Little, Anderson, Ervin, Worthington-Roberts, & Clarren, 1989). Little et al., (1989) found that there was a direct relationship between the level of exposure to alcohol through the mother's milk and developmental delays on the infant's part.

Further, the more that the mother drank while breast-feeding, the greater the developmental delay that was measured in the infant. Further, maternal alcohol use in the woman who is breast-feeding her child may interfere with the normal development of the child's immune system (Gilbertson & Weinberg, 1992). These results would strongly suggest that alcohol use by the mother who is breast-feeding is indeed a risk factor for the infant and should be avoided.

Cocaine Use during Pregnancy

As recently as 1982, some medical textbooks claimed that maternal cocaine use did not have a harmful effect on the fetus (Revkin, 1989). Further, although the last wave of cocaine abuse began to peak in the early 1980s, there was virtually no research into the effects of maternal cocaine use on fetal development available to guide health care workers as they struggled to understand the dangers to both the mother and the fetus. The media began to circulate reports that large numbers of expectant women were using cocaine during their pregnancy, and health care workers began to face pointed questions from community leaders as to how maternal cocaine abuse might harm the fetus.

To complicate matters, there was little firm information available as to the scope of the problem of maternal cocaine abuse in the 1980s, a state of affairs that continues until the present day. The team of Scafidi et al. (1996) reported that 10% to 15% of all expectant mothers used cocaine either alone, or in combination with other drugs, during the course of their pregnancy. The National Institute on Drug Abuse (NIDA), however, reached a different conclusion. NIDA conducted a National Pregnancy and Health Survey, which was the first *national* survey of drug use during pregnancy, and found that only about 1.1% of the 4 million pregnant women, or just 45,000 women, used cocaine during their pregnancy (Mathias, 1995). Finally, the team of Hawley, Halle, Drasin, and Thomas (1995) offered an estimate of 100,000 babies born each year who were exposed to crack (the most common form of cocaine) before birth.

A possible explanation for these widely different estimates was offered by Karch (1996), who suggested that since "sidestream" smoke from cocaine smokers can cause others in the room to passively absorb significant amounts of cocaine, the "presence of the drug [in a woman's urine] just proves that there is [cocaine] in the environment" (p. 29), not that *she* used the cocaine. Since many of the early studies on the scope of maternal cocaine use during pregnancy were based on the results of urine toxicology testing, there is a chance that these studies may have detected women who were passively exposed to cocaine smoke, not active users.

Thus, even after more than a decade of study, scientists have yet to agree on a firm estimate of the number of women who use cocaine at some point during their pregnancy. To further complicate matters, early reports in the medical journals suggesting the possibility of an epidemic of cocaine-disabled children fueled speculation in the mass media as to the dangers of maternal cocaine abuse during pregnancy. The public, unaware of the controversy surrounding this topic, began to fear the worst. Even now, more than a decade after the last epidemic of cocaine abuse reached its peak, researchers are still unclear as to the impact of maternal cocaine use on fetal development.

How Do You Identify an Infant Exposed to Cocaine in Utero?

In adults, blood or urine toxicology tests will detect cocaine only for 24 to 48 hours following the drug use. However, the newborn child's immature liver is unable to produce normal amounts of the enzyme *pseudo-cholinesterase*, which biotransforms cocaine (House, 1990; Peters & Theorell, 1991). Thus, the newborn child will require longer to metabolize and excrete any cocaine that may be in his/her body. However, the mebabolites of cocaine might still be detected for only 4 to 6 days after the infant was exposed to the drug (Levy & Rutter, 1992). Thus, urine/blood toxicology tests will detect only *recent* maternal cocaine use (Volpe, 1995).[2]

To further complicate matters, there is no pattern of fetal deficits, or fetal malformations, specific to maternal cocaine abuse during pregnancy. Many of the fetal developmental problems initially attributed to maternal cocaine abuse might be caused by such noncocaine factors as maternal lifestyle, lack of prenatal care, concurrent use of drugs besides cocaine, and poor maternal nutritional habits. In a provocative study, Racine, Joyce, and Anderson (1993) compared birth records of children born to cocaine-using mothers who had seen a doctor at least four times during pregnancy with those of children born to cocaine-using mothers who had not received even this limited prenatal care. The authors found significant improvements in the birth weight of children born to those mothers who had seen a doctor at least

four times, even if the mothers used cocaine during pregnancy. The results of this study were interpreted as evidence that many of the developmental deficits attributed to maternal cocaine abuse might actually be caused by a lack of prenatal medical care.

Because of the social stigma associated with maternal cocaine use during pregnancy, there is a chance that at least some women who are pregnant and who use cocaine actively avoid seeking medical care (Irwin, 1995). The woman might fear loss of custody of her child, or legal sanctions, if her cocaine use should be discovered while she is pregnant.[3] The unfortunate outcome of this process is that the woman fails to benefit from routine prenatal examinations. In many cases, the first medical care that a cocaine-abusing pregnant woman receives is when she arrives at a hospital emergency room, in labor (Sexson, 1994). Thus, a lack of proper prenatal medical care might have actually caused some of the fetal growth problems that medical researchers initially attributed only to maternal cocaine abuse.

Concurrent use of other chemicals besides cocaine is an additional confounding factor in studies that attempt to isolate the effects of maternal cocaine use. Research has shown that fully 50% of the women who were using cocaine during pregnancy were also using alcohol (Sexson, 1994). Alcohol is a known risk factor for abnormal fetal development, and it is virtually impossible to isolate the effects of prenatal alcohol use from that of the mother's use of cocaine. In addition, an unknown (but significant) percentage of cocaine-abusing pregnant women also smoke cigarettes, a practice known to have a negative effect on prenatal growth and development. Finally, many cocaine-abusing mothers-to-be also engage in polydrug use, and there is no research on the impact of multiple recreational chemicals on fetal development.

Another problem that has made it difficult to understand the impact of prenatal cocaine use on fetal growth and development is that, until recently, researchers compared the growth and behavior of *full-term* infants born to cocaine-abusing mothers with

---

[2] Volpe (1995) suggested that it might be possible to detect evidence of maternal cocaine use through traces of cocaine found in the infant's *hair*, if the mother had used cocaine in the last two trimesters of pregnancy. However, this procedure is not in general use, and remains controversial.

[3] The failure of some cocaine-abusing women to seek prenatal care would thus seem to be an unanticipated side effect of society's decision to impose legal sanctions against women who abuse cocaine or other chemicals during pregnancy.

that of other full-term infants (Scafidi et al., 1996). Yet one complication of maternal cocaine use during pregnancy is premature labor, according to the authors. Thus, to better understand the impact of maternal cocaine use during pregnancy, it would be necessary to compare the behavior and development of premature infants who were exposed to cocaine with that of infants who were not exposed to cocaine in utero.

In addition to the factors identified thus far, there is the problem of prenatal infection. There is a high incidence of sexually transmitted diseases (STDs) among the women who are likely to have used cocaine during pregnancy (Sexson, 1994). Many of the pathogens that cause STDs are able to disrupt normal fetal development as well as cause damage to the mother's body. Because all these factors have the potential to influence the growth and development of the fetus prior to and following birth, it is difficult, if not impossible, to isolate the effects of just the mother's cocaine use during pregnancy from the effects of these other known maternal risk factors.

The Professional Bias

As researchers struggled to understand the effects that prenatal cocaine exposure might have on both the mother and the developing fetus, an unspoken anticocaine bias developed in many professional journals. As a result, articles that found an adverse effect from maternal cocaine use were more likely to be published than articles that failed to document a negative impact (Raskin, 1994; Volpe, 1995). The average health care worker, unaware of this bias, assumed that maternal cocaine abuse was indeed the cause of numerous birth defects:

- Spontaneous abortions.
- Abruptio placentae.[4]
- Poor fetal growth/low birth weight.
- Small head size at birth.

- Urinary tract abnormalities in the developing fetus.
- Fetal skull abnormalities.
- Possible strokes for both the mother and the fetus.
- Cardiac system abnormalities in the developing fetus.
- Kidney malformations in the developing fetus.
- Structural abnormalities in the brain of the developing fetus.
- Damage to small intestine of the developing fetus.

Further, maternal cocaine use during pregnancy was thought to be a cause of preterm delivery. In some communities, as many as 17% of the women who experienced preterm labor were found to have measurable amounts of cocaine in their urine (Cordero, 1990; Ney, Dooley, Keith, Chasnoff, & Socol, 1990). Some physicians went to far as to advocate routine urine toxicology testing for any woman who experienced preterm labor (Peters & Theorell, 1991).

Now that the cocaine use epidemic of the 1970s and 1980s is over, researchers have started to reexamine the effects of maternal cocaine use on fetal development. Despite the general expectation that prenatal cocaine use would be dangerous to the fetus, physicians have concluded that the "great majority of cocaine-exposed pregnancies did not result in fetal structural abnormalities" (Behnke & Eyler, 1993, p. 1366). There does not appear to be a "consistent pattern of congenital abnormalities . . . and no increased incidence of malformations" in children born to cocaine-using mothers (Behnke & Eyler, 1993, p. 1365; Richardson & Day, 1994). In contrast to the popular image painted by the mass media in the past 15 years, there is no typical cocaine baby syndrome (Day & Richardson, 1994; Hawley et al., 1995; Hopfensperger, 1995; Sexson, 1994).

The Current Theories

Current research suggests that maternal cocaine still should be considered a potential source of danger for the developing fetus. The team of Scafidi et al. (1996) examined 30 premature infants who were exposed to cocaine prior to birth, with a

[4]In this condition, bleeding starts between the placenta and the wall of the uterus. As the blood accumulates, it gradually separates the placenta from the wall of the uterus, cutting the fetus off from its supply of oxygen. The result may be fatal for both the mother and the fetus.

similar number of premature infants who had not been exposed to cocaine in utero. The authors found that premature infants who had been exposed to cocaine prior to birth had smaller head circumferences, had to spend a longer time in neonatal intensive care units following birth, had more sleep-wake cycle disturbances, and were at higher risk for certain forms of stroke than premature infants who had not been exposed to cocaine.

There is also mixed evidence that maternal cocaine use might be more likely to suffer "crib death" (sudden infant death syndrome, or SIDS). Perhaps as many as 15% of the infants whose mothers used cocaine during pregnancy were found to suffer from SIDS, a potentially fatal condition that is seen in only 0.3% of those children whose mothers did not use cocaine during pregnancy (Bell & Lau, 1995; Peters & Theorell, 1991). It should be noted that many other studies have failed to find this association between SIDS and maternal cocaine use during pregnancy (Plessinger & Woods, 1993; Weathers, Crane, Sauvain, & Blackhurst, 1993). One would expect that if an increased risk of SIDS was a consequence of maternal cocaine use during pregnancy, this would be repeatedly found in research studies examining the subject.

Thus, the possibility that children born to mothers who used cocaine during pregnancy are more likely to suffer SIDS has not been resolved by researchers. Kandall, Gaines, Habel, Davidson, and Jessop (1993) found only a *slightly* higher incidence of SIDS in children whose mothers had used cocaine during pregnancy. Until research answers the question one way or another, maternal cocaine use during pregnancy must be considered a *potential but still not proven* factor in the possible development of SIDS. The use of cocaine during pregnancy should be avoided, to be sure, but medical researchers are still divided on the question of whether maternal cocaine abuse predisposes the baby to SIDS following birth.

Which leaves the question of how maternal cocaine use during pregnancy might affect fetal development. The answer is that, after decades of study, we do not know. Research into the effects of maternal cocaine use on fetal brain development has only recently been started, and the results of this research will not be known for many years (Day

& Richardson, 1994). However, on the basis of animal research and what we know about the clinical effects of cocaine on the user's body, we can make an educated guess as to some of the ways cocaine might disrupt fetal development.

Animal research has demonstrated that cocaine use by the mother results in constriction of the blood vessels in the placenta and uterine bed. This will reduce the blood flow to the fetus for a period of time. The reduction in uterine blood flow is postulated to be a possible cause of poor intrauterine growth for the fetus of cocaine-using mothers. This is also thought to be the mechanism by which maternal cocaine abuse during pregnancy can result in premature labor and birth in humans (Behnke & Eyler, 1993; Chasnoff, 1991a; Glantz & Woods, 1993; Plessinger & Woods, 1993). Cocaine is suspected of being able to cause strong contractions in the uterus. These contractions may, in turn, initiate labor. Indeed, many "street" addicts believe that cocaine is capable of bringing on a late stage abortion, and there is reason to suspect that some women may use cocaine for this purpose (Burkett, Yasin, Palow, LaVoie, & Martinez, 1994; Sexson, 1994).

Cocaine's vasoconstrictive effects may also be the mechanism by which maternal cocaine abuse may result in injury to the developing bowel of the fetus (Cotton, 1994; Plessinger & Woods, 1993). Animal research suggests that maternal cocaine use causes damage to the mesenteric artery, which provides blood to the intestines, according to the authors. An alternative hypothesis is that cocaine is able to cause a reduction in blood flow to "nonvital" (p. 271) organ systems of the developing fetus, including the intestines. In either case, maternal cocaine use is a suspected cause of damage to the intestines of the developing fetus in humans.

The team of Mitra, Ganesh, and Apuzzio (1994) used ultrasound examinations to explore the impact of maternal cocaine use on the renal function of the fetus. The authors found evidence that, in the fetus of a cocaine-abusing mother, the renal artery did not function normally, reducing the blood flow to the kidneys of the fetus. Thus, it would appear that maternal cocaine use during pregnancy results in periods of reduced blood flow to a number of internal organs, including the intestines and the kidneys, which may contribute to problems for the developing fetus.

There is some evidence suggesting that infants born to mothers who use cocaine during pregnancy might suffer from small strokes prior to birth (Chasnoff, 1988; Levy & Rutter, 1992; Volpe, 1995). One research study found that 6% of cocaine-exposed infants had evidence of having had at least one cerebral infarction (Volpe). These small strokes are thought to be a result of the rapid changes in the mother's blood pressure brought on by the maternal cocaine use. Chasnoff postulated that such strokes are similar to those occasionally seen in adults who use cocaine and went on to note that there is evidence that cocaine use during pregnancy may also result in cardiac and central nervous system abnormalities in the fetus.

The danger of CNS developmental abnormalities for the fetus is hardly insignificant. Research has shown that more than one-third of the infants known to have been exposed to cocaine during pregnancy have structural abnormalities of the brain that may be detected by computer tomographic scans (CT scans) or ultrasound examination (Behnke & Eyler, 1993; Plessinger & Woods, 1993; Zuckerman & Bresnahan, 1991). But as noted earlier, no definitive pattern of maldevelopment has been identified as being caused specifically by maternal cocaine abuse. Thus, the role of maternal cocaine use in the evolution of these fetal developmental abnormalities is still not clear.

Researchers have determined that at least some of the cocaine in the mother's blood will cross the placenta and enter the fetal circulation. However, it is still not clear how much cocaine may enter the fetal circulation. Animal research suggests that, in some species, the placenta may be able to metabolize limited amounts of cocaine before it enters the fetal circulatory system. If true, this would limit the transfer of cocaine to the fetus from the mother's blood (Plessinger & Woods, 1993). But it must be pointed out that these findings are based on animal research, and that there is no clinical evidence at this point to suggest that the human placenta shares this ability with the placenta of various research animals.

Children who were exposed to cocaine during pregnancy usually score within the normal range on tests of global development (Hawley et al., 1995). The authors noted, however, there was evidence to suggest that these children also had subtle defects in language use skills and in organizational abilities. The authors also suggested that prenatal cocaine-exposed children tended to have problems in their interpersonal attachments and an increased tendency for emotional problems. Thus, while maternal cocaine use during pregnancy should be discouraged, the question of what the impact of the woman's use of cocaine might be on fetal growth and development remains to be answered.

Cocaine and Breast-Feeding

Cocaine, because it is highly lipid-soluble, may be stored in breast milk. Thus some of the drug may be passed on to the infant by the mother through breast-feeding (Peters & Theorell, 1991; Revkin, 1989). But the level of cocaine exposure for the child might be far higher than it was for the mother. Research has shown that cocaine levels in the maternal milk might be *eight times* as high as the level of cocaine in mother's blood (Revkin). If the cocaine-using mother were to breast-feed her infant, that child might be exposed to extremely high levels of cocaine through the mother's breast milk. For this reason, maternal cocaine use during the time when the mother breast-feeds her infant should be discouraged.

Amphetamine Use during Pregnancy

The effects of the amphetamines on the developing human fetus have not been studied in detail (Bell & Lau, 1995). Clinically, since the effects of the amphetamines are so similar to those of cocaine, it seems likely that maternal use of amphetamines during pregnancy may produce the same effects as maternal cocaine use (Pirozzolo & Bonnefil 1995).

On the basis of the limited information that is available, Bell and Lau (1995) suggested that infants who were exposed to amphetamines during pregnancy tend to be born with a decreased head circumference, length, and body weight. The authors also suggested that maternal amphetamine use during pregnancy was associated with a higher rate of premature births and congenital brain lesions.

There is virtually no research into the long-term effects of maternal amphetamine use on the growth patterns of the infant following birth (Bell & Lau, 1995; Catanzarite & Stein, 1995). There is evidence to suggest that maternal use of methamphetamine may result in premature birth, poor intrauterine growth, and a tendency for the placenta to separate from the wall of the uterus (Catanzarite & Stein). Other possible complications of maternal amphetamine use during pregnancy include meconium aspiration, placental hemorrhage, and neonatal anemia (Beebe & Walley, 1995).

Following birth, children born to mothers who abused amphetamines during pregnancy may experience abnormal psychosocial development (Bell & Lau, 1995) or frontal lobe dysfunction (Beebe & Walley, 1995). However, most normal developmental milestones are achieved on time, and there is little firm evidence of long-term damage to the fetus or neonate (Pirozzolo & Bonnefil, 1995).[5] Thus, it is difficult to predict what long-term effects maternal amphetamine use during pregnancy will have on the child following birth.

Narcotic Analgesic Use/Abuse during Pregnancy

If a pregnant woman were to use a narcotic, the drug would cross the placenta and enter the bloodstream of the fetus. Because of the ability of narcotic analgesics to cross over from the mother's circulation to that of the fetus, it is estimated that each year approximately 300,000 children are exposed to narcotics in utero in this country (Glantz & Woods, 1993).

Not all these children are exposed to illicit narcotics. Each year, it is estimated that 1% to 21% of expectant mothers will use a narcotic analgesic at least once during pregnancy (Behnke & Eyler, 1993). Most of these women are using narcotic pharmaceuticals under a physician's supervision, for medically necessary reasons, and their use of the narcotic analgesic is limited to periods of medical necessity. But, an estimated 650,000 women have used heroin at least once, and approximately 88,000 women use heroin on a regular basis (Bell & Lau, 1995). Some of these women will be of childbearing

age, and a significant percentage of those women who use heroin on a regular basis will do so while they are pregnant. In the United States, maternal heroin abuse accounts for almost a quarter of all cases of fetal exposure to illegal drugs (American Academy of Family Physicians, 1990b). Each year in this country, some 9000 (Bell & Lau, 1995; Glantz & Woods, 1993) to 10,000 (Zuckerman & Bresnahan, 1991) children are born to women who are addicted to narcotics.

Many of the early symptoms of pregnancy, feelings of fatigue, nausea, vomiting, pelvic cramps, and hot sweats, might be interpreted by the narcotics-addicted woman as early withdrawal symptoms, rather than possible pregnancy (Levy & Rutter, 1992). Even physicians experienced in the treatment of narcotics addiction find it difficult to diagnose pregnancy in the narcotics-addicted women, according to the authors. All too often, rather than to seek prenatal care for her unborn child, the woman herself will initially try to self-medicate what she believes is "withdrawal," by using even higher doses of narcotics. This results in the fetus being exposed to significant levels of narcotic analgesics (and the chemicals that are used to "cut" street narcotics) by a woman who is not yet aware she is pregnant.

Maternal narcotics abuse during pregnancy carries with it a number of serious consequences both for the mother, and for the developing fetus. In addition to the dangers associated with narcotics abuse, the pregnant woman who abuses opioids runs the risk of:

- Septic thrombophlebitis.
- Postpartum hemorrhage.
- Depression.
- Gestational diabetes.
- Eclampsia.
- Death.

Physical complications associated with narcotic abuse during pregnancy include (Chasnoff, 1988; Glantz & Woods, 1993; Hoegerman & Schnoll, 1991; Levy & Rutter, 1992):

- Stillbirth.
- Breech presentation during childbirth.

[5] Of course, there also is no evidence that suggests amphetamine use during pregnancy is safe, either. If only for this reason, amphetamine abuse by the pregnant woman should be discouraged.

- Placental insufficiency.
- Spontaneous abortions.
- Premature delivery.
- Neonatal meconium aspiration syndrome (which may be fatal).
- Neonatal infections acquired through the mother.
- Lower birth weight.
- Neonatal narcotic addiction.

In addition to all these potential complications to pregnancy, children born to women who are addicted to narcotics have a 2 to 3 times higher risk of suffering from SIDS than children whose mothers never used illicit chemicals (Kandall et al., 1993; Pirozzolo & Bonnefil, 1995). Volpe (1995) suggested that the risk of SIDS increased with the severity of the infant's withdrawal from narcotics.

Chronic use of narcotics during pregnancy results in a state of chronic exposure to opiates for the fetus. Such infants are physically dependent on narcotics at birth, because of their passive exposure to the drug. Following birth, the infant will no longer be able to absorb drugs from the mother's blood and will go through drug withdrawal starting 24 to 72 hours of birth. Depending on the specific narcotic(s) being abused by the mother, the withdrawal process may last for weeks, or even months, in the newborn (Hoegerman & Schnoll, 1991; Levy & Rutter, 1992; Volpe, 1995). Pirozzolo and Bonnefil (1995) suggested that the *acute* stage of the neonatal withdrawal syndrome subsides in 3 to 6 weeks, but that a *subacute* stage marked by such symptoms as restlessness, agitation, tremors, and sleep disturbance might continue for 4 to 6 months after the acute stage of withdrawal has ended.

Some of the most immediate symptoms of neonatal narcotic withdrawal include muscle tremors, hyperactivity, hyperirritability, a unique, high-pitched cry, frantic efforts to find comfort, sleep problems, vomiting, loose stools, increased deep muscle reflexes, frequent yawning, sneezing, seizures, increased sweating, dehydration, constant sucking movements, fever, and rapid breathing (Anand & Arnold, 1994). In years past, neonatal narcotics withdrawal resulted in almost a 90% mortality rate (Mirin et al., 1991). The mortality rate has dropped significantly in recent years, in response to increased

medical awareness of the special needs of the addicted infant and improved withdrawal programs for such children, according to the authors.

Surprisingly, in light of the dangers of maternal narcotics abuse to the fetus, it is not recommended that the mother be withdrawn from opioids during pregnancy. Hoegerman and Schnoll (1991) warned that, except in extreme circumstances, the dangers associated with maternal narcotics withdrawal during pregnancy outweigh the potential for harm to the developing fetus. The authors recognize that infants born to mothers who are addicted to narcotics present special needs, and require specialized care, to survive the first few days of life and beyond. But they cite evidence suggesting that maternal narcotics withdrawal during pregnancy may result in extreme stress for the fetus, possibly resulting in fetal death.

It has been recommended that the mother be maintained on methadone during pregnancy. Following delivery, both the mother and child can then be detoxified from narcotics through the use of methadone (Hoegerman & Schnoll, 1991; L. Miller, 1994). One reason this recommendation seems to make sense is that children exposed to narcotic analgesics prior to birth seem to suffer adverse developmental problems only when they are born into an environment with risk factors for developmental dysfunctions such as poverty or indifferent caregivers (Hawley et al., 1995). After following a sample of 330 children, 120 of whom were raised by heroin-dependent parents, researchers at the Hebrew University Medical School in Israel concluded that except for a small percentage of infants with neurological problems, developmental delays noted in children born to heroin-dependent mothers were more the result of environmental deprivation than the effects of prenatal heroin exposure (Fishman, 1996). Thus, with the proper environment, it appears possible for the child to outgrow most, if not all, of the negative effects of prenatal exposure to narcotic analgesics.

Narcotics and Breast-Feeding

The woman who is using narcotics and breast-feeding her child will pass some of the drug on to the infant, through the milk (Lourwood & Riedlinger, 1989). While the effects of a single dose of narcotics have only a minimal impact on the child, prolonged use of narcotics may cause the child to become sleepy, eat poorly, and possibly develop respiratory depression.

Because of the infant's "immature liver metabolizing functions" (Lourwood & Riedlinger, 1989, p. 85), there is a danger that narcotics will accumulate in the child's body if the mother is using a narcotic analgesic during breast-feeding. The baby who is breast-fed by an opiate-abusing mother might actually obtain sufficient amounts of narcotics through breast milk to remain addicted to narcotics (Zuckerman & Bresnahan, 1991).

Marijuana Use during Pregnancy

Some researchers believe that marijuana is the most commonly abused illicit substance by women (Mathias, 1995). In the United States, it has been estimated that 12% of the women who are pregnant in nonghetto urban areas use marijuana at least once during their pregnancy (Pirozzolo & Bonnefil, 1995). A lower estimate of the scope of marijuana use during pregnancy was offered by Mathias, who suggested that 2.9% of the estimated 4 million women who give birth in this country each year, or approximately 119,000 women, use marijuana at least once during pregnancy (Mathias).

Despite these facts, relatively little is known about the effects of marijuana use on either the pregnant mother or the fetus (Dreher, Nugent, & Hudgins, 1994). Research into the possible effects of maternal marijuana use on fetal growth and development often provides only conflicting or inconclusive results, and researchers have yet to uncover a consistent pattern of marijuana-induced effects on the developing fetus. Nahas (1986) concluded that marijuana use during pregnancy might contribute to "intrauterine growth retardation, poor weight gain, prolonged labor, and behavioral abnormalities in the newborn" (p. 83). However, other researchers (Behnke & Eyler, 1993; Day & Richardson, 1991) found conflicting evidence as to whether maternal marijuana use during pregnancy might result in poor intrauterine growth. Thus, it is not yet clear whether marijuana use during pregnancy has an effect on fetal growth.

Roffman and George (1988) reported that several research studies have found significant evidence that marijuana use by the pregnant woman might result in developmental problems such as lowered birth weight, and possible central nervous system abnormalities for the fetus. Bays (1990) reported that women who used marijuana at least once a month during pregnancy have a higher risk of premature delivery, lowered birth weight, and children who were smaller than normal for their gestational age.

On the other hand, Dreher et al. (1994) examined 24 babies born in rural Jamaica, where heavy marijuana use is common. These 24 infants were known to have been exposed to marijuana, and their development was contrasted with 20 infants who were not exposed to marijuana. The authors failed to find *any* developmental differences in the two groups that could be attributed to maternal marijuana use. Where the authors did observe differences between the two groups of infants, it was possible to explain these differences on the basis of the mother's social status.

Marijuana-using mothers were also found to have a greater number of adults living within the household, and to have fewer children within the home. These factors allowed for more care to be given to the newborn than was the case in the homes where the mother did not use marijuana, according to the authors. While these findings are suggestive, there is too little known about either the short-term or long-term effects of maternal marijuana use during pregnancy to allow researchers to reach any definite conclusions (Day & Richardson, 1991). Further, it is not possible at present to isolate the effects of maternal marijuana use from the effects of poor nutrition, maternal use of other drugs, poor prenatal care, or maternal health. However, given the potential lifelong consequences for the child if it should be determined that maternal marijuana use during pregnancy has an impact on the fetus, marijuana use during pregnancy should be discouraged.

Marijuana and Breast-Feeding

THC, the active agent of marijuana, will pass into human milk and be passed on to the infant during breast-feeding. Researchers have found that THC is concentrated in human breast milk, often reaching levels eight times as high as blood plasma levels (Hartman, 1995). This would suggest that maternal marijuana use might have some impact on the infant if the mother breast-feeds her child. Breast-feeding by mothers who smoke marijuana is thought to result in slower motor development for the child in the first year of life (Frank, Bauchner, Zucker-man, & Fried, 1992; Pediatrics for Parents, 1990). Admittedly, this is based on a preliminary study of the effects of the mother's use of marijuana on the infant's development, but it suggests a potential hazard that should be avoided, if at all possible.

Benzodiazepine Use during Pregnancy

There is some question as to whether women who are pregnant, especially those in the first trimester of pregnancy, should use any of the benzodiazepines. In the 1970s, clinical reports began to surface that suggested the benzodiazepines might contribute to the formation of cleft palates in children. However, this conclusion was not supported by further research (L. Miller, 1994).

Nevertheless, benzodiazepine use during pregnancy has continued to be challenged. The team of Laegreid et al. (1990) concluded that there was sufficient evidence of benzodiazepine-induced damage to the developing fetus that these drugs should be used only with extreme caution by pregnant women.

In contrast to this conclusion, however, Miller (1994) suggested that "If there is a link between diazepam and oral clefts, it is a weak one" (p. 69). The author reported that only 0.4% of the children born to mothers who had used benzodiazepines during pregnancy suffered from facial development problems, and that most of these could be corrected through surgery. However, the author noted, animal research did suggest *possible* neurological changes in the offspring who were exposed to benzodiazepines prenatally. Thus, until further research determines whether there is potential danger to the fetus, the benefits of benzodiazepine use during pregnancy should be weighed against the potential for harm before these drugs are used.

Benzodiazepine Use during Breast-Feeding

Since the benzodiazepines are found in the nursing mother's milk, Graedon & Graedon (1996) suggests that nursing mothers also not use benzodiazepines. Lourwood and Riedlinger (1989) concluded that nursing mothers should not use any of

the benzodiazepines since these drugs are metabolized mainly by the liver, an organ not fully developed in the infant.

Hallucinogen Use during Pregnancy

There is only limited research into the effects of maternal hallucinogen abuse on fetal growth and development.

PCP Abuse during Pregnancy

Tabor, Smith-Wallace, and Yonekura (1990) compared the birth records of 37 children born between 1982 and 1987, whose medical records indicated that the mothers had used PCP during pregnancy. The authors then compared the birth records against those of infants born to mothers who had abused cocaine during pregnancy. It was concluded that the majority of the women in both groups had minimal prenatal care, a factor that might influence the growth and development of the fetus, and most of the women in the study were polydrug users. However, on the basis of their study, the authors concluded that infants who were exposed to PCP in utero had a high incidence of intrauterine growth retardation and premature labor, and often required extended hospitalization following birth. Infants born to women who had used PCP during pregnancy also seemed to experience abrupt changes in the level of consciousness, fine tremors, sweating, and were irritable, according to Tabor et al. (1990).

Buspirone Use during Pregnancy

Buspirone has not been studied in sufficient detail to determine whether there is a potential for harm to the human fetus (L. Miller, 1994). Animal research involving rats found an increased risk for stillbirth when buspirone was used at high dosage levels, but there did not appear to be any effect on the speed with which newborn rats were able to learn, their level of motor activity, or their emotional development, according to the author.

Bupropion Use during Pregnancy

The effects of bupropion on the developing fetus has not been studied in detail (L. Miller, 1994).

Disulfiram Use during Pregnancy

Disulfiram is not recommended for use in pregnant women (Miller, 1994). Animal research suggests that the combination of alcohol with disulfiram is potentially dangerous for the fetus, according to the author. Further, there is evidence, based on animal research, that suggests that a metabolite of disulfiram, diethyldithiocarbamate, may bind to lead, allowing this metal to then cross the blood-brain barrier and reach the central nervous system. Lead is a known toxin, which may cause neurological disorders and mental retardation. There is a need for further research into this potential danger, to determine whether disulfiram may contribute to higher lead levels in humans.

Cigarette Use during Pregnancy

Approximately 20% of the estimated 4 million women who give birth in this country each year smoke during their pregnancy (Mathias, 1995). This figure translates into approximately 820,000 pregnant women each year in the United States who smoke. Byrd and Howard (1995) give an even higher estimate of 1 million infants each year who are exposed to cigarette smoke prenatally. This number translates into 29% of the infants born in the United States each year, according to the authors. An additional 22% of all infants are exposed to secondhand, or "environmental," cigarette smoke, although their mothers did not themselves smoke cigarettes (Byrd & Howard).

Prenatal exposure to cigarette smoke is a known risk factor for numerous fetal developmental problems. It has been suggested that, in terms of fetal development, maternal cigarette use during pregnancy might be *worse than maternal cocaine use* (Cotton, 1994). Medical researchers have long known that children born to mothers who smoke cigarettes during pregnancy are likely to weigh an average of 200 grams less at birth than children born to nonsmoking mothers (Bell & Lau, 1995; Byrd & Howard, 1995). The American Medical Association (AMA) (1993a) estimated that 20% to 30% of the problem of low birth-weight children could be traced to maternal tobacco use. Further, nicotine use during pregnancy seems to be associated with such problems as premature labor and delivery and stillbirth.

Pregnant women who smoke have a 30% higher risk of stillbirth. Indeed, even after the child is born there is a 26% higher risk of having the infant die within the first few days of life for the mother who smoked during pregnancy (Bell & Lau, 1995). Women who smoke (or who are exposed to cigarette smoke) during pregnancy are more likely to suffer spontaneous abortion, a decrease in the blood flow to the uterus, and an increased chance of vaginal bleeding (Lee & D'Alonzo, 1993). Women who smoke during pregnancy are also at risk for a premature rupture of membranes, and both delayed crying time, and decreased fetal breathing time, following birth (Graedon & Graedon, 1996).

There is also evidence that maternal cigarette smoking during pregnancy may contribute to neurological problems for the developing fetus, and, following birth, for cognitive developmental problems for the child (Olds, Henderson, & Tatelbaum, 1994). The authors found in their study that children born to mothers who smoked 10 or more cigarettes a day during pregnancy scored an average of 4.35 points lower on a standardized intelligence test at ages 3 to 4 years than did children born to nonsmoking mothers. The authors concluded that the observed effects were due to maternal cigarette use during pregnancy.

There is also a growing body of literature that suggests maternal cigarette use during pregnancy is a risk factor for the development of attention-deficit/hyperactivity disorder (ADHD) (Milberger, Biederman, Faraone, Chen, & Jones 1996). Maternal cigarette use during pregnancy has also been linked to such neurodevelopmental problems as impulsiveness, although it is not clear what role cigarette smoking plays in the development of these problems (Day & Richardson, 1994). Finally, after examining the records of some 1.57 million births in Hungary over a 10-year period, Czeizel, Kodaj, and Lenz (1994) concluded that maternal cigarette smoking was a risk factor for the condition known as *congenital limb deficiency* (a failure for the limbs of the fetus to develop properly). The authors hypothesized that nicotine's ability to disrupt blood flow patterns to the uterus might be the cause of this developmental abnormality.

Infants born to smoking mothers appear to suffer from reduced lung capacity, with such infants experiencing an average of a 10% reduction in lung function (Byrd & Howard, 1995). Finally, infants who are exposed to cigarette smoke suffer a significantly higher rate of SIDS than infants who are not exposed to this environmental hazard. Researchers in England have found that for each hour that a newborn infant is exposed to cigarette smoke, his/her risk of SIDS increases 100% ("Tobacco Smoke," 1996). Thus, as these various studies suggest, maternal cigarette use during pregnancy carries with it a number of risks for the infant before and after birth.

Cigarette Smoking during Breast-Feeding

Medical research would suggest that the mother abstain from cigarette use during the period that she is breast-feeding the infant. Nicotine tends to concentrate in breast milk, with a half-life in breast milk of 1.5 hours (Byrd & Howard, 1995). The total concentration of nicotine in the woman's breast milk is dependent on the number of cigarettes she smokes, and the time between the last cigarette and the time she breast feeds the infant, according to the authors. Nicotine itself has been shown to interfere with the process of breast-feeding, reducing the amount of milk produced and the process of milk ejection (the "let down" reflex) (Byrd & Howard). Infants who are breast-fed by cigarette-smoking mothers tend to put on weight more slowly than breast-fed infants whose mothers do not smoke.

Over-the-Counter Analgesic Use during Pregnancy

Aspirin

Women who are, or who suspect that they might be, pregnant should not use aspirin except under the supervision of a physician (Shannon et al., 1995). Aspirin has been implicated as a cause of decreased birth weight in children born to women who used it during pregnancy. There is also evidence that suggests that aspirin may be a cause of

stillbirth and increased perinatal mortality (United States Pharmacopeial Convention, 1990).

Briggs, Freeman, and Yaffe (1986) explored the impact of maternal aspirin use on the fetus, and on the infant whose mother was breast-feeding. The authors reported that the use of aspirin by the mother during pregnancy might produce "anemia, antepartum and/or postpartum hemorrhage, prolonged gestation and prolonged labor" (p. 26a). Aspirin has also been implicated in significantly higher perinatal mortality and retardation of intrauterine growth when used at high doses by pregnant women (Briggs et al., 1986).

The authors noted that maternal use of aspirin in the week before delivery might interfere with the infant's ability to form blood clots following birth. The United States Pharmacopeial Convention (1990) went further than this, warning that women should not use aspirin in the last two weeks of pregnancy. Aspirin has been found to cross the placenta, and research has suggested that maternal aspirin use during pregnancy might result in higher levels of aspirin in the fetus than in the mother (Briggs et al., 1986).

Chasnoff (1988) noted that since the liver of the fetus is not fully developed, it is often difficult to predict the fate and effect of any drug in the fetus's body. Furthermore, the fetus often lacks the highly developed renal function of the mother, making it difficult for a drug to be excreted even if the fetus could metabolize the drug into an excretable form. Shannon et al. (1995) do not recommend any use of aspirin by pregnant women, especially those in the last trimester of pregnancy.

Briggs et al. (1986) observed that, in addition to the more traditional forms of aspirin, many "hidden" forms of this drug are also consumed during pregnancy. Chasnoff (1988) reported that between 50% and 60% of pregnant women use some form of analgesic during their pregnancy. Such a large number of women using various chemicals, under poorly controlled conditions, makes it most difficult to assess the impact of aspirin use on the fetus or nursing mother, according to Briggs et al. (1986).

However, the authors warn that pregnant women should not use aspirin or products that contain aspirin on the grounds that the benefit/risk ratio of such drug use has not been established. Although there have been no proven problems in women who breast-feed their children, the use of aspirin in women who choose to breast-feed is also not recommended (Briggs et al., 1986; United States Pharmacopeial Convention, 1990). Lourwood and Riedlinger (1989) recommended that nursing mothers on "high continuing doses" (p. 84) of aspirin should not breast-feed, but did not warn against occasional use of aspirin by breast-feeding women.

Acetaminophen

Acetaminophen was found to be "safe for short-term use" at recommended dosage levels by pregnant women (Briggs et al., 1986, p. 2a). There have been no reports of serious problems in women who have used acetaminophen during pregnancy. The authors noted, however, that the death of one infant from kidney disease shortly after birth was attributed to the mother's continuous use of acetaminophen at high dosage levels during pregnancy. However, there is a need for further research into the effects of this analgesic during pregnancy.

Although acetaminophen is excreted in low concentrations in the mother's breast milk, Briggs et al. (1986) found no evidence suggesting that this had adverse effects on the infant. However, since acetaminophen is metabolized mainly by the liver, which is still quite immature in the newborn child, Lourwood and Riedlinger (1989) suggested that the mother who breast-feeds during the immediate postpartum period not use this drug. However, the authors did not warn against the occasional use of acetaminophen in women who are breast-feeding their children after the postpartum period.

Ibuprofen

It is not recommended that ibuprofen be used during pregnancy. When used at therapeutic dosage levels, this drug was not reported to cause congenital birth defects (Briggs et al., 1986). However, similar drugs have been known to inhibit labor, prolong pregnancy, and potentially cause other problems for the developing child.

Research suggests that ibuprofen does not enter into human milk in significant quantities when used at normal dosage levels (Briggs et al., 1986) and is considered "compatible with breast feeding" (p. 217i). Lourwood and Riedlinger (1989) reported that ibuprofen was "felt to be the safest" of the nonsteroidal antiinflammatory drugs for women who are breast-feeding a child.

Inhalant Abuse during Pregnancy

Virtually nothing is known about the effects of the inhalants on the developing fetus. Although only a small percentage of those who experiment with inhalants go on to abuse these chemicals on a chronic basis, more than 50% of those persons who chronically abuse inhalants are women "in their prime childbearing years" (Pearson, Hoyme, Seaver, & Rimsza, 1994, p. 211). It is thus safe to assume that some children are being exposed to one or more of the inhalants during gestation.

Researchers have just started to study the effects of toluene inhalation on the developing fetus. Toluene is found in many forms of paint and solvents. It is known to cross the placenta into the fetal circulation when the mother inhales toluene fumes. In adults, about 50% of the toluene inhaled is biotransformed into hippuric acid, and the remainder is excreted unchanged (Pearson et al., 1994). But neither the fetus, nor the newborn child, has the ability to metabolize toluene. There is thus some question as to whether the effects of toluene exposure for the fetus or newborn would be the same as it would be for the adult who inhaled toluene fumes.

To attempt to answer this question, Pearson et al. (1994) examined 18 infants who were exposed to toluene through maternal paint sniffing during pregnancy. It was found that there were several similarities between the effects of toluene on the developing fetus and the effects of alcohol on the fetus. The authors found that like the FAS, toluene exposure during pregnancy may cause a wide range of problems, including premature birth, craniofacial abnormalities (abnormal ears, thin upper lip, small nose, etc.), abnormal muscle tone, renal abnormalities, developmental delays, abnormal scalp hair patterns, and retarded physical growth.

To explain the similarity between the effects of toluene abuse and alcohol abuse on the developing fetus, the authors hypothesized that toluene and alcohol might both result in a state of maternal toxicity. This state of maternal toxicity would, in turn, contribute to the fetal malformations seen in cases of toluene and alcohol exposure during pregnancy. While the authors' work is only preliminary, it appears that toluene exposure during pregnancy may have lifelong consequences for the developing fetus. Until proven otherwise, it would be safe to assume that maternal abuse of the other inhalants would have similar destructive effects on the growing fetus.

Blood Infections

The woman who abuses injected drugs such as the narcotics or cocaine, and who shares intravenous needles, runs the risk of contracting any of a number of infections from other addicts. If the woman becomes infected and is pregnant, the fetus may be exposed to the same infection. The children born of mothers who use intravenously administered drugs may develop any of the blood infections commonly found in addicted persons.

It is quite possible for the fetus to acquire AIDS through the mother's blood. Pope and Morin (1990) reported that in New York City, 2% of the babies born have HIV antibodies in their blood at the time of birth. Almost one-third of the children born to a woman infected with HIV will themselves be infected with the virus (Glantz & Woods, 1993). It is not possible to determine which children are infected with HIV at the time of birth. Only 30% to 50% of the children who test positive for HIV at birth actually are infected (Revkin, 1989). The other children are "false positives" caused by maternal antibodies that normally circulate in the blood of the fetus before delivery.

These antibodies from the mother's blood may remain in the child's system for up to a year following delivery (McCutchan, 1990). During this period, the mother will not know whether she has a healthy child, or a child infected with HIV. This makes it difficult for the mother to bond with the child, since, in addition to having to struggle with the reality of her own infection with HIV-1, she will not know whether the child is infected or not.

The transmission of blood-borne infections from mother to child is often thought of as an uncommon problem. Yet, in some populations, a significant percentage of the children born have been exposed to one or more infections as a result of the mother's use of intravenous drugs. These children are indeed hidden victims of drug addiction.

Summary

If a substance abusing woman is pregnant, the fetus that she carries becomes an unwilling participant in the mother's chemical use/abuse. However, the impact of the chemical use is often much greater on the growing fetus than it is on the mother. Because of this fact, infants born to women who have used chemicals of abuse during pregnancy represent a special subpopulation of alcohol/drug users. The child who was exposed to recreational chemicals did not willingly participate in the process of chemical use, yet his/her life might be profoundly affected by the effects of alcohol/drugs.

An extreme example of the unwilling participation of infants in maternal alcohol or drug use is when the child is born already addicted to the chemicals which the mother used during pregnancy. Other fetal complications of maternal chemical abuse might include stroke, retardation, or lower weight at birth, as well as a number of other drug-specific complications. The over-the-counter analgesics present a special area of risk, for the effects of these medications on fetal growth and development are not understood well. However, available research suggests that the OTC analgesics should be used with caution by pregnant or nursing women. Finally, the transmission of blood infections between the mother who shares hypodermic needles with other addicts and the fetus was discussed.

CHAPTER TWENTY-ONE

Hidden Faces of Chemical Dependency

There are many faces to chemical dependency. There is the stereotype of the "typical" skid row alcoholic, drinking a bottle of cheap wine wrapped in a plain brown paper bag. Another popular image is that of the young male heroin addict, with a belt wrapped around his arm, pushing a needle into a vein. A popular stereotype of the chemically addicted woman is of the "fallen" woman, who is immoral, often a neglectful parent, and most certainly not of the middle or upper social classes.

As Schneiderman (1990) observed, popular stereotypes of the person who is addicted to chemicals are persistent and often grossly inaccurate. Further, popular stereotypes serve to limit our vision. If the addicted person deviates from our expectation, we may not recognize the chemical dependency hiding behind the social facade. For example, how many of us would expect to meet a white, middle-class, well-groomed heroin addict at work? How many people would recognize the benzodiazepine-dependency behind the smiling face of a day-care worker?

This chapter explores some of the hidden faces of chemical dependency, so that the reader may become more sensitive to the many forms that substance abuse can take.

Women and Addiction: An Often Unrecognized Problem

Although health care professionals have struggled to come to terms with the growing problem of alcohol/drug abuse in the United States for more than a generation, women with substance use problems continue to form an invisible minority. To protect ourselves from the reality that alcohol/ drug addiction can strike any person, the woman with a substance use problem is viewed as being "poor or sexually available or weak and stupid" (Lawson, 1994, p. 138). All too often, she is viewed as being defective in some ill-defined way.

It has only been since the mid 1980s that substance abuse rehabilitation professionals have paid much attention to the problem of recreational chemical use/abuse among women (Blume, 1994; Brady, Grice, Dustan, & Randall, 1993; Griffin et al., 1989; Lawson, 1994). With the growing awareness that significant numbers of women have developed substance use problems, many of the popular misconceptions have fallen. But, there is still much to learn about the impact of chemical abuse on women and the most effective treatment methods for this population.

The "Convergence" Theory

Most people in "polite" society did not accept the fact that substance misuse was a very real problem for women in the United States in the last century. The truth is, that by the last years of the 19th century, the ratio of men to women who were addicted to chemicals was 1 : 2 (Lawson, 1994). It is only now, a century later, that health care professionals in the United States are starting to become more receptive to the possibility that women were abusing/becoming addicted to chemicals in numbers similar to that seen in males.

In the 1980s drug abuse rehabilitation professionals began to speak of a "convergence" in alcohol use patterns, and suggested that greater numbers of women were abusing, or becoming addicted to, alcohol with each passing year. Health care professionals began to speak about the possibility that an equal number of men and women had substance use problems. Fortunately, there is little empirical evidence to support the concept of "convergence" in alcohol use rates (Anthony, Arria, & Johnson, 1995). The percentage of women who have chemical use problems appears to be relatively stable and far lower than the percentage of men with substance use problems, according to the author. Thus, while the "convergence" theory was a popular myth in the 1980s and early 1990s, there is little evidence to suggest that it is more than a myth.

Statement of the Problem

It is believed that fully 40% of those who are physically dependent on chemicals are women (D. Anderson, 1993; Lawson. 1994). One of every three alcohol-dependent individuals is a woman (North, 1996). Yet, even though women make up such a large percentage of those who are addicted to chemicals, they are underserved both in terms of the number of treatment programs designed to meet their needs, "and of quality of service" by the treatment industry (Levers & Hawes, 1990, p. 528). For example, while many treatment program directors would dispute this claim, fewer than one-third of the treatment programs surveyed were found to have specialized treatment components for women (Wilsnack, 1991). D. Anderson (1993) arrived at an even more depressing figure, stating that only 10% of the treatment programs in this country are designed with the woman's special needs in mind. Yet 25% of those admitted for treatment for alcohol addiction are women ("Study: Cocaine Treatment," 1994).

These are inadequate resources to offer rehabilitation programs for all of the women who abuse or are addicted to chemicals. This situation is so dismal that some authors have concluded that that treatment industry as a whole has failed to meet the needs of women who are addicted to chemicals (M. Alexander, 1996; Levy & Rutter, 1992). Even now, more than a decade after rehabilitation professionals have concluded that women present special needs during treatment for substance use problems, they remain underserved, and their needs are virtually ignored.

Gender and the Rehabilitation Process

In the past 20 years, researchers have discovered significant differences in the way that an addictive disorder evolves for men and women. Women who are addicted to chemicals also present special needs in a rehabilitation setting (Kauffman, Dore, & Nelson-Zlupko, 1995). Women who are addicted to chemicals are more likely to present a history of having been exposed to some form of interpersonal violence than are men who are addicted to chemicals (Del Boca & Hesselbrock, 1996; Miller & Downs, 1995; O'Connor, Samet, & Stein, 1994).

Women who are dependent on alcohol are also more likely to suffer from problems with their self-esteem than men who are alcohol-dependent (M. Alexander, 1996; Beckman, 1994; North, 1996). There is some evidence to suggest that drug abuse represents an attempt on the part of the woman to self-medicate her feelings of low self-worth (M. Alexander). Further, alcohol-dependent women are 4 times more likely to be living with a partner who also has an alcohol use problem (Miller & Cervantes, 1997). Because of this, many women report that they receive less support from their partner for efforts to abstain from chemical use than do men (Kauffman et al., 1995).

Women who are addicted to a chemical(s) tend to have fewer social supports than their male counterparts (Kauffman et al., 1995). For example, it is not uncommon for the woman to be granted custody of the children following divorce, on the grounds that the children should live with their mother. Few substance abuse rehabilitation programs have provisions for taking care of the children while the parent is in treatment. Thus, if a woman needs to enter an inpatient rehabilitation program for a substance use problem, she could find that having custody of the children is a barrier to her participating in the treatment that she needs (Beckman, 1994; Kauffman et al., 1995; Raskin, 1994).

Further, women often feel inhibited in mixed groups, especially if they have been victimized in some way (M. Alexander, 1996). The language used by many men in the therapeutic setting intimidates many women, and in some cases may even revictimize them as memories of past abuse surface. Women have been found to speak less in mixed-group treatment settings than if they are in a unisex group. Indeed, it has been found that women who have been sexually abused are more likely to drop out of mixed-group treatment settings than if they are treated in women-only facilities.

Treatment staff must be alert to the subtle ways that the issues of substance abuse, gender identification, and victimization issues might intertwine in order to effectively work with the woman with a substance use problem. They must be able to help the woman establish a support system that will encourage her to remain abstinent from chemicals. Further, to work effectively, rehabilitation professionals must also understand how a woman's self-esteem might influence not only her chemical use pattern, but, the treatment process. Finally, rehabilitation staff need to understand the differing role of social expectations on the evolution of substance use disorders in men and women (Del Boca & Hesselbrock, 1996). Yet, as stated earlier, few treatment settings have gender-specific programs designed by, and for, women.

As a general rule, when women who are addicted enter into the rehabilitation system, they do so in a far different manner than do their male counterparts (M. Alexander, 1996; Weisner & Schmidt, 1992). When compared with male addicts, women are less likely to enter treatment as a result of a physician, employer, or court referral (Beckman, 1994). Rather, women tend to enter treatment programs through advertisements in the media or on the referral of a friend, according to the author. Once in treatment, women tend to present different needs than do male clients. For example, alcohol-addicted women are far more likely to suffer from a primary depression than are men who are addicted to alcohol (Blume, 1994). Further, the impact of a depressive disorder is different for alcohol-dependent men than it is for women addicted to alcohol (Hill, 1995). There is, according to Hill, significant evidence to suggest that the presence of a depressive disorder is usually associated with a more favorable outcome for alcohol-dependent women, and just the opposite for male alcoholics.

The team of Schutte, Moos, and Brennan (1995) examined the symptoms of depression and alcohol use in a sample of 621 women and 951 men, all of whom were in middle adulthood. The authors followed their research sample for 3 years and found that, for the women, alcohol use seemed to reflect a process of self-medication. The authors concluded that the depressed women in their sample were using alcohol to reduce their depression-induced emotional distress. The symptoms of depression would then serve as drinking cues, which would result in further alcohol use.

For the men in the sample (Schutte et al., 1995), however, depression seemed to be associated with a *decrease* in alcohol use. This suggests that (a) the men were less likely to try to self-medicate a depressive disorder through alcohol use, and (b) there are different pathways to alcohol dependence for men and women. Women initially tend to seek help from mental health rather than substance abuse rehabilitation professionals (Weisner & Schmidt, 1992). Men who are addicted to chemicals, on the other hand, are less likely to attempt to self-medicate emotional distress and thus tend to become involved with substance abuse treatment professionals immediately.

Finally, the resources that the addicted woman can call on in her effort to abstain from chemicals are often different from the resources available to the male addict. Thus, to work effectively with a woman addicted to alcohol or drug(s), staff must carefully assess her social support system to identify potential barriers to treatment, as well as individual traits that might contribute to relapse.

Work, Gender, and Chemical Abuse

At one point, it was thought that women who enter the workforce were thought to be 2 to 3 times as likely to develop problems with alcohol as those who do not (Kruzicki, 1987). Subsequent research, however, failed to document such a relationship between employment status and alcoholism (Wilsnack & Wilsnack, 1995; Wilsnack, Wilsnack, & Hiller-Sturmhoffel, 1994). In fact, the increased social status, social support, and improved self-esteem that go along with full-time paid employment seem to help reduce the chances that the working woman will abuse or become dependent on alcohol, according to the authors.

An employment variable that does seem to be associated with an increased risk of alcohol abuse for women is working in a nontraditional, male-dominated profession (Wilsnack & Wilsnack, 1995; Wilsnack et al., 1994). Women employed in a profession where more than 50% of their co-workers are males tend to report higher levels of alcohol use problems, according to the authors. However, male alcohol use patterns do not seem to be affected by the gender of their co-workers, again suggesting that there are different pathways to alcohol use problems for men and women.

Many women in the workforce are working below their potential work capacity, often in low status-high frustration positions. Because of this, it is often more difficult to detect problem chemical use in the working woman who has a substance use problem (Pape, 1988). Being underemployed, their chemical use is less likely to interfere with their job performance than it is for a man (Kruzicki, 1987). This makes it more difficult to detect the woman whose job performance is impaired by drug or alcohol use.

Also, the threat of loss of employment if the addicted woman does not seek treatment is not as effective as it is for men, since many women work only to supplement their husband's income. It is often easier for such a women to simply quit her job than to give in to a threatened loss of employment if she does not seek treatment (Pape, 1988).

Victimization Histories and Substance Use Patterns

Research has shown that women who are addicted to alcohol are 2.5 times as likely to report having been sexually abused in childhood as nonalcoholic women (Miller & Downs, 1995). Further, up to 85% of the women in treatment for alcohol dependence give a history of having been an incest victim (Beckman, 1994). As these statistics suggest, there appears to be a tendency for those women who are treated for a substance use problem to have been the victim of some form of interpersonal violence (M. Alexander, 1996).

Gender and Substance Use Patterns

Within the past generation, researchers have discovered that women usually obtain their drug of choice in different ways than do men. Unlike male addicts, many women who are addicted to chemicals obtain the drugs from their own physician. Indeed, it has been suggested that sedatives and "diet pills" have become "women's drugs" (Peluso & Peluso, 1988, p. 10). Nearly 70% of all prescriptions for psychotropic medications are written for women (Cohen et al., 1996). But, because these women obtain their drug of choice through a physician's prescription and the local pharmacy, their drug abuse problem, all too often, has "been rendered invisible" (Peluso & Peluso, 1988, p. 9).

Differing Effects of Common Drugs of Abuse on Men and Women

As medical researchers learn more about the effects of various drugs on men and women, they are discovering significant differences in the responses of each gender to specific chemicals. Not surprisingly, there are also differences in how men and women react when they use one or more of the popular drugs of abuse.

Narcotics Abuse and Gender

Griffin et al. (1989) found that the woman who was addicted to narcotics was likely to have started using opiates at a significantly older age than her male counterparts. But as a general rule, the typical narcotics-addicted woman will have a history of heavier drug use than male addicts, according to the authors. At the same time, the authors found that women addicted to narcotics were approximately the same age as men at the time of their first admission into drug treatment.

There appear to be differences in how male and female narcotics addicts use their drug of choice. In England, the team of Gossop, Battersby, and Strang (1991) found that male narcotics addicts were more likely to inject their drug, while female narcotics addicts were more likely to inhale narcotic powder. Female addicts were also more likely to be involved in a sexual relationship with another drug user than were male narcotics addicts. Finally, just under half of the female narcotics addicts studied by the authors had received drugs as a present from a sexual partner, according to the authors. These facts suggest that narcotics addiction follows dissimilar courses for men and women.

Cocaine Abuse and Gender

Research has also revealed contrasting cocaine use patterns between men and women. Although women make up approximately 50% of those addicted to cocaine (Lawson, 1994), Griffin et al. (1989) found that female cocaine abusers started drug use at an earlier age than did male cocaine abusers.

Further, the authors found that the typical woman cocaine addict was significantly younger at the time of her first admission to a drug treatment program than her male counterpart. The authors also found that male and female cocaine addicts were introduced to the drug in different ways. Again, these findings suggest that cocaine abuse follows a distinct course for each sex. Yet, research into narcotic and cocaine addiction has failed to compare the diverse effects of chemicals on women and men.

Alcohol Abuse and Gender

In the past generation, it has gradually been accepted that alcohol affects men and women differently. For example, the blood alcohol level (BAL) of a woman would be up to 40% higher than that of a man who had consumed a given amount of alcohol (North, 1996). Thus, as a general rule, women tend to require less alcohol to become intoxicated than

do men. Further, the monthly variations in estrogen levels can affect the speed with which the woman's body absorbs alcohol, while oral contraceptive medications used by women can slow the biotransformation of the alcohol already in the body (North, 1996).

There is significant evidence suggesting that women may be more sensitive to the destructive effects of alcohol than are men (Nixon, 1994). One begins to see alcohol-related physical problems in female alcohol abusers at just one-third the level of alcohol intake necessary for the typical male alcohol abuser to experience similar problems (North, 1996). Further, women appear to be more sensitive to the toxic effects of alcohol on striated muscle tissues such as the tissues of the heart than are male alcohol users (Urbano-Marquez et al., 1995). Thus, it should not be surprising that women with alcohol-use problems tend to develop alcohol-related health problems earlier in their drinking history than is generally the case for male alcohol abusers.

Alcoholic women develop cirrhosis of the liver about 13 years after they become addicted to alcohol, while it might take the typical male alcoholic 22 years to develop the same disorder (Blume, 1994; Hennessey, 1992). In addition, there is a known association between alcohol abuse and infertility, miscarriage, amenorrhea, uterine bleeding, dysmenorrhea, osteoporosis and, possibly, breast cancer (Cyr & Moulton, 1993; Hennessey, 1992). Despite this known association between alcohol abuse/addiction and illness, physicians often fail to recognize the signs of alcohol addiction in female patients (Kitchens, 1994; North, 1996).

Gender group membership is now considered a major variable in defining the developmental pathway of different subtypes of alcohol abuse/addiction (Del Boca & Hesselbrock, 1996). Research has uncovered at least two subforms of alcohol dependence in women (Hill, 1995). The first group, comprising a minority of women drinkers, appears to include those women whose alcoholism finds full expression between the ages of 18 and 24 years of age. These women might be said to have "early-onset" (Hill, 1995, p. 11) alcohol dependence, and their drinking pattern tends to be atypical. In contrast, however, is the larger group of alcohol-dependent women, classified as the "later-onset" (Hill, p. 11) drinkers, whose drinking seems to reach its peak between the ages of 35 and 49 years of age. However, the relationship between the two subtypes of female alcoholics identified by Hill, and the Type I–Type II typology of alcoholism in males (discussed in Chapter 17), is still not clear.

In their examination of the subtypes of alcoholism, Del Boca and Hesselbrock (1996) concluded that at least two of the four subtypes of alcoholism that they identified were strongly influenced by the individual's gender. On the basis of their data, the authors concluded that there were a number of possible developmental pathways that could result in alcoholism for men and women. While the authors do not explore possible etiologies of these different subforms of alcoholism, their data suggest that the expression of alcoholism for men and women follows traditional gender role expectations in the United States.

However, Miller and Cervantes (1997) suggested a positive note, observing that evidence suggests that women with alcohol use problems are more likely to respond positively to minimal interventions. Further, according to Beckman (1993):

> Women are often first to recognize their drinking problem, while men are more likely to have confrontations, especially with authorities, that bring them involuntarily into contact with treatment caregivers. (p. 236)

Thus, according to the author, women are more accepting of the treatment process, as well as the need for treatment. There is evidence to suggest that one catalyst that helps to bring the substance-abusing woman in for treatment is her responsibility for her children (Kline, 1996).

There are strong social barriers between the recovering woman and community resources such as Alcoholics Anonymous. In addition, significant evidence suggests that when women first enter treatment for alcoholism, their addiction is usually more severe than what one would expect for a man with the same drinking history (Weisner & Schmidt, 1992). Finally, young women apparently are starting to drink alcohol at an earlier age, and in far greater quantities, than did their older counterparts

(Weisner & Schmidt). These facts again suggest that the course of alcoholism is different for men and women.

But just at the time when society is starting to develop an awareness of the impact of alcohol/drug use problems:

> . . . there is evidence that the alcoholic beverage industry has targeted women as a "growth market," with advertising designed to make drinking more acceptable to women and to change their drinking patterns. (Blume, 1994, p. 9)

This is lamentable. It has been argued that, because of the important role women hold as the primary caretaker of the children, society has hesitated to recognize the problem of alcohol/drug addiction in women (Peluso & Peluso, 1988). At the same point in history where society is able to accept that significant numbers of women have substance use problems, new forms of advertising are emerging aimed at making alcohol use more attractive to women. The danger is that by making the use of alcohol seem more attractive to younger generations of women, future generations might witness the convergence in the percentages of men and women with substance use problems originally anticipated in the 1980s. One might only hope that society will learn to face the problem of drug addiction in both men and women with openness, compassion, and unrestricted access to proven treatment methods.

Addiction and the Elderly

As the latest wave of cocaine abuse peaked in the mid-1980s, behavioral scientists began to explore the scope of recreational chemical use/abuse in the general population. They discovered that large numbers of adults were using one or more recreational chemicals in ways that could be defined as abusive. Further, researchers discovered that rather than the later years of life being a time of peace and reflection, recreational chemical use/abuse was a significant problem in old age.

Scope of the Problem

It is difficult to obtain an accurate picture of substance use patterns among the elderly (Cohen et al.,

1996). Nevertheless, researchers believe that alcohol abuse is the third most common form of psychiatric dysfunction in the elderly, surpassed only by the various forms of dementia and anxiety disorders (J. Campbell, 1992). In the typical hospital, 14% of elderly patients seen in the emergency room, 23% to 44% of elderly patients seen in an inpatient psychiatric treatment center, 18% of the patients in general medical beds, and 11% of the elderly patients admitted to a nursing home, have alcohol use problems (Goldstein, Pataki, & Webb, 1996). Estimates of the scope of alcohol abuse/addiction in the general population of older adults runs from a low estimate of 2% to 4% (Brennan & Moos 1996), to a high estimate of 10% to 15% (Zimberg, 1996). In terms of actual numbers, Hyman and Cassem (1995) suggested that 1.5 million individuals over the age of 65 in the United States are alcohol-dependent.

Elderly alcohol abusers are overrepresented in the population of those who are seeking health care for one reason or another. Researchers estimate that between 5% to 15% (Dunne, 1994; Vandeputte, 1989) and 49% (Blake, 1990) of elderly patients seeking medical treatment for one reason or another also have an alcohol/drug-related problem. These estimates are consistent with that of Dunlop, Manghelli, and Tolson (1989) who suggested that 25% of the elderly population might be suffering from alcohol-related problems. Zimberg (1995) suggested that 10% of the men and 20% of the women might be classified as "escape drinkers" (p. 413), who have an alcohol use problem.

Older adults do not experience just alcohol use problems, but also experience problems caused by the abuse of other chemicals. Abrams and Alexopoulos (1987) suggested that "more than 20 percent of patients over 65 years old admitted to a psychiatric hospital in one year could be considered drug dependent" (p. 1286). Szwabo (1993) suggested that 15% to 20% of older adults abuse chemicals other than alcohol. The team of Cohen et al. (1996) suggested that 15% of older adults might be classified as having a drug abuse problem.

Researchers have found that older alcoholics take up a disproportional part of the health care resources in the United States. For example, the team of Adams, Yuan, Barboriak, and Rimm (1993)

examined discharge diagnosis statistics from across the United States, and found that between 19 and 77 of every 10,000 elderly patients admitted to acute care hospitals had an alcohol use disorder. The authors also found that the number of elderly patients being treated for myocardial infarction was between 17 and 44 per 10,000 patient admissions in the same age group. Their figures suggest that the rates of hospital admission for alcohol-related health problems in the elderly was "similar to those for myocardial infarction" (p. 1224) and may even have exceeded that for this form of heart disease in the elderly. This finding is consistent with the finding that families with an alcoholic member have health care costs 21 times as high as similar families without an alcoholic member. Nor is the problem of substance abuse in the older population limited only to alcohol. If these figures are accurate, then it would appear that chemical use problems are commonly found in the elderly.

Why Is the Detection of Substance Use Disorders in the Elderly So Difficult?

Alcohol/drug use problems are often unrecognized among older people (D. Anderson, 1989b; Dunne, 1994; Kitchens, 1994; Rains, 1990). Although this group tends to have more medical problems than do younger adults, physicians are ill-prepared to recognize the signs of substance abuse/addiction in the elderly. First, as discussed in Chapter 1, few physicians are adequately trained in the area of addiction medicine. But, the issue is more complicated than just a lack of physician training. For reasons that are not well understood, older alcoholics appear to be less likely to visit their physician than their nondrinking peers (Rice & Duncan, 1995).

There are many possible reasons why, as a group, older adults with alcohol use disorders are less likely to go to a physician on a regular basis. The older drinker may try to avoid seeing a physician to avoid the danger of having his/her alcohol use disorder discovered by the physician. Also, older drinkers, like their physicians, tend to attribute physical complications caused by their drinking to the aging process, rather than to alcohol use. Thus, older drinkers may avoid seeing a physician because they do not understand the true cause of their medical problem(s).

Another reason alcohol use disorders are so difficult to detect in the older drinker is that the traditional symptoms of excessive drinking, such as the number of drinks consumed, is a poor indicator of alcoholism in the elderly. Older adults tend to consume less alcohol in a given period of time than younger adult drinkers (Zimberg, 1996). At the same time, research has shown that older alcoholics are less able to withstand the physical impact of drinking (Blake, 1990; Rains, 1990). For the typical 60-year-old, just three beers or mixed drinks may have the same effect as 12 beers/mixed drinks at age 21 (D. Anderson, 1989b). Thus, although older drinkers typically consume less alcohol, they are also more affected by the alcohol that they consume than are younger adult drinkers.

This is because the brain becomes more sensitive to the toxic effects of alcohol in the later years (Goldstein et al., 1996). Because of age-related changes in the bodies of older individuals, a given amount of alcohol might cause up to a 20% higher blood alcohol level than would be the case if the drinker were in early adulthood (Goldstein et al.). For an elderly alcohol user, even social drinking might contribute to cognitive deterioration (Abrams & Alexopoulos, 1987; Rains, 1990). Thus, it should not be surprising to discover a "high association between alcoholism and dementia" (Goldstein et al., p. 941).

Although alcohol use/abuse is a known risk factor for the development of a wide range of psychosocial impairments, these problems are not as obvious in the older alcohol-dependent person as in the young adult (Abrams & Alexopoulos, 1987). All too often, alcohol-induced problems such as blackouts, financial problems, and job loss are often attributed to medical or age-related psychosocial problems, not to alcohol (Szwabo, 1993). Many of alcohol's effects on the cognitive abilities of older adults mimic changes associated with normal aging. Even trained physicians find it difficult to differentiate between late-onset Korsak-off's syndrome and forms of senile dementia such as Alzheimer's disease and multiinfarct dementia (D. Anderson, 1989b; Blake, 1990; Rains, 1990).

Another factor that makes the detection of alcoholism in the elderly more difficult than in younger drinkers is that older alcoholics rarely announce their plan to drink in advance (Peluso & Peluso, 1989; Vandeputte, 1989). Just imagine the shock in the family if grandmother, or grandfather, were to announce at the dinner table, "I'm going out tonight and get wasted!" Also, older drinkers tend to be steady drinkers, whereas younger alcohol users tend to be binge drinkers. Finally, because older drinkers tend to consume alcohol in private, rather than in a public setting such as a bar, they rarely get into situations where their drinking is obvious, such as barroom fights. Since their drinking is less obvious, alcohol-related problems such as blackouts are often attributed to a nonalcohol medical problem (Peluso & Peluso).

A final reason alcoholism or drug abuse in the elderly is so difficult to detect and treat is the problem of shame. The older addicted individual, his/her family, and friends may be ashamed, feel hurt, or feel guilty about the problem (Goldstein et al., 1996; Peluso & Peluso, 1989; Vandeputte, 1989). For this reason, family or friends may hesitate to seek help for the person.

What Are the Consequences of Alcohol/Drug Addiction in the Elderly?

Alcohol use/abuse may either directly/indirectly cause, or contribute to, accidental injuries in older adults. In one study, 14% of the elderly patients seen for injuries suffered in motor vehicle accidents were found to have a positive blood alcohol screen (Higgins, Wright, & Wrenn, 1996). In addition, alcohol and/or drug misuse is a major factor in causing older adults to lose their balance, fall, and experience bone fractures (Council on Scientific Affairs, 1996). Thus, one consequence of alcohol use/abuse is that the older drinker is at increased risk of accidental injury as a result of his/her drinking.

In addition, alcohol use may either complicate the treatment of other diseases, or even cause the individual to develop new, possibly life-threatening, medical problems (Vandeputte, 1989). The use of alcohol may alter the way an older individual's body responds to any of the other medications the person might be using for the treatment or control of disease (Goldstein et al., 1996). As a group, the elderly make up 12% of the population, and use 40% of all prescription and over-the-counter medications (Szwabo, 1993). Yet, despite the danger of alcohol-drug interactions, few health care providers search for alcohol use problems in the elderly. The result is, all too often, potentially deadly combinations of medications and alcohol (Peluso & Peluso, 1989).

Further, because they are more vulnerable to the negative effects of alcohol, older drinkers are more likely to experience medical complications as a result of alcohol use than are younger adults (Dunne, 1994; Hurt, Finlayson, Morse, & Davis, 1988; Rains, 1990). Alcohol use in the elderly may either influence the development of, or actually cause, such medical problems as myopathy, cerebrovascular disease, gastritis, diarrhea, pancreatitis, cardiomyopathy, and sleep disorders (Liberto, Oslin, & Ruskin, 1992). Other disorders that might be caused by alcohol use by older individuals include hypertension, diminished resistance to infections, peripheral muscle weakness, electrolyte and metabolic disturbances, and orthostatic hypotension (Szwabo, 1993).

As noted, older drinkers are less likely to seek medical attention for their distress, at least until the complications caused by their drinking become severe enough to require hospitalization. Even when their drinking is identified, few elderly alcoholics receive treatment for their drug addiction (Vandeputte, 1989). Treating these alcohol-induced problems results in increased medical costs for both the individual, and ultimately society.

Although few people stop to consider the possible impact of alcohol/drug use on the mental health of older individuals, substance abuse extracts a terrible toll on the older user's peace of mind. Depression, a common problem in old age, is also a common consequence of alcohol/drug abuse, and it has been estimated that 7% to 30% of all elderly suicide victims have alcohol use problems (Goldstein et al., 1996). If the individual is suffering from a substance-induced depressive episode, a misdiagnosis may result in inappropriate treatment of the individual's mental health problem (Council on Scientific Affairs, 1996; Szwabo, 1993; Vandeputte, 1989). As these studies suggest, alcohol/drug abuse problems are not uncommon in the older population, and are a cause of significant hardship for the addicted individual.

Different Patterns of Alcohol/Drug Abuse in the Elderly

Many older individuals develop alcohol use problems only in their later years (Zimberg, 1996). This phenomenon has been termed *late-onset alcoholism* by Hurt, Finlayson, Morse, and Davis (1988), or "reactive alcoholism" (Peluso & Peluso, 1989). Perhaps as many as 30% to 50% of the elderly alcoholic population actually began to have problems with alcohol only in either middle or late life (Brennan & Moos, 1996; Liberto et al., 1992).

Zimberg (1995) suggested that there were three subgroups of older alcoholics. The first group was made up of those individuals who had no drinking problem in young or middle adulthood, but who developed late-life alcoholism. These individuals could be said to have late-onset alcoholism, according to the author. The second subgroup of older alcoholics had a history of intermittent problem drinking over the years, but developed a more chronic alcohol problem only in late adulthood. This group of individuals could be said to have *late-onset exacerbation* drinking, according to Zimberg. Finally, there were those individuals whose alcohol problems started in young adulthood and continued into the later part of the individual's life. This group is identified as having *early-onset* alcoholism, according to Zimberg.

Drug misuse by the elderly is another form of drug abuse. J. Campbell (1992) estimated that 10% of the elderly misuse prescription medications. Drug misuse was found to take several forms by Abrams and Alexopoulos (1987): (a) intentional overuse of a medication, (b) underuse of a medication, (c) erratic use of a prescribed medication, or (d) the failure of the physician to obtain a complete drug history, including over-the-counter medications. Intentional misuse of prescribed medications was the largest category of drug abuse in the elderly (Abrams & Alexopoulos). However, the authors found that the elderly were far more likely to engage in the *under*utilization as opposed to the overutilization of prescription medications, mainly because of financial limitations.

The Treatment of the Older Alcoholic

Only a minority of elderly persons with a drug or alcohol problem are currently receiving help for that problem. Alcohol/drug addiction in the elderly is simply underrecognized and underreported. Further, in an era of shrinking resources, public health agencies are often overwhelmed with the task of dealing with younger alcohol/drug abusers. Consequently, substance use problems are undertreated in the elderly age group.

Even when older alcoholic/drug abusing patients are referred to treatment, they will present special treatment needs rarely found in younger addicts. Yet few treatment programs are geared to meet their needs (Goldstein et al., 1993). Dunlop et al. (1989) recommend that treatment programs that work with the elderly include the following components:

1. A primary prevention program to warn about the dangers of using alcohol as a coping mechanism for life's problems.
2. An outreach program to identify and serve older alcoholics who might be overlooked by more traditional treatment services.
3. Detoxification service providers trained and experienced in working with the elderly, who frequently require longer detoxification periods than younger addicted persons.
4. Protective (i.e., structured) environments for the elderly that allow the individual to take part in treatment while being protected from the temptation of further alcohol use.
5. Primary treatment programs for those who could benefit from either inpatient or outpatient short-term primary treatment programs.
6. Aftercare programs to help the older alcoholic with the transition between primary care and independent living.
7. Long-term residential care for those individuals who suffer from severe medical and/or psychiatric complications from alcoholism.
8. Access to social support services.

Older alcoholic or drug-abusing patients may require weeks or even months, to fully detoxify from alcohol or drugs (D. Anderson, 1989b). Rains (1990) suggested that older alcoholics may require up to 18 months of abstinence to fully recover from the effects of drinking. Thus, a standard 21- to 28-day inpatient treatment program might not meet the needs of elderly clients, who would hardly have completed the detoxification process before being discharged as "cured." Further, older adults may require more help than younger clients to build a non-alcoholic support structure (D. Anderson, 1989b). Further, older clients often have a slower physical and mental pace than younger individuals, present a range of sensory deficits rarely found in younger clients, and very often dislike the profanity commonly encountered with younger individuals in treatment (Dunlop et al., 1989).

Unless these special needs are addressed, older alcoholics are unlikely to be motivated to participate in treatment. Treatment professionals must help these patients deal with more than the direct effects of chemical addiction. For example, health care professionals need to be aware that, in addition to the drinking problem, older alcoholics may also experiencing age-specific stressors such as retirement, bereavement, loneliness, and the effects of physical illness (Dunlop et al., 1989; Zimberg, 1996).

On the bright side of the coin, however, there is evidence suggesting that late-onset drinkers respond better to treatment than do younger alcoholics (Brennan & Moos, 1996). Group therapy approaches that included a problem-solving and social-support component were thought to be useful in working with the older alcoholic, especially if such programs included exposure to the Alcoholics Anonymous 12-Step program (Dunlop et al., 1989; Rains, 1990; Zimberg, 1978).

The Homosexual and Substance Abuse

Homosexual men and women constitute a hidden minority (Fassinger, 1991, p. 157) within this society. Estimates of the percentage of the population that is "gay" or lesbian vary; high estimates suggest that 20% of adult males have had a homosexual experience, and between 1% to 6% have had a homosexual encounter in the past year (Seidman & Rieder, 1994). Society's response to individuals who have adopted a nontraditional form of sexuality has frequently been less than supportive, and many gay/lesbian individuals feel ostracized by a culture that neither understands, nor encourages, a homosexual lifestyle.

The homosexual may thus live on the fringes of society. Within the gay community, the gay bar assumes special significance, where one may socialize without fear of ridicule, meet potential partners, or simply escape from society in general (Paul, Stall, & Bloomfield, 1991). Further, the homosexual bar continues to play a crucial role in the process of discovering one's sexuality, for both gay men and lesbian women. While the homosexual bar thus might be said to serve a useful function, its central importance within the gay community may contribute to alcohol or drug problems.

There has been very little research into the frequency of alcohol/drug use problems among gay/lesbian individuals (Hughes & Wilsnack, 1997). The limited data available suggest that there is a significantly higher alcoholism rate for gay men/ lesbian women than for the general population. It has been estimated that 25% to 35% of the homosexual population meet the criteria for a formal diagnosis of alcohol/drug dependency (Klinger & Cabaj, 1993). Indeed, evidence suggests that more than half of all lesbians have alcohol use problems, a rate 5 to 7 times higher than that seen in nongay women (North, 1996).

There are several reasons for this association between homosexuality and alcohol abuse. Some individuals, uncomfortable with their sexual orientation or who may anticipate rejection once their sexual preference becomes known, may use alcohol or drugs to self-medicate shame or guilt feelings (Paul et al., 1991). The authors noted that individuals who experienced negative feelings surrounding their sexual orientation tended to use alcohol to reduce internal tension. Also, as noted, the homosexual bar plays an important role within the gay community, often providing the only safe environment within which the individual might explore his/her sexuality.

However, it has been suggested that research samples drawn from the gay bar scene may also have served to *inflate* estimates of alcoholism among the gay/lesbian population (Friedman & Downey, 1994). Many researchers have utilized the gay bar to recruit subjects for their research because the bar serves many homosexual clients and thus offers the researcher a chance to reach a number of potential volunteers at once. However, statistically, those people who are most likely to frequent the bar are also more likely to have alcohol/ drug problems. Since individuals who were not alcohol/drug users would be underrepresented in such a research sample, drawing samples from these settings might overestimate the prevalence of alcohol/drug use problems among homosexuals.

On the other hand, Hughes and Wilsnack (1997) concluded that lesbians may have higher rates of alcohol use problems than their heterosexual counterparts. However, because of the lack of adequate research studies, and the fact that many of the estimates of alcohol use problems among lesbians are extrapolated from studies done on male homosexuals, the authors call for more research into alcohol/drug use patterns among homosexual women. Thus, it is virtually impossible to determine the actual prevalence of alcohol/drug use problems among the gay/lesbian population (Friedman & Downey, 1994). There also is little research into the special health care needs of the gay/lesbian client, and virtually no research into what treatment methods are effective for the substance-abusing gay/lesbian client. However, based on estimates stating that gay/lesbian individuals make up 10% to 15% of the population (Fassinger, 1991) as well as the estimate that approximately one-third of homosexuals abuse chemicals, it seems likely that a significant percentage of those in treatment for substance-abuse problems live a nontraditional lifestyle.

In contrast to this fact, the development of specialized treatment services for gay/lesbian clients has been "slow" (Hughes & Wilsnack, 1997, p. 31). The vast majority of substance abuse professionals believe that their training in meeting the needs of gay/lesbian clients was "fair" at best. Almost 40% of the substance abuse counselors received no formal training in how to effectively work with the gay/ lesbian client (Hellman, Stanton, Lee, Tytun, & Vachon, 1989). Only a small number of specialized treatment programs exist to meet the needs of the gay/lesbian community, according to the authors, and these programs are usually located in major metropolitan areas.

While there is a growing trend to set up specialized AA groups oriented toward the special needs of gay/lesbian members (Paul et al., 1991), these groups are not widespread. There is thus a significant need for substance abuse counselors to recognize the special treatment needs of gay/lesbian clients, and for treatment professionals to arrange for the specialized training necessary to effectively meet these needs.

Substance Abuse and the Disabled

There has been very little research into the problem of substance abuse among the disabled (Tyas & Rush, 1993). The limited research that does address this topic, however, suggests that substance abuse is a significant problem among those who are physically challenged. For example, Nelipovich and Buss (1991) suggested that 15% to 30% of the 33 to 45 million Americans with disabilities abuse alcohol or drugs, a rate that is generally between 1.5–3 times higher for the disabled compared with the physically able.

Although substance use problems are thus quite common for those who have a disability, the treatment resources are few. It is safe to conclude that as a group "this is a highly underserved population" (Nelipovich & Buss, 1991, p. 344). Cavaliere (1995) noted that many treatment programs have videotapes of lectures with closed captions, and utilize sign language interpreters during group therapy sessions, for the hearing-impaired client. But few programs utilize sign language interpreters outside group/individual therapy sessions so that the hearing-impaired client might participate in the give-and-take of informal discussions. Thus, even within the treatment setting, the hearing-impaired client continues to be isolated.

Rather than being identified as a special needs subgroup, the disabled are often "perceived as isolated occasional cases, only remembered because of the difficulty and frustration they present to the professionals trying to serve them" (Nelipovich & Buss, 1991, p. 344). The authors call for "creativity" (Nelipovich & Buss, 1991, p. 345) on the part of rehabilitation staff who are attempting to meet the needs of the disabled, substance-abusing client.

Unfortunately, only a minority of treatment programs have the special resources necessary for working with the disabled (wheelchair ramps, etc.).

Indeed, because of the unique needs of this subgroup of substance abusers and their relatively small numbers (when compared to the general population), many programs would rather not serve the disabled client (Tyas & Rush, 1993). In contrast, drug *dealers* are only too happy to offer their services to the disabled. For example, there are hints that at least some drug dealers are specifically targeting hearing impaired individuals, going so far as to learn sign language, or recruit assistants who know sign language, in order to sell drugs to the hearing impaired (*Associated Press*, 1993).

To further complicate the problem, family members often come to believe that the disabled person is "entitled" to use recreational chemicals, even to excess. A common attitude is that the hearing-impaired person should be allowed to use chemicals, because of his/her disability (Cavaliere, 1995). Family and friends often rationalize the substance abuse on the grounds that "I'd drink, too, if I were deaf!" In this manner, significant others may overlook signs that substance use is starting to interfere with the hearing-impaired person's life.

Thus, the physically disabled form an invisible subgroup of those who abuse, or are addicted to, chemicals in the United States. As such, they are hidden victims of the world of drug abuse/addiction.

Substance Abuse and Ethnic Minorities

Virtually nothing is known about the natural history of substance abuse in the various minority groups that make up this nation. Franklin (1989), for example, found that of 16,000 articles on alcoholism published between 1934 and 1974, only 11 "were specifically studies of blacks" (p. 1120). Virtually no research has been done on the subject of alcoholism and the black woman, and little is known about this area. The author noted that, when compared with white alcoholics, blacks "have a higher incidence of medical complications from alcoholism" (p. 1120), possibly as much as ten times as high as would be seen from a similar group of white alcoholics. Alcoholics Anonymous (AA) has become a significant part of the treatment and recovery process within the black community, according to the author.

Along these same lines, it should be noted that there is virtually no research on the subject of alcohol/substance abuse within such minority groups as the American Indian, Chinese American, Japanese American, or Asian Americans. What little is known, or thought to be known, about alcohol or substance abuse patterns within these subgroups is based on studies involving mostly white alcohol- or substance-using samples. There is a need for research into how substance use has impacted these subgroups and what treatment methods might be of value in working with members of each minority group.

Summary

We all have imagined what the "typical" addict looks like. For some, this is the picture of the skid row alcoholic, while for others the picture associated with "addiction" is that of a heroin addict, hidden in the ruins of an abandoned building with a belt around his arm, ready to inject the drug into his vein. These images of addiction are correct, yet each image fails to accurately reflect the many many hidden faces of addiction.

There is the grandfather, who is quietly drinking himself to death, or the mother who exposes her unborn child to staggering amounts of cocaine, heroin, or alcohol. There is the working woman whose chemical addiction is hidden behind a veil of productivity, or whose drug use is sanctioned by the unsuspecting physicians who are trying to help her cope with feelings of depression or anxiety. There are faces of addiction so well hidden that, even today, they are not recognized. As professionals, we must learn to look for, and identify, the hidden forms of addiction.

CHAPTER TWENTY-TWO

The Dual-Diagnosis Client

Chemical Addiction and Mental Illness

The destruction that can result from a substance abuse problem, or from one of the many forms of mental illness, can literally tear a person's life apart. When these problems coexist in an individual, the potential for harm is multiplied a thousandfold. Yet despite the potential for harm when someone suffers both from mental illness and a substance use disorder, the typical substance abuse rehabilitation professional or health care worker usually has an "inadequate understanding of the complex relationship between other psychiatric illnesses and substance use disorders" (Decker & Ries, 1993, p. 703).

There are many reasons for this lack of insight into the combined impact of a psychiatric illnesses and a substance use disorder. For decades, mental health workers were taught that if a person suffered from a form of mental illness and also a substance use disorder, the chemical use problem was secondary to the "primary" mental illness. Once the mental illness was cured, the theory went, the substance use disorder should resolve itself. This theory was taught to generations of mental health professionals, many of whom still think in terms of primary and secondary disorders.

In reality, substance use disorders are rarely secondary to mental illness issues. Rather, substance abuse and mental illness in the same individual represent separate, coexisting disorders. At least half of all patients seen for a psychiatric emergency also have a substance use problem (Beeder & Millman,

1995). The fact that substance use disorders often co-exist with mental illness has made it difficult for health care professionals to understand the relationship between these two conditions. In this chapter the problem of substance use problems among those individuals who also suffer from a form of mental illness is examined.

Definitions

Patients who suffer from a form of mental illness, and who also abuse chemicals, are often said to be "dual-diagnosis" clients. This term has been applied to a wide range of coexisting problems, including combinations of substance abuse/addiction and anorexia, bulimia, gambling, spouse abuse, and AIDS. Mental health professionals often use the term *dual diagnosis* to refer to substance-abusing psychiatric patients. In this text, the term dual diagnosis, or "MI/CD" (mentally ill/chemically dependent) will be used to denote individuals with a *coexisting* psychiatric disorder and substance abuse problem.

The important point is that the individual's substance use disorder and psychiatric problem are *independent disorders that coexist*. Recreational chemical use can either magnify preexisting psychiatric disorders or bring about a drug-induced disorder that simulates any of a wide range of psychiatric problems (S. Cohen, 1995; Washton, 1995). But, unlike the patient with dual disorders, these drug-induced symptoms will usually diminish, or entirely disappear, within a few days, or weeks, after the patient stops taking recreational chemical(s) (Falls-Stewart & Lucente, 1994; Woody, McLellan, et al., 1995).

When mental health professionals use the term dual diagnosis, or MI/CD, they are speaking of a substance-using patient who suffers *both* from a mental illness and a separate substance use disorder. The concept really is not all that difficult to understand. Consider, for example, an alcohol-dependent person who also suffers from a medical problem. Perhaps the alcohol-dependent individual has a kidney dysfunction or a genetic disorder of some kind. The patient's medical condition did not *cause* him/her to become alcohol-dependent, nor did his/her alcohol dependence bring about the medical condition. Yet each disorder, once it develops, is intertwined with the other. The prudent physician treating this hypothetical patient would need to consider the impact of the patient's alcohol use problem on the possible treatment methods under consideration for the kidney disorder. At the same time, substance abuse rehabilitation professionals would need to consider the impact that the patient's kidney disease might have on his/her life, when they explore possible treatment interventions for the chemical use problem.

In much the same way, MI/CD clients have two separate disorders: substance abuse/dependence and mental illness. Each disorder has an independent, often chronic, course. Yet although they are separate, either disorder is able to influence the progression of the other (Carey, 1989; Woody, McLellan, et al., 1995).

Limitations of the Available Literature

In researching dual-diagnosis patients, scientists have discovered that there is a great deal more to discover about this fascinating group of individuals. Until now, much of the literature has been limited to those individuals with the most severe forms of mental illness (usually schizophrenia), who also have a substance abuse problem. But there is a dearth of information on substance-abusing patients who have only a mild or moderately severe form of mental illness. A review of the literature has failed to find any significant amount of research into the possible interactions between many significant forms of mental illness, and substance use disorders.

For example, Wender (1995) suggested that individuals who had attention-deficit/hyperactivity disorder (ADHD) were at increased risk for alcoholism. Yet, virtually nothing is known about how ADHD affects the evolution of alcohol use disorders in the individual. Further, although researchers know that personality disorders are a form of psychiatric disability, there is little information on how a substance use disorder might interact with dysfunctional personality patterns (Ryglewicz & Pepper, 1996). Thus, there is a great deal that we still must learn about the many possible interactions of substance abuse and mental illness.

Dual-Diagnosis Clients: A Diagnostic Challenge

For a number of reasons, dual-diagnosis clients present a special challenge to treatment professionals (N. Miller, 1994; Riley, 1994). One reason is that it is difficult to correctly diagnose concurrent problems such as mental illness and substance abuse (Twerski, 1989). Up to two-thirds of those patients admitted to substance abuse treatment programs have symptoms of psychiatric problems at the time of admission (Falls-Stewart & Lucente, 1994). But these psychiatric problems often remit after the patient has been alcohol/drug-free for a period of time, suggesting that the presenting symptoms are often alcohol/drug-induced.

But, because recreational drug abuse can cause symptoms that mimic psychiatric disorders does not mean that the patient has a coexisting form of mental illness. To identify those individuals with a dual diagnosis, treatment professionals are often forced to wait days, weeks, or even months, in the hope that the patient has only a substance-induced disorder (Carey, 1989; Evans & Sullivan, 1990; Rado, 1988; Wallen & Weiner, 1989). It might be necessary for the patient to be drug-free for *up to 6 weeks* before an accurate diagnosis can be made (Director, 1995; Nathan, 1991).

To further complicate the problem of making an accurate diagnosis, there is evidence suggesting that many MI/CD clients actively attempt to hide that they engage in recreational chemical use from health care professionals (Shaner et al., 1993). Even when dual-diagnosis clients admit that they engage in recreational chemical use, they may underreport the frequency and severity of their substance use problems (Carey et al., 1996). As discussed in Chapter 26, this makes the use of collateral information sources imperative.

MI/CD clients may attempt to hide their recreational alcohol or drug use from health care professionals for a number of reasons. In some cases, the dual-diagnosis client may be unable to discuss his/her chemical use because of ongoing psychiatric problems (Kanwischer & Hundley, 1990). For example, the schizophrenic patient may be too disorganized to discuss his/her chemical use, while the patient suffering from a phobia may be unwilling to give up what seems to have been an effective coping mechanism for anxiety.

Other MI/CD patients hesitate to discuss their substance use problems with health care professionals because direct questions about alcohol or drug use contribute to feelings of defensiveness or shame (Pristach & Smith, 1990). Other dual-diagnosis patients fear that, by admitting to having a substance use problem, they will experience the loss of entitlements (such as Social Security or welfare payments), or be afraid that they will be denied access to psychiatric treatment (Mueser, Bellack, & Blanchard, 1992). But denial is also a trait found in people who are addicted to chemicals. Thus, some MI/CD clients deny their substance-use problem for the same reasons other addicts do: they want to avoid the reality of admitting that they are abusing, or are addicted to, recreational chemicals.

Why Worry about the Dual-Diagnosis Client?

Research now suggests that even limited recreational chemical use by a client with a form of mental illness may exacerbate the psychiatric disorder and cause treatment for either disorder to become much more complicated (Cohen & Levy, 1992; Drake, Osher, & Wallach, 1989; Evans & Sullivan, 1990; Pristach & Smith, 1990; Ries & Ellingson, 1990; Rubinstein, Campbell, & Daley, 1990). The research team of Drake et al. (1989) found that drinking even in amounts clearly not abusive by traditional standards, was one factor that predicted those clients who had

schizophrenia would require rehospitalization within a year. In another study, psychiatric patients who abused chemicals on a regular basis were found to have hospitalization rates 250% higher than those individuals who rarely or never abused chemicals (Kanwischer & Hundley, 1990).

Thus, recreational chemical use is now viewed by mental health professionals as a negative influence on the course of a patient's psychiatric disorder (Kivlahan, Heiman, Wright, Mundt, & Shupe, 1991; Miller & Tanenbaum, 1989; Osher et al., 1994; Rubinstein et al., 1990; Stoffelmayr, Benishek, Humphreys, Lee, & Mavis, 1989). As a group, MI/CD patients tend to make less progress in therapy, and, to suffer a greater number of problems while in treatment (Osher & Drake, 1996; Woody, McLellan, et al., 1995).

In addition to exacerbating the individual's psychiatric problem, substance abuse by individuals who suffer from schizophrenia places an additional economic strain on the family (R. Clark, 1994). The author attempted to calculate the cash value of direct cash contributions, time spent with the client, lost career opportunities for the parents, and stress-related illness for family members with, and without, dual-diagnosis clients. R. Clark found that the estimated level of family assistance to dual-diagnosis clients was between $9,703 and $13,547 a year, while the value of family assistance to adult children without a chronic mental illness was, at most, $3,547 per year.

Further, substance abuse may contribute to family conflicts. As the family withdraws from the patient as a result of the increased level of conflict, his/her available social support base becomes smaller. This, in turn, makes it harder for the patient to cope with the demands of life. Since psychiatric patients with weaker social support systems tend to require longer, and more frequent, periods of hospitalization, the negative impact of substance abuse on the individual's psychiatric condition becomes more clear.

When one stops to consider the level of pain experienced by the mentally ill, the cost of lost productivity, and the cost of hospitalization and treatment, and then adds on the financial, social, and personal cost of substance abuse by mentally ill clients, the need to address this problem becomes understandable.

probs in assessment!

The Scope of the Problem

The twin problems of substance abuse by those individuals with some form of mental illness has resulted in a significant amount of personal, and economic suffering in the United States. It has been estimated that substance abuse by persons with mental illness causes a loss of productivity of $273 billion per year in the United States, and by the year 2001, it is estimated that this figure will be close to $300 billion a year (Riley, 1994).

Although different researchers have found that substance use/abuse is a significant problem for varying percentages of those with a mental illness, they all agree that it is a major problem. Kivlahan et al. (1991) concluded that substance use disorders are seven times as common among the mentally ill as among the general population, while alcohol use disorders are ten times as prevalent among the mentally ill as among the general population. In contrast, N. Miller (1994) reported that 30% of those psychiatric patients with a depressive disorder, 50% of those patients with a bipolar affective disorder, 50% of those patients with some form of schizophrenia, 30% of the patients with some form of anxiety disorder, and 25% of those patients with a phobic disorder have abused alcohol and/or recreational drugs at some point in their lives.

Other researchers have found that substance abuse is at least twice as common in the mentally ill as in the general population (Brown, Ridgely, Pepper, Levine, & Ryglewicz, 1989; Regier et al., 1990). There is evidence to suggest that between one-third and one-half of psychiatric patients also have a substance use problem (Carey, 1989; Carey et al., 1996; Regier et al., 1990). The team of Shaner et al. (1993) found that more than one-third of the sample of schizophrenic patients admitted to the abuse of CNS stimulants in the 6 months prior to their study.

The tendency to abuse alcohol or chemicals has been reported to be more common among younger clients who have some form of mental illness (Drake et al., 1989), especially young adult male psychiatric patients (Szuster, Schanbacher, & McCann, 1990). However, this might be an artifact, in the sense that younger people are more likely to have been exposed to a drug-using subculture than are older individuals (Kovasznay et al., 1993). Thus, it is not clear whether the tendency for younger mentally ill patients to have abused chemicals reflects a specific form of psychopathology or the tendency for younger individuals to have used chemicals in general within this society.

What is clear from the literature is that a significant percentage of those with some form of mental illness have abused chemicals. Brown et al. (1989) estimated that, in the younger mentally ill population, the "substance abuse rate approaches or exceeds 50%" (p. 566), a conclusion supported by others (Evans & Sullivan, 1990; Kanwischer & Hundley, 1990; Miller & Tanenbaum, 1989). Psychiatrists are ill equipped to detect substance abuse problems, especially in the mentally ill (Cohen & Levy, 1992). Lacking a pattern to look for, mental health professionals often fail to recognize that a mentally ill client may also have a substance abuse problem (Cohen & Levy, 1992; Peyser, 1989). To illustrate this point, consider the findings of the team of Ananth et al. (1989). The authors reevaluated a sample of 75 psychiatric patients, each of whom had already been seen by, and received a diagnosis from, mental health professionals. None of these patients had been diagnosed as having an alcohol or drug abuse problem at the time of admission.

The authors found that 54 of the 75 subjects should also have received a diagnosis of either drug abuse, or drug dependence, in addition to their psychiatric diagnosis. Ten of the 54 subjects found to use drugs were also found to either abuse or be addicted to alcohol, while two additional subjects were found to meet the diagnostic criteria for only alcohol abuse/dependence. Thus, of the 75 patients who had been admitted for psychiatric treatment, three-quarters had an undiagnosed alcohol or drug abuse problem.

Characteristics of Dual-Diagnosis Clients

Although researchers speak of the substance-abusing mentally ill clients as if they were all the same, this is a gross oversimplification. There is no single clinical model of the MI/CD client. Rather, there are various combinations of substance use problems, substance-induced problems, and psychiatric symptoms, which vary from individual to

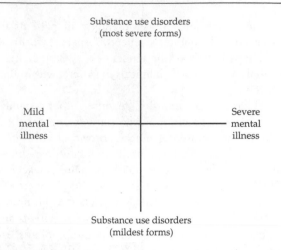

Substance use disorders
(most severe forms)

Mild
mental
illness

Severe
mental
illness

Substance use disorders
(mildest forms)

FIGURE 22.1 Interaction between substance use and mental health disorders.

individual. Further, each category—substance use, substance-induced problems, and symptoms of mental illness—can vary in severity or the impact on the individual's life. Thus:

> The dually diagnosed are not a uniform clinical entity, but a heterogeneous group who differ in psychiatric disorder, level of functioning, social support, and capacity for independent living. (Director, 1995, p. 377)

Assume, for a moment, that it would be possible to chart the severity of a person's substance use problem, and his/her mental illness. Such a graph would illustrate that are almost an infinite number of different MI/CD clients (see Figure 22.1).

As this diagram illustrates, there are many different forms of dual-diagnosis client, one set of characteristics will not apply to every client. Researchers have studied different sample populations of substance-abusing patients with some form of mental illness. Each researcher has found that his/her sample had unique characteristics. Thus, the reader should keep in mind that the following list of characteristics of the MI/CD client is based on several sample groups of clients:

- The MI/CD client has been found to be less impaired, but with more suicidal, homicidal, and impulsive behaviors than other psychiatric patients (Kay, Kalathara, & Meinzer, 1989; Szuster et al., 1990).

- These clients were less severely psychotic, and more intelligent, than the typical psychiatric patient (Mueser, Yarnold, & Bellack, 1992; Zisook et al., 1992).

- Schizophrenic patients who abused alcohol were found to have poor social adjustment; be more delusional, disruptive, and assaultive; experience more treatment noncompliance; have more housing instability and homelessness; experience higher rates of rehospitalization; and be more depressed (Osher et al., 1994).

- MI/CD patients were found to be at higher risk for suicide (Osher & Drake, 1996; Osher et al., 1994).

- Psychiatric clients who also have substance use disorders seem to have more trouble staying sober (Osher & Drake, 1996).

- MI/CD clients are less likely to be able to use alcohol on a social/recreational basis for extended periods of time (Drake & Wallach, 1993).

- MI/CD clients seem to be more vulnerable to the effects of the recreational drugs (Brown et al., 1989; Drake et al., 1989).

- Dual-diagnosis clients tend to be "binge" users of recreational chemicals (Osher & Drake, 1996; Riley, 1994).

- MI/CD clients tend to be more manipulative than traditional psychiatric patients (Mueser, Bellack, & Blanchard, 1992).

- Although their risk factors for psychiatric complications is reduced when they abstain from chemicals, as a group MI/CD clients are less likely to work for total abstinence than traditional substance-abusing clients (Drake, Mueser, Clark, & Wallach, 1996).

Psychopathology and Drug of Choice

A popular theory is that the MI/CD patient is attempting to self-medicate emotional pain through chemical use. Some researchers believe that the client is using chemicals in an attempt to treat, or at least control, the symptoms of his or her psychiatric condition. In support of this hypothesis are studies such as the one conducted by Test, Wallisch, Allness, and Ripp (1990). The authors found that alcohol was the most frequently abused chemical in their sample, followed by marijuana. When asked why they used the chemical(s) that they did, the authors found that the drug-abusing schizophrenic patients in their sample reported that their drug of choice helped them to deal with feelings of anxiety, insomnia, boredom, depression, and the side effects of prescribed antipsychotic medications.

But this research has not been replicated in other studies. The research team of Kivlahan et al. (1991) found that 71% of their sample of 60 volunteers being treated at an outpatient community support program for schizophrenia would qualify for a diagnosis of a "substance abuse disorder" at some point in their lives. Surprisingly, the authors found that marijuana, not alcohol, was the most frequently abused drug for their sample. The authors found that 88% of their sample used marijuana at least occasionally, with the other drugs being abused by their sample being amphetamines (used by 30% of their sample at some point), alcohol (22%), hallucinogenics (18%), cocaine and narcotics (both used by 13% of the total sample at some point).

The conflicting results of these two investigations might be explained by the results obtained by the research team of Cuffel, Heithoff, and Lawson (1993) in their recent study. The authors examined the drug usage of 231 individuals who were diagnosed as having schizophrenia and found that their sample tended to follow one of three patterns.

First, there were those individuals who did not abuse chemicals; this group made up 54% of the total sample. In the second group were those individuals with schizophrenia who tended to abuse alcohol, marijuana, or both. This subgroup made up 31% of the sample. The last group were individuals with schizophrenia who were "polysubstance" abusers, a group that made up only 14% of the overall sample.

While Cuffel et al. (1993) found that while individuals with schizophrenia tend to most commonly abuse alcohol, and/or marijuana, there was no apparent relationship between drug of choice, and psychiatric diagnosis. The authors did find a weak statistical association between depressive symptoms and substance abuse, but not between schizophrenia and substance abuse patterns. This study suggests that there might not be any specific relationship between form of psychiatric illness and the individual's drug of choice.

In a pair of unrelated studies, Mueser et al. (1992), and Kovasznay et al. (1993) also failed to find any significant pattern between the drug of abuse, and the patient's diagnosis. Although the authors found a weak trend for patients with a diagnosis of bipolar affective disorder to abuse alcohol, they failed to find other consistent trends for drug use among the mentally ill patients that they studied.

Yet another alternative to the self-medication hypothesis of drug of choice for MI/CD clients was offered by Mueser et al. (1992). The authors suggested that *availability* was the key factor that most strongly influenced the pattern of chemical use, not the individual's specific form of psychiatric illness. This is why alcohol was the most popular drug of abuse for patients with schizophrenia who admitted to using drugs: it is the most available, most frequently abused chemical in this society (Mueser et al., 1992; Test et al., 1990). If this theory is correct, then presumably the pattern of substance use/abuse by dual-diagnosis patients will parallel the community's pattern of recreational drug use. This hypothesis has never been tested.

The team of Dunn, Paolo, Ryan, and Van Fleet (1993) found evidence to suggest that more than 41% of the patients sampled might also experience some form of a dissociative disorder. The dissociative disorders are marked by episodes in which the individual loses touch with reality. In its most extreme form, the individual may develop more than one personality, a condition known as *multiple personality disorder* (MPD). However, most patients who suffer from a dissociative disorder do not develop MPD, although they do have episodes in which they "disconnect" from reality.

There appears to be a relationship between patients with dissociative disorders, and, substance abuse (Dunn et al., 1993; Kolodner & Frances, 1993). Although the diagnosis of a dissociative disorder is complex, Kolodner and Frances (1993) suggested two diagnostic signs for the patient with coexisting substance abuse and dissociative disorders. First, unlike other patients addicted to chemicals, patients with dissociative disorders do not feel better after completing the detoxification stage of treatment. Rather, patients with dissociative disorders tend to experience significant levels of emotional pain, after detoxification from chemicals.

Kolodner and Frances (1993) also suggested that patients who suffer from dissociative disorders tend to relapse at times of "relative comfort and clinical stability" (p. 1042). This is in contrast to other substance-abusing patients, who are thought to relapse when under stress (see Chapter 27). The authors suggested that these situations might alert the clinician to the possibility of the patient having a dissociative disorder, which could then be addressed in treatment.

As mentioned, the most serious form of a dissociative disorder is multiple personality disorder. Perhaps one-third of these patients are thought to also abuse chemicals (Putnam, 1989). They tend to utilize CNS depressants and alcohol although stimulants are also frequently abused, according to the author. Hallucinogenics, possibly because of the nature of dissociative disorders, did not seem to be a popular drug of abuse for this subgroup (Putnam). Exactly why chemicals are so popular among individuals with dissociative disorders is not clear. However, these clients may be using chemicals to self-medicate their internal distress (Putnam).

It has been observed that obsessive-compulsive disorder (OCD) is the fourth most common psychiatric disorder in the United States (Falls-Stewart & Lucente, 1994). The authors suggested that OCD is four or five times as common among substance abusers as in the general population, although the reason for this is not clear.

Problems in Working with Dual-Diagnosis Clients

The first step for the substance abuse specialist who works with MI/CD clients is to examine his/her own attitudes toward psychopharmacology. Some individuals in the recovering community are uncomfortable with a patient's use of medications to control his/her psychiatric disorder (Evans & Sullivan, 1990; Fariello & Scheidt, 1989; Penick et al., 1990; Riley, 1994). Many of those recovering from chemical use problems equate any *use* of drugs as substituting one addiction for another, despite the legitimate function of the psychotropic medications. These individuals should examine their attitude toward prescribed use of psychotropic

medications, and if they are unable to accept this, not work with MI/CD clients.

For a number of reasons, the outlook for dual-diagnosis clients has traditionally been thought to be quite poor. One of the most common problems encountered in working with a dual-diagnosis client is that the treatment philosophies of substance abuse counselors and mental health professionals often conflict (Carey, 1989; Howland, 1990; Osher & Kofoed, 1989; Wallen & Weiner, 1989). In addition, dual-diagnosis clients have trouble recognizing that substance abuse is a personal problem, do not see the relationship between chemical use and their problems, and do not accept abstinence as a viable treatment goal. These factors may bring about a significant degree of confusion and frustration for both the client and treatment professionals.

Kofoed, Kania, Walsh, and Atkinson, (1986) noted that more severe levels of psychopathology have been associated with an unfavorable outcome for substance abusers, in part because "coexisting thought or affective disorders may exacerbate denial of substance abuse" (p. 1209). Denial of substance abuse is a significant problem in the dual-diagnosis client, which contributes to the difficulty of working with such clients.

Although denial is a characteristic of dual-diagnosis clients, the added dimension of a psychiatric disorder will cause their denial of drug addiction to express itself in different ways. It is not uncommon for clients, when in a counseling session with substance abuse rehabilitation professionals, to focus almost exclusively on their psychiatric disorder. When these patients are being interviewed by medical staff, they may focus exclusively on their chemical dependency treatment issues. Patients may do this consciously, or unconsciously, to avoid confronting the substance abuse problem. Finally, once the psychiatric condition is controlled, such clients are likely to self-terminate (i.e., drop out) from treatment.

This is the process of "interchangeable" or "free-floating" denial, in which clients tell the mental health professional that most of their problems are drug related, while telling the substance abuse counselor that most of their problems are caused by the mental illness. It is not uncommon for clients to use one disorder as a shield against intervention for the other disorder. As noted in Chapter 5, individuals who have multiple personality disorder often attribute their loss of memory (experienced when one personality is forced out of consciousness and another takes over) to the use of chemicals. This is far less threatening to these clients than the acceptance of their mental illness.

The mentally ill, chemically dependent client is often a "crisis user" (Rubinstein et al., 1990, p. 99) of medical and chemical dependency services. This makes it hard for treatment staff to become motivated to invest a great deal of time and energy into working with MI/CD clients. To complicate this problem of treatment dropout, chemical dependency professionals often view dual-diagnosis clients as being primarily psychiatric patients, while mental health professionals often view MI/CD clients as being primarily substance abuse cases.

In the 1970s and early 1980s, federal drug treatment initiatives resulted in the establishment of a number of agencies devoted to the identification and rehabilitation of the substance user (Osher & Drake, 1996). At the same time, rehabilitation efforts for patients with psychiatric problems were assigned to a different series of federal agencies. Interdepartmental communication/cooperation was virtually nonexistent, and as a result of this political (Layne, 1990, p. 176) atmosphere, the treatment of substance abuse cases became separated from traditional psychiatric care.

This division in treatment philosophy is most clearly seen with dual-diagnosis clients. When the MI/CD client comes into contact with a treatment center, the staff frequently views the patient as "not our problem" and will refer the patient elsewhere. All too often, the outcome of this refusal-to-treat philosophy is that clients are bounced like a ping-pong ball between psychiatric and chemical dependency treatment programs (Osher & Kofoed, 1989; Wallen & Weiner, 1989).

Staff psychiatrists in traditional psychiatric hospitals usually lack training and experience working with addicted individuals (Howland, 1990; Riley, 1994). So, when such patients are admitted to a psychiatric facility, they may receive potentially addictive substances as part of their care, prescribed by psychiatrists who are more experienced in working with nonaddicted clients. This practice is often contraindicated when working with the MI/CD client (Drake, Mueser, Clark, & Wallach, 1996).

The MI/CD Client and Medication Compliance

There appears to be a relationship between substance use/abuse and medication noncompliance for MI/CD clients (Owen, Fischer, Booth, & Cuffel, 1996). The team of Kivlahan, Heiman, Write, Mundt, & Schupe (1991) concluded that MI/CD clients were 12.8 times more likely to be noncompliant as the traditional psychiatric patient. That is, the dual-diagnosis client is more than 12 times as likely not to take medications as prescribed as non-drug-abusing psychiatric patients. This might include not only refusing to take prescribed medications but also continuing to use drugs of abuse even after admission to inpatient psychiatric treatment (Alterman, Erdlen, LaPorte, & Erdlen, 1982). Some MI/CD clients will even stop taking prescribed medication in anticipation of recreational drug use, to avoid potentially dangerous chemical interactions (Ryglewicz & Pepper, 1996).

Many MI/CD clients use recreational drugs in an attempt at self-medication (Caton, Gralnick, Bender, & Simon, 1989; Rubinstein et al., 1990). They may possibly do this because they mistrust prescribed medication (Evans & Sullivan, 1990). Further, some psychiatric medications have a significant abuse potential of their own. It is not uncommon for patients who receive anticholinergic medications, which are often prescribed to help control the side effects of antipsychotic agents, to abuse their anticholinergic medications. The anticholinergics may potentiate the effects of alcohol or the amphetamines (Land, Pinsky, & Salzman, 1991). Even when used alone, the "buzz" from anticholinergic medications is often substituted for the effects of other chemicals when supplies run short. Thus, treatment center staff must keep in mind that MI/CD clients may resort to abusing their psychiatric medications.

Urine toxicology testing is a useful tool to help determine whether the patient is taking his/her antipsychotic medications as prescribed. Urine toxicology testing is also valuable to detect illicit chemical use, since MI/CD clients often test positive for recreational drugs even when they have openly denied the use of such agents (Drake et al., 1996). Another approach to the problem of noncompliance is the use of long-term injectable forms of some phenothiazines currently available, rather than the more traditional short-term preparations, for control of the thought disorder and agitation often found in dual-diagnosis clients (Fariello & Scheidt, 1989).

Hatfield (1989) provided a graphic description of the internal world of schizophrenic patients, noting that these individuals "suffer high levels of stress and anxiety as they struggle to negotiate between the world as others know it and the world of their inner reality" (p. 1142). Those who are able to perceive the pain and suffering inherent in many forms of mental illness find it understandable that mentally ill individuals often strive to cope with the lack of internal structure and predictability by substituting external structure and predictability.

Self-administered drugs are one way to substitute external structure and predictability on internal chaos, since the chemicals provide an illusion of control over one's feelings (Brown, 1985). Even if the drugs cause the schizophrenic patient to experience additional hallucinations, at least the individual has the illusion of controlling these hallucinations by deciding whether or not to take the chemical. This is an important consideration for those whose internal lives seem out of control because of their mental illness.

Treatment Approaches

While it is becoming apparent that dual-diagnosis clients require specialized treatment programs to meet their needs, few such programs exist (Howland, 1990). The traditional approach to dual-diagnosis clients has been to address the client's mental illness first, and after psychiatric stabilization has been achieved, to begin to explore the client's chemical use pattern (Rado, 1988). Usually, different professionals work with the client, in turn, to first achieve a reduction in the patient's psychiatric symptoms, and then to address the substance use problem. This approach is an example of the *Serial Treatment model* (N. Miller, 1994).

The decision which to treat first—the psychiatric condition or the drug dependency—is often quite arbitrary (Howland, 1990; Kofoed et al., 1986). Indeed, there is little research data to suggest which treatment format works best with the dual-diagnosis client (Evans & Sullivan, 1990; Osher & Kofoed, 1989). One alternative, suggested by Layne (1990), was to treat both disorders *concurrently*, a possible alternative to the either/or approach utilized by other treatment centers.

N. Miller (1994) identified two subtypes of concurrent treatment models. In the first, which he termed the *Parallel Treatment model*, the patient shuttles between treatment facilities, dealing with mental health concerns on one unit and substance use issues on another unit. There are a number of disadvantages to this form of treatment, according to the author. First, communications between staff on different units may be difficult, especially if the psychiatric rehabilitation staff is not used to working with substance abuse rehabilitation professionals. Second, the need to physically move from one unit to another may prove to be a source of stress to vulnerable patients, resulting in an exacerbation of their psychiatric problems. Finally, parallel treatment facilities tend to experience significant problems of patient attrition (Drake et al., 1996).

The second subtype of concurrent treatment, which N. Miller (1994) termed the *Integrated Treatment model*, is clearly the most efficient. In an integrated treatment setting, there are both mental health and substance abuse rehabilitation professionals on the staff. By coordinating their treatment goals, staff are able to address the psychiatric and chemical use issues at the same time, in the same treatment facility. In such a treatment model, interstaff communications and cooperation are essential, according to the author. However, this treatment approach offers the advantage of dealing with the client's substance use and psychiatric issues simultaneously, while reducing the potential for conflict between treatment professionals.

In all three preceding models, the team approach is a basic requirement. The rehabilitation team provides a forum where the different treatment philosophies of psychiatric and chemical dependency professionals can be synthesized into a unified whole to be utilized in working with the individual client (Evans & Sullivan, 1990; Osher & Kofoed, 1989; Riley, 1994).

Chemical detoxification is a necessary first step to treatment of a dual-diagnosis client (Layne, 1990; Wallen & Weiner, 1989). This requires psychiatric support from professionals who are knowledgable in both psychiatry and chemical dependency (Evans & Sullivan, 1990). Once detoxification has been achieved, the treatment team would be in a position to identify which problems are a result of the client's chemical use, which ones are manifestations of the client's psychiatric disorder, and in what order the problems need to be addressed.

The Treatment Setting

The general psychiatric unit is usually unsuited to the needs of a dual-diagnosis client (Kofoed & Keys, 1988; Howland, 1990). Kofoed and Keys suggested that psychiatric units might do best if treatment goals were limited to (a) detoxification from drugs of abuse, (b) psychiatric stabilization, and (c) persuasion of the client to enter chemical dependency treatment. The clinician must be patient, often waiting years until conditions are right to finally persuade a dual-diagnosis client to enter treatment.

The ideal program for a dual-diagnosis client would have facilities for working with both the psychiatric and the chemical use problems. This would allow the staff to utilize the treatment resources most needed by the dual-diagnosis patient at that moment. This would, obviously be easier in a facility that followed the Integrated Treatment model discussed earlier. Such a program might be either an outpatient (Kofoed et al., 1986) or inpatient (Pursch, 1987) basis, depending on (a) the client's needs and (b) the available resources. In more difficult cases, however, long-term inpatient treatment may be the only option for effectively working with the MI/CD client (Caton et al., 1989).

The Stages of Treatment

The dual-diagnosis client usually will come to the attention of mental health or chemical dependency professionals as a result of a crisis situation such as repeated hospitalizations, legal problems, psychiatric decompensation, or eviction from his/her apartment (Fariello & Scheidt, 1989; Rubinstein et al., 1990). It is at this point that treatment might be initiated. Durell, Lechtenberg, Corse, and Frances (1993) pointed out that a crisis "can provide the motivation for overcoming addiction" (p. 428). Thus, the therapist might be able to use such a crisis to help the client face the reality of his/her addiction.

Director (1995) called this first phase of treatment that of *Initial assessment/Engagement*, while Lehman, Myers, and Corty (1989) used the term *acute treatment and stabilization* (p. 1020). Minkoff (1989) termed this part of treatment the phase of *acute stabilization*. It is during this phase of treatment that the client's psychiatric condition is stabilized and detoxification is carried out. The possibility of a dual diagnosis is also weighed by the clinician during this phase. If the symptoms of a psychiatric disorder completely clear during detoxification, then the possibility that the client is not a dual-diagnosis patient should be considered (Layne, 1990).

If the symptoms persist after detoxification, however, then the diagnosis of a dual-diagnosis client becomes more likely (Lehman et al., 1989). In either case, during this second phase of treatment staff should focus on helping the individual to understand the relationship between the crisis, and his or her untreated psychiatric problem(s). Staff will try to break "the cycle of substance abuse, noncompliance, decompensation, and rehospitalization once the patient is sober and psychiatrically stable" (Fariello & Scheidt, 1989, p. 1066). This process might include the introduction of money management programs, psychoeducational materials or lectures, and social support.

During this phase, staff attempt to break through the denial that surrounds both the individual's mental illness and his or her addiction. Both the team of Osher and Kofoed (1989) and Minkoff (1989) termed this phase of treatment that of *engagement*. Layne (1990) used the term *early engagement* while Director (1995) classified the period as one of *Primary care*.

The goal here is for the professional staff to strive to establish a therapeutic relationship, arrive at an accurate diagnosis, and convince the client that treatment has something to offer him/her. Staff members should attempt to work with family members or legal representatives during this period, to bring the client into treatment on an involuntary basis if this should become necessary.

In their work with dual-problem clients, Kofoed and Keys (1988) concluded that peer group therapy offered "a more acceptable source of support and confrontation than is usually available . . . on a general psychiatric ward" (p. 1209). Group therapy may be an important element in working with the dual-diagnosis client although such groups should be held on the psychiatric unit, rather than in the substance abuse unit (Kofoed & Keys, 1988; Layne, 1990).

During this phase of treatment, which Lehman et al. (1989) termed *maintenance and rehabilitation,* the clinician should work toward the goal of preventing a recurrence of both the chemical abuse and the psychiatric disorder. This is the same process that Fariello and Scheidt (1989) identified as *breaking the cycle of addiction.*

Osher and Kofoed (1989) called this phase of treatment that of *persuasion.* The treatment staff will, during this phase of treatment, attempt to convince the client to accept the need for abstinence. Kofoed and Keys (1988) identified the therapeutic goals here as persuading clients (a) to accept the reality of their drug dependency, and (b) to seek continued treatment for the drug dependency.

The third phase of treatment, that of *active treatment* (Osher & Kofoed, 1989), attempts to help the client learn "the attitudes and skills necessary to remain sober" (p. 1027). Director (1995) called this phase of treatment *Continuing Care.* Many of the same techniques utilized in general drug addiction treatment groups are useful in working with dual-diagnosis clients. Most certainly, Osher and Kofoed (1989) argued against lower treatment expectations, or the acceptance of relapse as being inevitable, for dual-diagnosis clients. Layne (1990) suggested that treatment staff might need to teach clients specific life skills to help them learn how to function in society without abusable drugs, despite ongoing delusions.

However, the very nature of the client population offers unique challenges, and requires modification of techniques used in traditional chemical dependency work. It has been suggested that, when confrontation is utilized with dual-diagnosis clients who are in treatment, the confrontation should be less intense than the confrontation used with traditional personality-disordered clients (Carey, 1989; Penick et al., 1990; Riley, 1994).

As with the nonpsychiatric addict, dual-diagnosis clients will utilize denial as a major defense. The danger is that once the psychiatric condition is controlled, the client's drug-related defenses again begin to operate (Kofoed & Keys, 1988). Dual-diagnosis clients will often express a belief that, once their psychiatric symptoms are controlled, they are no longer in danger of being addicted to chemicals. These clients are often unable to see the relationship between their chemical abuse, and the psychiatric symptoms that they experience.

Another form of denial that is frequently found in traditional clients is evident when the client informs the drug rehabilitation specialist that he/she has discontinued all drug/alcohol use. In effect, the client enters into a period of trying to "tell the counselor what he wants to hear" to avoid confrontation. This evasion is frequently encountered with all clients, including those who suffer from mental illness.

MI/CD clients are often unable to utilize support systems such as Alcoholics Anonymous or Narcotics Anonymous because they tend to feel out of place in traditional self-help group meetings (Fariello & Scheidt, 1989; Wallen & Weiner, 1989). This is especially true in the earlier stages of rehabilitation (Drake et al., 1996). For this reason, a group of peers is most effective in working with the dual-diagnosis client (Kofoed & Keys, 1988). In such a group, other members, who may have once dropped out of treatment after their own psychiatric disorder was controlled, can now share their own experiences with the group.

The group provides an avenue through which clients may share their experiences with even limited recreational drug use and discuss the need for a twelve-step group, both for support and as a place to discuss problems (Fariello & Scheidt, 1989; Kofoed & Keys, 1988; Rado, 1988). When the group is effective, dual-diagnosis clients tend to achieve a lower rehospitalization rate (Kofoed & Keys, 1988) and function better in society. However, the few limited follow-up studies suggest that MI/CD clients tend to continue to abuse alcohol and/or drugs despite the best efforts of staff (Drake et al., 1996).

Summary

The dual-diagnosis client presents a difficult challenge to the mental health and the chemical dependency professionals. Many of the syndromes that may result from the chronic use of chemicals are virtually indistinguishable from organic or psychiatric problems. This makes it most difficult to arrive at an accurate diagnosis. Further, MI/CD clients often use defenses, such as an interchangable system of denial, that further complicate the diagnostic process.

Dual-diagnosis clients are also difficult to work with in the rehabilitation setting. When they are in treatment, dual-diagnosis clients often talk about their psychiatric problem with drug addiction counselors, while talking about their drug abuse or addiction with mental health professionals. Because of these characteristics, it has been found necessary to modify some of the traditional treatment methods used when working with the chemically dependent client. For example, the degree of confrontation useful in working with a personality-disordered client is far too strong for working with a dual-diagnosis client who suffers from schizophrenia or another form of mental illness. However, gentle confrontation often works with the mentally ill and drug-dependent client who is not personality disordered.

CHAPTER TWENTY-THREE

Chemical Abuse by Children and Adolescents

Childhood and adolescence are periods of special concern for substance abuse rehabilitation professionals. Researchers have discovered that vulnerability for developing a substance use problem peaks between the ages of 15 and 19 years, while the median age for developing an alcohol use problem is approximately 21 years (Chatlos, 1996). Further, researchers have learned that many of the attitudes and values that support substance use problems in later life are developed in childhood or early adolescence. These discoveries, combined with the awareness that significant numbers of children and adolescents are using recreational chemicals, have made the childhood and adolescent periods of life of special interest to substance abuse rehabilitation professionals.

Although the news media speak of the problem of substance use/abuse by children and adolescents as if it were a new phenomenon, the truth is that this problem has been with us for a long time. During the early 1800s, alcoholism was rampant among the youth of England (Wheeler & Malmquist, 1987). Although social reformers attempted to intervene during the 19th and 20th centuries to eliminate the problem of recreational chemical use by children and adolescents, there has always been experimental drug and alcohol use by minors. Fifty years ago just under half of the adolescents entering high school had already used alcohol at least once (Takanishi, 1993).

However, recreational chemical use by children and adolescents appears to be more widespread, and more accepted, now than perhaps in any earlier age. Further, researchers are only now starting to identify the consequences of substance use disorders on young people's later growth and development. For this reason, this chapter focuses on chemical use/abuse by children and adolescents.

Problems in the Assessment of Child and Adolescent Drug Use Patterns

Surprisingly, very little is actually *known* about the problem of substance use/abuse in childhood or adolescence (Bukstein, 1995; Evans & Sullivan, 1990; Y. Kaminer, 1994). Many of the estimates of childhood/adolescent substance abuse are little more than watered-down versions of the assumptions that are made about chemical abuse in adults (Bukstein).

Researchers are only now starting to identify the characteristics of those who will abstain from recreational drug use during childhood and adolescence, those who will only use chemicals as part of a phase of experimentation, and those individuals who will go on to develop a problem with drug abuse/addiction. There is still much to be discovered. For example, there is virtually no research whatsoever into possible chemical use patterns by children (Newcomb & Bentler, 1989). This lack of information makes it difficult to determine what the implications of drug use during childhood might be for the individual's subsequent growth and development.

Furthermore, the lack of information makes it extremely difficult to identify criteria by which experimental and problem chemical use by children might be identified. Is chemical use in childhood automatically a cause for concern, or are there patterns of experimental chemical use that one might expect to see in childhood? What chemicals will children use most often? The truth is that nobody really knows the answers to these questions.

On a similar note, the research into teenage drug use patterns is quite limited (Bukstein, 1995; Evans & Sullivan, 1990; Newcomb & Bentler, 1989). Much of what is known about adolescent drug use patterns is based on studies that use students in school as research subjects. But since 15% to 30% of adolescents drop out of school prior to graduation (Eccles et al., 1993), school-based studies are of limited value in the understanding of adolescent chemical use patterns. This lack of data makes it quite difficult to determine current drug abuse trends. The lack of a comprehensive database also makes it difficult to identify forces that motivate the adolescent to begin to use chemicals, or when this chemical use is just part of a normal phase of experimentation. Mental health workers have little information about when adolescent chemical use might be a symptom of a serious problem, or the impact that drug use might have on the adolescent's emotional adjustment.

A third factor contributing to the confusion surrounding child and adolescent drug use is that there is a tendency for some to equate virtually any use of a chemical during adolescence as being a sign of a serious drug abuse problem (Newcomb & Bentler, 1989; Peele, 1989). This viewpoint both causes some confusion into what exactly constitutes "drug abuse" by an adolescent, and overlooks that, for many adolescents, limited episodes of chemical use might reflect only a phase of experimentation or exploration (Greenbaum, Foster-Johnson, & Petrila, 1996; Shedler & Block, 1990).

Finally, drug use patterns among children and adolescents may show rapid fluctuation and variation. Some of the variables that influence adolescent drug use trends include the individual's geographic location, peer group, and the current drug use trends. The phenomenon of inhalant abuse is one such drug use fad, which rapidly waxes and wanes in a given geographic area as individuals embrace and then discard the use of these

substances. Yet without an adequate database, it is virtually impossible to identify drug use trends among adolescents.

Scope of the Problem

Any researcher who attempts to understand the scope of alcohol/drug use problems among children/adolescents in the United States will quickly become lost in a sea of statistical information. This is unavoidable. However, if a large enough pool of data is examined, it is possible to begin to form some general impressions of the scope of chemical use/abuse in children and adolescents in the United States.

Childhood Chemical Abuse Patterns

Surprisingly, alcohol use during childhood seems to be more common than most parents are willing to admit. In England, 80% of the 13-year-old students surveyed reported that they had ingested a "proper drink" (Swadi, 1993, p. 341) at least once. Using a different methodology, the team of Johnston et al. (1996) found that 55% of eighth graders in the United States who were surveyed in 1995 admitted to having used alcohol at least once.

Statistically, the average age of the first drink is between 12 and 13 years (Novello & Shosky, 1992). Boys tend to begin drinking earlier than girls, with an average age for the first drink of alcohol being 11.9 years for boys, compared with 12.7 years for girls (Alexander & Gwyther, 1995; Morrison et al., 1995). Thus, by the time they reach adolescence, most children have had at least limited experience with alcohol use. Fortunately, despite isolated reports of alcohol abuse problems in children as young as 11 years of age, problem drinking (as opposed to experimental alcohol use) would seem to be quite rare in preadolescence (Rogers, Harris, & Jarmuskewicz, 1987).

But alcohol is not the only recreational chemical that children or adolescents are likely to experiment with. There is strong evidence that suggests many children use inhalants as their first mood-altering chemical (Newcomb & Bentler, 1989). As discussed in Chapter 14, adolescent inhalant abuse is a serious problem that, while it might not be the norm for childhood, is still quite common. For

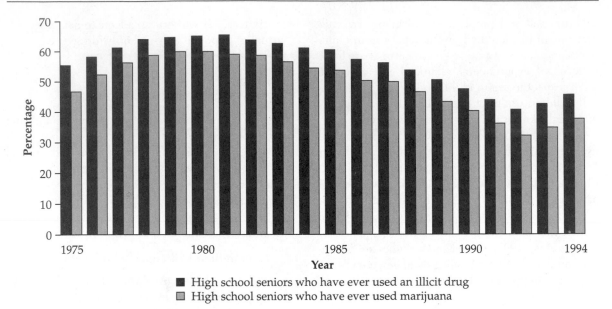

FIGURE 23.1   Illicit drug use and marijuana use by high school seniors.

example, 22% of the eighth graders surveyed in 1995 had used an inhalant at least once (Johnston et al., 1996).

As noted in Chapter 14, inhalant abuse is usually a phase. Most adolescents will engage in rare, episodic episodes of inhalant abuse over a 1- to 2-year span of time, after which most users will have abandoned the use of inhalants. But in about one-third of the cases, the individual goes on to "graduate" to more traditional forms of drug abuse (Brunswick, 1989). For these children, inhalants serve as a gateway chemical that leads to other forms of drug abuse. Another possible gateway substance is marijuana, according to Millman and Beeder (1994).

The team of Kandel, Yamaguchi, and Chen (1992) examined the theory that some chemicals function as gateway drugs. The authors interviewed 1160 subjects aged 15 to 35 years. Their results suggested that, over time, the individual's substance use progressed through the use of legal substances (alcohol, cigarettes) to marijuana, and from there on to "hard" drugs. On the basis of their findings, the authors concluded that there is evidence of a progression from the gateway chemicals to other, more serious, forms of substance use. When viewed in

this light, child/adolescent inhalant abuse seems to suggest that the individual is potentially at risk for more serious forms of chemical abuse later in life.

Adolescent Chemical Abuse Patterns

The available research suggests that adolescent drug use peaked sometime around the year 1981, slowly declined for about a decade, and has gradually been increasing since the mid-1990s (Edwards, 1993; Johnston et al., 1996). This gradual increase in the number of adolescents who admit to the use of alcohol and/or illicit chemicals is a matter of some concern for health care professionals (see Figure 23.1).

Not surprisingly, adolescent drug use patterns tend to mirror those of the society in which they live (Callahan, 1993). Thus, in a society where alcohol is the most popular recreational chemical, it should not be surprising to learn that alcohol is by far the most popular chemical of choice for adolescents (Johnston, O'Malley, & Bachman, 1993, 1994; Morrison, Rogers, & Thomas, 1995). The percentage of high school seniors who have experimented with alcohol has remained fairly stable over the past several years. For example, slightly under 90% of the class of 1990 had used alcohol

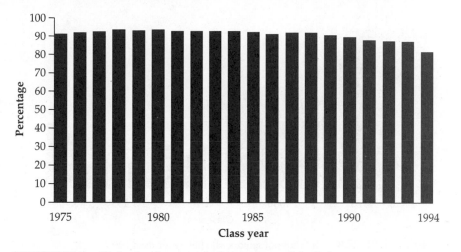

FIGURE 23.2 High school seniors who have ever used alcohol.

at least once (Johnston et al., 1993; Novello & Shosky, 1992). Eight-eight percent of the seniors from the class of 1992 questioned admitted to having used alcohol at least once, according to the authors, while 81% of the seniors of the class of 1995 admitted to having used alcohol at least once (Johnston et al., 1996). Thus, with a moderate degree of variation, it would appear that approximately 90% of graduating high school seniors will have used alcohol at least once (see Figure 23.2).

Although this statistic is frightening by itself, there is evidence to suggest that a sizable percentage of high school seniors use alcohol fairly heavily. Approximately 30% of the graduating seniors of the high school class of 1995 claimed to have consumed five or more drinks at least once in the 2 weeks preceding the survey (Johnston et al., 1996). Although a majority of the adolescents studied in 1990 experimented with alcohol, the heaviest alcohol use was confined to 500,000 students, who consumed five or more drinks at a time at least once a week (Novello & Shosky, 1992).

The most popular form of alcohol for the adolescents surveyed is beer, although wine coolers are increasing in popularity (Novello & Shosky, 1992). Few adolescents seem to be drawn to hard liquor. Indeed, so rare is adolescent use of vodka, gin, whiskey, or bourbon that even occasional experimentation with these liquors should be considered a

sign of an alcohol abuse problem (Rogers et al., 1987). Although many parents worry about possible alcohol use by their adolescent children, they are poor sources of information about their teenagers' use of this chemical. It has been found that parents tend to underestimate their teenagers' alcohol consumption by a factor of at least ten to one (Morrison et al., 1995; Rogers et al., 1987; Zarek, Hawkins, & Rogers, 1987).

Alcohol is not the only recreational chemical used by adolescents. By the time of graduation, 48% of the seniors from the class of 1995 admitted to the use of an illicit chemical at least once (Johnston et al., 1996). Marijuana was the most frequently used illicit chemical, and by the time of graduation, 42% of the seniors of the class of 1995 admitted to having used marijuana at least once, according to the authors.

For eighth graders, alcohol is the most commonly used mood-altering chemical, with 55% of the eighth-grade students surveyed in 1995 admitting to having used alcohol at least once (Johnston et al., 1996). However, inhalants have replaced marijuana as the most frequently used mood-altering illicit chemical, with 22% of the eighth graders surveyed in 1995 admitting to the use of inhalants at least once (Johnston et al.). A small percentage of adolescents have used hallucinogenics (Gold et al., 1994). In their survey of 522,000 high school juniors and seniors, the authors found that only 5.3% of the students surveyed in 1993

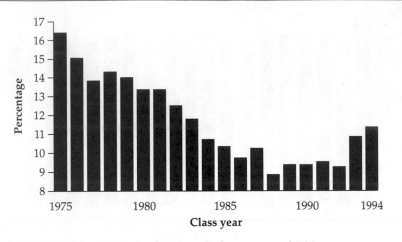

FIGURE 23.3   High school seniors who have ever used LSD.

admitted to having used hallucinogens at least once, up from 4.9% the previous year. Johnston et al. offered an even higher percentage of seniors who admitted to the use of hallucinogens at least once. The authors reported that 13% of the seniors from the class of 1995 surveyed admitted to having used a hallucinogenic substance at least once. There is evidence to suggest that LSD is also growing in popularity among adolescents. The National Institute on Drug Abuse (1994) reported that 8.6% of the seniors in the class of 1992, 10.3% of the seniors in the class of 1993, and 10.5% of the seniors in the class of 1994 all claimed to have used LSD at least once (see Figure 23.3).

Those adolescents who develop substance use problems seem to show a definite progression in their substance use (Kandel & Davies, 1996). In the first stage, the adolescent will use a chemical normally reserved for adults (i.e., tobacco and/or alcohol). Most adolescents do not progress beyond this stage. For example, Newcomb (1996) suggested that only 8% of all adolescents in the United States will ever have a substance use disorder. But, for those who do progress, the next step is the use of an illicit chemical. Kandel and Davies noted that this substance is usually marijuana. Again, of those adolescents who reach this stage, most do not proceed further. However, the use of marijuana precedes the use of hard drugs such as cocaine, according to the authors. Thus, the progression of substance

abuse first identified in the 1970s seems to continue to apply to adolescent chemical use patterns at the turn of the 21st century (see Figure 23.4).

College students form a unique subpopulation. Traditionally, college is viewed as spanning the period from late adolescence to early adulthood. However, now that the legal definition of "adulthood" has been lowered to 18 years of age, most college students are considered legal adults. Yet, at the same time, these individuals are still below the age of 21, which is the age at which an adult can purchase alcohol in most states.

Although most college students cannot legally purchase alcohol, the abuse of this chemical is the most significant problem found on the campus (Wechsler, Davenport, Dowdall, Moeykens, & Castillo, 1994). The authors mailed questionnaires to 28,709 college students across the country, of which 17,592 were correctly filled out and returned. On the basis of the information in the questionnaires, the authors concluded that despite most college students being unable to legally purchase alcohol, 44% of all college students were "binge" drinkers. A binge was defined by the authors as a period in which an individual consumed five or more drinks in an evening.

Further, Wechsler et al. (1994) found that most of those students in their sample followed the same drinking pattern in high school as they did in college.

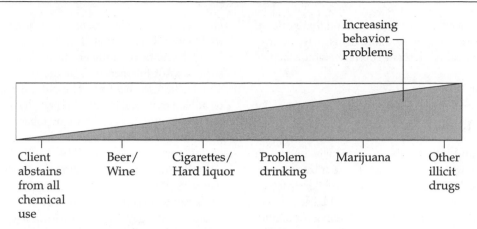

FIGURE 23.4 Continuum of adolescent substance abuse problems.

Thus, although the majority of those who consumed alcohol in college did not consider their drinking to be indicative of a problem, the roots of college binge drinking often seem to extend back to the student's high school years.

A factor that may contribute to the tendency for many college students to use alcohol in an abusive manner is a pattern of social misperception that contributes to the tendency to abuse chemicals. As a group, college students tend to overestimate both their peers' acceptance of the individual's drunken behavior and the number of their peers who are drinking heavily (DeAngelis, 1994b). Further, there is a tendency among heavy drug/alcohol users to equate substance use with fun, according to the author. It is not clear whether these misperceptions are found in younger adolescents or develop during the college years. However, such social misperceptions seem to contribute to the tendency for college students to abuse recreational chemicals.

Do Adolescent Drug Use Surveys Give Us the Whole Picture?

The answer to this question is "no." Frequently, adolescent drug use surveys focus on the greatest concentration of adolescents: those who are still in school. However, adolescents who use hard drugs on a regular basis are more likely to drop out of school. Thus, these individuals are less likely to be included in school-based surveys, and school-based adolescent substance use surveys might not provide a complete overview of adolescent chemical use patterns (Bukstein, 1995; Oetting & Beauvais, 1990).

There appears to be a relationship between academic performance and recreational drug use. Those students who encounter academic problems in middle to late elementary school grades are more likely to engage in alcohol/drug abuse than students who achieve satisfactory grades (Board of Trustees, 1991). Adolescents who are not interested in academic achievement are considered to be at risk for both using recreational chemicals and for dropping out of school (Board of Trustees, 1991). Thus, surveys of adolescent drug use patterns that are based on student responses may actually underestimate chemical use patterns by failing to question those individuals who are most likely to engage in substance use/abuse.

Another shortcoming of national surveys is that regional variations may exist in terms of the drug(s)-of-choice, or patterns of use, which might not be reflected in a national survey of student substance abuse behaviors (Oetting & Beauvais, 1990). For example, Moncher, Holden, and Trimble (1990) concluded that adolescent Native Americans were two to three times as likely to be "at least moderately involved with alcohol" (p. 408) as were non-Indian urban adolescents. But, in most school districts, Native American students are only a small minority of the student body. It is only in school districts with a large proportion of Native American students that this ethnic variation in substance abuse rates would be detected.

Thus, the reader must keep in mind that *national* drug use patterns among adolescents may, or may not, reflect local adolescent substance abuse behavior patterns.

Tobacco Use by Children and Adolescents

Cigarettes and other tobacco products occupy a unique place within this society. These substances are known to be both addictive and terribly destructive, and yet they may be legally purchased by adults. Tobacco use problems are also a very real part of childhood and adolescence. Since the mid-1970s, researchers have discovered that the roots of nicotine addiction lie in childhood or adolescence. For example, by the age of 12, fully one-half of the schoolchildren in Canada have already experimented with cigarette smoking (J. Walker, 1993). In the United States, the *average* age at which smokers begin to smoke is thought to be 14.5 years (Roberts & Watson, 1994).

These discoveries are a cause for concern for many reasons, not the least of which is that cigarette manufacturers have apparently used this knowledge to try to manipulate adolescents into starting to smoke cigarettes. At least one major tobacco company has conducted research into the phases of adolescent cigarette smoking, apparently to better understand how to help the individual make the transition to regular cigarette smoking (Hilts, 1996). Another major tobacco company referred to adolescents in an internal memo as an "up and coming new generation of smokers" (Phelps, 1996, p. 1A).

There is significant evidence that cigarette smoking by adolescents may interfere with the normal development of the lungs, which may have lifelong consequences for the individual (Gold et al., 1996). Also, as a general rule, adolescents tend to underestimate the addictive potential of nicotine (Benowitz & Henningfield, 1994). Few adolescents plan to smoke for the rest of their lives, according to the authors, but start out with the intention of quitting in a few years. But, as discussed in Chapter 15, "a few years" is more than enough time for the individual to become addicted to nicotine. Further, once a person is addicted to nicotine, it is difficult to quit. This makes the fact that each day in the United States an estimated 3000

children or adolescents *begin* to smoke especially frightening (Bhandari et al., 1996; Kessler, 1995).

Adolescents are unlikely to understand the consequences of tobacco use, or the risk of developing an addiction to nicotine. The natural rebelliousness of adolescents makes them especially vulnerable to the image, encouraged by many tobacco companies' advertising, that cigarette smoking is a way to rebel against parental authority (Hilts, 1996). When adult cigarette smokers are questioned, it becomes clear that 90% (Pierce et al., 1991) of adult cigarette smokers began to smoke before the age of 21. MacKenzie et al. (1994b) gave an even earlier age, stating that 80% to 90% of all smokers begin before the age of 18.

Individuals who use smokeless tobacco also begin to do so at an early age. There are an estimated 1.5 million people under the age of 19 who use smokeless tobacco (Kessler, 1995). Researchers believe that 73% of those who use smokeless tobacco started to do so by the time that they were in the ninth grade (Barker, 1994). Further, 90% of cigarette smokers are already *addicted* to nicotine by the age of 20 (J. Walker, 1993). These figures underscore the need to address the use of tobacco products during childhood or adolescence.

In support of this observation, by the time of graduation from high school, 22% of the students surveyed admitted to smoking at least once each day (Johnston et al., 1996). Further, the authors found that just under 64% of the seniors surveyed in 1995 had used cigarettes at least once. These figures are very similar to that obtained by DiFranza and Tye (1990), who found that 18.1% of high school seniors smoke cigarettes on a daily basis. The American Heart Association estimated that 2.2 million children between the ages of 12 and 17 smoke cigarettes (Associated Press, 1994a), while Mead (1993) offered a figure of 3 million children and adolescents in this country who either smoke, or use smokeless tobacco products. An estimated 100,000 of the adolescents who smoke are thought to be below the age of 13 (Bhandari et al., 1996).

Are Children/Adolescents Being Targeted by the Tobacco Industry?

Despite strident public denials from cigarette manufacturers, there is strong evidence that tobacco companies have targeted children and adolescents in order to introduce them to the practice of cigarette smoking (Hilts, 1996). Consider the following: if, as research has shown, 75% of those people who smoke do so on a regular basis by the age of 17, and, if cigarette manufacturers conduct research studies on "presmokers" (Hilts, p. 73), then what age group is being targeted? The conclusion, which few people want to discuss, appears obvious.

In an internal memo that originated in one major tobacco company in the United States, the tobacco company and a law firm had discussed the possible impact of taxation on the price of cigarettes. In this memo, which became available to the public only 30 years after it was written, it was concluded, *"The price affects the ability of young people to buy cigarettes"* (Glantz et al., 1996, p. 249, italics in original).

The truth is that, given the high mortality rates associated with tobacco smoking, the tobacco industry is dependent on recruiting children to replace smokers who either stop or who die for one reason or another (Kessler, 1995). To this end, it has been suggested that tobacco advertising techniques have been developed that specifically target children and adolescents (DiFranza et al., 1991; Glantz et al., 1996; Hilts, 1996; Kessler, 1995; Pierce et al., 1991). Publicly, tobacco companies deny this charge. But, in an internal memo that became available to the public 23 years after it was written, the assistant general counsel of one tobacco company expressed concern to the director of public relations of the same company over the National Cancer Institute's development of *"educational programs to prevent young, non-smokers taking up the practice of smoking"* (Glantz et al., p. 247, italics in original). If his tobacco company did not target children and adolescents to encourage them to smoke cigarettes, why would they worry about the National Cancer Institute's program to help them not begin?

Given this apparent internal interest in young smokers on the part of at least one major tobacco company, it should not be surprising to learn:

> If sales to children account for 3.3% of cigarette sales, these six . . . companies share an annual $703 million in revenues and $221 million in profits from the sale of cigarettes to children. (DiFranza & Tye, 1990, p. 2786)

Each year in the United States, children and adolescents smoke an estimated 1.1 billion packs of cigarettes (Bhandari et al., 1996). These figures raise disturbing doubts about current sales and advertising tactics used to promote tobacco use, especially to children and adolescents. The authors observe that many of the children or adolescents who begin to use tobacco before the age of 21 will go on to become addicted. This fact will provide "an 'investment' that will pay dividends into the future" (p. 2786) in the form of a new generation of smokers.

Males (1992) challenged the conclusion that tobacco advertising was a major factor in adolescent cigarette smoking. He concluded that a more important factor is that 75% of all teenagers who smoke had parents who also smoked. According to the author, the evidence points toward the fact that "teenage smoking is largely the active continuation of a childhood of passive smoking" (p. 3282). This theory is certainly consistent with research suggesting that the transition from a nonsmoker to smoker in childhood or adolescence appears to pass through several stages (Holland & Fitzsimons, 1991):

1. *Preparatory phase.* The child forms attitudes accepting of cigarette smoking.
2. *Initiation phase.* The person smokes for the first time.
3. *Experimentation phase.* The child or adolescent learns how to smoke.
4. *Transition.* The person smokes regularly.

Thus, the attitudes supportive of, or at least accepting of, smoking are formed in childhood, prior to the initiation of actual smoking behaviors. Thus, it should not be surprising that 75% of the adolescents who smoke were raised by parents who also smoked cigarettes. But, this research does not explain why more cigarette advertising is displayed at convenience stores within 1000 feet of schools than at convenience stores further away from such high concentrations of children/adolescents (Hilts, 1996).

Hints for Successful Intervention

Given the progression from forming attitudes accepting of smoking through the addictive use of tobacco, attempts at intervention need to be aimed at children who have not yet started to form pro-smoking attitudes (Holland & Fitzsimons, 1991). Attempts at intervention should focus on helping children learn social skills that will enable them to resist smoking, according to the authors, on the grounds that if the adolescent reaches 16 to 18 years of age without having initiated smoking, he/she is unlikely to do so. For example, fully 90% of those who *begin* to smoke cigarettes after the age of 21 are unlikely to continue the habit, according to Hilts (1996).

Why Do Adolescents Use Chemicals?

The initial factor that seems to influence adolescent experimentation with recreational chemical use seems to be curiosity. Some adolescents begin to experiment with chemicals as a form of rebellion. Others will begin to engage in chemical use in response to peer pressure (Bukstein, 1995). Indeed, there is a strong relationship between the individual's substance use and the substance use patterns of an adolescent's peers, according to the author. However, the individual's substance use is also influenced by his/her cognitive level. For example, many adolescents do not see themselves as being vulnerable to the negative effects of alcohol or drugs of abuse (B. Alexander, 1991).

For some adolescents, recreational chemicals offer the promise of relief from internal discomfort, such as feelings of depression (Joshi & Scott, 1988). It was found that chemically dependent adolescents were three times as likely to be depressed as were their non-drug-using counterparts (Deykin, Buka, & Zeena, 1992). So strong was the relationship between affective disorders such as anxiety or depression and substance abuse that Burke, Burke, and Rae (1994) suggested that these conditions identified adolescents who were at high risk (p. 454) for later drug use disorders. Thus, there is strong evidence to suggest that adolescents use chemicals to self-medicate painful feelings.

Other reasons adolescents are thought to use chemicals is their attempt to fit in, as a rite of passage, or as a way to deal with the stress of interpersonal conflict (Evans & Sullivan, 1990; Morrison et al., 1995). Chemical use may offer some adolescents a

way to rebel against parental authority, a way to fit in a social group, or the means to prove sexual prowess (Morrison et al., 1995; Rhodes & Jason, 1990). The specific reason(s) for any given individual's chemical use is often influenced by the person's emotional maturity, available intrapersonal and interpersonal resources, and his/her social support systems.

The evolution of child/adolescent substance use patterns and values takes place in a swirling mixture of forces that vary in intensity at different points in the individual's early years. During the childhood years, parental influence on subsequent drug use behavior is the strongest. The child will accept parental guidance as to how to behave, but will also be very aware of parental modeling behaviors (Cohen, Richardson, & LaBree, 1994; Rogers et al., 1987).

Thus, there is evidence to suggest that parental substance use is associated with subsequent use of chemicals by the adolescent (Alexander & Gwyther, 1995; Chassin, Curran, Hussong, & Colder, 1996; Y. Kaminer, 1991). Most certainly, adolescent substance use patterns are consistent with the individual's attitudes and beliefs (Bukstein, 1995). If the parents of the adolescent use recreational chemicals, it would be easier for the child/adolescent to form beliefs and attitudes supportive of recreational substance use. However, the relationship between parental chemical abuse and drug use by the teenager is complex and involves other factors than simply whether the adolescent's parents have used chemicals.

Cohen et al. (1994) noted that several factors seem to be associated with problem adolescent alcohol use, including:

1. Parental modeling behaviors.
2. Parental efforts to shape behavioral standards and values.
3. The quality of the family's affectional interactions.

In their examination of the factors that might influence adolescent smoking and alcohol use behaviors, the authors found that children who reported that their parents spent more time with them, and who made greater efforts to communicate with them, had lower rates of alcohol/tobacco use in the months preceding the study. On the basis of their findings, the authors called for greater efforts to include the parents of the children deemed at risk for later chemical use in any intervention program.

Chassin et al. (1996) also concluded that parent-child communication was an important element in the child's subsequent chemical use/abuse. This team of researchers noted that parents who use recreational chemicals tend to engage in fewer "parental control practices" (p. 70) with their adolescent. Decreased monitoring of the adolescent's activities, possibly brought on by the parents' own use of recreational chemicals, then allows the teenager greater opportunities to join social groups likely to engage in recreational drug/alcohol use.[1]

Thus, recreational chemical abuse by the parents contributes to a tendency for the parents to fail to fulfill their role to supervise the adolescent's social contacts, allowing him or her to select a peer group that might support drug/alcohol abuse. The adolescent's peer group is another important factor in shaping the individual's chemical use patterns (Adger & Werner, 1994; Bukstein, 1995). Peer group influences have been termed "crucial" (Y. Kaminer, 1991, p. 330) in the development of adolescent substance use patterns. It is hypothesized that because they lack adequate sources of nurturance within the family of origin, some adolescents may be vulnerable to *any* display of acceptance, no matter how dysfunctional its source. According to this theory, these adolescents find that the use of chemicals brings a form of acceptance from other drug-using teens, whose companionship then seems desirable. Only later do the adolescents seeking nurturance discover that they have become physically dependent on the drugs or alcohol because of their addictive potential.

Other researchers have suggested, however, that peer groups might not be a major factor in adolescent alcohol abuse (Bauman & Ennett, 1994; Novello & Shosky, 1992). Novello and Shosky noted that of the 10.6 million adolescents who consume

alcohol, almost one-third do so when alone, rather than in groups. The authors interpreted this data as evidence that the theory that adolescents use chemicals in response to peer pressure must be accepted only as a theory and may not be true in all cases.

Bauman and Ennett (1994) identified several factors that might distort the relationship between adolescent peer group membership and substance use patterns. One such factor was the influence of friend-selection. According to the authors, individual friendship patterns evolve, in part, because of a congruence of substance use patterns. In other words, drug-using adolescents tend to form friendships mainly with other drug-using adolescents, a pattern that might lead to researchers overestimating the influence of peer groups on substance use patterns.

A second factor that might distort the apparent relationship between substance use patterns and peer group membership was the possibility of *projection* on the part of the research subjects. In other words, when asked about their friends' substance use, drug-using adolescents are more likely to respond on the basis of *their own* drug use behavior, rather than on the basis of what they know about their friends' chemical use. In support of this theory, Bauman and Ennett (1994) pointed out that adolescents who do not use chemicals were more likely to be judged as using recreational drugs by their drug-using friends than they were by their non-drug-using friends. On the basis of their research, Bauman and Ennett suggested that the factor of adolescent peer use on substance abuse patterns was "overestimated" (p. 820).

A factor that seems to be related to later substance abuse is that of having been victim of some form of abuse (Fuller & Cavanaugh, 1995). Adolescents might turn to alcohol/drugs as a way of coping with the anxiety, emotional pain, and the shame of having been victimized earlier in life. Another group of adolescents who are vulnerable to the effects of recreational chemicals are those individuals who become aware of homosexual urges within themselves. According to Fuller and Cavanaugh, the homosexual adolescent might use alcohol and/or drugs in an attempt to self-medicate feelings of guilt, inadequacy, or self-depreciation. Admittedly, the early adolescent years appear to be a time of special vulnerability for

---

[1]An interesting point to consider is whether the parents do not engage in adequate supervisory behaviors because they are using chemicals, or, if they are using recreational chemicals because they are dysfunctional, and thus unable to fulfill their parental roles in the first place.

later drug abuse. During this period, many adolescents begin to experiment with gateway chemicals that open the door to later drug abuse problems (Pentz et al., 1989):

> The more extensive, the more intensive and the longer one uses drugs such as marijuana, the more likely it is that a person will begin to use drugs such as cocaine or heroin. (Cattarello et al., 1995, p. 152)

Thus, researchers and rehabilitation professionals pay special attention to adolescents' possible use of gateway chemicals such as tobacco, alcohol, and marijuana. Brunswick (1989) suggested that inhalants also collectively serve as gateway chemicals of abuse.

As mentioned, a number of factors interact to shape the average adolescent's recreational substance use pattern. In the next section, we examine the question of whether chemical use is a natural part of adolescence.

The Adolescent Abuse/Addiction Dilemma: Or, How Much Is Too Much?

After more than a decade of study, researchers still do not have a proven method to determine which adolescents are in need of professional help because of their abuse of chemicals (Bukstein, 1994). Such variables as low socioeconomic status, a lack of religious commitment, low self-esteem, and disturbed families, have all been suggested as helping to identify the adolescent drug abuser (Newcomb & Bentler, 1989). As noted, another factor that has been suggested to be a strong influence on adolescent drug use is that peer group (Joshi & Scott, 1988; Newcomb & Bentler, 1989).

However, Shedler and Block (1990) reported that their longitudinal study of a group of adolescents who have been followed by investigators since they were young children, suggests that certain personality traits seem to predispose the individual to abstain from recreational chemical use or drug abuse during adolescence. The authors found that extremes of behavior (i.e., total abstinence or serious drug abuse) were found in adolescents who were most maladjusted, while the healthiest group

were those who had only occasionally experimented with chemicals.

These findings, although surprising at first glance, seem to make clinical sense. The emotionally healthy adolescent might experiment with recreational drug use, but ultimately would have the interpersonal and intrapersonal skills necessary to cope with life. However, as Shedler and Block (1990) reported, those adolescents who used drugs on a frequent basis demonstrated poor impulse control, a pattern of social alienation, and emotional distress, all signs that these individuals lack the emotional resources of the first group.

Further, those individuals who totally abstained from chemical use were found to be anxious, emotionally constricted, and lacking in social skills. These individuals seem to lack the self-confidence to allow them to explore their environments, which would include an exploration of the possibility of recreational drug use. The authors concluded that the individual's chemical use pattern (i.e., abstinence, experimental drug use, or frequent drug abuse) could only be interpreted in light of the individual's emotional adjustment.

Adolescent chemical use/abuse must be considered in terms of the individual's developmental stage (Bukstein, 1995; Cattarello et al., 1995; Steinberg, 1991). For example, although experimental chemical use might be a normal part of the adolescent experience, chemical use/abuse or the use of alcohol to the point of intoxication, in the early part of adolescence, appears to indicate adolescents who are at risk for later drug use problems (Bukstein). However, in later adolescence, which is to say after the age of 15, the experimental use of alcohol or drugs might not reflect serious problems so much as society's more liberal attitude toward recreational substance use, according to the author.

Thus, for the majority of adolescents, especially for those in later adolescence, recreational substance use seems to be a phase of experimentation (Miller, Westerberg, & Waldron, 1995). During this phase of experimentation, the individual is exploring new forms of behavior that are commonly found in his/her culture. However, for a small percentage of adolescents, recreational substance use is the first step to a chemical use problem. Mental health and substance abuse professionals are often called on to identify, and treat, these individuals.

Problems in Diagnosis and Treatment of Adolescent Drug Abuse

The diagnosis of adolescent drug abuse/addiction is difficult, and the diagnostic criteria are arbitrary (Alexander & Gwyther, 1995; Bukstein, 1994). Indeed, researchers are unsure what criteria to use to define a substance use disorder in adolescence and often rely on the same diagnostic signs used with adult substance abusers (Bukstein, 1995; Greenbaum et al., 1996).

One way to improve the accuracy of an assessment of an adolescent's chemical use pattern is to establish an extensive database about the individual, and his/her substance use patterns (Evans & Sullivan, 1990). For example, the occasional use of alcohol or marijuana at a party, say once every 6 months, is not, automatically, a sign of a drug abuse problem (Newcomb & Bentler, 1989). It may reflect only isolated episodes of alcohol or marijuana use.

Referrals for a chemical dependency evaluation on an adolescent come from many potential sources. The juvenile court system frequently refers an offender for an evaluation, especially when that individual was under the influence of chemicals at the time of arrest. School officials may request an evaluation on a student suspected of abusing chemicals. Treatment center admissions officers will frequently recommend an evaluation, although this is usually referred to in-house staff rather than to an independent professional. Some parents, especially those who have "religious, restrictive families" (Farrow, 1990, p. 1268) will also request an evaluation and/or treatment after the first known episode of alcohol or drug use.

One important point to remember in evaluating the adolescent's chemical use pattern is that his/her developmental stage may prevent the adolescent from being able to understand the implications of drug use. Adolescents frequently feel that they are invulnerable, and their normal narcissism prevents them from being able to understand the long-term consequences of substance abuse. Unlike older addicts, the adolescent will not have had time to "hit bottom" and may have a rather immature view of life.

Their simplistic outlook on life and continued chemical use may mistakenly be interpreted by treatment staff not as emotional immaturity, but as resistance. The authors recommended a multidisciplinary team approach to assessment in cases of suspected adolescent substance abuse, to allow for the accurate identification of the client's strengths, weaknesses, and, adaptive style.

Even when the legitimate need for treatment is identified, several factors may interfere with the treatment process. Kaminer and Frances (1991) identified these factors as being (a) unrealistic parental expectations for treatment, (b) hidden agendas for treatment by both the adolescent and the parents, (c) parental psychopathology, and (d) parental drug or alcohol abuse. Another factor is parental refusal to provide consent for treatment (Y. Kaminer, 1994). Often, combinations of these problems are found in the family of an adolescent drug or alcohol abuser who fails to enter, or complete, treatment.

Several factors seem to identify adolescents who are at risk for alcohol abuse problems (Adger & Werner, 1994; Alexander & Gwyther, 1995; Fuller & Cavanaugh, 1995):

- Family history of alcoholism or drug abuse.
- Depression or other psychiatric illness.
- Loss of loved one(s).
- Low self-esteem.
- Poor social skills.
- Problems in relationship with parents (parents are either too permissive or too authoritarian).
- Feelings of alienation.
- School problems, or limited commitment to school.
- Low expectations for school.
- Family tolerance for deviant behavior.
- Peer tolerance for deviant behavior.
- Attitude accepting of drug use.
- Antisocial behavior.
- Early sexual experience.
- Early experimental drug use.

The team of Wills, McNamara, Vaccaro, and Hirky (1996) followed a group of 1184 adolescents from the seventh to the ninth grade, to identify those factors that might be used as predictors of adolescent substance use. They concluded that those adolescents who initiated, and then rapidly escalated, their substance use, seemed to have a greater number of predictor variables than adolescents whose substance use was low to minimal. Such variables included:

1. Greater level of life stress.
2. Lower level of parental support.
3. Higher levels of parental substance use/abuse.
4. A greater number of deviant attitudes and maladaptive coping mechanisms.
5. Lower levels of self-control.
6. Higher levels of engagement with drug-using peers.

Although adolescent "problem behavior" (Robert Haggarty, quoted in Kirn, 1989, p. 3362) such as substance use/abuse has long been viewed as a warning sign of potential adolescent chemical use problems, there are a number of reasons for adolescents to engage in such behavior. For example, they may do so because of economic problems, or because they have a pessimistic view of the future. Other such problem behaviors include teen pregnancies and delinquency; in Haggart's opinion, these are all non-specific problems that suggest present unhappiness and pessimism about the future.

There is an apparent relationship between the adolescent's substance use, and his/her participation in other forms of socially deviant behavior (Cattarello et al., 1995). Because of the relationship between adolescent substance abuse, and socially deviant behaviors, Jones (1990) suggested that adolescents who were depressed, who run away from home, or who were school behavior problems, should be evaluated for possible substance abuse problems. Further, adolescents who experienced any form of legal problems, suicidal behaviors, delinquency problems, or recurrent accidents, should be considered to be abusing chemicals "until proved otherwise" (Jones, p. 680, italics in original deleted).

The Stages of Adolescent Chemical Use

For adolescents who abuse chemicals, there is a progression that leads, ultimately, to more serious substance use problems. The individual's progression from experimental substance use to a substance use problem might be viewed as passing through four different stages (Jones, 1990). Chatlos (1996), on the other hand, suggested a five-stage model of adolescent substance use/abuse. These two models are contrasted in Table 23-1.

Each model suggests that the adolescent substance user must first be exposed to the chemical(s) he/she will abuse, and learn what to expect from the use of that substance. Each model suggests that for those adolescents who continue to engage in recreational chemical use there is a change in friendship patterns as the adolescent begins to drift away from his/her former peer group, toward a new peer group that is more accepting of chemical use. Other new behaviors that might develop during this stage include erratic school performance, unpredictable mood swings, and manipulative behaviors, all in the service of continued substance abuse.

When the individual becomes preoccupied "with the mood swing" (Jones, 1990, p. 680), non-drug-using friends are avoided, family fights and confrontations develop, there is a loss of employment, expulsion from school, consistent lying, and daily use of mood-altering chemicals. Ultimately, some individuals will continue to the final stage of substance use, where they must use drugs just "to feel normal" (Jones, p. 680). During this stage, the individual will experience physical complications from drug use, memory loss and/or flashback experiences, paranoia, anger, and drug/alcohol overdoses.

Adolescence and Addiction to Chemicals

It was once thought that adolescents were unlikely to have had the opportunity to use a drug(s) long enough to develop physical dependence on that chemical (Kaminer & Frances, 1991). Thus, adolescents were thought to be unlikely to develop withdrawal symptoms when the chemical was discontinued. If symptoms of chemical dependency are encountered in the adolescent, they are usually much less severe than these same symptoms are in the adult who has been abusing drugs, according to Kaminer and Frances. The authors believe: (a) it is unlikely that adolescents might actually become addicted to chemicals, but (b) if the adolescent *did* become addicted to chemicals, the symptoms of the addiction would be less pronounced than those seen in an adult addicted to the same chemical.

Other clinicians disagree with this assessment, however. Many clinicians believe that adolescents may become addicted to alcohol and chemicals, although they usually have used drugs only for a short period. Hoffmann, Belille, and Harrison (1987) found, for example, that more than three-quarters of their sample of 1000 adolescents, all of whom were in treatment at the time, reported having developed tolerance to alcohol or other drugs. Further, one-third of their sample reported withdrawal symptoms from drugs or alcohol.

Chassin and DeLucia (1996) reported that, like their adult counterparts, chronic adolescent alcohol abusers show evidence of liver damage on blood chemistry studies, suggesting that it is possible for the adolescent to use alcohol extensively enough to cause physical damage to their bodies. It is not clear whether this is a common occurrence. But Farrow

(1990) challenged the concept of adolescent addiction. The author concluded, "The number of teenagers who are truly chemically dependent is less than 1% of all users" (p. 1268). Another 10% to 15% might meet the diagnostic criteria for drug or alcohol abuse, while a full 10% to 15% of all teenagers have little or no experience with either alcohol or drugs. The remainder are occasional users of alcohol/drugs, and will likely adjust "their use in nonproblematic ways as they grow older" (p. 1268). As these conflicting study results suggest, there is a need for more research into the possible indicators of adolescent problem substance use patterns.

Adolescent Substance Use: A Cause for Optimism?

On the bright side, significant evidence suggests that the majority of those adolescents who engage in recreational chemical use will not go on to develop a drug dependency problem (Jones, 1990; Y. Kaminer, 1994). Rather, one phase of development that many

TABLE 23-1 Comparison of Two Theories of the Stages of Adolescent Substance Abuse

Jones's (1990) theory	*Chatlos's (1996) theory*
Learning the Mood Swing The adolescent is exposed to substance use, and learns from more experienced users what to expect from the use of recreational substances.	*Initiation* Individual begins the use of mood-altering chemicals.
Seeking the Mood Swing The young substance user begins to center his/her life around chemical use (e.g., changing his/her circle of friends to those people who use chemicals), and also increases use of recreational chemicals.	*Learning the Mood Swing* The new substance user must learn what effects to expect from his/her chemical use, and why these effects are desirable.
Being Preoccupied with the Mood Swing Person stops relationships with nonusing friends; may lose job or be expelled from school; uses mood-altering drugs daily; may lie to friends/family to protect continued use of drugs.	*Regular Use/Seeking the Mood Swing* The adolescent continues to seek what are now viewed as the positive benefits from recreational chemical use.
Using Just to Feel Normal Drug/alcohol use has reached the point where the individual must engage in use of chemicals just to feel "normal" and to be able to function. Person experiences some consequences of chronic chemical abuse, may become paranoid, have memory loss, or experiences flashbacks.	*Abuse/Harmful Consequences* Negative effects of recreational chemical use begin to make themselves felt on the user's life (poor academic performance, etc.), but the individual continues to use recreational chemicals.
	Substance Dependence/Compulsive Use The adolescent is now physically addicted to chemicals, or at least is trapped in a cycle of compulsive use, despite serious consequences of this behavior.

adolescents go through seems to involve experimental chemical use. Of those adolescents who enter into this phase of experimental drug use, only a small percentage develop a more serious drug abuse problem (Chatlos, 1996).

The Financial Incentive for Overdiagnosis

The admissions officers of many treatment centers, hold that the use of chemicals by adolescents automatically means a drug abuse problem is present. Such treatment professionals, perhaps with an eye more on the balance sheet than on the individual's needs, frequently recommend treatment on the basis of any adolescent drug use. Harold Swift, president of the world-famous Hazelden Foundation, was quoted by Iggers (1990) as asking "what harm has been done?" (if a teenager was mistakenly told that he/she was addicted to chemicals).

Newcomb and Bentler (1989) recognized that the treatment of chemical dependency has become a multimillion-dollar industry, where, on occasion, the client's needs are placed after those of the treatment center. Almost a decade after they issued their warning, the words of the authors continue to ring true:

> There is growing concern that for various reasons, not the least of which is the profit motive, treatment programs are purposefully blurring the distinction between use and abuse (any use equals abuse) and preying on the national drug hysteria to scare parents into putting their teenager in treatment with as little provocation as having a beer or smoking a joint. (p. 246)

The annual bonus for the director and staff of many inpatient treatment programs is based on the average daily census (Dr. Norman Hoffmann, quoted in Turbo, 1989). Because there is a financial incentive for the clinical staff to keep as many beds occupied as possible, it is advantageous for the treatment center staff to find as many cases of "addiction" as possible. One must wonder, in this situation, how much effort the treatment center staff invests in excluding the possibility of drug abuse in an adolescent (or even an adult) being evaluated for possible admission.

Forcing the individual—even if this person is "only" an adolescent—into treatment when he/she does not have a chemical addiction may have lifelong consequences (Peele, 1989). Such action may violate the rights of the individual, and in some states, it is illegal to force an adolescent into treatment against his/her will, even with parental permission (Evans & Sullivan, 1990).

The reader should keep in mind that, to date, diagnostic criteria have not been developed that allow for the accurate identification of those adolescents who are—and are not—addicted to chemicals. Nevertheless, drug rehabilitation programs continue to:

> . . . aim . . . to convince children they are perpetually debilitated. Only after making this concession, treatment personnel contend, can children begin to make progress through life, albeit now convinced that they can never really be whole or lead a normal existence. (Peele, 1989, pp. 103–104)

There is no research into how this treatment approach may affect the individual's subsequent emotional growth. Nor is there research to determine if there might be a negative consequence to telling the adolescent that he/she is forever an addict at such a young age, especially when the literature does not support this extreme view.

A possible solution to this dilemma is offered by Beeder and Millman (1995), who suggested that when working with adolescents who have a substance use problem:

> After one year or more of abstinence and *appropriate social adjustment*, young people may be encouraged to think of themselves as similar to their peers, though with the recognition that they continue to be at increased risk. (p. 79, italics added for emphasis)

Thus, the authors neatly sidestep the issue of whether the adolescent is/is not "addicted" to chemicals. From this perspective, the goal of treatment should be to help the client to achieve a state of appropriate social behavior, one aspect of which is abstinence from recreational chemicals on the grounds that the individual might be "at risk" for further substance use problems.

Although many adolescents will experience substance use problems at some point in their lives, the majority will adopt a more acceptable pattern of chemical use in young adulthood (Evans & Sullivan, 1990; Peele, 1989). Statistically, the peak period of substance use problems is between ages

18 and 22 years, after which the average individual tends to return to a more appropriate pattern of chemical use (Bukstein, 1995). Of those adolescents identified as heavy drinkers at age 18, half were not judged to be heavy drinkers 12 years later, according to Bukstein (1994). Thus, the adolescent who might have abused chemicals on a regular basis may, or may not, go on to develop a problem with chemicals in young adulthood.

The Risks of Underdiagnosis

The diagnosis of adolescent drug/alcohol abuse is complicated partly because adolescents, as a general rule, do not develop the characteristic withdrawal symptoms often found in adults addicted to alcohol (Chassin & DeLucia, 1996). If the assessor were to look for these "adult" symptoms of addiction in the child or adolescent who was using alcohol, it is possible that the individual's chemical abuse might be entirely overlooked.

However, there are also risks associated with failing to treat those adolescents for whom drug use is a serious problem (Evans & Sullivan, 1990). First, there is evidence that protracted chemical use may interfere with the adolescent's ability to develop age-specific coping mechanisms (Y. Kaminer, 1994). Further, by the time that the individual's drug use has resulted in serious physical changes, or when he/she has acquired a blood infection from dirty needles, the individual is scarred for not just the rest of adolescence, but for life. Once a brain cell has died, it will never regrow. AIDS is forever. Thus, there are very real reasons to identify adolescents who have a chemical use problem, before it is too late to avoid lifelong damage.

As researchers have explored the factors associated with suicide during the adolescent years, it has been discovered that alcoholism, or drug dependence, is one of the factors associated with an increased risk of suicide in the adolescent population (Bukstein, 1995; Callahan, 1993). The exact nature of this relationship is not clear. But researchers do know that chemical use is a factor in 70% of all adolescent suicide (Bukstein et al., 1993; Group for the Advancement of Psychiatry, 1990).

The team of Bukstein et al. (1993) attempted to identify the factors associated with successful adolescent suicide attempts and uncovered several risk factors. While no single risk factor seemed to identify those who were to ultimately take their own lives, the authors suggested that some of the factors associated with a successful adolescent suicide attempt included (a) the individual actively abused chemicals, (b) the individual was suffering from a major depression, (c) the individual had thoughts of suicide within the past week, (d) a family history of suicide and/or depression, (e) the individual was facing legal problems, and (f) the adolescent had access to a handgun within the home.

Adolescent substance use is also considered a factor in accidental injury (Chassin & DeLucia, 1996; Loiselle, Baker, Templeton, Schwartz, & Drott, 1994). After receiving parental permission, Loiselle et al. (1994) conducted urine toxicology tests on 65 adolescents admitted to a major hospital for the treatment of traumatic injuries. It was found that 34% of these individuals tested positive for alcohol and/or drugs. Because alcohol/drug use was so common for the patients seen for traumatic injuries, the authors suggested that urine toxicology tests be a standard part of the treatment protocol for such cases. Along the same lines, Morrison (1990) observed that the first sign of an adolescent substance use problem might be his/her visit to a hospital emergency room, for treatment of injuries or substance-induced physical problems.

Thus, the chemical dependency treatment professional who works with adolescents must attempt to find the middle ground between the underdiagnosis, with all the dangers associated with teenage drug/alcohol abuse, and overdiagnosis, which may leave the individual with a false lifelong diagnosis of chemical dependency.

Possible Diagnostic Criteria for Adolescent Drug/Alcohol Problems

Given these arguments, are there indicators of adolescent chemical problems? The Committee of Substance Abuse (1995) suggested that some of the signs of adolescent alcohol use problems include (a) the experiencing of withdrawal symptoms following periods of alcohol use, (b) tolerance to the effects of alcohol, (c) unsuccessful attempts to cut back on the amount of alcohol consumed, (d) unsuccessful attempts to stop using alcohol, (e) the development of alcohol-related blackouts, (f) continued alcohol use despite adverse social, educational, physical, or psychological consequences, and/or (g) alcohol-related injuries.

Zarek, Hawkins, and Rogers (1987) identified six criteria as indicators of adolescent drug abuse:

1. The use of chemicals to get "smashed."
2. Going to parties where drugs other than alcohol are in use.
3. Refusing to attend parties where drugs are not present.
4. Drinking liquor, as opposed to beer or wine.
5. Using marijuana.
6. Being drunk at school.

The authors concluded that the adolescent who has a drug abuse problem is likely to be "enrolled in school, but is experiencing behavior problems related to school, such as being sent to the principal, or skipping classes" (p. 485).

Nunes and Parson (1995) offered a series of potential risk factors that might suggest adolescent substance use: (a) poor parent-child relationships; (b) psychiatric disorders, especially depression; (c) a tendency to seek novel experiences or take risks; (d) family members and peers who use substances; (e) low academic motivation; (f) acting-out behaviors; (g) absence of religious beliefs; (h) early cigarette use; (i) low self-esteem; (j) being raised in a single-parent or blended family; (k) high level of stress within the family; and (l) engaging in health-compromising behaviors. As the number of risk factors increases, so does the probability that the adolescent has a substance use problem, according to Nunes and Parson. Those adolescents who simultaneously have five or more of these risk factors are virtually guaranteed to also have a substance use problem, according to the authors.

As adolescents become more and more preoccupied with chemical use, or demonstrate an interest in an expanding variety of chemicals, they might be said to have developed the adolescent equivalent to the progression of chemical use often seen in adults (Evans & Sullivan, 1990). They will also demonstrate a loss of control, which is expressed through violations of personal rules about drug use (e.g., "I

will only drink at weekend parties"). Thus, those adolescents who are preoccupied with substance use, or who wish to experiment with a wide range of chemicals, should be evaluated and referred to treatment, if necessary.

According to Newcomb and Bentler (1989), the signs of adolescents who are experiencing problems with alcohol or drugs include: (a) repeatedly using chemicals, (b) using chemicals at an inappropriate time, or whose (c) becoming involved in legal, school, or social problems as a result of chemical use. This drug abuse problem may either be acute, episodic, or chronic, depending on how often the individual has engaged in the drug use.

The Special Needs of the Adolescent in a Substance Abuse Rehabilitation Program

The adolescent who has been found to be in need of rehabilitation because of a substance use problem presents special needs to treatment staff. First, as noted earlier, staff should be sufficiently aware of the developmental process that is taking place during adolescence to understand the adolescent's cognitive abilities, strengths, and, defensive style.

Second, the treatment center should be able to offer a wide variety of services, including the ability to work with the student's educational needs, recreational needs, and possible coexisting psychiatric disorders (Bukstein, 1994). The staff should also address peripheral issues, such as AIDS, birth control, and the individual's vocational needs, according to the author.

Further, treatment center staff should be sensitive to the adolescent's cultural beliefs, and, the social status of the adolescent and his/her family (Bukstein, 1994, 1995). A diverse staff helps to ensure that the adolescent is able to find at least one member of the staff to identify with during treatment. Further, staff sensitivity to the cultural and social beliefs of the individual adolescent, and his/her family, will enhance communication between staff members and the patient.

Next, rehabilitation center staff should attempt to engage family members in the treatment process (Bukstein, 1994). Some of the goals that might be addressed with family members include improving communications between family members, the development of problem resolution skills, resolution of discipline problems, and the identification of problems within the family unit that might undermine the efforts of the treatment center staff (such as undiagnosed substance use by one or both parents).

Next, the treatment process should be of sufficient duration to ensure a meaningful change in how the adolescent, and his/her family, cope with life's problems (Bukstein, 1995). In that behavioral change takes time, and time is also necessary for a person's attitudes to change, the treatment process should be sufficiently long, and intense enough, to allow for these necessary components of recovery to take place.

The next component of an adolescent treatment program should be that the treatment center staff should have access to a wide range of specialized social service agencies. In addition to their own work with the adolescent, treatment center staff might need to make referrals to juvenile justice, child welfare, and social support agencies (Bukstein, 1994, 1995). As part of the rehabilitation process, involvement in AA/NA might be useful for the adolescent, especially if there is a young persons group in the area. Al-anon might prove to be a valuable support for the family members who question their role in the adolescent's substance use. Finally, the goal of the rehabilitation effort should be for the adolescent to achieve a chemical-free lifestyle (Bukstein, 1994, 1995).

While adolescents offer treatment center staff unique challenges, there are also rewards that are earned through effectively working with a younger substance abuser. Adolescents are less entrenched in their pathology, and thus more responsive to rehabilitation efforts, in many cases. Thus, when substance abuse does become an issue for adolescents, rehabilitation offers the opportunity to help them turn their life around.

Summary

Children and adolescents are often hidden victims of drug addiction. Yet there is a serious lack of research into the problem of child or adolescent drug use/abuse. While mental health professionals acknowledge that peer pressure and family environment influence the adolescent's chemical use pattern, the exact role that these forces (or the media) play in shaping the adolescent's behavior is still not known.

There are many unanswered questions surrounding the issue of child and adolescent drug use, and in the years to come one might expect to see significant breakthroughs in our understanding of the forces that shape chemical use beliefs and patterns of use in the young.

In the face of this dearth of clinical research, the treatment professional must steer a cautious path between the underdiagnosis of chemical dependency in the younger client, and overdiagnosis. Just as surgery carried out on a child or adolescent will have lifelong consequences, so will the traumatic experience of being forced into treatment for a problem that may, or may not, exist. As with surgery, the treatment professional should carefully weigh the potential benefits from such a procedure against the potential for harm to the individual.

During this phase of experimentation, an adolescent might demonstrate repeated and regular use of one or more chemicals, only to settle down in young adulthood to a more acceptable pattern of chemical use (Evans & Sullivan, 1990; Peele, 1989). One study, for example, found that of identified "problem drinkers" during adolescence, fully 53% of the men and 70% of the women were not judged to still be problem drinkers 7 years later (Zarek et al., 1987). Thus, the adolescent who might have abused chemicals on a regular basis may, or may not, go on to develop a problem with chemicals in young adulthood.

Although treatment professionals understand that chemical use during adolescence is a factor in a wide range of emotional and physical problems that develop during this phase of life, the diagnostic criteria needed to identify those adolescents who are at risk for subsequent problems as a result of their chemical use are still evolving. Thus, treatment professionals have no firm guidelines as to what symptoms might identify the adolescent who is passing through a phase of experimental chemical use or the adolescent whose chemical use reflects a serious problem.

CHAPTER TWENTY-FOUR

Codependency and Enabling

Scientists who specialize in the behavioral sciences are often faced with a bewildering array of behaviors that they must both categorize and try to understand. To help them with this task, behavioral scientists utilize *constructs* to help them express complex ideas to others more easily. An example of a construct is the symbol of a weather "front" on a meteorological map: in reality there are no lines between different weather cells, or firm boundaries between different bodies of air. But, by using the analogy of battle lines from World War I, it is possible for meteorologists to quickly summarize data and communicate that information to others.

In the late 1970s, substance abuse rehabilitation professionals developed a series of new constructs to help them understand the dynamics of the interpersonal relationships of the substance abuser. This was necessary because each identified person with a substance use problem either directly or indirectly touches the lives of many, many other people. Some of those people affected by an individual's use of alcohol or chemicals are total strangers, as in the case of the victim of a drug-related burglary, or an alcohol-related motor vehicle accident. While these episodes are sometimes tragic, the individual victim is not usually involved in an ongoing relationship with the addicted person. Rather, the drug-related burglary, or an alcohol-related accident, is an isolated incident, not a part of an unhealthy relationship with a substance-abusing individual.

Rehabilitation professionals have also found that there are those who, while sickened by the addicted person's behavior, actually behave in ways that *enable* him/her to continue to drink or use drugs. Other researchers have suggested that some family members seem to enter into a relationship pattern with the alcohol/drug abuser that appears to have certain predictable elements. Indeed, some researchers have noted that the significant other often enters into a *codependent* relationship with the person with the substance use problem. In the past decade, thousands of pages of text have been devoted to these constructs, which have come to have a life of their own. In this chapter, the constructs of enabling and codependency are examined.

Enabling

One of the most important theoretical concepts to emerge in the late 1970s and early 1980s was that of *enabling*. Essentially, to enable someone means to *knowingly* behave in such a way as to make it possible for another person to continue to use chemicals without having to pay the natural consequences for that behavior. The concept of enabling emerged in the early 1980s, when some therapists suggested that within some families there almost seemed to be a conspiracy in which at least some family members supported the continued use of chemicals by the individual with a substance use problem.

According to the prevailing theory, the actions of at least some family members became part of the problem, not a part of the solution. The enabler came to be viewed as behaving in ways that prevented the person with a chemical use problem from taking advantage of the many opportunities to discover firsthand the cost and consequences of his/her chemical abuse. The spouse, for example, might call the partner's workplace with the excuse that the substance-abusing partner was "sick," when he/she actually was actually under the influence of chemicals.

A popular misconception is that only family members might enable a substance abuser. The truth is that you do not have to be a family member to enable a person with a chemical use problem. An enabler might be a parent, sibling, co-worker, neighbor, or even a supervisor. Other potential enablers include a well-meaning friend, a trusted adviser, a teacher, a therapist, or even a drug rehabilitation worker. Any person who *knowingly* acts in such a way as to protect the alcohol/drug abuser from the natural consequences of his/her behavior is an enabler.

For example, in speaking of alcoholism, the booklet *The Family Enablers* (Johnson Institute, 1987) defined an enabler as *any* person who "reacts to an alcoholic in such a way as to shield the alcoholic from experiencing the full impact of the harmful consequences of alcoholism" (p. 5). The same criteria can be applied to those who enable people who are addicted to other drugs of abuse. Thus, the enabler is any person who knowingly shields the user from the harmful consequences of his/her behavior.

One does not need to be involved in an ongoing relationship with a person who abuses/is addicted to chemicals, in order to be an enabler. A person who refuses to provide testimony about a crime that he/she witnessed out of a wish not to become involved, or, out of fear, has enabled the perpetrator of that crime to escape. But the clinical theory suggests that the enabler is usually involved in an ongoing relationship with a person with a substance use problem.

Enabling Behaviors in the Workplace

It is difficult to fathom the multitude of ways in which one person might enable another to continue his/her compulsive use of chemicals. For example, in the hospital setting, operating room staff, for a number of reasons, might hesitate to confront a surgeon

suspected of being under the influence of chemicals. They might engage in denial, or, fear reprisal from the surgeon, or simply desire not to become involved in what promises to be a messy situation within the workplace (Hyde, 1989). In this case, the health care professionals are enablers of the surgeon's continued use of chemicals.

Enablers in the workplace have several characteristic behaviors (Hyde, 1989):

1. Doing the individual's work, because he/she is unable to do it.
2. "Covering" for the impaired individual's poor performance.
3. Accepting excuses, or making special arrangements for the impaired individual.
4. Overlooking frequent absenteeism or tardiness.
5. Overlooking evidence of chemical use.

Admittedly, it is difficult to deal with the problem of substance use/abuse in the workplace, especially if the person with a chemical use problem is a supervisor or administrator. To further complicate matters, the person with a substance use problem will actively manipulate the interpersonal environment to force others to continue enabling his/her chemical use. It is not uncommon for an alcohol-dependent person to treat the enabler as if he/she was being granted a favor for the privilege of taking responsibility for him/her! The temptation here is for the other person to go along with the myth that "none of this conflict is caused by your use of chemicals."

For example, when confronted by his/her supervisor for being late to work again, the employee might respond, "You are lucky that I work here in the first place!" The supervisor may, perhaps out of a fear of legal or union action, or simply overwork, agree that the company is indeed lucky to have that person as an employee. Without taking any firm action, the supervisor might warn darkly that the errant employee should not let "it" happen again. If the employee was late because of chemical use, then the supervisor has become an enabler.

The same signs of enabling found in the workplace also are apparent in other environments, such as the home. Because of the multitude of intrapersonal and interpersonal defenses that operate within a family, however, it is often easier (and less threatening) to identify enabling behaviors in a more neutral setting such as the work environment, than it is within a home setting.

Styles of Enabling

Over the years, a number of different patterns of enabling have been suggested. Ellis et al. (1988) offered one system of classification, which offered the reader a framework within which to understand the different styles of behavior that enabled another to continue to use chemicals. According to the authors, some people could be called *joiners* (p. 109). The joiner actively supports the use of chemicals by another person, and might actually use alcohol/drugs with that person, according to the authors. A classic example of a joiner is the woman who asked for marital counseling, because her husband would not limit his cocaine use to the $100 a week that she set aside in the family budget for his drug use!

Another, all too common, example of the joiner is the spouse who drinks or who uses chemicals along with the addict, in the hope of somehow controlling his or her chemical use. For example, substance abuse rehabilitation professionals know that it is quite common for a spouse to go to a bar with the alcohol abusing/dependent partner, in the hopes of teaching the partner how to drink in a "responsible" manner. Such efforts are usually doomed to failure.

A second type of enabler suggested by the authors is the *messiah* (Ellis et al., 1988, p. 109). The messiah fights against the addict's chemical use, but does so in such a way that the addict is never forced to experience the consequences of his/her behavior. For example, the father of an opiate-dependent young adult woman explained to a mixed group of family members and other opiate-addicted patients that he had taken out a personal loan more than once to pay off his daughter's drug debts. The father had admitted this tearfully to illustrate how much he loved his daughter.

Another group member, who had been in recovery for some time, asked why the father would do this. After all, the second person said, if the father paid off her debts, she would not have to worry about having to pay her drug debts herself. The father responded that, if he did not, his daughter

"might leave us!" Several group members then suggested to this parent that the daughter might need to suffer some consequences on her own, in order to "hit bottom" and come to terms with her addiction. The father was silent for a moment, then said "Oh, I couldn't do that! She's not ready to assume responsibility for herself, yet!"

Ellis et al. (1988) suggested a third form of enabler, which they termed the *silent sufferer* (p. 109). The silent sufferer almost seems to live by the philosophy, "As long as I suffer, I *am* somebody!" In a very real sense, silent sufferers live the life of a martyr. They will live with an alcohol/drug abusing family member, despite the pain they suffer in this troubled environment. Silent sufferers are unwilling to leave, according to the authors, almost as if they believe that they would not have a life if they should do so. Silent sufferers lock themselves into a cycle of continued pain and suffering, by refusing to leave the substance-abusing partner.

With the best of intentions, silent sufferers prevent the alcohol/drug abuser from suffering the consequences of his/her behavior by "always being there and pretending that nothing is wrong" (Ellis et al., 1988, p. 109). The authors viewed the goal of this relationship pattern as being *security*. Rather than to risk the loss of what little emotional security the partner might offer, silent sufferers try not to "rock the boat." They will say nothing, in an attempt to keep family conflict from breaking out. Indeed, persons in this role might act as a lightning rod, drawing all the pain and suffering away from the disturbed family members to themselves, in an attempt to defuse family conflict.

The Relationship between Enabling and Codependency

The key concept to remember is that an enabler knowingly behaves in a manner that protects the addicted person from the consequences of his/her behavior. We all behave in ways that, in retrospect, may have enabled someone to avoid consequences that he/she would otherwise have suffered as a result of drug use. The intertwining of these constructs is often confusing to the student of addiction. Codependency and enabling may be, and often are, found in the same person. However, one may also enable an addicted person without being codependent on that person. Enabling refers to *specific behaviors*, while codependency refers to *a relationship pattern*. Thus, one may enable addiction without being codependent. But the codependent individual, because he/she is in an ongoing relationship with the addict, will also frequently enable the alcohol/drug-abusing person. Enabling does not require an ongoing relationship. A tourist who gives a street beggar a gift of money, knowing that the beggar is likely addicted and in need of drugs, has enabled the beggar. But, the tourist is hardly in a meaningful relationship with the addicted person.

Codependency and enabling are *overlapping* issues that may, or may not, be found in the same individual. A diagram of this relationship is shown in Figure 24.1. Although these two forms of behavior may overlap, it is important to keep in mind that enabling and codependency are separate patterns of behavior that may, or may not, be found in the same person.

Codependency

The concept of codependency has emerged in the past two decades to become one of the cornerstones of rehabilitation. When one stops to remember that codependency is a theoretical construct, it is easy to understand why, despite all that has been said and written about it, there is no standard definition of *codependency* (Heimel, 1990; Tavris, 1990). Indeed, mental health professionals have yet to agree on such a basic issue as whether to hyphenate the term (i.e., co-dependency) or spell it as one word (codependency) (Beattie, 1989).

Although there is no standard definition for the concept and it is only a theoretical construct, many families and friends of addicted persons believe that they have suffered, and often continue to suffer, as a result of having "a relationship with a dysfunctional person" (Beattie, 1989, p. 7).

According to Wegscheider-Cruse (1985), codependency can be defined as a condition:

> . . . that is characterized by preoccupation and extreme dependence (emotionally, socially, and sometimes physically) on a person or object. Eventually, this dependence . . . becomes a pathological

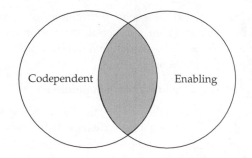

FIGURE 24.1   Relationship between codependency and enabling behaviors.

condition that affects the co-dependent in all other relationships. (p. 2)

Yet even this definition does not fully capture the flavor of codependency. O'Brien and Gaborit (1992) viewed codependency as being a relationship in which:

> . . . the needs of two people are met in dysfunctional ways. The chemical dependent's need for a care taker, caused by an increasing inability to meet basic survival needs as the drug becomes increasingly intrusive . . . is met by the codependent's need to control the behavior of others who have difficulty caring for themselves. (p. 129)

In contrast, Gorski (1992) provided a definition of codependency as a general term:

> . . . describing a cluster of symptoms or maladaptive behavior changes associated with living in a committed relationship with either a chemically dependent person or a chronically dysfunctional person either as children or adults. (p. 15)

Perhaps the most radical definition of the term codependency is offered by Brown and Lewis (1995):

> The term *codependence* defines a reactive, submissive response to the dominance of another. (p. 281)

Although these definitions are both similar and dissimilar, they identify different core aspects of codependency: (a) the *overinvolvement* with the dysfunctional family member, (b) the *obsessive* attempts on the part of the codependent person to control the dysfunctional family member's behavior, (c) the extreme tendency to use *external sources of self-worth* (i.e., approval from others, including the dysfunctional person in the relationship), and (d) the *tendency to make personal sacrifices* in an attempt to "cure" the dysfunctional family member of his/her problem behavior.

The Dynamics of Codependency

In an early work on the subject, Beattie (1987) spoke of codependency as a process wherein the individual's life becomes unmanageable because of being involved in a committed relationship with an addict, making it impossible to simply walk away. Often, part of this commitment involves the codependent individual coming to believe that somehow the addict's behavior is a reflection on the codependent person. In response to this threat to self-esteem (i.e., *"Your* behavior is a reflection of *me"*) the codependent person comes to feel obsessed with the need to control the behavior of the person who is addicted to chemicals (Beattie). In so doing, the codependent will assume responsibility for decisions and events not actually under his/her control, such as the significant other's recreational chemical use. Codependent spouses often blame themselves for "causing" the alcoholic to go out on a binge, after having a fight. The drinking spree "is all my fault" a common belief of the codependent partner.

As noted, one symptom of codependency is a *preoccupation* (Wegscheider-Cruse, 1985), or an *obsession* (Beattie, 1989) with controlling the behavior of the significant other. This obsession with controlling another's behavior might extend to the point where the codependent will try to control the addict's drug use, or even all of the addict's life. An excellent example of this obsessive attempt to control the significant other's behavior took place several years ago. A staff psychologist, at a maximum security penitentiary for men in the Midwest, received a telephone call from an elderly mother of an inmate. She asked the psychologist to "make sure that the man who shares my son's cell is a good influence" on her son, because "there are a lot of bad men in that prison, and I don't want him falling in with a bad crowd!"

The woman in this case overlooked the grim reality that her son was not simply in prison for singing off-key in choir practice, and that he had been to prison on several different occasions for various crimes. Rather than let him live his life, and try to get on with hers, she continued to worry about how to

"cure" him of his behavior problem. She continued to treat him as a child, was overinvolved in his life, and was upset at the suggestion that it might be time to let her son learn to *suffer* (and perhaps learn from) *the consequences of his own behavior.* This woman had yet to learn how to *detach* from her son's behavior. *Detachment* is one of the cornerstones of the recovery process (Brown & Lewis, 1995). By learning to detach and separate from her dysfunctional son, this woman could learn to "let go" and cease attempting to control his life. But, with the best of intentions, she remains overinvolved in her son's life.

The Rules of Codependency

Although the codependent person often feels as if he or she is going crazy, an outside observer will notice that there are certain patterns, or "rules," to codependent behavior. Beattie (1989) identified six of these unspoken rules of codependency:

1. It's not okay for me to feel.
2. It's not okay for me to have problems.
3. It's not okay for me to have fun.
4. I'm not lovable.
5. I'm not good enough.
6. If people act bad or crazy, I'm responsible.

These rules are actively transmitted from one partner in the relationship to the other, setting the pattern for codependency. "If you weren't so unreasonable, I would never have gone out drinking last night!" is a common example of Rule 6. "You shouldn't have tried in the first place!" might enforce Rules 2, 3, 4, and 5.

Are Codependents Born, or Made?

Proponents of the concept of codependency suggest that codependency is a *learned behavior.* It is often passed from one generation to another. In a real-life example of how one unhealthy generation helps the next to be codependent, a parent might confront a child who wants to go to college with the taunt, "You're too dumb to go to college! The best that you can hope for is that somebody is stupid enough to marry you, and take care of you!"

Scarf (1980) pointed out that people tend to try to resolve "unfinished business" with their parents, by recreating these all-important early relationships in their adult lives. Frequently, especially for those who struggle with feelings of low self-esteem as a result of having been raised in a dysfunctional home, this means being drawn to unhealthy partners as part of the process of trying to resolve their original parent-child conflicts. These adults are trying to recreate their original families through their pattern of adult relationships and are attempting to resolve any unresolved childhood conflicts through these surrogates. Depending on how healthy or unhealthy these surrogates may be, this process can be a positive one or one that traps the person into unhealthy cycles.

Heimel (1991) provided a beautiful capsule summary of this process when she realized that she was reacting to a boyfriend's rejection with the same depression that she experienced as a child, growing up:

> . . . when my mother turned her back and wouldn't speak to me, when my father, my beloved father, shook his head and said, "After all we've done for you." This is how I felt when I was turning myself inside out trying to get my parents to love me, something they couldn't quite manage. (p. 42)

Because of this earlier rejection, Heimel (1991) saw herself as being vulnerable to being rejected again, in adulthood. She lacked sufficient self-esteem to weather the crisis of being rejected, although on one level she understood that there was never a serious relationship with the young man in question.

Another example of how people attempt to resolve past conflict through their adult relationships is seen in the development of children who have been exposed to physical, sexual, or emotional abuse. These individuals are frequently left with feelings of low self-esteem and, in adulthood, struggle to affirm the self. The survivors of childhood abuse often come to believe that they are not valuable, lovable, or capable individuals. Such individuals are vulnerable to repeatedly being drawn to unhealthy partners, in their unconscious attempt to resolve the past trauma. It is almost as if they are trapped in a never-ending cycle.

Further, as the dysfunctional elements in the relationship develop, the codependent will frequently come to also feel "imprisoned" in the relationship. All relationships have some dysfunctional elements. In a healthy relationship, however, the partners confront these unhealthy components and work on

resolving them to the satisfaction of both partners. For example, one partner might express an opinion to the other that their finances are getting a little tight, and that perhaps they should look at cutting back on unnecessary spending for a couple of weeks. But, in the codependent relationship, this working-through process is stalled. If one partner does express concern over a possible problem, the other partner will move to prevent the problem from being clearly identified or, if it is identified, resolved.

As part of the attempt to avoid displeasing the partner with the substance use problem, the codependent person is thought to restrict his/her communications, to avoid people or topics of conversation that might displease the significant other. Eventually, the codependent person is afraid to say the "wrong" thing, afraid to talk to the "wrong people," and is afraid to assert selfhood. According to the theory of codependency, the person becomes afraid to leave, believes that he/she has nobody but the alcohol/drug-abusing partner, and yet is not satisfied in this relationship, either.

Codependency and Self-Esteem

In an attempt to live up to the unspoken rules of codependency, the codependent experiences a great deal of emotional pain. The core of codependency, as viewed by Zerwekh and Michaels (1989), is "related to low self-esteem" (p. 111) on the part of the codependent person. The authors go on to conclude:

> Co-dependents frequently appear normal, which in our culture is associated with a healthy ego. Nevertheless, they also describe themselves as "dying on the inside," which is indicative of low self-worth or esteem. (p. 111)

Lacking sufficient self-esteem to withstand the demands of the addicted partner, the codependent persons often come to measure personal worth by how well they can take care of the dysfunctional partner. Another way that codependent individuals measure self-worth is through the sacrifices they make for significant others (A. Miller, 1988). In this way, codependent individuals substitute an external measure of personal worth for their inability to generate *self*-worth.

Drug rehabilitation workers are often surprised at the amount of suffering and pain that codependent family members suffer, but confused as to why they do not do something to end the pain. There is a reward for enduring this pain! Many people feel a sense of moral victory through suffering at the hands of another (Shapiro, 1981). By suffering at the hands of a dysfunctional spouse, the codependent individual accuses "the offender by pointing at his victim; it keeps alive in the mind's record an injustice committed, a score unsettled" (p. 115). For some people, such suffering is "a necessity, a principled act of will, from which he cannot release himself without losing his self-respect and feeling more deeply and finally defeated, humiliated, and powerless" (Shapiro, 1981, p. 115).

The trials and suffering imposed on the codependent person become almost a badge of honor, a defense against the admission of personal powerlessness, or worthlessness. The codependent person, in many cases, comes to affirm personal worth by being willing to "carry the cross" of another person's addiction or dysfunctional behavior.

The Relationship between Codependency and Emotional Health

There is a tendency for some to *overidentify* with the codependency concept. As Beattie (quoted in Tavris, 1992), pointed out, there are those who believe that codependency is "anything, and everyone is codependent" (p. 194). This extreme position overlooks that many of the same characteristics that define the codependency are also found in healthy human relationships. Only a few "saints and hermits" (Tavris, 1990, p. 21A) fail to demonstrate at least some of the characteristics of the so-called codependent individual.

Even Wegscheider-Cruse and Cruse (1990), strong advocates of the codependency movement, admitted that "co-dependency is an exaggeration of normal personality traits" (p. 28). But in some cases these traits become so pronounced that the individual "becomes disabled (disease of codependency)" (p. 28). Codependency is thus a matter of degree. But, whereas in some personality patterns people isolate themselves from interpersonal feedback, the codependent person tends to be extremely dependent on feedback from the significant other. The whole goal of codependents seems to be that of winning love, approval, and acceptance from the

object of their affection. Codependents appear to be unable to affirm the self, and as a substitute, seek to win this affirmation from the significant other.

Remember that a central theme of alcohol/drug addiction is *control*. The alcohol/drug-abusing partner's need for control extends beyond his/her use of chemicals, to the marital partner, and the family. One method of control is emotional withdrawal. The addicted partner uses the threat of abandonment to control the behavior of his/her partner, or the other family members. In turn, the codependent becomes exquisitely sensitive to the slightest sign of disapproval or rejection from the alcohol/drug-abusing partner. The dysfunctional partner, sensing this, often uses this fear to control the codependent member of the marital unit. The codependent partner, on the other hand, may lose touch with his/her own feelings because of being so invested in pleasing the addicted partner. Thus, on one hand, there is a total insensitivity toward interpersonal feedback on the part of the addicted partner, while on the other there is a supersensitivity to external feedback on the part of the codependent member of the marital unit.

In between these two extremes is an *interdependency* that is the hallmark of healthy relationships. The extremes between isolation and codependency are shown in Figure 24.2.

The point to remember is that codependency is not an all-or-nothing phenomenon. *There are degrees of codependency*, just as there are degrees of isolation from interpersonal feedback. Few of us are at either extreme, and the majority of us tend to fall somewhere in the middle: exhibiting tendencies both to behave in codependent ways and to be overly isolated from feedback from others.

How to Build a Codependent

Substance abuse professionals often speak of a "cycle" of codependency. This is to say that, once the cycle of codependency, has started, it takes on a life of its own. A graphic representation of the cycle of codependency appears in Figure 24.3.

On the chart outlining the steps involved in the growth of codependency, there are two necessary components. First, that one partner, the codependent, suffers from low self-esteem. If one partner *does*

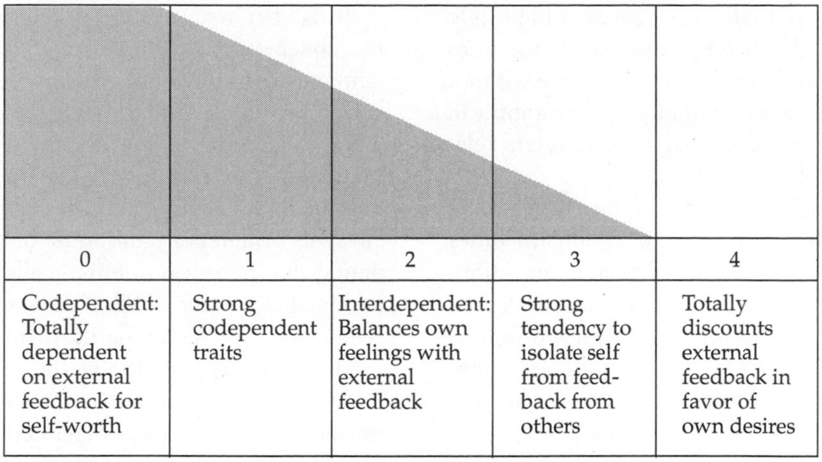

0
1
2
3
4
Codependent: Totally dependent on external feedback for self-worth
Strong codependent traits
Interdependent: Balances own feelings with external feedback
Strong tendency to isolate self from feed-back from others
Totally discounts external feedback in favor of own desires

FIGURE 24.2 The continuum between isolation and dependency.

Person suffers from poor self-esteem: unable to affirm "self"
External sources of support and affirmation are substituted for self-acceptance
Significant other proves to be dysfunctional
Person believes "self" to be un-able to withstand rejection by partner
Person tries to avoid issues that might threaten relationship
Person feels powerless—self-esteem is lost

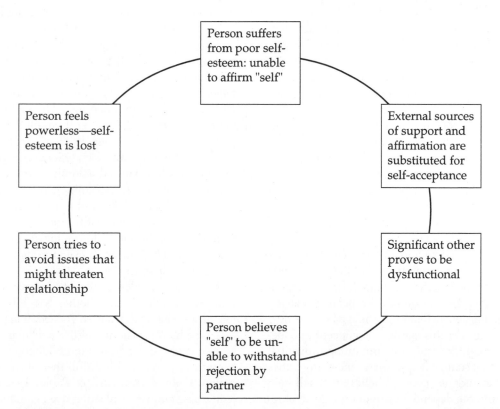

FIGURE 24.3 The circle of codependency.

not suffer from low self-esteem, he /she would be able to affirm "self." Such a person would back away from a dysfunctional partner or find a way to cope without depending on the dysfunctional partner's approval. In such a case, it is unlikely that a codependent relationship would evolve.

Second, the "significant other" must prove to be dysfunctional. The dysfunctional significant other is necessary, for if the partner were to be emotionally healthy, he or she would affirm the codependent. Such an atmosphere would enhance psychological growth on the part of the codependent partner, who would, in time, come to be able to affirm self without the need for external supports, pulling down the house of cards on which codependency rests. Thus, codependency rests on an interaction between the pathology (for want of a better word) of the two partners.

Reactions to the Concept of Codependency

At least 21 different self-help books are available that address the problem of codependency (McCrady & Epstein, 1995). The very fact that there are this many titles devoted to this topic would suggest it is a serious problem, at least in the minds of some people. However, many people suggest that codependency is a *pseudo*problem more than a legitimate mental health concern. For example, some argue that, rather than serving to "empower" the client, *the concept of codependency takes away from the individual's power*. The codependent person is then told that the "disease" of codependency is progressive, and that he/she can never come to terms with codependency alone (W. Kaminer, 1992; Tavris, 1990).

Victims of codependency are constantly reminded that only through the aid of the appropriate self-help group can the individual face codependency. Further, the individual member is repeatedly encouraged to accept that he or she is powerless over this condition. For this reason, the concept of codependency might be said to maintain the individual in a perpetual state of helplessness, and many critics of the codependency concept believe that self-help groups "promote dependency under the guise of recovery" (Katz & Liu, 1991, p. xii).

It has been suggested (W. Kaminer, 1992) that the codependency literature, in a subtle manner, demands not individual growth and autonomy, but, conformity to a standard recipe for salvation and grace. According to the codependency model, no matter how trivial or serious the trauma, there is just one model for recovery. If the individual resists the "insights" offered by different books on codependency, that person is automatically viewed as being in denial (Kaminer, 1992; Katz & Liu, 1991). There is no room for individuality in the codependency model, as it is applied to therapeutic situations.

Adherents to this theory, view codependency as a universal condition. Indeed, it often seems that much of the literature on codependency strives to convince the individual that he or she is "doomed to suffer as a result of the trauma of childhood travails" (Japenga, 1991, p. 174). However, there is little research to support this position. The literature on codependency seems to discount the possibility that the individual might have successfully weathered the storm of childhood trauma to become a well-adjusted adult.

Detractors from the codependency theory point out that the literature on codependency suggests that up to 99% of all people are raised in a "dysfunctional" home, and that because of this, they *automatically* have deep emotional scars from childhood. They are "encouraged to see themselves as victims of family life rather than self-determining participants" (W. Kaminer, 1992, p. 13). Those who challenge the concept of codependency point out that the family is viewed as nothing more than an "incubator of disease" (Kaminer, p. 12) by proponents of this theory. Within this incubator, the helpless child is infected with one or more dread conditions that he/she will have to struggle with forever, unless salvation is achieved through the appropriate self-help group.

Yet research evidence suggests that even if a child is raised in a dysfunctional home, that child is not automatically doomed to suffer. Indeed, it appears that many, perhaps a majority, of those who are exposed to even extreme conditions in childhood find a way to adjust, survive, and to fulfill their life goals (Garbarino, Dubrow, Kostelny, & Pardo, 1992). Admittedly, some children will suffer deep emotional scars, as a result of childhood trauma. But, the evidence does not suggest children are automatically doomed to suffer if their homelife is less than perfect.

Researchers now believe that some children are able to develop a natural resilience to even extreme forms of psychological trauma (Werner, 1989; Wolin & Wolin, 1993, 1995). This natural resilience seems to help them weather the emotional storms not only of childhood, but of later adult life as well. Indeed, the very fact that the child's environment *is* dysfunctional might serve as an impetus toward the development of positive emotional growth in many cases (Garbarino et al., 1992; Wolin & Wolin, 1993, 1995). However, the codependency model does not accept the possibility of individual resilience. Rather, its proponents suggest that *all* children raised in a dysfunctional environment have emotional scars that need to be addressed.

Another challenge to the concept of codependency is based on the theory (frequently advanced in different books on the subject) that all suffering is relative. But, as W. Kaminer (1992) pointed out, it is hard, to equate degrees of suffering. Consider the case of two hypothetical children in two different families. Both were the oldest boys in a family of three children, with an alcoholic father. In the first family, the father was a "happy" drunk, who would drink each evening after work, tell a few "funny" jokes, watch television, and fall asleep in his favorite chair. In the second family, the father would drink each evening after work and become violently angry. He would physically abuse his wife and children, and on occasion fired a rifle at family members.

The impact that each father would have on the family would be far different. Yet, in the literature on codependency, both events are treated as being of equal importance. This example also underscores another criticism of the concept of codependency. The theory could be said to excuse the addicted individual from all responsibility for his/her behavior (Roehling, Koelbel, & Rutgers, 1994; Tavris, 1990). In effect, through the "disease" of codependency, blame is shifted from the individual with the substance use problem to his/her significant other, who is said to "enable" the unhealthy behaviors of the afflicted person to continue.

Still other detractors from the construct of codependency, at least as this theory now is applied to substance abusers and their families, point out that it excuses codependent individuals from all responsibility for his/her own life. As Kottler (1992) observed:

> By subscribing to a codependency model we reinforce the idea that the client is not responsible for her behavior, that she was born or made into "a woman who loves too much," a "woman who loves men who hate women," or who has a "doormat syndrome," or any number of other euphemisms that explain the disease invading the "codependent psyche." (p. 138)

In this way, the individual is excused from responsibility for his/her life. After all, they have a "disease": codependency. So, they cannot be held accountable for whatever decisions he/she make because it is just his/her codependency asserting itself.

Another challenge to the concept of codependency is that family members are judged not because of their own accomplishments, but on whether another person in the family is able to abstain from chemicals. In other words, they are guilty of "addiction by association" (Katz & Liu, 1991, p. 13). For example, in their text on the impact of alcoholism on the family, Steinglass, Bennett, Wolin, and Reiss (1987) asserted that the *entire family* can have "alcoholism" because one member is a problem drinker. Notice the shift in responsibility inherent in this line of reasoning: the problem is not that one parent is alcohol-dependent, physically and/or sexually abusive, or possibly both emotionally inappropriate and absent. Rather, the problem is that the *family* members suffer from the disease of codependency.

Detractors from the concept of codependency point out that it is an outgrowth of the theory (popular in the 1950s) that the spouse of the alcoholic was a "co-alcoholic" (Sher, 1991; Simmons, 1991). This theory assumed that the co-alcoholic was as much in need of treatment as the alcoholic, on the assumption that he/she (a) helped to bring about the other's alcoholism, (b) was continuing to support it, and (c) must thus, as a general rule, be quite disturbed. The spouse of the alcoholic has "traditionally" (Imhof, 1995, p. 6) been viewed as being a dysfunctional individual.

As appealing as this theory might be, in the past 40 years the concept of the co-alcoholic has been discredited by mental health professionals. Researchers have found virtually no evidence to support the assumption that the spouse of the alcoholic has any predictable form of psychopathology (Tavris, 1992). But, according to some detractors of codependency, the theory of co-alcoholism has apparently found new life as "codependency." For example, although there is little evidence to support the theory of the co-alcoholic, much of what was once said about the co-alcoholic in the 1950s is repeated as gospel "truth" about the codependent of the 1990s.

Another weakness of the concept of codependency is that this term has been modified to serve as a noun or an adjective, with a definition that has "been broadened to include anyone who has ever been involved with anyone who has ever had a problem around which a Twelve Step program has been, is being, or should be built" (Simmons, 1991, p. 26A). It is a term that ultimately fails to communicate anything meaningful about the individual. The defining characteristics of the codependent person virtually guarantee that any given individual will meet at least one of the defining criteria (Tavris, 1992; S. Walker, 1996).

In the past decade, the term codependent has been applied to so many people, for so many behaviors, that it is almost a secret language, a "recoveryspeak" (Simmons, 1991, p. 26A). Codependent is a trendy word that might serve as a noun or an adjective, depending on the person using the word and the situation it is applied to. Simmons went so far as to define "recoveryspeak" as a form of secret handshake, that might be used to bring a sense of security to people in an insane, overpowering world.

Nor is codependency limited to the world of addiction. It has even been suggested (O'Brien & Gaborit, 1992) that codependency is a separate condition that may, or may not, actually involve a substance-abusing marriage. The authors suggested that codependency it is a clinical syndrome in its own right. From this perspective, if codependency does exist in a marriage where one/both partners are abusing chemicals, that is only a coincidence. The hypothetical "disease" of codependence might also be found in a variety of non-substance-abusing relationships, according to O'Brien and Gaborit.

Another challenge to the concept of codependency rests on the lack of firm parameters. The term appears to be vague, without foundation. Consider M. Scott Peck's definition of codependency as "a relationship in which the partners cater to—and thereby encourage—each other's weaknesses" (1997a, p. 180). This would certainly seem to be an apt definition of virtually all relationships, not just those that are "codependent," since we all tend to encourage others to behave in unhealthy ways from time to time.

Although the belief that there is such a thing as codependence is quite strong among some mental health professionals—and much of the general population—there is no consensus among professionals that the condition even exists (Roehling et al., 1994). This is not to say that excessive dependency is not a clinical problem, but that *codependency* might not exist as a separate disorder. Further, in reading many of the books and articles on codependency, one is left with the impression that it rests on a foundation of "new age" sand. For example, the husband-and-wife team of Wegscheider-Cruse and Cruse (1990) speak knowingly of how codependency results from the:

> . . . interaction between one's own manufactured "brain chemicals" (having to do with our reinforcement center) and one's behavior that stimulates the brain to establish compulsive and addictive behavior processes. (p. 12)

The authors go on to conclude that codependency is a disease of the brain, on the grounds that:

> . . . we have a brain that gives us an excessive rush, (and) we get into self-defeating behaviors that keep the rush coming (co-dependency). (pp. 12–13)

What the authors overlook is that there is no scientific evidence to support this theory. Science has failed, to date, to find evidence of "an excessive rush" (what would be a "sufficient rush"?). Nor have scientists found evidence to suggest that people tend to "get into self-defeating behaviors that keep the rush coming." Such a position tends to be a contradiction, in the sense that if human beings, as a species engaged in self-defeating behaviors simply for the rush, how would *homo sapiens* ever have survived long enough to learn how to become "codependent"?

In considering the construct of codependency, there is a need for a sense of balance. Admittedly, there are those people who experience significant hardship because of their involvement in an ongoing relationship with an addict. But, not *every* person in such a relationship is necessarily codependent. Indeed, there is little evidence to support the concept of codependency, according to its detractors. Further, according to the codependency model, the victim must somehow come to terms with his/her emotional pain, without blaming the substance abuser for virtually anything he/she might have done:

> According to adherents of this theory, families of alcoholics cannot . . . hold them responsible for the abuse. Somehow the victim must get well by dint of pure self-analysis, meditation and prayer, without reference to the social, economic, legal and psychological forces that create dysfunctional families in the first place. (University of California, Berkeley, 1990a, p. 7)

For many people, this is an impossible task.

Summary

In the late 1970s, substance abuse professionals were introduced to a new way of viewing the substance-abusing person, and his/her support system. The constructs of codependency and enabling were introduced to explain how the members of the substance abuser's support system behave. Since that time, however, the fact that they are just theoretical constructs has been forgotten. Proponents have seized on these theoretical entities and suggested that they are real manifestations of a new "disease"—"codependency." In the past decade, a battle has raged over whether these constructs are indeed real entities, and, the applicability of this new disorder to the problem of substance-related interpersonal dysfunctions.

A number of challenges to the constructs of codependency and enabling have been suggested over the years. For example, some researchers point out that the construct of codependency is only a revised term for the 1950s' theory that the alcoholic's spouse was a "co-alcoholic." Although this theory was discredited in the 1960s, it seems to have found new life under the guise of codependency, at least according to some who challenge the theory. These constructs may still be evolving, and the role that they will play in the understanding and rehabilitation of substance abusers remains to be determined.

CHAPTER TWENTY-FIVE

Addiction and the Family

There has been very little research into the impact of even the most common drug of abuse, alcohol, on the evolving marital unit (Leonard & Roberts, 1996). On the basis of their research, researchers are starting to realize that the role of alcohol—and, by extension, the other recreational chemicals—on the young adult during the premarital and early years of marriage is far more complex than was once thought. It is not uncommon for individuals who drink alcohol to reduce their alcohol intake not only during the engagement period, but also in the first year following marriage (Leonard & Roberts). Following marriage, young adults often also change not only the context within which they drink alcohol, but, also the people that they drink with (Leonard & Roberts). The role of recreational chemicals within the marital unit, and the family, is thus much more complex than was once imagined.

From time to time, chemical abuse/addiction becomes intertwined with marital/family units. The phenomenon of substance abuse/addiction does not exist in isolation. Individuals who are, or who become, addicted to chemicals are often married. Sometimes they are married when they begin down the road to addictive use of drugs. Another possibility is one marital partner is unaware of his/her future mate's addiction prior to the marriage. All too often, one partner is aware that the other has a substance use problem, but mistakenly believes that he/she can somehow "fix" the substance-abusing partner.

If there are children, they will also become involved in the dance of addiction, to a greater or lesser degree. But it is difficult to speak of the impact of addiction on the family unit, because there are so many different potential ways that the family can be affected by alcohol or drug dependency. Consider the following examples:

- A man becomes addicted to alcohol as an adult, then, at a later point in time, he marries. This is the first marriage for each partner, and neither has any children from previous relationships.
- A man becomes addicted to alcohol as an adult, then marries. It is the first marriage for him, but she was previously married, and the wife brings a daughter from her previous marriage to the relationship.
- A man addicted to alcohol marries a woman that he met at a rehabilitation center. She is also addicted to alcohol. This is the second marriage for each, and they both have a son from their first marriage who lives with their former spouse, but who will come to visit on weekends.
- A couple who have been married for 18 years are discovered to be social users of cocaine when the husband's employer carries out a random urine toxicology test to detect illicit drug use. When confronted with the evidence of his chemical use, the husband makes a full confession, without first discussing this with his wife.
- A couple who have been married for 18 years discover that the husband's father, who lives in the same town, has been abusing alcohol in the past

2 or 3 years. There is evidence that he might be alcohol-dependent. But, there was never any hint that the husband's father might have had an alcohol use problem earlier in life. Now the adult son is faced with the reality that his father has, in the later stages of life, developed an alcohol use problem.

This list is hardly an exhaustive review of all the combinations of chemical use problems and how they might affect the family. For example, consider how the family's discovery that a 16-year-old adolescent is using marijuana might be received in a home where the parents have alcohol use problems, as opposed to how this same 16-year-old's use of marijuana might be received in a home where neither parent uses recreational chemicals.

Alcohol/drug use is not always an unwelcome part of the marital or family unit. It is not uncommon for an addicted person to marry another addicted person. Such a marriage of convenience brings with it a "using partner," who will be an additional source of chemicals, provide excuses to authorities when the spouse's chemical use has caused absenteeism from work, and so forth.

Scope of the Problem

Chemical use/abuse within the marital unit is hardly a minor issue, but researchers have no accurate way of estimating the interrelationship between marriage and substance use problems. To illustrate the difficulty, consider a marriage where one partner drinks alcohol, but the other does not. If, while intoxicated, the alcohol-using spouse were to lash out and strike his/her partner just once in 25 years of marriage, should this be cited as an example of alcohol impacting on the marriage, a momentary indiscretion that is unlikely to be repeated, or an example of spousal abuse? What was the role of the individual's alcohol use in the abuse of his/her partner?

Yet, it is known that there is a reciprocal relationship between alcohol/drug use and marital problems (O'Farrell, 1995). Further, individuals who have chemical use patterns often go on to have children. It has been estimated that *one of every six individuals* in the United States was, or is being, raised in a

home with at least one alcohol-dependent parent (Kelly & Myers, 1996). An estimated 28 million people in the United States have at least one alcoholic parent (Kelly & Myers). While there is little information about the number of people who were raised in a home where the parental drug of choice was something other than alcohol, it is safe to say that for many, many years significant numbers of children have been raised in homes where some form of addiction is present.

Addiction and Marriage

Very little is known about the role that chemicals play within the marital relationship (Leonard & Roberts, 1996). What little information that is available deals almost exclusively with the "alcoholic marriage," which is to say the marriage where one partner is abusing/dependent on alcohol. The impact of one partner's alcohol use on the marital relationship is difficult to examine, if only because the two are so closely intertwined (McCrady & Epstein, 1995).

At one point in time, it was automatically assumed that alcohol use/abuse prior to marriage suggested that alcohol would prove to be a problem for the marital unit. Researchers have now discovered that, for many individuals, the act of marriage seems to stimulate a change in his/her alcohol use pattern (Leonard & Roberts, 1996). It is not clear at this time whether this change in alcohol use patterns is a result of the act of marriage itself, or reflects the multitude of changes that seem to occur in the individual's life status at about the time of marriage (stable employment, independence, growing involvement in the world of adulthood, etc.). However, it is known that many adults modify their alcohol use pattern into a more socially acceptable direction, following the decision to marry and in the first year of marriage (Leonard & Roberts).

The act of marriage provides the individual with an opportunity to form a "drinking partnership" (Leonard & Roberts, 1996, p. 194) with his/her partner. Not only does alcohol use seem to play a role in the individual's choice of a marital partner, but in the majority of cases, the individual will adjust his/her alcohol use until it is more consistent with that of the partner. However, in a minority of cases, a wide discrepancy evolves between the amount of alcohol used by each partner in the marital unit. The possibility then exists that the individual's alcohol abuse/addiction will have a negative impact on the marital relationship. In many alcohol-impacted marital units, the partners undergo a "role reversal" (Ackerman, 1983). The alcohol-dependent member of the marital unit may give up some of the power and role(s) he/she would normally hold within the marriage, or, if there are children, within the family. This role reversal might, eventually, also involve other family members, and could span two, or even three, generations. Over time, an unhealthy state of dependency will evolve between the alcoholic and the other family members, who, in turn, may become involved in a dysfunctional relationship with the alcohol-dependent member.

The Family Systems Perspective

To understand how family members might exchange roles, it is necessary to view the family from a "systems" perspective. As a general rule, people tend to marry those who have achieved similar levels of "differentiation of self" (Bowen, 1985, p. 263). The concept of differentiation is "roughly equivalent to the concept of emotional maturity" (Bowen, p. 263). A primary developmental task, is for the individual to separate from one's parents (*individuate*), and to resolve certain emotional attachments to the parents that emerged during childhood.

Over time, the relationship pattern between the parent and the child should evolve, as the child becomes more and more independent. A primary force in this process of change within the family is the pattern of communications. For example, at birth, and for the first few years, the child is almost totally dependent on his/her parents. But, the maturing child becomes less and less dependent on his/ her parents. The child communicates this growing independence by a variety of means to the parents, who, in a healthy relationship, gradually withdraw their control as the child becomes more capable of independent living. This process of separating from one's parents is known as *individuation* (Bowen, 1985).

Inherent in the struggle to individuate is the person's need to separate from his/her parents and family of origin. The parents may either encourage the child's emotional growth, or they may inhibit it. Inherent in Bowen's (1985) theory was the belief that it is possible for the child to fail to resolve the multiple conflicts found in childhood and adolescence, and thus fail to individuate. Family therapists who operate from a "Family Systems" model suggest that this often happens in the alcoholic home.

Communication patterns within the alcohol-impacted home are often poor (McCrady & Epstein, 1995). One reason for this is parental psychopathology. Because of their own lack of emotional maturity, the parents are unable to provide the proper guidance and support to their children as they mature. Indeed, it is possible that, unlike what happens in the healthy family, the parents might affirm their increasing control over their children. This makes it more difficult for children to make the appropriate emotional break necessary to individuate, because they lack guidance and support from the parents. In such a case they would remain emotionally dependent on the parents for feedback and support. As they mature, these children would view themselves as being weak and, very possibly, incompetent.

An individual raised in this environment would remain dependent on external sources of feedback and support, which might be provided either by continued dependency on the parents or a parental substitute. This is because we all tend to select for a marital partner a person with a similar level of emotional independence as our own (Bowen, 1985). If neither partner has achieved a significant degree of individuation, each would look to his/her partner to meet emotional needs, according to Bowen. While this marriage, like every marriage, might bring with it the potential for further emotional growth for both partners, the marriage also brings with it the risks inherent in such growth. For some, this risk is too great, and they turn away from the potential for growth to the pseudointimacy and the illusion of control offered by alcohol or chemicals.

Characteristics of the Alcohol-Abusing Marriage

Within the dysfunctional marriage, issues of control often become important, as each person struggles to achieve some sense of order within the marital unit. Control often becomes a central theme within the marriage, and *conditional* love becomes one of the weapons each will use to try and control the other. Such conditional love finds expression in demands like these: You must behave in a certain way, if you want to be (a) loved by me, (b) supported by me, and so forth. If you don't meet my demands, I will (a) leave you, (b) withdraw my love from you, (c) not give you money, (d) go out and get drunk, or (e) abuse you physically.

For the alcohol-dependent spouse, the goal of these control "games" is to make sure that family members do not stray too far from the alcoholic fold. To regain emotional health, family members must learn to *detach* from the behavior and threats of the alcohol/drug addicted member. Detachment thus becomes both an expression of *unconditional* love and the vehicle that transports one away from the *enmeshment* found in the dysfunctional family. Through detachment, each spouse allows the other the freedom to make his/her decisions, without conditions. In working with the codependent individual, it is often necessary to teach him/her the difference between *concern* for another, and *responsibility* for that person. In effect, the individual must learn that it is possible to "have feelings for another person, but I am not responsible for living that person's life."

Often it is also necessary to help the codependent person learn appropriate interpersonal *boundaries*. The alcoholic home, resting as it does on the unstable sands of addiction, is in constant danger of being washed away. Each family member develops an unnatural involvement in the lives of the other. As part of the natural growth process that results in individuation, the child must learn to establish boundaries between self and other, but in the alcoholic home the child learns to become *enmeshed* in the lives of others. Each person has been trained to feel responsible for every other member of the family.

Addiction and the Family

There is actually little information available about the effects of parental drug addiction other than alcohol on different members in the family constellation. Researchers have much to learn about how, for example, the mother's heroin addiction might affect the emotional growth of her children.

From the Family Systems perspective, the treatment of an addictive disorder involves the identification, and ultimately the modification of the dysfunctional family system that allowed the development and maintenance of the addiction in the first place (Bowen, 1985). In the alcoholic marriage, for example, it has long been known that the alcoholism becomes a "secret partner" first of the marriage, and ultimately of the family. In time this "family secret" becomes the dominating force around which the family's rules and rituals are centered (Brown, 1985).

The parents, because of their special role in the family, often set the tone or themes around which the family will center their lives. They do this through the use of parental *injunctions*. In the alcoholic home, however, the parental rules that come to dominate the family's life are those of the alcoholism. The parental injunctions in the addicted home are often: (a) there is no addiction in this home, and (b) don't you dare talk about it!

One of the developmental tasks facing a new child is to learn to adapt to the environment into which he/she was born. If the child were born into a family where one or both parents were abusing alcohol, this task is more difficult. The whole family must learn to adapt to the demands of an alcohol-dependent parent (Ackerman, 1983). One of the ways that the family might come to terms with parental alcoholism is to structure itself in such a way that the alcoholic parent is actually allowed to continue drinking.

At first glance, it might seem strange that the family would maintain the drinking behavior of the alcoholic member. But there is a reward for this behavior! Rather than to fight with the alcohol-dependent member, to force him/her to carry out the role that he/she *should* occupy, it becomes easier just to redistribute the power and responsibilities within the family. The family system changes to accommodate the alcohol-dependent member, and in so doing other family members may find themselves holding unusually powerful positions within the new family constellation.

The process of adaptation to the family's rules, values, and beliefs is a normal part of family life (Bradshaw, 1988b). However, when the family's rules, values, and beliefs are warped by dysfunctional behavior on the part of one of the parents, then the entire family struggles to adapt to the unhealthy family themes. But, the family struggles to adapt to the addiction without guidance or, often, external support. Often, family members come to use the very same defense mechanisms so characteristic of addicts: denial, rationalization, and projection, although the Johnson Institute (1987) termed "denial" as "avoiding."

As the other family members come to assume responsibilities formerly held by the addicted member of the family, the addict becomes less and less responsible for his/her family duties, and less involved in the family life. An older brother assumes the responsibility for discipline of the children, or a daughter assumes responsibility for making sure that the younger children are fed each night before they go to bed. In each case, one of the children has assumed a parental responsibility left vacant, perhaps because of alcoholism.

Thus, within the alcoholic family a paradox often comes to exist: the family is uncomfortable with the addiction but may be quite happy with the current distribution of power and responsibility. However, if the family allows the alcoholism to continue, they may rather quickly fall into the trap of actually becoming a part of the individual's support system, making it easier for the alcohol-dependent partner to drink. In so doing, the family members enable the addict's sick behavior to continue, as they feed into the addicted member's dependency.

Although adaptation allows the family to survive in the short term, the ability to adapt to parental alcoholism is not without its cost. The adaptation that accommodates the alcoholic's drinking is often based on fear. According to Brown and Lewis (1995), the family with an alcoholic parent "is now recognized as one of chaos (covert or overt), inconsistency, unpredictability, blurring of boundaries, unclear roles, arbitrariness, changing logic, and perhaps violence and incest" (p. 285).

Within such a dysfunctional home, fear, often in combination with guilt and threats (both real and imagined), might even be used by the alcoholic parent to control the family: "If you don't do what I want, I will start drinking, and it will be *your* fault!"

Further, within the new family constellation, different individuals may assume roles that they are not emotionally ready to handle. For example, the young child may assume responsibility for setting limits on the parent's behavior, rather than the other way around. While this might achieve a short-term adjustment to the parental alcoholism, such accommodation is achieved only at the cost of long-term emotional growth. In this way, families pass pathology from one generation to another.

For this reason, many professionals who work with chemical dependency view addiction as a multigenerational, family-centered disorder. Parental alcoholism becomes "a governing agent affecting the development of the family as a whole and the individuals within" (Brown & Lewis, 1995, p. 281). The alcohol addiction within one parent thus becomes a defining characteristic that shapes the growth of both the family as a whole and the individual members of that family.

Without professional intervention, it is difficult for the individual members of the family to learn how to detach from the member who is addicted to chemicals. Further, without professional intervention, family members are unlikely to learn how to let the addicted individual suffer the natural consequences of his/her behavior (Johnson Institute, 1987). Rather, the entire family assumes responsibility for the pathology of a single member, living their lives in an attempt to somehow "cure" the disturbed family member. In so doing, the addicted person is relieved of responsibility both for his/her substance use problem and, all too often, the problems of everyday living.

As the individual's substance use disorder progresses, the chemical assumes a position of greater and greater importance in his/her life. Family commitments become less important than opportunities to engage in the use of the drug of choice. Activities that interfere with the chemical use are dropped, in favor of drug-centered activities. Thus, a long awaited visit to the grandparents' house is postponed because Dad had a chance to go "fishing" with his drinking buddy.

Examples of familial accommodation to parental alcoholism are almost too numerous to count: a son keeps silent when the teacher asks for volunteer drivers for an upcoming school trip, knowing that Mom is unlikely to be sober enough to drive that day. The children stop bringing friends over to visit any more, to avoid the embarrassment of having their friends see their substance-abusing parent. The daughter joins every after-school activity she possibly can, to have excuses for not going home to an alcoholic, abusive parent.

The Cost of Parental Addiction

Until recently, clinicians did not understand the impact of parental alcoholism on the development of the children. Current theory holds that parental alcoholism will create a disturbed home environment that is similar to the home where there is physical, emotional, or sexual abuse (Treadway, 1990). Thus, in theory, it appears that children raised by alcoholic parents are at risk for the development of any of a number of stress-related disorders (Kelly & Myers, 1996; Owings-West & Prinz, 1987).

It has even been suggested that the damage caused by parental alcoholism might reach beyond the children, to the *grandchildren* of the alcoholic (Beattie, 1989; Stein, Newcomb, & Bentler, 1993). Even if we limit our investigation to the immediate consequences of addiction, the suspected impact of parental substance abuse and dependency is staggering.

In the early to mid-1980s, clinical case studies suggested that children of alcoholic parents were prone to a number of different disorders. For example, in their review of the impact of parental alcoholism on the psychological development of children, Owings-West and Prinz (1987) concluded that parental alcoholism contributed to conduct problems, poor academic performance, and inattentiveness. Silverman (1989) suggested that one expression of these conduct problems might be the development of an antisocial personality disorder, or even an addictive disorder later in life.

Webb (1989) thought that some of the children who are raised in an alcoholic home will become "addicted" to excitement. They might, for example, engage in fire-setting behaviors, according to the author. Also, some clinicians suggested that children raised by a substance-abusing parent might become "superresponsible," by assuming roles far beyond their abilities or maturity. For example such an overly mature child would ". . . spend an inordinate amount of time worrying about the safety of the whole (family) system" (Webb, p. 47), a responsibility that, in a healthy family, would be assumed by one or both parents.

Further, the author suggested that, as adolescents these children would stay awake while the alcoholic parent is out drinking, check on the safety of sleeping siblings, and develop elaborate fire escape plans that might involve returning time and time again to the burning house to rescue siblings, pets, and valuables. In response to this distorted family system, many adolescents would become overly mature, serious, and well organized, behaviors that develop in an attempt to maintain control of their home environment.

Webb (1989) suggested that adolescents raised in an alcoholic home were forced to spend so much time and energy meeting basic survival needs that they were unlikely to establish a strong self-concept. Because of the atmosphere of "chronic trauma" (Brown & Lewis, 1995, p. 285), a significant percentage of the children raised in the alcoholic home were thought to develop long-lasting emotional injuries.

Thus, clinical lore and legend hinted that children raised in an alcoholic home suffered some form of psychological harm. But, since the 1980s, researchers have discovered that parental alcohol/drug use problems do not automatically result in problems for the growing child. A number of factors shape the impact of parental alcoholism on the developing children in the family (Ackerman, 1983). For example, there is the sex of the substance-abusing parent. Each parent plays a different role within the family, and an alcoholic mother will have a far different impact on the family than will an alcoholic father.

A second factor that influences the impact of parental substance abuse on the family is the length of time that the parent has actively been abusing/addicted chemicals. For example, an alcoholic father who has used chemicals for "only" three years will have a far different impact on the family than an alcoholic father who has been physically dependent on alcohol for 15 or 16 years.

A third factor that influences the impact of parental substance use problems on the individual child's growth and development is the sex of the child. A daughter will be affected differently by an alcohol-dependent father than would a son (Ackerman, 1983). Also, the specific family constellation plays a role in how parental alcoholism will affect each child.

This is a difficult point for many people to understand. To help illustrate it, consider two different families. In the first family, the father has a 3-month relapse when the third boy in a family of six children is 9 years old. Contrast this child's experience with that of the oldest child in a family of six children whose father relapsed for 3 months when the child was 9 years old. Both of these children would experience a far different family constellation than would the only child, a girl, whose father relapsed for 3 months when she was 9 years old. All three children would have a far different experience in life than would the third boy in a family of six children whose mother was constantly drinking until he turned 14 years of age.

Finally, as Ackerman (1983) observed, it is possible for the child to escape from the brunt of the impact of parental alcoholism, if he/she is able to find a *parental surrogate*. It has been found that, if the child is able to find a parental substitute (uncle, neighbor, real or imagined hero, etc), it may be possible for that child to find a way to avoid the worst of alcoholic parenting (Ackerman). This alternative is discussed in a later section of this chapter.

The Adult Child of Alcoholics (ACOA) Movement

As discussed, earlier, many researchers believe that the effects of growing up in an alcoholic home often last beyond the individual's childhood years. Within the past generation, a large number of adults have stepped forward, to claim that they were hurt by a parent's alcoholism. These individuals are known as "adult children" of alcoholics (ACOA). An entire treatment industry has evolved, to meet their perceived needs.

Estimates of the number of adult children of alcoholics (ACOAs) in this country range between 22 (Collette, 1990) and 34 (Mathew, Wilson, Blazer, & George, 1993) million adults. As stated earlier, the alcoholic home shares many characteristics with other forms of dysfunctional home environments that leave scars on the developing child. Woititz (1983), an early pioneer in the field of therapeutic intervention with ACOAs, reported that the adult child of alcoholic parents has several distinctive characteristics, including:

- The need to "guess" at what normal adult behavior is like, including the tendency to have trouble in intimate relationships.
- The tendency to have difficulty following a project through from beginning to end.
- A tendency to lie in situations where it is just as easy to tell the truth.
- A tendency not to be able to relax, but to always judge themselves harshly and feel the need to always keep busy.
- A tendency to not feel comfortable with self, but to constantly seek affirmation from significant others.

Other researchers have also explored the impact of parental alcoholism on the later adjustment of the children. Berkowitz and Perkins (1988) found, for example, that ACOAs are more critical of themselves, and depreciate themselves more, than do adult children of nonalcoholic parents.

Hunter and Kellogg (1989) argued that the traditional view of the adult child of alcoholic parents is too narrow. In addition to the expected forms of psychopathology, the authors suggested that ACOAs might also develop personality characteristics that are the *opposite of those expected of a child raised in a dysfunctional home*. For example, as noted, one characteristic thought to apply to ACOAs is that they tend to have trouble following a project through from start to finish. Yet Hunter and Kellogg (1989) suggested that some ACOAs might actually be compulsive workaholics, who struggle to carry out a project despite feedback that this work is no longer necessary, or that the work is actually counterproductive.

The research team of Sher, Walitzer, Wood, and Brent (1991) explored the differences between young adults who had been raised by alcoholic parents and young adults who had not been raised by alcoholic parents. The authors used a volunteer sample of college students, whose parental drinking status was confirmed by extensive interviews. Their findings suggested:

- College freshmen with an alcoholic father tended to drink more and to have more symptoms of alcoholism, when compared with freshmen who were not raised by an alcoholic father.

- Women who were raised by an alcoholic parent or parents reported a greater number of alcohol-related consequences than their nondrinking counterparts.

- Children of alcoholic parents have an increased risk of using not only alcohol, but other drugs of abuse as well.

- Adolescent children of alcoholic parents had more positive expectancies for alcohol than did adolescent children of nonalcoholic parents.

- As adults, children raised by alcoholic parents tended to have higher scores on test items suggesting "behavioral under-control" (p. 444) than did those individuals who were not raised by alcoholic parents.

- As college students, children raised by alcoholic parents tended to score lower on academic achievement tests than did their non-ACOA counterparts.

The authors thus identified several areas where parental drinking status appeared to affect the college student's adjustment and academic performance. But this study also failed to answer the question of what shape this assumed relationship between the parental drinking pattern and the student's academic performance might take. The study *did* suggest, however, that parental alcoholism had a strong impact on the subsequent growth and adjustment of the children raised in that family, thus providing support for the theoretical model advanced by Ackerman (1983).

Drawing on data collected as a study of the prevalence of psychiatric disorders in a selected area, Mathew et al. (1993) examined the differences between the mental health of adults raised by alcoholic parents, and adults who were not raised by alcoholic parents. They concluded that, as a group, "Adult children of alcoholics had higher rates of dysthymia, generalized anxiety disorder, panic disorder, simple phobia, agoraphobia and social phobia than did matched comparison subjects" (p. 795).

There are other ways in which adult children of alcoholic parents have suffered, beyond the development of psychiatric problems. During childhood, many children of alcoholic parents blame themselves for their parent's drinking (Freiberg, 1991). Sometimes, this self-blame continues well into adulthood. Collette (1988, 1990) spoke of how she blamed herself for her father's pain, and was close to the point of suicide until she became involved in an Adult Children of Alcoholics self-help group. Sanders (1990) related how he felt responsible for his father's drinking, and how he "paid the price" for his father's drinking through nights of fear and dread, as his father threatened to leave time after time, or argued with his mother night after night.

Thus, a number of theoretical models have suggested that adult children of alcoholic parents suffer from emotional distress. A number of research studies have revealed higher levels of psychiatric problems in samples of adult children of alcoholic parents, providing some support for the theoretical models advanced in the late 1970s and early 1980s. In response to this pain, many ACOA children banded together, and formed self-help groups.

The Growth of ACOA Groups

In a survey text such as this book, it is not possible to examine the self-help movement for adult children of alcoholic parents in great detail. However, the reader should be aware that the historical growth of ACOA groups has been phenomenal. Although this movement only started in the 1970s and 1980s, it is now thought that 40% of the adults in this country belong to some kind of a twelve-step self-help group such as the groups for adult children of alcoholics (Garry, 1995).

This number reflects many different factors. It is a reflection, first, of how many people have been hurt by a parent's alcoholism, and, second, of the desire of these hidden victims of addiction to find peace by working through the shame and guilt left over from childhood (Collette, 1990).

Criticism of the ACOA Movement

The ultimate goal of the ACOA movement is to provide a self-help group format for those who believe that they were hurt by being raised in a dysfunctional environment. However, there are those who are critical of the ACOA movement or who question whether the ACOA movement could achieve its goal.

Elkin (quoted in Collette, 1990), pointed out, "We all want to feel like victims" (p. 30). But as the author points out:

> If you identify yourself as a survivor of incest or abuse, you are making an existential and self-hypnotic statement that defines you by the most destructive thing that ever happened to you. In the short term, its important to say it, but you can get stuck there. (p. 30)

Further, therapies that focus on traumatic events such as childhood abuse, or rape, tend to keep the focus on the trauma, not on the individual's strengths and potential for further growth (S. Walker, 1996). This might account for the phenomenon in which the individual seems to become dependent on the ACOA program, almost as if "addicted" to being in an ACOA recovery group (May, 1991).

Another danger is that, as Treadway (1990) noted, the process of attaching a label to the "adult child" may simply "perpetuate the process of blaming in a new language" (p. 40). The format of the ACOA movement simply allows the adult children to continue to blame their parents for whatever problems they might have encountered in life. Thus, while the ACOA group may help meet the ever-present need within this culture for "a sense of community, empowerment, and spiritual renewal" (Treadway, p. 40), one must ask at what cost this sense of belonging is achieved.

Further, the whole concept of ACOA limits the individual by keeping the focus *on the previous generation* (Peele et al., 1991). Admittedly, some children are raised in terrible, abusive, environments. But, the central thesis of the ACOA movement rests on the impact of past parental behavior (often, years past) on the individual's *current* life problems. The

ACOA movement tends to encourage the individual to define self on the basis of parents' problems and choices, according to Peele et al.

The possibility exists that the ACOA movement is based on a mistaken assumption—that "healthy," conflict-free, families really exist. While the traditional view of the American family has been one of peace and security, the reality is far different. "Family historians" wrote Furstenberg (1990, p. 148) "have been unable to identify a period in America's past when family life was untroubled." Familial conflict has been the norm within this culture, not the exception. Thus, one must question the degree to which the ACOA group movement is based on a conflict-free family model that simply has never existed in this country.

Another criticism of the ACOA model is that it rests on an assumption that Wolin and Wolin (1993, 1995) term the *Damage model*. This model holds that children raised in a dysfunctional environment will *automatically* suffer psychological harm. Claudia Black (1982), a strong proponent of the ACOA model, stated for example, that "All children are affected" (p. 27) if they are raised in an alcoholic home. Another example of this position is seen in the work of Brown and Lewis (1995), cited earlier. These authors assume that *all* children raised in a home where one or both parents are alcoholic will suffer emotional harm.

Another proponent of this belief is Daniel Anderson, who is one of the fathers of the Minnesota Model of treatment. According to Anderson (1995), if a person was raised in a home where there was alcohol, he/she automatically suffered some form of emotional damage. Children raised by an alcoholic parent never had the chance to express their "anger or outrage in a healthy manner" (p. 4Ex), a statement that assumes all children raised by a parent who is addicted to alcohol will feel anger or outrage at their fate.

Essentially, the Damage model assumes that people are simply "passive vessels whose dysfunctional histories inhabit and control them like so many malignant spirits" (Garry, 1995, p. 10A).

Yet the Damage model has never been established as being the result of having been raised in a disturbed home, and research studies have generally failed to support this model. Tweed and Ryff (1991), who examined the emotional adjustment of 114 ACOAs and 127 adults from nonalcoholic families, found no clear differences between the emotional adjustment of the adults raised in homes with an alcoholic and the adjustment of those raised in nonalcoholic homes.

The team of Senchak, Leonard, Greene, and Carroll (1995) examined a group of 82 adult children of alcoholic parents, 80 adult children of divorced parents, and 82 control subjects, whose parents were neither divorced nor alcoholic, to determine what impact being raised in a dysfunctional home might have on later adjustment. The authors found that "negative outcomes among adult children of alcoholics are neither pervasive nor specific to paternal alcoholism" (p. 152).

Indeed, after allowing for confounding variables such as parental depression and low socioeconomic status, the authors failed to find any significant difference between adult children of alcoholic, divorced, or control parents.

The team of D'Andrea, Fisher, and Harrison (1994) administered the California Psychological Inventory (CPI) to 97 self-identified ACOA volunteers. The authors found three different subgroups within the ACOA sample that they used. A minority (16%) of their sample of volunteers had CPI profiles suggestive of serious psychopathology. But the largest subgroup, almost half of their sample, had a normal CPI profile, according to the authors.

Another study that failed to find evidence that ACOAs are different from "normal" adults was the study conducted by Giunta and Compas (1994). The first author, as part of a doctoral dissertation research project under the direction of the second author, examined the responses of 184 women between the ages of 25 and 35 to a questionnaire, a modified form of the Michigan Alcoholism Screening Test (MAST), and the Symptom Check List-90. No special attempt was made to identify this as a study on ACOAs. Rather, the subjects in this study were told that the study was on women's relationships. The authors concluded that there was no evidence to suggest that the adult daughters of alcohol-abusing parents were more distressed than were adult female children of nonalcoholics. Further, the authors failed to find evidence suggesting that the ACOAs in their sample were more afraid of intimacy or that all children of alcoholic parents are in need of treatment.

Finally, Kelly and Myers (1996) administered the Beck Depression Inventory (BDI) to a sample of 20 volunteer ACOA female undergraduate college students, and, a control group of 20 female undergraduate college students whose parents were not alcohol-dependent. Although there was a statistically significant difference in the measured levels of depression between these two groups, according to the authors, the average BDI score for both subgroups fell within the normal range. In other words, as a group, neither the ACOA sample nor the control sample seemed to be significantly depressed. These findings cast doubt on the Damage model, which serves as the foundation of the ACOA movement. Indeed, in contrast to the Damage model, it appears that many individuals are able to avoid significant emotional scars, despite being raised in a "dysfunctional" environment (Peele et al., 1991; Wolin & Wolin, 1995).

Perhaps a more appropriate model for how children respond to having an alcoholic parent might be called the *Challenge model* (Wolin & Wolin, 1993). This model takes into account the possibility of individual resiliency, something the Damage model fails to do. Werner (1989) is a strong advocate of resiliency. She studied a number of children who were at risk because of social or biological trauma. Surprisingly, these children often went on to succeed in life, despite adverse childhood conditions. Those children who were able to overcome their early environmental handicaps seemed "to be particularly adept at recruiting . . . surrogate parents when a biological parent was unavailable . . . or incapacitated" (p. 108D).

This conclusion was supported by the team of Parker, Barrett, and Hickie (1992), who stated "childhood adversity is not always associated with a poor outcome" (p. 883), especially if the child is able to form stable, supportive relationships later in life. Indeed, the quality of subsequent interpersonal relationships may moderate, or overcome, the impact of poor parenting (Parker et al., 1992; Werner, 1989). These studies would seem to provide at least partial support for Ackerman's (1983) assertion that if the child finds a suitable parental substitute, it is possible for him/her to escape from the full consequences of parental alcoholism. At the same time, these studies seem to raise questions as to the validity of the ACOA model.

Further evidence that suggests a dysfunctional environment might not have lasting consequences for the individual was provided by the team of Garbarino et al. (1992). The authors examined the effects of extreme psychological trauma on children, especially those children raised in the inner cities or war zones. It was found that for a majority of these children, perhaps as many as 80%, no permanent scars are caused by the stress of being raised in the inner city, or a war zone. The authors suggested that for many children, the challenge of meeting the demands of living in such an environment might enable them to become stronger. However, one factor that the authors concluded was essential for the child to survive, and not be scarred, by the experience of growing up in such an environment was a stable, mature relationship with at least one adult.

Another criticism of the ACOA movement is that the ACOA model rests on the unproven assumption that, as a group, children raised by an alcoholic parent(s) manifest a unique kind of pathology. There is research that suggests children of alcoholic parents are likely to experience some psychological problems, such as depression, more often than children raised in the nonalcoholic home. However, these reports are inconclusive, often fail to be replicated in follow-up studies (Goodwin & Warnock, 1991; Wolin & Wolin, 1995), and fail to suggest that children of alcoholic parents demonstrate a *unique* form of psychological trauma as a result of parental alcoholism.

Thus, the research literature has failed to support some key components of the ACOA model. For example, D'Andrea et al. (1994) found little evidence to support the theory that adult children of alcoholic parents shared similar characteristics in their research. Indeed, after reviewing their data, the authors concluded, "There is a danger in assuming . . . that growing up in an alcoholic home inevitably leads to dysfunction in adulthood" (p. 580).

The team of Domenico and Windle (1993), who examined the intrapersonal and interpersonal functioning of 616 middle-aged women, also failed to find evidence that supported the theory of ACOA psychopathology. The authors compared the adjustment of women who were adult children of an alcoholic parent with that of women who were not raised by an alcoholic parent. While they found that the ACOA women seemed to have higher levels of depression, and lower levels of self-esteem, as a group the ACOA women scored in the normal range on the tests used in this study. These findings were apparently consistent with those of Seilhamer, Jacob, and Dunn (1993), who failed to find any consistent impact, either positive or negative, of parental alcoholism on parent-child interactions.

One is left with the impression that, in the absence of hard research data, the literature on which the ACOA movement is based rests on a foundation of nothing more than "assertions, generalizations and anecdotes" (University of California, Berkeley, 1990a, p. 7). A very real shortcoming of the ACOA literature is that it is "long on rhetoric and short on empirical data" (Levy & Rutter, 1992, p. 12). Yet it is based on this literature that many have labeled significant portions of society as diseased—dysfunctional—in the jargon of the ACOA movement.

Another criticism of the ACOA movement is based on the fact that the self-help movement, of which the ACOA movement is a part, has become something of a growth industry in this country (Blau, 1990; C. Boyd, 1992). It has been suggested that the publishing industry, armed with the knowledge that the majority of those who purchase self-help books are women, slant their titles and design their covers to attract the attention and activate the insecurities of women (Boyd). One could very well argue that the ACOA movement is the stepchild of the publishing industry, which has used the movement to develop a market for a new line of self-help books.

When the ACOA movement began in the early 1980s, it focused upon the survivors of extreme abuse, according to Blau (1990). However, over the years, the definition of what constitutes "abuse" has become blurred, to the point where the tendency to blame "parents for what they did or didn't do has become a national obsession—and big business" (Blau, 1990, p. 61; W. Kaminer, 1992).

But, because of the lack of diagnostic rigor, and the vague language of the ACOA movement, virtually *96% of the population might be said to have been raised in a dysfunctional family* (Garry, 1995; Peele et al., 1991). Indeed, many proponents of the self-help movement quote this 96% figure even though there has never been any research to suggest that it is accurate (Hughes, 1993). Given this fact, one must wonder to what degree the characteristics identified by the proponents of the ACOA movement reflect, not some form of pathology, but simply the problems-in-living that we all experience in today's society. But now, thanks to an overabundance of self-help books, we have the "language" for which to blame our parents and grandparents for all our problems-in-living.

In reality, there has been very little research into the psychological dynamics of families of alcoholics, or other forms of addiction (D'Andrea et al., 1994; Goodwin & Warnock, 1991; Sher, 1991; University of California, Berkeley, 1990a). Further, very little is known about what constitutes a "normal" family, or the limits of unhealthy behaviors (which we all have) that may be tolerated in an otherwise "normal" family.

Blau (1990) challenged the very concept of ACOA, on the ground that the entire theory of the "adult child" is a reflection of the "baby boomer's" resistance to accepting that they are now adults, who are themselves entering middle adulthood. Developmentally, the adults of the baby-boomer generation are no longer the children of their parents, at least in the same sense that they were three decades ago. They are now middle-aged adults, who are now discovering that they will not fulfill all the dreams of young adulthood. Perhaps, as Blau suggested, the ACOA movement is a reaction by the baby-boomer generation against growing older.

From this perspective, it is understandable that the ACOA movement places great emphasis on the so-called inner child. However, the inner child concept is not a part of any single therapeutic theory. Rather, the theory behind the ACOA concept of the inner child is a complex blend of: "[Carl] Jung, New Age mysticism, holy child mythology, pop psychology, and psychoanalytic theories about narcissism and the creation of a false self" (W. Kaminer, 1992, p. 17).

Another challenge to the ACOA emphasis on the inner child comes from Hughes (1993). The pursuit of the "Inner Child," he writes, comes:

> . . . just at the moment when Americans ought to be figuring out where their Inner *Adult* is, and how that disregarded oldster got buried under the rubble of pop psychology and short-term gratification. (p. 29, italics added for emphasis)

Finally, when one stops to consider that the idea of the inner child is based on a phase of life when the individual was developmentally, socially, psychologically, and neurologically immature, one must wonder the degree to which this construct is able to meet the demands of adult life.

As Levy and Rutter (1992) point out, the ACOA movement is essentially a white, middle-class invention. It is not known whether this model applies to inner-city children, whose parents may be addicted to heroin or cocaine, or who may come from a single-parent family, and so forth. As the authors note, children of heroin and cocaine addicts are "primarily nonwhite, minority members who live in poverty. They have no national movement . . . do not write books and make the rounds of the talk shows" (p. 5).

Thus, virtually nothing is known about them. However, as the authors remind us, many children are raised by parents who are addicted to chemicals other than alcohol, in environments other than the white, middle-class world. There is no research as to whether the ACOA model applies to these other children of addiction.

Summary

This chapter explored the family of the addicted individual, and the impact that one individual's addiction to chemicals is thought to have on the rest of the family. There are few research studies that actually explore the impact of one member's alcohol/drug addiction on the other members of the family. Much of what is assumed to be true about the family in which one or more persons is addicted to alcohol/drugs is based on theory, not established fact.

The theory of codependency assumes that the individual who is codependent is "trained" by a series of adverse life events to become dependent on the feedback and support of others. Further, it is assumed that family members come to assume new roles, as the addicted person gives up the power and responsibility that he/she would normally hold within the family. In this manner, the family comes to "accommodate," or adapt to, the individual's chemical addiction.

From the perspective of the codependency model, the individual's substance abuse is viewed as a family-centered disorder, which is passed on from one generation to the next. The self-help group movement of "adult children" of alcoholics is viewed as a logical response to the pain and suffering that the family members experienced because of their participation in a "dysfunctional" family. However, the adult child concept has met with criticism. Some health care professionals stress that the theory behind the adult children movement places too much emphasis on past suffering, at the expense of possible resilience on the part of the individual or his/her future growth.

Further criticism has been made of the adult children movement on the grounds that it automatically assumes the individual has experienced some lasting psychological trauma as a result of parental alcoholism or drug addiction. This theory has never been tested, and thus much of the ACOA self-help movement rests on a series of unproven assumptions.

Research is needed to begin to understand how chemical addiction affects the growth and development of both the individual family members and the family unit.

CHAPTER TWENTY-SIX

The Evaluation of Substance Use Problems

For those individuals with a suspected substance use/abuse problem, the process of assessment forms the cornerstone (Bukstein, 1995, p. 95) first of the *detection* of alcohol/drug use problems and, ultimately, of *rehabilitation*. For many who abuse/are addicted to chemicals, the first step in the direction of recovery is a complete, accurate, alcohol/drug use evaluation (Donovan, 1992). In this chapter, evaluating a client's drug/alcohol use pattern and relating the assessment to rehabilitation are briefly explored.

The Theory behind Alcohol and Drug Use Evaluations

As Cohen and Marcos (1989) observed, mental health professionals are increasingly being called on to determine those individuals "whose criminal ('bad') behavior is not necessarily attributable to being mentally ill ('mad')" (p. 677). Chemical dependency professionals are being asked to make the same determination for those thought to be addicted to chemicals. Some of those who come to the attention of the criminal justice system have committed crimes because of their addiction. For these individuals, treatment may be a more viable option than legal sanctions. It is often the task of the substance abuse professional to determine whether a given individual will benefit from treatment for substance abuse.

In addressing this issue, Lewis et al. (1988) warned:

Merely walking into a substance abuse treatment facility does not, in and of itself, warrant a diagnosis of "chemical dependency" or "alcoholism." Rather, clinicians must carefully evaluate the client and only then make decisions concerning diagnosis and treatment. (p. 75)

Along the same lines, Miller et al. (1995) warn that *screening* a patient (to determine whether there are indications of a specific condition being present) is *not* the same as making a formal *diagnosis*. In the case of chemical dependency, the diagnosis should be made only after an extensive evaluation of the client, not just because one or two symptoms of a substance use disorder are present.

This is a timely warning because there are those who would like to excuse their antisocial behavior behind the shield of an "illness" such as chemical dependency. As discussed in Chapter 34, extreme chemical abuse is often able to "short circuit" the legal system, enabling many individuals to avoid paying the full consequences of their behavior. Therefore, it is the first duty of the assessor to establish a firm basis either for or against a diagnosis of chemical dependency.

It is only after the diagnosis has been established—*if it is established*—that the need for treatment should be considered. Treatment centers with the philosophy that "this person *must* have a problem with chemicals, or else he/she would not be here!" do not serve the client's interests, only their own. Thus, the need for treatment *must be proven*, and the reasons for recommending treatment *documented in sufficient detail* to justify this recommendation.

If all drug/alcohol dependent individuals were carbon copies of each other, there would be no need for an assessment to proceed beyond determining whether the individual was abusing chemicals. However, each person who is abusing/addicted to alcohol/drugs presents the clinician with a unique combination of hopes, strengths, needs, fears, and past experiences. Therefore, to "the extent that treatment is selected and individualized to address clients' differing needs and problems, comprehensive evaluation provides an information foundation upon which to plan treatment" (Miller et al., 1995, p. 64).

It is through the process of evaluation that the therapist can identify problem areas that need to be addressed (Lehman, 1996). On the basis of the information uncovered during a careful evaluation, the substance abuse rehabilitation professional is able to identify appropriate goals and treatment strategies for each client. The opposite outcome is also predictable: without a careful evaluation of the client's strengths, experiences, and needs, it is difficult to identify appropriate goals for the person, or, to effectively intervene. The evaluation process itself consists of three interrelated phases: *screening*, *assessment*, and *diagnosis*.

Screening

The first step in assessment is to identify those individuals who might have a chemical abuse/addiction problem. This process is known as *screening* and is analogous to the *triage* system in a hospital emergency room/trauma center setting. Through the screening process, the treatment professional attempts to identify the patient's individual strengths, needs, and areas of weakness, and to determine whether professional intervention is warranted for a substance use problem.

The screening phase can be relatively simple and straightforward, or complicated and time consuming. The individual who arrives in a hospital emergency room with alcohol-induced liver disease, alcohol-induced gastritis, a history of five prior admissions for alcohol-related disorders, and a blood alcohol level of .230 at the time of the current admission, would present few questions as to the possibility that the patient has an alcohol use disorder. However, every case is not as simple and easy to screen as this hypothetical example.

The first step in the screening interview is to rule out the possibility that the client might go into, or actually be in, alcohol withdrawal. A valuable tool in measuring the client's intoxication/withdrawal potential is the Clinical Institute Withdrawal Assessment for Alcohol Scale-Revised (CISA-Ar). This noncopyrighted scale measures 15 symptoms of alcohol withdrawal such as anxiety, nausea, and visual hallucinations. The CISA-Ar takes 3 to 5 minutes to administer. It has a maximum score of 67 points, with each symptom being weighted in terms of severity. A score of 0–4 points indicates minimal withdrawal discomfort, while a score of 5–12 points indicates alcohol withdrawal of mild severity. Patients who earn a score of 13–19 points on the CISA-Ar are likely to be in moderately severe alcohol withdrawal; a score of 20+ points is indicative of severe alcohol withdrawal. The CISA-Ar can be repeatedly administered over time, to provide a baseline measure of the patient's recovery from alcohol withdrawal.

To aid in the screening process, researchers have devised a number of paper-and-pencil tests, or questionnaires, to help detect those individuals who might have a substance use problem. These instruments are either filled out by the client (and as such are known as *self-report* instruments), or by the assessor as he/she asks questions of the person being evaluated. Self-report instruments offer the advantages of being inexpensive and possibly less threatening to the client than a face-to-face interview (Cooney, Zweben, & Fleming, 1995).

One of the most popular screening instruments for alcohol use disorders is the Michigan Alcoholism Screening Test (MAST) (Selzer, 1971). This test consists of 24 questions that the respondent may answer either "yes" or "no." Test items are weighted with a value of 1, 2, or in some cases 5 points. A score of 8 points or more suggests an alcohol use problem. The effectiveness of this screening instrument has been demonstrated in clinical literature, and it is a popular tool for detecting individuals with a possible alcohol use disorder (W. Miller, 1976).

But the MAST has some drawbacks. First, this instrument addresses *only* alcoholism (Lewis et al.,

1988). Further, it is useful only as a "crude general screen" (Miller et al., 1995, p. 62) for alcohol use problems. Also, the MAST does not detect binge drinking, and it does not shed light on the individual's drinking pattern (Smith, Touquet, Wright, & Das Gupta 1996). The current consensus is that the MAST is best at the detection of those individuals with severe alcohol use problems (Saunders, Aasland, Babor, de la Fuente, & Grant, 1993). It is of limited value if the person uses other chemicals and is not sufficient by itself to diagnose alcoholism The questions on the MAST tend to be weighted toward the detection of severe alcohol dependence, and thus it is ill-suited to "problem" drinkers who are not alcohol-dependent.

Another screening tool for alcoholism that is growing in popularity is the "CAGE" questionnaire (Ewing, 1984). CAGE is an acronym for the four questions that make up this test:

1. Have you ever felt you ought to **CUT DOWN** on your drinking?
2. Have people **ANNOYED** you by being critical of your drinking?
3. Have you ever felt bad or **GUILTY** about your drinking?
4. Have you ever had a drink first thing in the morning to steady your nerves, or to get rid of a hangover (**EYE-OPENER**)?

A "yes" response to one of these four questions suggests the need for a more detailed inquiry by the assessor. Affirmative answers to two or more items suggests that the client has an alcohol use problem. The CAGE questionnaire has been found to have an accuracy of 80% to 90% in detecting alcoholism, when the client answers "yes" to two or more of these questions. But, like the MAST, the CAGE is most effective in detecting alcohol-dependent individuals rather than alcohol *abusers* (Saunders et al., 1993). It is also relatively insensitive to binge drinking (Smith et al., 1996).

There are other screening tools available. The team of Saunders et al. (1993) developed the Alcohol Use Disorders Identification Test (AUDIT) to detect individuals whose alcohol use problems had not progressed to the point of alcohol dependence. The AUDIT was found to be over 90% effective in

detecting alcohol use disorders (Brown, Leonard, Saunders, & Papasoulioutis, 1997). Roffman and George (1988) provided examples of a self-report instrument used in the evaluation of marijuana use patterns. Washton, Stone, and Hendrickson (1988) discussed the use of the Cocaine Abuse Assessment Profile in their essay on the evaluation of cocaine users. Each of these tests, while useful, is of limited value in the assessment of polydrug users since they focus on the use of only one chemical of abuse.

The team of Brown et al. (1997) suggested the use of a simple, two-item question set to detect possible substance use disorders:

1. In the last year, have you ever drank or used drugs more than you meant to?
2. Have you felt you wanted or needed to cut down on your drinking or drug use in the last year?

Despite its brevity, the authors claimed that a "yes" answer to one item indicated a 45% chance that the individual had a substance use disorder, while a "yes" response to both items indicated a 75% chance that the respondent had a chemical use problem (Brown et al., 1997). Although these results are promising, the authors also pointed out that their two-item test might result in false-positive results in some cases and that their initial findings needed to be replicated in follow-up studies. However, this two-item test shows promise as a screening tool for health care workers.

Another screening tool often used in health care settings is urine toxicology testing. This process, discussed in more detail later in this chapter, detects *current* or *recent* substance use by the individual. However, even if the individual does test positive for alcohol or illicit drugs, this information does not provide the assessor with any data as to the individual's substance use pattern. Urine toxicology testing will only provide evidence that the patient has used alcohol/drugs during a variable detection window (discussed later in this chapter).

An instrument that is often mistakenly considered to be a screening/assessment tool is the Minnesota Multiphasic Personality Inventory (MMPI). The original MMPI was introduced almost 65 years ago. In 1965, the *MacAndrew Alcoholism Scale* (also known as the "Mac" Scale) was introduced, after an item analysis suggested that alcoholics tended to answer 49 of the 566 items of the MMPI differently than nonalcoholics. A cutoff score of 24 items out of 49 answered in the "scorable" direction correctly identified 82% of the alcoholic and nonalcoholic clients, in a sample of 400 male psychiatric patients (J. Graham, 1990).

In 1989, after seven years of research, an updated version of the MMPI, the Minnesota Multiphasic Personality Inventory-2 (MMPI-2), was introduced. The Mac Scale was modified slightly, but was essentially retained in its original form. However, in the time since it was first introduced, research has revealed that the Mac Scale has several inherent problems. First, it has been discovered that black clients tend to score higher on the Mac Scale than do white clients. Further, rather than being specific for alcohol use problems, research has suggested that the Mac Scale might measure a general tendency toward addictive behaviors (J. Graham, 1990). Also, clients who are extroverted or exhibitionistic, who experience blackouts for *any* reason, who are assertive, or who enjoy risk-taking behaviors, all tend to score higher on the Mac Scale, even if they are not addicted to chemicals (J. Graham).

Although the Mac Scale was designed to detect alcoholics, in working with the original MMPI, Otto, Lang, Megargee, and Rosenblatt (1989) discovered that alcoholics might be able to "conceal their drinking problems even when the relatively subtle special alcohol scales of the MMPI are applied" (p. 7). This is because personality inventories in general, including the MMPI/MMPI-2, are vulnerable to both conscious and unconscious attempts at denial, self-deception, and distortion (Isenhart & Silversmith, 1996). Thus, although the MMPI Mac Scale was designed as a subtle test for alcoholism, it is possible to obtain either false positive or false negative results from it. Until proven otherwise, counselors should assume that the revised Mac Scale on the MMPI-2 shares this same weakness with the original Mac Scale.

Unlike many of the other assessment tools, the MMPI offers an advantage of having five "truth" scales built into it. These scales offer insight into how truthful the individual taking the test may have been, and are discussed in more detail by J. Graham

(1990). A major disadvantage of the MMPI is that it is possible for the individual taking the test to "intentionally diminish . . . the level of pathology evident in overall MMPI profiles" (Otto et al., 1989, p. 7). Furthermore, although truth scales are built into the MMPI, individuals who are attempting to project an image of themselves as being well adjusted may still accomplish their goal and reduce measured levels of distress. Finally, the length of the MMPI/MMPI-2 makes it difficult to justify its use in the screening process. This instrument might better be used during the *diagnosis* phase of assessment (discussed later in this chapter).

The goal of the screening process is the identification of those individuals who seem to have a substance use problem. Once these individuals are detected, they then move on to the next stage of the evaluation process: *assessment*.

Assessment

During the *assessment* phase of the evaluation process, the assessor attempts to measure the severity of the individual's substance use problem. One of the most useful tools in assessment is the clinical interview, which forms the cornerstone of the drug/alcohol use evaluation. Clients are an important source of data about their current and previous chemical use. It is important to keep in mind, however, that clients may either consciously or unconsciously distort the information they provide. Thus, other sources of data should also be utilized in the evaluation of a person suspected to have a chemical use problem.

The first part of the interview process is an introduction by the assessor, who explains that he/she will be asking questions about the client's possible chemical use patterns, and that *specific* responses are most helpful. It is explained that others may have asked many of these questions in the past, but that this information is important. The assessor asks whether the client has any questions, after which the interview begins.

The assessor should review the diagnostic criteria for chemical use problems utilized in the *Diagnostic and Statistical Manual of Mental Disorders* (fourth edition) *(DSM-IV)* (American Psychiatric

Association, 1994). This manual provides a framework for making the diagnosis of chemical dependency and provides a standard language that is understood by most treatment professionals. The *DSM-IV* criteria for alcohol/drug use problems are discussed in more detail in the next section.

Many of the questions in the clinical interview are designed to explore the same piece of information from different perspectives. For example, at one point, the client might be asked, "In the *average* week, how many nights would you say that you use drugs/alcohol?" Later in the interview, this same client might be asked, "How much would you say, on the average, that you spend for drugs/alcohol in a week?" The purpose of this redundancy is not to "trap" the client so much as provide different perspectives on the client's chemical use pattern. It is often wise to consider the *percentage of the client's income spent on recreational chemicals* (Washton, 1995).

Consider the case of a client who claimed using alcohol one or two nights a week and spending $60 per week on beer. This person's alcohol use would be seen as excessive in anybody's eyes. But, if the client's only source of income was an unemployment check for $120 each week, this person would be devoting fully 50% of that income to buy alcohol. This information reveals more about the individual's chemical use pattern, helping the evaluator better understand the client.

A number of assessment instruments are available to aid the professional conducting an alcohol/drug use evaluation.[1] Perhaps the most popular for individuals over the age of 16 is the *Alcohol Use Inventory* (AUI). The AUI is a copyrighted instrument made up of 228 items and takes 30 to 60 minutes for the individual to complete. The answers to the test items provide data for 24 subscales that the assessor can analyze to better understand the client's alcohol use pattern. But, the AUI is limited to alcohol use problems.

A popular research instrument, which is gaining popularity as an assessment tool, is the *Addiction Severity Index* (ASI). The ASI is administered to adults during a semistructured interview with the client. The fifth edition, which contains 161 items, which requires approximately an hour to complete. The administrator asks the questions of the client and records the answers on the answer form. The ASI is "public domain," which is to say that it is not copyrighted, and it provides a severity rating score based on the impressions of the person who administers the test. Unlike the AUI, the ASI can be used for evaluating the severity of other forms of drug abuse such as cocaine and opiates.

Diagnosis

The final stage in the evaluation process is *diagnosis*. Abel (1982) identified four elements as being necessary to the diagnosis of alcohol/drug addiction. These are the interrelated elements of (a) a compulsion to continue use of the drug, (b) the development of tolerance, (c) major withdrawal symptoms following withdrawal from the drug, and (d) adverse effects from drug use both for the individual, and for society. A more standardized conceptual model is presented in the *DSM-IV* (American Psychiatric Association, 1994), which suggests that some of the signs of alcohol/drug addiction include:

1. *Preoccupation* with use of the chemical between periods of use.
2. *Using more of the chemical* than had been anticipated.
3. *The development of tolerance* to the chemical in question.
4. A *characteristic withdrawal syndrome* from the chemical.
5. Use of the chemical *to avoid or control withdrawal symptoms*.
6. *Repeated efforts to cut back or stop* the drug use.
7. *Intoxication at inappropriate times* (e.g., at work), or when *withdrawal interferes with daily functioning* (e.g., hangover makes person too sick to go to work).
8. A *reduction in social, occupational, or recreational activities* in favor of further substance use.

---

[1] It is not possible to review all the assessment instruments currently in use, especially since new tools are constantly being introduced. This section discusses only some of the more popular instruments.

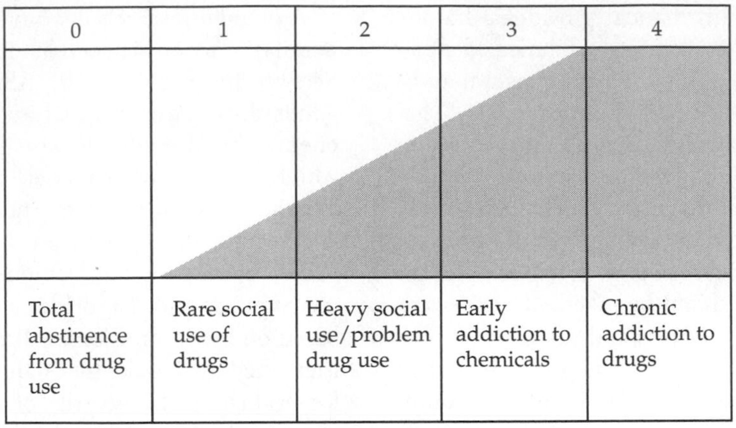

0	1	2	3	4
Total abstinence from drug use	Rare social use of drugs	Heavy social use/problem drug use	Early addiction to chemicals	Chronic addiction to drugs

FIGURE 26.1   The continuum of addiction.

9. Chemical use continues despite the individual having suffered social, emotional, or physical problems related to drug use.

Any combination of four or more of these signs are used to identify the individual who is said to suffer from an addiction to one or more recreational chemicals.

In Chapter 1, the concept of a substance use continuum was introduced. Figure 26.1 illustrates that continuum of drug use/abuse, with the different points on the continuum ranging from total abstinence from chemicals to the stage of chronic addiction.

If the *DSM-IV* criteria are applied to this continuum, then the individual who meets four or more of the *DSM-IV* criteria would fall in Level 3 or 4 of the continuum introduced in Chapter 1.

Shaffer and Robbins (1995) offered a different continuum of substance abuse:

1. *Initiation.* The person starts the use of the chemical(s).
2. *Positive consequences.* The person enjoys the drug-induced pleasure.
3. *Beginning of adverse consequences.* The person starts to suffer some of the adverse consequences associated with recreational chemical use.
4. *Turning points.* The individual begins to question whether he/she can continue to use chemicals.

5. *Active quitting.* The person begins a recovery program.
6. *Relapse prevention.* The person works to set up a program to enhance recovery while minimizing the chances of returning to chemical use.

Of these various diagnostic systems, the one offered by the American Psychiatric Association in its *DSM-IV* (1994) provides a standardized framework within which a professional can make a diagnosis of substance dependence. It is through the evaluation process that the professional gathers the data on which to make such a diagnosis as to where on any of the preceding continuums the individual being assessed might fall. A second part of the evaluation process is the determination, to the degree that this is possible, of the client's motivation. The vast majority of those individuals who are abusing/addicted to chemicals are unready/unwilling to pursue abstinence (Miller et al., 1995). Thus, in addition to the determination of whether the individual has a substance use problem, his/her motivation for change should also be assessed. However, the assessor must always remember to work within the framework of state and federal "data privacy" regulations.

The Assessor and Data Privacy

The client *always* has a right to privacy: the assessor does not automatically have access to personal information about the client. The client may refuse to answer a specific question or refuse permission for another person to reveal specific information to the assessor. This is the client's right, and the assessor should respect the client's right to control access to this information.

Both federal and state data privacy laws often apply when working with individuals who are thought to be addicted to drugs or alcohol. If these clients agree to the assessment, they are then willingly providing information about themselves during the assessment process. Clients still retain the privilege to refuse to answer any question. If information is required from persons other than a client, *the professional should always obtain written permission* from the client authorizing him/her to contact *specific* individuals to obtain information about the client's chemical use, or any other aspect of the client's life. This written permission is recorded on a form known as a *release of information authorization form.*

Occasionally, the client will refuse such permission. The client retains this right and can refuse to allow the assessor to speak with *any* other person. This refusal in itself may say a great deal about how open and honest the client has been with the assessor, especially if the evaluator has explained to the client exactly what information will be requested. A possible solution to this problem advocated by some professionals is to have the client sit in on the collateral interview. The drawback to this solution is that the client's presence may inhibit the collateral information source from freely discussing his/her perception of the client. If this happens, a potentially valuable source of information about the client is unavailable to the assessor. Thus, it is rarely productive to have the client, or the client's representative, sit in on collateral interviews.

When the client is being referred for an evaluation by the court system, the court will often provide referral information about the client's previous legal history. The courts will often also include a detailed social history of the client, which was part of the presentence investigation. If asked, the evaluator should acknowledge having read this information, but should not discuss it. Such discussions are to be avoided for two reasons.

First, the purpose of the clinical interview is to assess the client's *chemical use patterns.* A discussion of information provided by the court does nothing to further this evaluation. Second, the client has access to this information through his/her attorney. Thus, the client who wants to review the information provided by the court may do so at another time through established legal channels.

Clients occasionally ask to see the records provided by the court during the clinical interview. Frequently, these clients are checking to see what information has been provided by the courts, to decide how much and what they should admit to during the present interview. This often reflects the philosophy of "let me know how much *you* know about me, so that I will know how 'honest' I should be!" The solution to this dilemma is a simple statement to the effect that the client may obtain a copy of the court record through the established legal channels. Those persistent clients who demand to see their court records on the grounds that "it is about me, anyway" are to be reminded that the purpose of this interview is to explore the client's drug and alcohol use patterns, not to review court records. However, under no circumstances should the chemical dependency/mental health professional let the client read his/her referral records. To do so would be a violation of the data privacy laws, since the referral information was released to the professional, *not* to the client.

When the final evaluation is written, the evaluator should identify the source of the information summarized in the final assessment. Collateral information sources should be advised that the client, or his/her attorney, has a right to request a copy of the final report before the interview. It is *extremely* rare for a client to request a copy of the final report, although technically the client does have the right to do so after the proper release-of-information authorization forms have been signed.

Diagnostic Rules

Many, perhaps most, clients initially resist a diagnosis of chemical dependency (Washton, 1990). Because of this, two diagnostic rules should be followed as closely as possible in the evaluation and diagnosis of a possible drug addiction. Occasionally, it is not possible to adhere to each of these diagnostic rules for one reason or another; however, the assessor should always attempt to carefully evaluate each individual case in light of these guidelines, even in special cases. Then, even if the rule is not followed, the professional making the diagnosis should identify why one guideline or another could not be met in a given situation, to avoid missing important information.

Rule 1. Gather Collateral Information

Traditional belief holds that one characteristic of the alcohol/drug dependent individual is deceptiveness. This belief is only a half-truth. Research has shown that, *as a group*, alcohol-dependent individuals will, when sober, be reasonably accurate as to the amount and frequency of their alcohol use. But there are exceptions. For example, one major exception to this rule is when the individual is facing some kind of legal problem (Donovan, 1992; McCrady, 1993). Further, individuals who have both a mental illness problem, and a substance use problem also tend to underreport the extent of their substance use problems (Carey et al., 1996).

But because of the importance of the diagnostic process, the individual attempting to make a diagnosis of addiction should *utilize as many sources of information as possible*. Do not "ever diagnose using information based only on the client's presentation at the time of assessment" (Evans & Sullivan, 1990, p. 54). Rather, the assessor should use other sources of information besides the client's self-report (McCrady, 1993). To illustrate the importance of collateral information, every chemical dependency professional has encountered cases where the individual being evaluated claims to drink "once a week . . . no more than a couple of beers after work." The spouse of the person being evaluated often reports, however, that the client is intoxicated "five to seven nights a week."

Collateral information sources might include (Slaby et al., 1981):

- Patient's families.
- Friends of the patient.
- Employer or co-workers.

- Clergy members.
- Local law enforcement authorities.
- Primary care physician.
- Psychotherapist (if any).

The time restrictions imposed on the assessment process might prevent the use of some of these collateral resources. If the assessment must be completed by the end of the week, and the professional is unable to contact the client's mother, it may be necessary to write the final report without her input. In addition, the other people involved may simply refuse to provide any information whatsoever. It is the assessor's responsibility, however, to *attempt* to contact as many of these individuals as possible and to include their views in the final evaluation report.

Rule 2. *Always* Assume Deception, until Proven Otherwise

As noted, evidence suggests that, *as a group*, alcoholics are quite accurate in their self-report as to the amount of alcohol consumed, and the frequency of their alcohol use. But, clinicians still cling to the belief that the nature of addiction is deception. There is a reason for this belief! For example, Sierles (1984) found that substance abusers were one of the two groups of patients most likely to attempt to deceive assessors (individuals with a history of sociopathic behaviors composed the other subgroup). Cunnien (1988) went so far as to state that the addict will be "persistent" (p. 25) in attempts to deceive others.

There are many different ways of expressing this deception. Some alcohol-dependent individuals will minimize the amount of alcohol that they drink, or the frequency of their drinking. Opiate addicts who are admitted for detoxification, on the other hand, will often exaggerate the amount of drugs that they use in the hopes of obtaining more drugs from detoxification center staffs. Cocaine addicts may also exaggerate their drug use, although this is not consistent. Some cocaine addicts, instead of exaggerating their drug use report, may initially deny or minimize it.

Thus, when evaluating another person's alcohol/drug use pattern, always expect deception unless proven otherwise. On more than one occasion, professionals have encountered a person who claims to be using a given amount of heroin or cocaine, only to later find out from friends of the client that the person has *never* used opiates or cocaine but is just attempting to impress the evaluator, the courts, or drug-using friends.

It is not uncommon for a person who is addicted to alcohol to only admit to drinking "once or twice a week" until reminded that their medical problems are unlikely to have been caused by such moderate drinking levels. At this point, these individuals sometimes admit to more frequent drinking episodes. However, even when confronted with evidence of serious, continual alcohol use, many alcoholics have been known to deny the reality of their alcoholism.

Clients have been known to admit to "one" arrest for driving under the influence of alcohol or possession of a controlled substance. Records provided by the court at the time of admission into treatment have often revealed that the person in question was arrested in two or three different states for similar charges. When confronted, these clients might respond that they thought that the evaluator "only meant in *this* state" or that "since that happened outside this state, it doesn't apply." Thus, to avoid the danger of deception, the assessor *must use as many different sources of information as possible.*

The Assessment Format

The assessor's diagnosis usually is recorded on a standardized record form, often with the title "Alcohol and Drug Use Evaluation Summary." Although each individual is unique, there is a general assessment format that professionals use for record keeping. This assessment format is modified as necessary to take into account the differences between individuals and provides a useful framework within which to evaluate the individual and his/her chemical use pattern. This format is utilized in this chapter.

Area 1. Circumstances of Referral

The first step in the diagnostic process is to examine the circumstances under which the individual is seen. For example, the patient who is seen in a hospital alcohol detoxification (or "detox") unit for the first time is far different from the patient who has

been in the detox unit 10 times in the past 3 years. Thus, the first piece of data for the chemical dependency assessment is a review of the circumstances surrounding the individual's referral.

The manner in which the client responds to the question "what brings you here today?" can provide valuable information about how willing a participant the individual will be in the evaluation process. The individual who responds with "I don't know, they told me to come here" or "You should know, you've read the report" obviously is being less than fully cooperative. The rare client who responds "I think I have a drug problem" is demonstrating some degree of cooperativeness with the assessor. In each case, the manner in which the client identifies the circumstances surrounding his/her referral for evaluation provides a valuable piece of information to the assessor.

Area 2. Drug and Alcohol Use Patterns

The next step is for the evaluator to explore the individual's drug and alcohol use patterns *both past and present.* All too often, clients will claim to drink "only once a week, now" or to have had "nothing to drink in the last six months." Treatment center staff are not surprised to find out that this drinking pattern has been the rule *only* since the person's last arrest for an alcohol-related offense.

From time to time, every assessor encounters a person who proudly claims not to have had a drink, or to have used chemicals, in the past 6 to 12 months, or perhaps even longer. This person may forget to report having been locked up in the county jail awaiting trial during that time, or that he/she was under strict supervision after being released from jail on bail, with little or no access to chemicals. This is a far different situation from the client who reports that he/she has not had a drink or used chemicals in the past year, is not on probation or parole, and has no charges pending.

Thus, the evaluator should explore the client's living situation to determine whether there were any environmental restrictions on the individual's drug use. Environmental restrictions exist when a person is incarcerated, in treatment, or is required by a probation officer to undergo both frequent and unannounced supervised urine screens. In such a case, a report of having "not used drugs in six months" may be the literal truth, but fall far short of the facts.

The individual's chemical use pattern and *beliefs about his/her drug use* should then be compared with the circumstances surrounding referral. For example, the client may state that he/she does not have a problem with chemicals. Earlier in the interview, he/she may also have admitted being recently arrested on the charge of possession of a controlled substance for the second time in 4 years. In this situation, the client has provided two important, but discrepant, pieces of information to the evaluator.

Several important areas should be explored at this point. The evaluator needs to consider whether the client has ever been in a treatment program for chemical dependency, and whether the individual's drug or alcohol use has ever resulted in legal, family, financial, social, or medical problems for the person being evaluated. The assessor also needs to consider whether the client ever demonstrated any signs of either psychological dependency or physical addiction to drugs or alcohol.

To understand this point, consider two hypothetical clients who were seen following their recent arrest for driving a motor vehicle while under the influence of alcohol/drugs. The first person might claim (and have collateral information sources to support his claim) that he only drank in moderation once every few weeks. Furthermore a background check conducted by the court revealed that this client never had any previous legal problems of any kind. The evaluation also revealed that, after receiving a long awaited promotion, the client celebrated with some friends. The client was a rare drinker, who uncharacteristicly drank heavily with friends to celebrate the promotion and apparently misjudged the amount of alcohol that he had consumed.

In contrast to this person is the client who also was arrested for driving a motor vehicle under the influence of chemicals. This individual's collateral information sources seemed to suggest a more extensive chemical use pattern to the evaluator than she admitted during the interview. A background check conducted by the police at the time of the individual's arrest revealed several prior arrests for the same offense.

In the first case, one might argue that the client simply made a mistake. Admittedly, the person in question was driving under the influence of alcohol. However, he had *never* done so in the past, and does not fit the criteria necessary for a diagnosis of even heavy social drinking. The report to the court would outline the sources of data examined, and in this case provide a firm foundation for the conclusion that this individual made a mistake in driving after drinking.

But, in the second case, the individual's drunk driving arrest was the tip of a larger problem, outlined in the report to the court. The assessor would detail the sources of information that supported this conclusion, including information provided by family members, the individual's physician, the patient, and the county sheriff's department, as well as friends of the client. The final report in this case would conclude that the client has a significant addiction problem requiring treatment in a chemical dependency treatment program.

Area 3. Legal History

Part of the assessment process should include an examination of the client's legal history. This information is based on the individual's self-report, or on a review of the client's police record as provided by the court, the probation/parole officer, or other source. *It is important to identify the source of the information on which the report is based.* Identify:

- What charges have been brought against the client in the past, by the local authorities, and their disposition.
- What charges have been brought against the client in the past, by authorities in other localities, and their disposition.
- The nature of current charges (if any) against the individual.

There are many cases on record where the individual was finally convicted of a misdemeanor charge for possession of less than an ounce of marijuana. However, all too often, a review of the client's police record reveals that the individual was *arrested* for a felony drug-possession charge, and that the charges were reduced through plea bargaining agreements. In some states, it is possible for an arrest for the charge of driving a motor vehicle under the influence of alcohol (a felony in many states) to be reduced to a misdemeanor charge such as public intoxication, by plea bargaining agreements.

The assessor needs to determine *both the initial charge, and the ultimate disposition* by the court of these charges. The assessor should specifically inquire whether the client has had charges brought against him/her in other states, or by federal authorities. Individuals may admit to *one* charge for possession of a controlled substance, only to have the staff later find out that the same client has had several arrests, and also convictions, for the same charge, in other states. Or clients may admit to having been *arrested* for possession charges in other states, but may not mention that they left the state before the charges were brought to trial.

Many clients reason that, since they were never *convicted* of the charges, they do not have to mention them during the assessment. These clients overlook that the charges were never proven in court because they were fugitives from justice (as well as that interstate flight to avoid prosecution is a possible federal offense).

Past Military Record

An important, and often overlooked, source of information is the client's *military history, if any.* Many clients with a military history will report only on their civilian legal history, unless specifically asked about their military legal record. Clients, who may have denied any drug/alcohol legal charges whatsoever, may on inquiry admit to having been reprimanded or brought before a superior officer on charges of chemical use while in the military.

The assessor must specifically inquire whether the individual was ever in the service. If the client denies military service, it might be useful to inquire *why* the client has never been in the service. Often, this question elicits a response to the effect that "I wanted to join the Navy, but I had a felony arrest record," or "I had a DWI (driving while under the influence of alcohol) on my record, and couldn't join." These responses provide valuable information to the assessor and open new areas for investigation.

If the client has been in the military, was the client's discharge status "Honorable," a "General" discharge under honorable conditions, a "General" discharge under dishonorable conditions, or a "Dishonorable" discharge? Was the client ever brought up on charges while in the service? If so, what was the disposition of these charges? Was the client ever referred for drug treatment while in the service? Was the client ever denied a transfer or promotion because of drug/alcohol use? Finally, was the client ever transferred because of drug/alcohol use?

The client's legal history should be verified, if possible, by contacting the court or probation/parole officer, especially if the client was referred for evaluation for an alcohol/drug-related offense. The legal history will often provide significant information about the client's lifestyle, and the extent to which drug use has (or has not) resulted in conflict with social rules and expectations.

Area 4. Educational/ Vocational History

The next step in assessment is to determine the individual's educational and vocational history. This information, which is based on the individual's self-report, school, or employment records, provides information on the client's level of function, and on whether their chemical use has interfered with their education or vocation. As before, the evaluator should identify the source of this information.

For example, the client who says that she dropped out of school in the 10th grade "because I was into drugs" presents a different picture than does the client who completed a bachelor of science degree from a well-known university. The individual who has had five jobs in the past 2 years is unlike the individual who has held a series of responsible positions and received regular promotions with the same company for the past 10 years. Thus, the assessor should obtain the client's educational/vocational history, to determine educational level, potential, and degree to which chemical use has started to interfere with educational or work life.

Area 5. Developmental/Family History

The assessor can often uncover significant material through an examination of the client's developmental and family history. The client might reveal that his/her father was "a problem drinker" in response to the question "were either of your parents chemically dependent?" but hesitate to call that parent an alcoholic. How the client describes parental or sibling chemical use might reveal how the client thinks about his/her own chemical use.

For example, the client who says that his/her mother "had a problem with alcohol" might be far different from the client who says "My mother was an alcoholic." Clients who hesitate to call a sibling alcoholic but are comfortable with the term "problem drinker" might be hinting that they are also uncomfortable applying the term alcoholic to themselves. But they may have accepted the rationalization of being a problem drinker, just like the brother or sister. Information about either parental or sibling chemical use is important for another reason, as well. As noted in Chapter 4, there is significant evidence suggesting a genetic predisposition toward alcoholism. By extension, one might expect that future research will uncover a genetic link toward other forms of drug addiction, as well. Thus, a sibling who is perceived as being addicted to alcohol/drugs by the individual being assessed *hints* at the possibility of a familial predisposition toward substance use disorders.

In addition, the reviewer will be able to explore parental alcohol/drug use in the home while the client was growing up. Did the client view this chemical use as normal? Was the client angry or ashamed about the parents' chemical use? Does the client view chemical use as being a problem for the family? Thus, it is important for the assessor to examine the possibility of either parental or sibling chemical use either while the client was growing up, or at the present time. Such information will offer insights into the client's possible genetic inheritance, especially whether he/she might be at risk to develop an addiction. Furthermore, an overview of the family environment provides clues as to how the client views drug or alcohol use.

As discussed in Chapter 25, family environments differ. The client whose parents were rare social drinkers would have been raised in an environment unlike that of the client whose parents where drug addicts. The client who reported that he never knew his mother because she was a heroin addict who put her children up for adoption when they were little might have a different view of drugs than the client who reported that she was raised to believe that hard work would see a person through troubled times, and whose parents never consumed alcohol.

Area 6. Psychiatric History

Often, as was discussed earlier in this book, chemical use will result in either outpatient or inpatient psychiatric treatment. A natural part of the assessment process should be to discuss with the client whether he/she has ever been treated for psychiatric problems on either an inpatient or an outpatient basis. A natural part of this part of the assessment should be a review of the patient's alcohol and drug use patterns (Beeder & Millman, 1995).

For example, clients have been known to admit to having been hospitalized for observation, because they were hallucinating, had attempted suicide, were violent, or depressed. On admission to chemical dependency treatment, perhaps months or years later, these same individuals might reveal that they were using drugs at the time of their hospitalization for a "psychiatric" disorder. It is not uncommon for substance abuse rehabilitation professionals to discover that clients, during hospitalization, failed to mention their substance abuse to the staff of the psychiatric hospital. This happens because clients lie to the hospital staff, or because the hospital staff simply do not ask the appropriate questions.

The assessor should always ask whether the client:

- Has *ever* been hospitalized for psychiatric treatment.
- Has ever had outpatient psychiatric treatment.
- Had revealed to the mental health professional the truth about his/her drug use during the former hospitalization.

If possible, the assessor should obtain a release-of-information form from the client, and send for the treatment records, and the discharge summary from the treatment center where the client was previously hospitalized. The possibility that drugs contributed to the psychiatric hospitalization or outpatient treatment should be either confirmed, or ruled out if possible. This information then will allow the assessor to determine whether the client's drug use has resulted in psychiatric problems serious enough for professional help to be necessary.

As noted earlier, it is not uncommon for chronic use of amphetamines or cocaine to cause a drug-induced psychosis which is, at least in its early stages, very similar to paranoid schizophrenia. A client who reports having spent a short time in a psychiatric hospital for a "brief psychosis" may well have developed such a drug-related problem, whether it was recognized as such by the hospital staff or not.

Area 7. Medical History

Clients who are chemically dependent will often present a history of numerous hospitalizations for the treatment of accidents or injuries. These periods of hospitalization might be for drug-related injuries, such as one client who reported having been hospitalized many times after rival drug dealers had tried to kill him. He had accumulated an impressive assortment of knife wounds, gunshot wounds, and fractured bones from these "business transactions" that had, in his words, "gone bad" over the years.

However, he had never been hospitalized for a drug overdose. An assessor who asked the question "Have you ever been hospitalized because of a drug overdose?" would miss out on the details of these hospitalizations, since the client viewed them as the results of business transactions, not personal drug use. On a similar note, alcoholics who drive while under the influence of alcohol are often hospitalized following accidents that may or may not be alcohol-related.

The assessor should inquire about periods of hospitalization *for any reason*. Then, the assessor should explore whether these were alcohol/drug-related. For example, a client who was hospitalized following an automobile accident may contract hepatitis B (discussed in Chapter 32) following a blood transfusion. If that accident was caused by the person's drinking, then indirectly he/she might be said to have contracted hepatitis B as a result of drinking.

Another area of inquiry is the *client's current medical problems*. What prescriptions and over-the-counter medications is the client taking? How often is the client taking these medications? When were the medications prescribed? Who prescribed the medications for the client, and why were the medications needed? It is not uncommon to find a client who has seen three or four doctors for prescriptions for the same condition. Patients with opiate use problems have been known to use the same medical condition as a pretense to obtain narcotic analgesics from three, four, or even more doctors.

It is up to the assessor to try and determine, if possible, whether the person's chemical use was a causal agent in any period of hospitalization that the client might have experienced. While the assessor is usually not a physician, it is also up to the assessor to identify possible medication use patterns that *should* be discussed with the patient's doctors, to help the assessor gain a better understanding of the client's chemical use, and the consequences that the patient has had to face as a result of the chemical use.

Area 8. Previous Treatment History

In working with a person who may be addicted to chemicals, it is helpful for the evaluator to determine whether the client has ever been in a treatment program for chemical dependency. This information, which may be based on the client's self-report, or on information provided by the court system, sheds light on the client's past, and on the client's potential to benefit from treatment.

The man who has been hospitalized three times for a heart condition, but continues to deny having any heart problems, is denying the reality of his condition. Likewise, the woman who says that she does not think she has a problem with chemicals, but has been in drug treatment three times, may not have accepted the reality of her drug problem. The problem then becomes one of making a recommendation in light of the client's previous treatment history and current status.

The assessor should pay attention to the discharge status from previous treatment programs, and to the period of time after treatment that the person maintained their abstinence. Clients often claim to have been sober for three months, but on close questioning may admit that they were in treatment (or in jail!) for these same three months. Further, clients may admit that they started to use drugs shortly after they were discharged, if not before. The discouraging report of a client who used chemicals on the way home following treatment is well known to chemical dependency treatment professionals.

A client, who admits using chemicals throughout the time that he was in treatment is providing valuable information about his possible attitude toward *this* treatment exposure, as well. The prognosis for this client would differ from that of a client who had maintained total sobriety for three years following her last treatment exposure and who then relapsed.

In questioning clients, the evaluator should pay attention to the past treatment history, the discharge status from these treatment programs, and the total period of sobriety *after* finishing treatment. Specific questions should be asked as to *when they entered treatment, how long they were there,* and *when they started to use chemicals following treatment.*

Other Sources of Information: Medical Test Data

Laboratory test data is of only limited value in the assessment of a person who is suspected of being addicted to chemicals. There are no blood/urine tests specific for alcohol/drug addiction that a physician can use for general screening purposes. It was suggested that elevations in certain blood tests such as liver function tests might serve as "alerting factors" (Hoeksema & de Bock, 1993, p. 268) to the physician for possible alcohol dependence. Thus, laboratory test data does provide one important piece of information to the assessor: the results of blood/urine studies may provide important hints about a person's chemical use status. For example, if a patient being assessed admitted that his/her personal physician had warned him/her about alcohol-related liver damage 3 years ago, this would suggest that the problems caused by the patient's alcohol use date back at least that long, and provide strong evidence that the client is alcohol-dependent.

Medical personnel and laboratory test data can often shed further light on the client's chemical use pattern at the time of the evaluation by detecting actual traces of alcohol or illicit drugs in the patient's body. It is for this reason that Washton (1995) recommended that urine toxicology testing be a routine part of a drug or alcohol use assessment. Consider the case of the client who claimed never to have used marijuana, only to have a supervised blood or urine toxicology test be positive for THC. This would strongly suggest that the patient was using marijuana, in addition to whatever drugs of abuse he/she might have been using.

Medical tests or the patient's physician can often:

- Confirm the presence of certain chemicals in the client's blood or urine samples.
- Identify the *amount* of certain chemicals present in a person's blood/urine sample (e.g., the BAL).
- Determine whether the drug levels in the blood or urine sample have increased (suggesting further drug use), remained the same (which also might suggest further drug use), or declined (suggesting no further drug use since the last test).

Finally, the patient's medical history can often offer hints as to how long the patient has been using chemicals.

The detection of chemical use by laboratory testing is a highly technical procedure that is affected by many variables (Verebey & Turner, 1991). Furthermore, both blood and urine toxicology testing involves an element of intrusiveness (Cone, 1993). At the very least, urine toxicology testing involves an invasion of privacy, while obtaining a blood sample for toxicology screening is physically invasive, according to the author. However, medical test data is often useful to the assessor. It is not uncommon, for example, for a client who was involved in an automobile accident to claim to have "only had two beers" prior to when he/she started to drive. A blood alcohol (BAL) test conducted within an hour of the accident may reveal, however, that the client's BAL was far higher than what would be achieved from two beers. This information would suggest some distortion on the client's part.

Clients who had tested negative for marijuana on one occasion, may very well test positive for this same chemical only a few days later. Subsequent inquiry will often reveal that he/she used drugs sometime after the first test, thinking that he or she was "safe" and would not be tested for drugs again for a long time. Such drug use would be detected by *frequent* and *unannounced* urine tests, which are *closely supervised* to detect illicit drug use.[2]

Thus, medical test data is often a valuable source of objective information about a client's drug use. Clients might appear sleepy simply because they did not sleep well the night before, or because they used drugs/alcohol in the past few hours. The laboratory test data often is valuable in making this determination, or in the detection of continued drug use while clients are in treatment.

For these reasons, the assessor should always attempt to utilize medical test information where possible, to further establish a foundation for the diagnosis of a chemical use problem.

Psychological Test Data

There are a number of psychological tests that, either directly or indirectly, may be useful in the diagnosis of chemical dependency. A major disadvantage of paper-and-pencil tests is that they are best suited to situations where the client is unlikely to fake (the technical term is "positively dissimulate") his/her answers on the test, in order to appear less disturbed (Evans & Sullivan, 1990). A common problem, well known to chemical dependency professionals, is that these instruments are subject to the same problems of denial, distortion, and outright misrepresentation often encountered in the clinical interview setting.

As noted, clients have been known to initially deny the use of a chemical, say marijuana, only to subsequently test positive for THC on a urine toxicology test conducted at the time of admission. Clients have also been known to either overestimate the amount or the frequency of their drug use, or to underestimate the amount or frequency. Such distortion may be unintentional (e.g., the person simply forgets an episode of chemical use), or it may be quite intentional. Another source of distortion encountered by assessors is that clients often do not know the level of potency of the drug(s) that they use (Roffman & George, 1988). Such clients might not know how to answer questions such as how the

drug(s) interfered with their ability to work or to drive a motor vehicle. Lacking a valid yardstick by which to measure the drug's effects, a client might honestly believe that he/she was only mildly intoxicated, whereas an outside observer might express the belief that the client was barely able to function.

A technique that may be useful in the detection of intentional dissimulation is to review the test results with the client when the client's spouse or significant other is also present. The assessor then reviews the test item by item, stating the client's response. Often, the spouse or significant other will contradict the client's response to one or more test items, providing valuable new data for the assessment process. For example, on the Michigan Alcoholism Screening Test (MAST), clients often answer "no" to the question inquiring whether the client had ever been involved in an alcohol-related accident. The client's spouse, if present, may speak up at this point, asking about "that time when you drove off the road into the ditch a couple of years ago." If the client then points out that the police ruled the cause of the accident as being ice on the road, the spouse may respond "but you told me that you had been drinking, earlier that night."

Another technique to detect dissimulation is to administer the same test, or ask the same questions, twice during the assessment process. For example, the MAST may be administered during the initial interview and again at the follow-up interview a week or so later. If there are significant discrepancies, these are explored with the client to determine why there are so many differences between the two sets of test data. For example, if a client scored 13 points when he/she first took the MAST, but afer taking the same test just a month later his/her score was only 9 points, an assessor might assume that the client was actively denying his/her alcohol use problem.

Psychological test data can often provide valuable insights into the client's personality pattern, and chemical use. Many such tests require a trained professional to administer and interpret the test to the client. However, when used properly, psychological test data can add an important dimension to the diagnostic process.

[2] The use of urine, hair, and saliva samples for toxicology testing is discussed in more detail in Chapter 30.

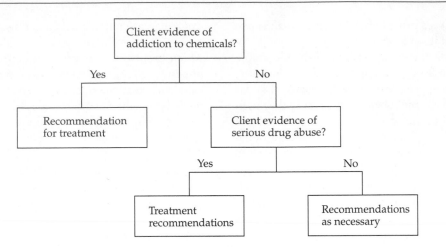

FIGURE 26.2   A flowchart of the assessment process.

The Outcome of the Evaluation Process

At the end of the assessment, the chemical dependency professional should be in a position to answer four interrelated questions: (a) whether the client seems to have a substance use problem, (b) the *severity* of that individual's substance use problem, (c) the individual's *motivation to change,* and (d) the *factors that seem to contribute to further substance use* by the individual (McCrady, 1993). Based on this assessment, the professional should then be able to decide whether treatment is necessary as well as the level of care that appears necessary to help the client, and make some recommendations as to the disposition of the client's case. Figure 26.2 is a flowchart that outlines the assessment process.

If the client is found to be addicted to one or more chemicals, a recommendation to enter treatment would be appropriate. The detection of a substance use problem is of little value if there is no recommendation for treatment (Paton, 1996). The form of treatment, however, would be determined by the assessor's opinion as to the *appropriate level of care.* Treatment programs are ranked by their *intensity.* For example, a medical inpatient treatment program is considered more intense than a day outpatient treatment that meets on a 5-days-a-week basis, and both of these programs are considered more intense than an evening outpatient treatment program that meets

once a week. The deciding factor is the client's need for treatment.

For example, if the client is found to be only an abuser of chemicals, but is not addicted to recreational drugs, the decision might be to recommend participation in a self-help group such as Alcoholics Anonymous or Narcotics Anonymous. However, it is possible that the client will be found not to present a substance drug use problem but still be in need of professional support. Even if there was no evidence of a substance use problem, if there is a marital problem, a referral to a family/marriage counselor or a community mental health center may be in order. The assessor might still make an appropriate referral based on the client's assessed needs, even if there is no evidence of alcohol/drug addiction.

Summary

The evaluation process involves three phases: screening, assessment, and diagnosis. Each of these phases was reviewed. The application of various tools such as the Addiction Severity Index, the Minnesota Multiphasic Personality Inventory (MMPI), and the Michigan Alcoholism Screening Test (MAST), as aids to the evaluation process were discussed. The goal of each phase of the evaluation process, was discussed, as was the need for a wide database to provide the most comprehensive picture of the client's chemical use pattern. Data sources discussed include the client; and the advantage of collateral information as well as the application of medical test data was discussed as possibly providing information that would aid the evaluation process.

Medical personnel, who are in a position to evaluate the client's physical status, can often provide valuable information about a client, and the role that drugs have had on his/her life. Finally, psychological test data may reveal much about the client's personality profile and drug use pattern. However, psychological test data suffers from the drawback that it is easily manipulated by a client who wishes to dissimulate.

The outcome of the assessment process should be a formal report outlining the evidence to support the conclusion that the client is/is not abusing, or dependent on chemicals. The recommendations that result from the evaluation process might include suggestions for further treatment, even if the client is found not to be addicted to chemicals.

CHAPTER TWENTY-SEVEN

The Process of Intervention

Substance abuse rehabilitation processionals used to believe that, before a person could benefit from any form of treatment, he/she had to "hit bottom." Then, in the 1970s, Vernon Johnson, a minister who worked with alcoholics, suggested that it was possible to "raise" the "bottom" through the process of *intervention*. Even the substance abusing client who was functioning poorly (McCrady, 1993), or the person who was ". . . not in touch with reality" (Johnson, 1980, p. 49) because of his/her chemical abuse, was viewed by Johnson as being ". . . capable of accepting some useful portion of reality, *if that reality is presented in forms they can receive*" (p. 49, italics in original). On the basis of this theory, the practice of intervention was born.

The goal of intervention is to present to the substance-abusing individual the truth about his/her chemical use problem in terms that he/she can understand, so that he/she will agree to enter into a rehabilitation program. In this chapter, the theory behind the process of intervention, and its application in clinical settings, will be examined.

A Definition of Intervention

It was once thought that, for addicts to accept the need for help, they had to "hit bottom," as it is called in Alcoholics Anonymous (AA). "Bottom" is the point where substance abusers have to admit utter, and total, defeat. When alcohol/drug dependent individuals reached this point in their lives, there was no question about the need to stop using recreational chemicals. But this passive approach to treatment meant that many alcohol/drug abusers died before reaching bottom, and many never accepted the need to stop using chemicals.

Vernon Johnson (1980), a pioneer in the intervention process, challenged the belief that it was necessary for addicts to hit bottom before they could accept help. Rather, he suggested that alcohol-dependent persons could learn to comprehend the reality of his/her addiction, *if this information was presented in language that he/she could understand*. Further, because of the physical and emotional damage that uncontrolled addiction could cause, Johnson did not recommend that concerned family/friends wait until the addicted person "hit bottom." Rather, he advocated *early intervention* in cases of alcohol/drug addiction.

In a later work, Johnson identified intervention as:

> [a] process by which the harmful, progressive and destructive effects of chemical dependency are interrupted and the chemically dependent person is helped to stop using mood-altering chemicals, and to develop new, healthier ways of coping with his or her needs and problems. (Johnson Institute, 1987, p. 61)

Twerski (1983), who also advocated early intervention for drug addiction, defined intervention as:

> a collective, guided effort by the significant persons in the patient's environment to precipitate a crisis through confrontation, and thereby to

remove the patient's defensive obstructions to recovery. (p. 1028)

Rothenberg (1988) who explored the legal ramifications of intervention, noted that the intervention process for alcoholism consisted of:

talking to the alcoholic, confronting his or her denials, and breaking down defenses so as to secure agreement to seek treatment. (p. 22)

A Final Definition

Drawing on these three definitions, it is possible to define an intervention project as being (a) an *organized* effort on the part of (b) *significant others* in the addict's environment, to (c) *break through the wall of denial, rationalization, and projection* by which the addict seeks to protect his/her addiction. The purpose of this collective effort, which is (d) *usually supervised* by a chemical dependency professional, is to (e) secure an agreement to *immediately* seek treatment.

A Consequence of Early Intervention Projects

A situation that sometimes occurs is that the person abusing chemicals may not view his/her alcohol/drug use as being problematic (McCrady, 1993). Individuals who have not hit bottom may not understand, or accept, the relationship between the problems that they have encountered and their chemical use. Thus, they may resist intervention efforts by concerned others.

Characteristics of the Intervention Process

A significant characteristic of intervention is that *no malice is involved.* This is not a session to allow people to vent pent-up frustration. The process is seen as a "profound act of caring" (Johnson, 1986, p. 65) through which significant others in the addict's social circle break the rule of silence surrounding the addiction. Each person confronts the addicted person with specific evidence that he/she has lost control of drug use, in language that the addicted individual can understand.

The participants also express their desire for the addict to seek professional help for the drug problem (Williams, 1989). In the process, all members affirm their concern for the addict, but each participant offers hard data showing how the addicted person is no longer in control of his/her life. The collective hope is that those involved will be able to break through the addict's system of denial. The goal is for the addict to accept the need for help with the drug problem. This is the central theme around which an intervention session is planned.

Johnson (1987) noted that effective intervention sessions are *planned in advance.* In addition, sessions are repeatedly *rehearsed* by the individual participants, to ensure that the information presented is appropriate for an intervention session. Behavioral rehearsals are necessary for the intervention project. Participants should be warned that the goal of intervention is not:

that persons "admit" to being addicted, or that they have behaved in a manner that has caused others pain, or that they were wrong, or even that they were under the influence of a drug (including, of course, alcohol) in any given situation. Diagnosing chemical dependency is not part of an intervention. The goal is to elicit an agreement from the person to be *evaluated* for possible chemical dependency and to follow the resulting recommendations. (Williams, 1989, p. 99, italics added for emphasis)

Although the intervention project may provide some families with a powerful tool through which they can intervene when a member develops an alcohol/drug use problem, there is little research into which types of families benefit most from intervention training (Edwards & Steinglass, 1995). Further, according to the authors, the period of preintervention training may be insufficient to help some, perhaps most, types of families.

The important point to keep in mind is that the intervention project is designed not to get the individual to admit that he or she has a problem with chemicals. Rather, the goal is to convince the individual of the immediate need to be evaluated and, if treatment is recommended, to follow through with this recommendation.

The Mechanics of Intervention

The intervention process is, as noted, *planned*, and should be rehearsed beforehand by the participants.

Usually, three or four sessions are held prior to the formal intervention session, so that participants might learn more about the process of intervention, and practice what they are going to say (O'Farrell, 1995). The intervention process should involve *every* person in the addicted person's life who might possibly have something to add, including the spouse, siblings, children, possibly friends, supervisor/employer, minister, co-workers, or others. Johnson (1987) suggested that the supervisor be included because addicts often use his/her perception of his/her job performance as an excuse not to listen to the others in the intervention project. Each individual is advised to bring forward *specific incidents* where the addicted person's behavior, especially the chemical use, interfered with their lives in some manner.

Individually confronting an addicted person is difficult at best, and in most cases is an exercise in futility (Johnson, 1987). Any person who has tried to talk to an addicted person can attest that addicts will deny, rationalize, threaten, or simply try to avoid any confrontation that threatens his or her continued drug use. The spouse who, individually, questions whether the alcoholic was physically able to drive the car home last night may meet with the response, "No, but my friend Joe drove the car home for me, then walked home after he parked the car in the driveway."

However, if Joe *also* is present, he can then confront the alcoholic by insisting he did *not* drive the car home last night, or any other night for that matter! The alcoholic's wife may be surprised to hear this, as the excuse "Joe drove me home last night" could very well have been a common one. But, quite likely, nobody ever asked Joe whether he did or did not drive the family car home last night. Before everybody was brought together for an intervention session, it was likely that nobody checked out the isolated lies, rationalizations, or episodes of denial. Denial, projection, and rationalization will often crumble when the addicted person is confronted with all the significant people in his/her environment. This is why a collective intervention session is most powerful in working with the person.

Twerski (1983) observed that it is common for the person for whom the intervention session was called to promise to change his/her behavior. These promises may be made in good faith, or, simply to avoid further confrontation. But the fact remains that since the disease of addiction "responds to treatment and not to manipulation, it is unlikely that any of these promises will work, and the counselor must recommend treatment as the optimum course" (Twerski, 1983, p. 1029).

If the person refuses to acknowledge the addiction, or acknowledges it but refuses to enter treatment, each participant in the intervention session should be prepared to detach from the addict. This is *not* an attempt to manipulate the addict through empty threats. Rather, each person should be willing to follow through with a specific action to help detach from the addicted person who refuses to enter treatment.

If the employer or supervisor has decided that the company can no longer tolerate the addicted individual's behavior, then as soon as it is the employer/supervisor's turn to speak at the intervention session, he/she needs to clearly state that termination is intended if the addicted individual does not seek treatment. Then, if the addicted person refuses treatment, the employer/supervisor should follow through with this action.

Family members should also have thought about, and discussed, possible options for detaching from the addict. This should be done prior to the start of the intervention session, and if the addicted person should refuse treatment (possibly by leaving the session before it ends), they should follow through with their alternative plan. The options should be discussed with the other participants of the intervention project, and during the rehearsal each participant should practice informing the addicted person what he/she will do if the addicted person does not accept treatment.

There is, again, no malice in the intervention process. There is a very real danger that, without proper guidance, the intervention session may become little more than a weapon used by some family members to control the behavior of another (Claunch, 1994). The participants in the intervention process do not engage in threats, to force the addicted person into treatment. While having the addicted person see and accept the need for treatment is one goal of the intervention process, it is not the only goal. An even more important goal of the intervention process is for participants to begin to break the conspiracy of silence that surrounds the subject of the addicted person's behavior, according to the author.

In the intervention process, each participant will learn that he/she has the right to *choose* how he or she will respond, should the addict choose to continue to use chemicals. The addicted person is still able to exercise his/her own freedom of choice, by either accepting the need for treatment or not, as the person sees fit. But, now the involuntary support system composed of friends and family members will not be as secure: people will be talking to each other and drawing strength from each other. While making sure the addict either accepts the need for treatment or fully understands the consequences of not going into treatment is one goal of the intervention session, an equally important goal is to ensure that all members of the family are *heard* when they voice their concern (Claunch, 1994).

Family Intervention

Family intervention is a specialized intervention process by which *all* concerned family members, under the supervision of a trained professional, gather together and plan on a joint confrontation of the individual. The family intervention session, like all other forms of intervention, is carried out to break through the addict's denial, allow the family members to begin to voice their concerns and, possibly, obtain a commitment from the addict to enter treatment. The focus is on the individual's drug-using behaviors and on the participant's concern for the addict.

An advantage of the intervention session is that through confrontation family members of the addicted person may begin to detach from the addict. The conspiracy of silence is broken, and family members may begin to communicate more openly and more effectively. Meyer (1988) identified the intervention process as an "opportunity for healing" (p. 7) for this reason. The participants in the intervention session can express both their love and concern for the addicted person, while rejecting the addict's drug-centered behaviors.

The family intervention process allows the members of the addict's social circle to come forward, compare notes, and express their awareness of the individual's lifestyle. Sometimes, the family members, friends, employers, or whoever is involved in the intervention process will write down detailed lists of specific incidents. The information reviewed during the intervention session is highly specific, to avoid as much confusion as possible.

During the stress of the moment, it can be helpful for the participants in the intervention process to have written notes they can refer to. These notes should include information about the specific episodes of drug use, dates, and the addict's response to these episodes. Sometimes, family members bring in a personal diary to use as a reference in the intervention session. The written notes help to focus the participant on specific information.

During the rehearsal, the professional who will coordinate the intervention session decides who will present information, and in which order. As much as possible, this planned sequence is followed during the intervention session itself. The participants do not threaten the addict. Rather, they present specific incidents and information that highlight the need for the addicted person to enter treatment. V. Johnson's (1980, 1987) work provides a good overview of the intervention process.

An Example of a Family Intervention Session

In this hypothetical intervention session, the central character is a patient named "Jim." Also involved are his parents as well as two sisters and a chemical dependency counselor. The intervention session is being held at his parents' home, where Jim has been living. During the early part of the session, Jim has asserted that he never drinks to the point of passing out. He also claims that he always drinks at home so that he won't be out on the roads while intoxicated. For these reasons, he does not believe that his drinking is as bad as everybody say it is, and sees no reason for everybody to be so concerned.

One of the Jim's siblings, a sister named "Sara," also lives at home with their parents. She immediately points out how, just 3 weeks previously, Jim ran out of vodka early in the evening, after having four or five mixed drinks. Sara says that Jim had hopped into the car to drive down to the liquor store, to buy a new bottle or two after having consumed the last of the vodka in the house.

Sara concludes that she is not calling Jim a liar, but that she *knows* that he drove a car after drinking, on this occasion. She is concerned about the possibility that he might have had an accident and still feels uncomfortable about this incident. She is afraid that he might do it again, and that the next time he might not be lucky enough to make it back home again in one piece.

Jim's mother then speaks. She explains that she has found her son unconscious on the living room floor twice in the past month. She identifies the exact dates that this happened, and observes that she felt uncomfortable with his sleeping on the floor, surrounded by empty beer bottles. So, Jim's mother picked up the empty bottles, to keep them from being broken by accident, and covered Jim up with a blanket while he slept. But, she also is convinced that her son is drinking more than he realizes.

As Jim's mother finishes, his other sister, Gloria, begins to present her information and concerns. She describes how she had to ask that Jim leave her house last week, which is news to the rest of the family. She took this step, she explains, because Jim was intoxicated, loud, and abusive toward his nephew. She adds that everybody who was present, including her son's friend who happened to be visiting at the time, smelled the alcohol on his breath and was repulsed by his behavior. Gloria concludes by stating that Jim is no longer welcome in her home, unless he (a) goes through treatment, and (b) abstains from alcohol use in the future.

At this point, the chemical dependency counselor speaks, pointing out to Jim that his behavior is not so very different from that of many thousands of other addicts. The counselor adds that this is about the point in the intervention session where the addict begins to make promises to cut back or totally eliminate the drug use, a prediction that catches Jim by surprise because it is true. His protests and promises die in his throat, even before he opens his mouth.

Before he can think of something else to say, the counselor goes on to state that Jim gives every sign of having a significant alcohol problem. The counselor lists the symptoms of alcohol addiction one by one, and stresses how Jim's family identified different symptoms of addiction in their presentations. "So now," the counselor concludes "we have reached a

point where you must make a decision. Will you accept help for your alcohol problem?"

If Jim says "Yes," family members will explain that they have contacted the admissions officer of two or three nearby treatment centers, which have agreed to hold a bed for him until the end of the intervention session. Jim will be given a choice of which treatment center to enter and will be told that travel arrangements have been taken care of. His luggage is packed in the car, waiting, and if he wishes, the family will escort him to treatment as a show of support.

If Jim says "No," the family members then will confront him about the steps they are prepared to take to separate from his addiction. His parents may inform him that they have arranged for a restraining order from the court, and present him with papers informing Jim that, if he should come within a quarter of a mile of his parents' home, he will be arrested. The other family members may then inform Jim that, until he seeks professional assistance for his drinking, he is not welcome to live with them, either. Had his employer been present, Jim might have been told that his job would no longer be there for him, unless he entered treatment.[1]

Jim may be told that, no matter what he may think, these steps are not being taken as punishment. Each person will inform him that, because of his drug addiction, they find it necessary to detach from Jim until such time as he chooses to get his life in order. Each person there will affirm his/her concern for Jim, but will also start the process of no longer protecting Jim from his addiction to chemicals.

These decisions have all been made in advance of the intervention session. Which option the participants take rests, in large part, on Jim's response to the question: "Will you accept help for your alcohol problem?" Through the process of intervention, the family members have been helped to identify boundaries, which are limits that they can enforce for their own well-being (Claunch, 1994).

---

[1] The employee has certain legal rights, and it is necessary for the employer to consult with an attorney to ensure that he/she does not violate the employee's rights by this process. See Kermani and Castaneda (1996) for a discussion of this issue.

Intervention and Other Forms of Chemical Addiction

The Johnson Institute (1987) addressed the issue of intervention when the person's drug of choice was not alcohol, but any of a wide range of other chemicals. The same techniques used in alcoholism also apply to cases where the individual's drug of choice is cocaine, benzodiazepines, marijuana, amphetamines, or virtually any other drug of abuse. Significant others will gather, discuss the problem, and review their data about the addict's behavior. Practice intervention sessions are held, and the problems are addressed during the practice sessions as they are uncovered.

Finally, when everything is ready, the formal intervention session is held with the addicted person. The addicted person might need to be tricked into attending the intervention session, but there is no malice in the attempt to help the addict see how serious his/her drug addiction has become. Rather, there is a calm, caring review of the facts by person after person, until the addict is unable to defend against the realization of being addicted to chemicals and in need of professional help.

The goal of the intervention session is, again, to secure an agreement for the individual to immediately enter treatment. During the preintervention practice sessions, arrangements are made to find a time when the addicted person would be able to participate. A family reunion might provide the opportunity to carry out an intervention session, for example. Although this might, at first glance, seem disruptive to a family holiday, would the intervention session be any more painful than the family's unspoken anger and frustration at the addicted member's behavior? Indeed, the intervention project might serve as a catalyst for change within the family constellation, opening the door for changes in other areas. However, the point being stressed here is that the timing of the intervention project must be such that the person who is the focus of the effort can participate for as long as the intervention session might last.

Arrangements are made in advance for the individual's admission into treatment. This may be accomplished by a simple telephone call to the admissions officer of the treatment center. The caller may then explain the situation, and ask if they would be willing to accept the target person as a client. Usually, the treatment center staff will want to carry out their own chemical dependency evaluation to confirm that the person is an appropriate referral to treatment. But, most treatment centers should be more than willing to consider a referral from a family intervention project.

The Ethics of Intervention

As humane as the goal of intervention is, questions have been raised concerning the ethics of this practice. Rothenberg (1988) noted that there is some question as to whether it is necessary to validate the diagnosis of chemical dependency before making an attempt at intervention. In other words, should there be an independent verification of the diagnosis of drug addiction before an attempt at intervention is carried out? If there is not, what legal sanctions can be brought against a chemical dependency professional who, in good faith, supervises an attempt at intervention?

This question becomes very important because some families attempt to use the intervention process as a weapon to control the behavior of a wayward individual (Claunch, 1994). To avoid this potential danger, the wise treatment professional may want to independently confirm the diagnosis before allowing the intervention process to proceed.

Furthermore, the question of whether chemical dependency professionals involved in an intervention project should tell the client that he/she is free to leave at any time has not been answered (Rothenberg, 1988). The possibility has been suggested that, by failing to state that the client is free to leave, current intervention methods might be interpreted as violating federal or state laws against kidnapping or unlawful detention.

Rothenberg's (1988) warning raises some interesting questions for the chemical dependency professional in both the moral and legal areas. In future years, the courts may rule that the professional is legally obligated to inform the client that he/she is free to leave the intervention session at any time. Furthermore, the courts may rule that the professional can make no move to hold the client either by physical force, or by threats, should he/she express a desire to leave.

Or, the courts may rule that intervention is a legitimate treatment technique, when used by trained professionals. The legal precedent for this area has not been established at this time. Legal counsel is necessary to guide chemical dependency professionals through this quagmire, and they are advised to consult with an attorney to discuss the specific laws that might apply in their area of practice.

Legal Intervention

Sometimes, the "intervention" comes in a much simpler form: through the courts. Individuals may have been arrested for driving while under the influence of alcohol (a "DUI," or "DWI," as it is called in some states), for possession of chemicals, or for some other drug-related charge. The judge might offer an alternative to incarceration: *either* you successfully complete a drug treatment program, *or* you will be incarcerated.

The exact length of time that the convicted persons might spend in jail would depend on the specific charges brought against them. However, either/or treatment situations are unique in that these individuals are offered a choice. They might elect to spend time in jail to fulfill their obligation to the courts. This is a matter of choice. However, they might elect instead to accept the treatment option. In so doing, they are not *ordered* into treatment, but have made a choice to enter treatment. The DUI offenders always have the choice of incarceration, if they do not believe treatment is necessary or will be helpful.

Such either/or treatment admissions are easier to work with than voluntary admissions to treatment. Court-sponsored intervention is viewed by some as a powerful incentive for the individual to complete a treatment program (Moylan, 1990). The very fact that there is a legal hold on the person means it is much less likely he/she will leave treatment when his/her denial system is confronted. Also, being admitted on an either/or basis is information that can be used to confront the individual about the addiction problem. After all, it is difficult for persons who have just been arrested for their second or third drug-related charge to deny that chemicals are a

problem for them, although this has been known to happen!

A pair of research studies have found that when the treatment programs of those individuals were "legally induced to seek treatment" (Collins & Allison, 1983, p. 1145) were compared with those who entered treatment on a voluntary basis, there were no significant differences in outcome (Collins & Allison, 1983; Ouimette, Finney, & Moos, 1997). Furthermore, those who were in treatment at the court's invitation were more likely to stay in treatment longer than were those who had no restrictions placed on them. Collins and Allison concluded:

> The use of legal threat to pressure individuals into drug treatment is a valid approach for dealing with drug abusers and their undesirable behaviors. Legal threat apparently helps keep these individuals constructively involved in treatment and does not adversely affect long-term treatment goals. (p. 1148)

In her review of the effectiveness of court-mandated treatment, Wells-Parker (1994) concluded that individuals who were mandated to treatment because of having been convicted of driving a motor vehicle while under the influence of alcohol/drugs were 8% to 9% less likely to have a subsequent DWI offense than were untreated offenders. Further, the author concluded that DWI offenders who were mandated to treatment had a 30% lower mortality rate than untreated offenders, although the exact mechanism through which treatment might reduce mortality is still not clear at this time. On the other hand, W. Miller (1995) suggested that individuals who were court-ordered into treatment only did about as well as those individuals who were self-referred into rehabilitation. Thus, even if the court should order an individual to treatment, this is still not a guarantee of success.

Three factors that have a significant impact on whether court-mandated treatment will be effective were recently identified by Howard and McCaughrin (1996). They examined 330 treatment programs that did not utilize methadone and accepted court-mandated treatment patients. The authors found that (a) those treatment programs where staff did not view the fact that the client was court-ordered into treatment as a hindrance had better client outcomes, (b) those programs with more than 75% court-mandated referrals had poor client outcomes, and (c) those treatment programs that allowed the court-mandated client some input into his/her length of stay, whether the employer would be notified that the individual was in treatment, the treatment goals, and treatment methods, seemed to have better client outcomes than programs that did not grant court-mandated clients these rights.

Again, there is significant evidence to suggest that those who accept treatment as an alternative to incarceration seem to do better than individuals who are not mandated to treatment. Legal intervention seems to be a viable alternative for some who, if left to their own devices, would not accept the need for treatment.

Peele (1989), on the other hand, views such either/or referrals as intrusive and counterproductive. He pointed out that individuals convicted of driving a motor vehicle while under the influence of chemicals respond better to legal sanctions (i.e., jail, probation) than to being forced into treatment. Peele argued strongly that people should be held responsible for their actions, *including the initial decision to use chemicals*, and that chemical use or abuse does not excuse individuals from responsibility for their behavior.

Thus, the use of legal sanctions to invite a client to take part in a treatment program has not met with universal approval. The final question of whether such legal sanctions are effective in the treatment of chemical abuse has not been settled at this time.

Treatment or Incarceration: When Is Treatment Appropriate?

Frequently, the courts offer the person convicted of a drug-related charge the opportunity to enter into a drug treatment program rather than to go to jail or prison. While many individuals have used this "last chance" to begin serious work on their recovery from drug addiction, in many cases the individual accepts treatment to avoid jail or prison.

Participation in a treatment program should not be substituted for incarceration, when incarceration is deserved. All too often, individuals are offered the opportunity to enter treatment, without an examination of their motivation. To cite a common example,

one must question the individual's motivation in the case of the alleged drug pusher who was arrested with several pounds of a controlled substance, but enters "treatment" prior to going to court.

The motivation of the person arrested for the fifth time while driving under the influence of chemicals, who also enters treatment on the advice of his/her attorney prior to going to court, must also be questioned. Some chronic drinkers openly admit that they plan to continue to drink and that their only motivation for entering treatment is to try to avoid the legal consequences of their alcohol use. "I am here because my attorney said that it would look good in court" is a frequent refrain heard by treatment center staff.

Chemical dependency treatment professionals encounter time and time again the situation where, after being admitted to treatment, the individual "suddenly remembers" having to go to court for a drug-related charge. This revelation often comes within the first or second week following admission. The treatment center staff is then placed in the uncomfortable position of having to allow the client to briefly leave treatment to go to court, secure in the knowledge that they have been used by the addict against the courts.

Likewise, chemical dependency professionals repeatedly find themselves faced with a narcotics addict in need of detoxification, who reports being due to go to court in 2 or 3 weeks. Discussion then reveals that the individual's attorney suggested that the person enter treatment to finish detoxification from opiates before going to court for some offense. Some addicts have openly boasted taking this step to make a better impression on the judge and jury.

Such situations do not suggest that these clients are willing to use treatment to learn how to come to terms with their addiction. One must, however, seriously question the benefit of using limited treatment resources on persons who openly admit they entered treatment to manipulate the courts. Another example of the way treatment can be abused is in the common situation where individuals enter treatment to stop their personal use of chemicals, while openly admitting that they plan to continue selling drugs to others.

In these all too common situations, how seriously the individual is going to participate in the treatment program, and how cost-effective will treatment be under these circumstances? This is a question that the courts often do not ask. It is easier for the overworked legal system to accept treatment as an option, without examining whether it is likely to be effective in helping the individual come to terms with his/her drug use.

A physician who indiscriminately prescribed antibiotics for every patient who came into the office, without an examination to determine the individual's needs, would quickly be brought up on charges of incompetence. The decision to use one medication or another is not one that should be taken lightly. The physician must weigh the potential benefits of each approach to the patient's problems against the anticipated risk for every possible treatment method.

The same is true for chemical dependency treatment. While the option of treatment in place of incarceration should certainly be considered by the courts, it must be remembered that the treatment program is *not* the answer to every drug-related problem. A most useful concept to help the professional identify when treatment is most appropriate is that *treatment should never stand between the individual and the natural consequences of his/her behavior.*

Other Forms of Intervention

Another form of either/or situation comes about when the spouse or even the alcoholic's employer, sets down the law. *"Either* you stop drinking, *or* I will _____." Often, the physician establishes the either/or situation by threatening to file commitment papers on the addict, unless he/she enters treatment. With the advent of worksite-mandated urine toxicology testing, the strong suggestion that a person should enter treatment may come from an employer. On occasion, the coercion comes at the hands of the spouse. More than one individual has entered treatment shortly after being confronted by a spouse's either/or proposition: either you stop using alcohol and drugs, or I will leave!

Employer-Mandated Treatment

Because of widespread urine toxicology testing and increasing sensitivity on the part of industry to economic losses related to employee substance abuse,

employer-mandated treatment referrals are becoming more and more common. But there is relatively little research data to provide hints as to which forms of intervention are most effective in the workplace (Roman & Blum, 1996).

It has been found that although employees who had to be coerced into treatment under threat of loss of employment tend to have more serious substance use problems, they also tend to benefit more from treatment (Adelman & Weiss, 1989; Lawental, McLellan, Grissom, Brill, & O'Brien, 1996). Employer-mandated treatment has been justified from an economic standpoint, on the grounds that employees with alcohol/drug use problems tend to be absent from work 16 times as often as nonabusing co-workers (Lawental et al., 1996). On the basis of the available evidence, it appears that employment settings utilizing such "constructive coercion" (Adelman & Weiss, 1989, p. 515) may actually provide a positive service to employees with substance use problems. However, a great deal of research is needed to determine which forms of intervention are most effective in the workplace (Roman & Blum, 1996).

Court-Ordered Involuntary Commitment

Individuals enter treatment through many avenues. In some states, it is possible for people to be committed to treatment against their will, if the courts have sufficient evidence to believe they are in imminent danger of harming themselves or others. "Harm to self" may include neglect, and more than one alcoholic who fell asleep in the snow while walking home has been surprised to be labeled a danger to "self" on the basis of this fact, and sent to treatment against his/her will.

The exact provisions of such a court-ordered commitment vary from state to state, and some states may have no provision for such commitments. Chemical dependency professionals in each state must consult with an attorney to review the exact legal statutes that apply in their respective state. However, the reader should be aware that the laws of many states allow for the courts to intervene, should the person's chemical use put his/her life, or the life of others, in danger.

As Johnson (1987) observed, occasionally, the individual will enter treatment on a voluntary basis although this is unusual. It is more common to learn that the substance-abusing person would continue to use chemicals if he or she could do so. Thus, external pressure of some kind—be it family, legal, medical, or professional penalties—is often necessary to help the addicted person see the need to enter treatment.

Summary

The intervention process is an organized effort on the part of significant others in the addicted person's social environment to break through the wall of defenses that protect the individual from the realization that his/her life is out of control. Intervention projects are usually supervised by a substance abuse rehabilitation professional and are held with the goal of securing an agreement for the individual to immediately enter treatment.

In this chapter, we discussed the mechanics of the intervention project and some of the more common forms that intervention might take. It was noted that the individual retains the right to choose to enter treatment or to refuse to enter treatment. Persons who participate in the intervention project must be prepared for either choice and to have alternate plans in hand, in case the addicted individual does not accept the need for treatment.

Also in this chapter, we discussed that the individual retains certain rights, even during the intervention process. It was pointed out that the individual may not be detained if he/she expresses the wish to leave the intervention session. Finally, we explored the question of when legal sanctions should be imposed and when treatment should be substituted for these legal sanctions.

CHAPTER TWENTY-EIGHT

The Treatment of Chemical Dependency

Questions about the effectiveness of substance abuse treatment no longer sparks fierce debate between health professionals. Overall, the success rate of substance abuse rehabilitation compares very well with that of other chronic, relapsing diseases such as diabetes or multiple sclerosis (Morey, 1996; D. Smith, 1997). When viewed in terms of economic risk analysis, treatment has been found to be *seven times as effective* in reducing cocaine use as law enforcement activities (Lewis, 1997; Scheer, 1994b). Other studies have found that alcohol-dependent persons who participate is some form of treatment had significantly lower health care costs than their untreated peers (McCaul & Furst, 1994). Further, treatment was found to enhance the health status not only of the drinker, but his/her family. Rice and Duncan (1995) found, for example, that health care costs for families with at least one alcoholic member were *21 times higher* than for families without an alcoholic member.

Unfortunately, in the United States, treatment programs for individuals with substance use problems developed in a haphazard manner, and for the most part the evolution of treatment formats was not guided by scientific feedback (Miller & Brown, 1997). A treatment industry emerged which became deeply entrenched, and resistant to change. As a result of this process, the most commonly utilized treatment methods in pharmacological interventions for the treatment of substance abuse. However, as discussed in Chapter 31, this approach has had only limited success. Finally, there are those who

recommend the "self-help group" approach of Alcoholics Anonymous, or similar groups. This approach to the treatment of drug dependency is discussed in a later chapter.

In this chapter, some of the basic elements of substance abuse treatment are explored. Specific treatment components vary from one program to another. For example, a treatment program that specializes in working with say alcohol-dependent businesspeople would have little use for a methadone maintenance component. Yet, there are also many common elements in the treatment process, and this chapter focuses on these aspects of treatment.

Characteristics of the Substance Abuse Rehabilitation Professional

The relationship between the client and the counselor is of central importance to the rehabilitation process (Bell, Montoya, & Atkinson, 1997). Indeed, the therapeutic relationship is of such critical importance that it has been likened to the individual's initial relationship with his/her parents, by the authors.

To effectively help persons with substance use disorders, the helper needs to have certain characteristics, one of the most important being that he/she have no pressing personal issues. Individuals who are dealing with chemical dependency or psychological issues of their own should be discouraged from actively working with persons in treatment, at least until they have resolved their own problems. This injunction makes sense: if the counselor is preoccupied with personal problems, including those of chemical addiction, he/she is unlikely to be able to help the client advance further in terms of personal growth.

In his work on the characteristics of the effective mental health counselor, Rogers (1961) suggested a number of characteristics that he thought were essential:

- Warmth.
- Dependability.
- Consistency.
- The ability to care for and respect the client.
- The ability to be separate from the client, which is to say the ability not to try and "live through" a client.
- The ability not to be perceived as a threat by the client.
- The ability to free one's self from the urge to judge or evaluate the client.
- The ability to see the client as a person capable of growth.

In a sense, clients who enter a rehabilitation program are admitting that they have been unable to change on their own (Bell et al., 1997). Being unable to make the desired change without professional assistance, these clients presumably need help from therapists with strong interpersonal skills. It is thus not surprising to learn that when Adelman and Weiss (1989) examined the personality attributes of successful treatment staff members at an alcoholism treatment center, they concluded that those staff members who possessed the highest level of interpersonal skills were best equipped to help their clients.

The authors based their conclusions on a study they designed that compared the treatment outcome of clients of alcoholism counselors with low interpersonal skills with those of counselors who had high interpersonal skills. The authors found that clients of low-skill counselors were twice as likely to relapse as were patients whose counselors had high interpersonal skill levels. Although Adelman and Weiss (1989) did not speak in the same terms that Rogers (1961) did, the implication is clear that the most effective counselor is one who is well adjusted and accepting of others.

The client's acceptance of the therapist's efforts is one of the most essential characteristics of a successful therapeutic relationship, according to Bell et al. (1997). The other characteristics that most strongly influence the client's efforts to change are the individual's ability to trust the therapist, to depend on the therapist, to be open with the professional, and to accept external help.

A point that needs to be clarified is that *these characteristics do not mean that the chemical dependency professional should be permissive.* Human service professionals occasionally confuse permissiveness with interpersonal warmth. Just as it is possible to be too confrontive, a subject to be discussed, it is also possible to be too permissive. *Caring for clients does not mean protecting them from the consequences of their behavior.*

Confrontation and Other Treatment Techniques

For a number of years, substance abuse rehabilitation counselors in the United States have used a "hard-hitting, directive, exhortational style" (Miller, Genefield, & Tonigan, 1993, p. 455) that serves to overwhelm the addict's defenses. Confrontation has been a central feature of this treatment approach and, in theory, helps clients begin to understand the reality of their addiction or the need for treatment (Twerski, 1983).

Admittedly, the *appropriate* use of confrontation may be useful in working with some clients. But, there is no evidence that confrontation is the method of choice in the treatment of alcoholism (Hester, 1994; Washton, 1995). Indeed, *inappropriate confrontation* may be somewhat counterproductive when directed toward addicted individuals (Miller et al., 1993). *Empathy* was found to be a more useful tool in working with the substance-abusing client, according to the authors. The research carried out by Miller et al. suggested that, as the therapist's level of confrontation increased, the client's level of resistance also increased.

It was suggested by the authors that a "supportive-reflective" (Miller et al., 1993, p. 455) style of therapy was more effective than the use of confrontation in working with substance-abusing clients. Thus, there is little evidence to support the extensive use of confrontation as a treatment technique (W. Miller, 1995; Miller et al., 1993; Miller & Rollnick, 1991).

The Minnesota Model of Chemical Dependency Treatment

To say that what has come to be called the "Minnesota Model" of chemical dependency treatment has been a success is something of an understatement. First designed in the 1950s by Dr. Dan Anderson, the Minnesota Model has long served as one of the major treatment formats in the fight against alcoholism and drug abuse.

To earn money to finish his college education, Dr. Anderson worked as an attendant at the State Hospital in Willmar, Minnesota (Larson, 1982). Following graduation, Anderson returned to the State Hospital in Willmar to work as a recreational therapist. He was assigned to work with the alcoholics who were in treatment at the State Hospital, the least desirable position at that time. Anderson was himself influenced by the work of Mr. Ralph Rossen, who was later to become the Minnesota State Commissioner of Health. At the same time, the growing influence of Alcoholics Anonymous (AA) was utilized by Dan Anderson and a staff psychologist by the name of Dr. Jean Rossi as a means of understanding and working with alcoholics. They were supported in this approach by the medical director of the hospital, Dr. Nelson Bradley (Larson).

These individuals joined together in an effort to understand, and treat, the patients sent to the State Hospital for treatment of their alcoholism. Coming from different professions, each person contributed a different perspective on addiction and the patient's needs. To this team was added the Rev. John Keller, who had been sent to Willmar State Hospital to learn about alcoholism in 1955. The staff then had "knowledge of medicine, psychology, A.A. and theology together under one roof to develop a new and innovative alcohol treatment program" (Larson, 1982, p. 35).

This new treatment approach, since called the Minnesota Model of treatment, was designed to work with dependency on alcohol ("ONDCP," 1990). Since its introduction, it has also been used as a model for the treatment of other forms of chemical addiction. The Minnesota Model utilizes a *treatment team* comprising chemical dependency counselors familiar with AA, psychologists, physicians, nurses, recreational therapists, and clergy, all of whom work with clients during the treatment program.

Stage 1 of the Minnesota Model treatment approach, the evaluation phase, involves each member of the treatment team meeting with the client, to assess his/her needs from the professional's own area of expertise. Each professional will then make recommendations for the client's *treatment plan.* Stage 2, the goal setting phase, the professionals then meet *as a team* to discuss the areas that they feel should be the focus of treatment. The treatment team meeting is chaired by the individual who is ultimately responsible for the execution of the treatment process. This is usually the chemical dependency counselor who will function as the client's case manager. The treatment team reviews and discusses each of the assessments, and the recommendations that come from these assessments. The team then selects those recommendations that the members, based on their training and experience, feel are most appropriate to focus on to help the client achieve and maintain recovery.

The client, his/her parole/probation officer, and interested family members, are all invited to participate in the treatment plan meeting. Both the client and family members are free to recommend additional areas of concern or to suggest specific goals for inclusion in the treatment plan. The case manager will review the treatment goals that were identified as of value to the client, and discuss the rationale for these recommendations.

On the basis of this meeting, the case manager and client enter Stage 3 of the treatment process. In this phase, the client and his/her case manager develop a formal *treatment plan.* The resultant treatment plan is multimodal and will offer a wide variety of potential treatment goals and recommendations. It will identify specific problem areas, behavioral objectives, methods by which one can measure progress toward these objectives, and a target date for each goal. The treatment plan is discussed in more detail in the next section of this chapter. A flowchart of the treatment plan process is shown in Figure 28.1.

The strength of the Minnesota Model of treatment lies in its redundancy, and in its multimember concept. The information provided by the client is

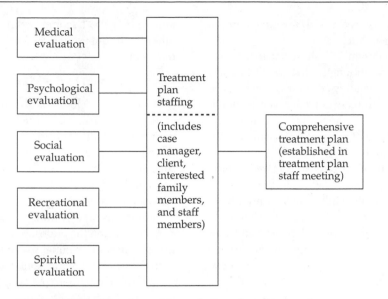

FIGURE 28.1 Flowchart of the evolution of a treatment plan.

reviewed by many different professionals, each of whom may on the basis of his/her training identify a potential treatment problem that others may have overlooked. This allows for the greatest possible evaluation of the client's needs, strengths, and priorities.

Another advantage of the Minnesota Model is that it allows for different professionals to work together in the rehabilitation of the client. The different professionals, with their training and experience, offer a wider range of services than any single chemical dependency counselor ever could. In addition to multidisciplinary intake evaluations, each professional on the treatment team can work with the client, *if that client presents special needs.*

The chemical dependency counselor does not need to try to be a "jack of all trades, master of none." Rather, if the client presents a need that one staff member cannot fulfill, a referral for specialized treatment can be made to another member of the team. This feature has helped make the Minnesota Model one of the dominant treatment program models in the field of chemical dependency rehabilitation, although few people are aware of its roots.

The Treatment Plan

No matter what approach the therapist elects to utilize, he/she should develop a *treatment plan* with the client. The treatment plan is "the foundation for success" (Lewis et al., 1988, p. 118) of the treatment process. It is a highly specific form, which in some states might be viewed as a legal document. Different treatment centers tend to use different formats, depending on the specific licensure requirements in that state, and the treatment methods being utilized.

However, all plans share several similarities. First, it should provide a brief summary of the problem(s) that brought the client into treatment. The second section provides a brief summary of the client's physical and emotional state of health. A third section contains the individual's own input into the treatment process; that is, what he/she thinks should be included in the treatment plan.

The fourth section is the heart of the treatment plan. This is where the specific goals of treatment are identified. The discharge criteria follow, which list the steps that must be accomplished to discharge the client from treatment. Finally, there is a brief summary of those steps that are to be made part of the client's *aftercare* program.

Because the heart of the treatment plan is where the specific treatment goals are outlined, this section is often identified as "Treatment Goals." Such goals should include (a) a *problem statement,* or brief description of the problem, (b) *long-term goals*, (c) *short-term objectives*, (d) *measurement criteria*, and (e) a *target date*.

The problem statement is a short statement, usually a sentence or two in length, that identifies a *specific problem* to be addressed in treatment. The *long-term goal* is the ultimate objective, and as such is a general statement of a hoped-for outcome. The long-term goal statement is usually also only one or two sentences in length.

Following the long-term goal is a *short-term objective*. The objective is *a very specific behavior, which can be measured*. The objective statement usually requires three sentences or less, and identifies the measurement criteria by which both the client and staff will be able to assess whether progress is being made toward this objective. Finally, there is the *target date*, which is usually a simple sentence that identifies a specific date by which this goal will be achieved.

An example of a treatment goal for a 24-year-old male polydrug addict (cocaine, alcohol, marijuana, and occasionally benzodiazepines) who has used chemicals daily for the previous 27 months might appear as follows:

- *Problem.* Client has used chemicals daily for at least the past two years, and has been unable to abstain from drug use on his own.
- *Long-Term Goal.* That the client achieve, and maintain, sobriety.
- *Short-Term Objective.* That the client not use mood-altering chemicals while in treatment.
- *Method of Measurement.* Random supervised urine toxicology screens, to detect possible drug use.
- *Target Date.* Scheduled discharge date.

The typical treatment plan might identify as many as five or six different problem areas. Each of these goals might be modified as the treatment program progresses, and each provides a yardstick of the client's progress. If the client is not making progress on *any* of the goals, it is time to question whether the client is serious about treatment. The goals become the heart of the treatment program.

The Minnesota Model of rehabilitation for substance abusers has long dominated the field of treatment for alcoholism/drug addiction. However,

although it has become a standard against which other treatment models are compared, it is not without its critics.

Reaction to the Minnesota Model

The Minnesota Model has been challenged for several reasons. First, this model was designed to work with cases of alcoholism. There has been no research into whether it is applicable to other forms of substance addiction. Yet the Minnesota Model has been utilized in the treatment of virtually every known form of substance abuse ("ONDCP," 1990).

Admittedly, the Minnesota Model of treatment draws heavily on the philosophy of Alcoholics Anonymous. Indeed, individual participation in AA is a required part of the Minnesota Model. Yet AA itself is not a form of treatment (C. Clark, 1995). Further, as discussed in Chapter 35, there is no clear evidence to suggest that AA is effective in cases where the individual is coerced into joining. Thus, there is an inherent contradiction in the Minnesota Model in that one of its central tenets is mandatory participation in AA.

Another challenge to the Minnesota Model involves its length. When it was developed, the client's length of stay at Willmar State Hospital was often arbitrarily set at 28 days. There is, however, little research data supporting a need for a 28-day inpatient treatment stay (Turbo, 1989). The optimal length of treatment for inpatient treatment programs has yet to be defined (McCusker, Stoddard, Frost, & Zorn, 1996). Yet, the 28-day treatment program has become something of an industry standard for Minnesota Model programs (Turbo), and at one time served as a guide for insurance reimbursement (Berg & Dubin, 1990).

Despite its widespread acceptance and use in the substance abuse rehabilitation field, there is also little evidence to suggest that the Minnesota Model is effective in helping people deal with their chemical use problems (Holder, Longabaugh, Miller, & Rubonis, 1991; McCrady, 1993).

Other Treatment Formats for Chemical Dependency

In recent years, health care professionals and mental health care workers have developed several treatment approaches to alcoholism rehabilitation that differ from the Minnesota Model. The guiding philosophy of these treatment programs is often notably different from that of the Minnesota Model. While it is not possible to do full justice to each treatment philosophy, this section briefly describes some of the more promising treatment models that have emerged in the past two decades.

Detoxification Programs

It is not possible to work effectively with an individual who is under the influence of alcohol or drugs. Thus, detoxification from alcohol/drugs is a prerequisite for treatment. As such, it is often the first step in the rehabilitation process. But detoxification from alcohol/drugs is not in itself considered a form of "treatment" for individuals with substance use problems (Mattick & Hall, 1996; Miller & Hester, 1986; National Academy of Sciences, 1990; "Treatment," 1995).

The goal of the detoxification process is to offer the patient a safe, humane withdrawal from alcohol/drugs of abuse (Mattick & Hall, 1996). The patient's safety is assured, to the degree that this is possible, by having the detoxification process carried out under the supervision of a physician who is both trained and experienced in this area of medicine (Miller, Frances, & Holmes, 1988). The physician will evaluate the patient's needs and resources, and then recommend that the process of detoxification be carried out either on an inpatient or an outpatient basis.

Although detoxification from alcohol/drugs has usually been carried out in a hospital setting, in recent years it has become apparent that the practice of automatically admitting the alcohol-dependent person into a hospital for detoxification might not be cost-effective (Berg & Dubin, 1990; Mattick & Hall, 1996). Depending on the patient's drug of choice, his/her available resources, and the patient's medical status, it is possible to carry out the detoxification process on an outpatient basis. For example, Abbott, Quinn, and Knox (1995) found that with careful screening, it was possible for more than 90% of the alcohol-dependent patients that they worked with to be detoxified on an outpatient basis. One recent study from Australia found that less than 0.5% of the alcohol-dependent patients *required* hospitalization for detoxification (Mattick & Hall).

Patients who are selected for outpatient detoxification, which is called "ambulatory detox" (National Academy of Sciences, 1990, p. 175), or "social detox" (Mattick & Hall, 1996), first are evaluated by a physician. Then, depending on the patient's medical status, he/she is sent home with instructions as to how to complete the detoxification process or referred to a special detoxification setting. In either case, the patient's progress after this point is monitored not by a physician, but by nurses or trained personnel. Once or twice a day, a nurse may stop by to check on the progress of patients who are sent home. In the detoxification center, the patient's progress and vital signs are monitored as often as necessary.

As long as the patient's physical status does not indicate there is danger of severe withdrawal-related distress, the patient is not referred to a more staff-intensive setting such as a general hospital. If, on the other hand, the patient's status indicates significant withdrawal-related distress, or inability to complete detoxification on an outpatient basis, then the person is transferred to a more suitable setting.

One of the factors to consider when making the decision to use an inpatient or outpatient detoxification program is the patient's drug of choice. Withdrawal from some drugs of abuse can cause severe, or even life-threatening, problems during detoxification. As discussed in Chapters 6 and 7, withdrawal from either the barbiturates or the benzodiazepines can result in life-threatening seizures for patients who are physically dependent on these drugs. While there is little evidence that detoxification from opiates can cause significant physical danger to the patient, there is strong evidence that opiate-dependent patients who are detoxified on an inpatient basis are more likely to complete the process (Mattick & Hall, 1996).

There is some debate as to whether detoxification programs should function as a funnel for guiding patients into the rehabilitation process. When detoxification is carried out at a freestanding clinic, many patients fail to go on to participate in rehabilitation programs (Miller & Rollnick, 1991). On the other hand, the charge has been made that detoxification programs housed in treatment settings are often little more than recruitment centers for the treatment program. To counter this danger, patients should be advised of their treatment options, including the possibility of seeking treatment elsewhere, to avoid a possible conflict-of-interest situation.

Whether detoxification is carried out on an inpatient or an outpatient basis, the patient being withdrawn from chemicals should be closely monitored by staff to detect signs of drug overdose or seizures, to monitor medication compliance, and to ensure abstinence from recreational chemical use (Miller et al., 1988). It is not uncommon for patients who are addicted to chemicals to "help out" the withdrawal process by taking additional drugs when they are supposedly being withdrawn from chemicals.

The process of detoxification is vulnerable to being abused in other ways. For example, there are addicted individuals who have gone through detoxification dozens, or perhaps even hundreds, of times to give themselves a place to live (Whitman et al., 1990). Other individuals "check into detox" to give themselves a place to hide because of drug debts, or to elude the police.

It is also not uncommon for narcotics addicts to seek admission to a detox program when they are unable to obtain drugs. Sometimes, opiate-dependent individuals seek admission to detox because they want to lower their daily drug requirement to a level they can more easily afford. At other times, a "panic" develops when the authorities arrest a major drug supplier or break up a major drug supply source. In such cases, large numbers of opiate-dependent patients may seek admission to detox to have a source of drugs while they wait for new supplies of opiates to become available through illicit sources. Thus, while detoxification programs provide a valuable service, they are also vulnerable to abuses.

Videotape/Self-Confrontation

Many programs draw on the potentials of videotaping clients while they are under the influence of chemicals, to allow them to see their own behavior while intoxicated. The goal of this procedure, according to Holder et al. (1991), is to allow the drinker's own drunk behavior to illustrate the need for treatment. After recovering from the acute effects of drinking, the individual is forced to watch a videotape of his/her behavior. The videotape is usually made in the emergency room of the local hospital. There is, however, no evidence that this brief treatment approach is effective.

Acupuncture

This form of alternative medicine is occasionally applied to the treatment of the addictive disorders. Treatment professionals are still divided as to how acupuncture works. Small sterile needles are inserted into specific locations on the individual's body, in an attempt to treat the patient's condition. There is limited evidence that this treatment technique is effective in the rehabilitation of substance abusers (Holder et al., 1991).

For example, Avants, Margolin, Chang, and Birch (1995) attempted to utilize acupuncture in the treatment of cocaine addiction. The authors used a treatment sample of 40 cocaine-dependent individuals, who were split into two groups: a treatment group, and a control group. Both subjects had acupuncture needles inserted into their bodies. However, the control group had needles inserted approximately 2 mm away from the active sites necessary for acupuncture to be accurate, according to theory. The authors concluded that there were no significant differences in treatment outcome for these two groups, suggesting that the benefits of acupuncture in the treatment of cocaine addiction has yet to be proven.

Family and Marital Therapy

Preliminary research has suggested that family therapy approaches are perhaps 4 to 5 times as effective as rehabilitation programs that focus on the individual (Alexander & Gwyther, 1995). For example, the defense system of the addicted member, and those of the other family members, tend to be *inter*-reinforcing (Williams, 1989). The family members come to develop defense mechanisms that interlock with, and reinforce, those of the addicted person. An effective family systems approach allows for the modification of the role that the drug-using behavior fills within the family. The alternative is that the family will, *as a unit*, resist any change in the addicted person's behavior.

In their review of the cost-effectiveness of treatment methods for alcoholism, Edwards and Steinglass (1995) concluded that marital therapy was potentially useful and effective as a treatment approach at some points in the treatment process. The authors conducted a meta-analysis of research articles on marital therapy as a treatment modality for alcoholism rehabilitation. They found that there was clear-cut evidence suggesting that family/marital therapy was effective during the intervention and aftercare phases of treatment for alcohol-dependent individuals. The authors found little evidence suggesting that marital therapy was useful during the treatment phase of recovery, but suggested that this might be because treatment goals during this phase of treatment are often quite vague.

Overall, Edwards and Steinglass (1996) concluded that marital/family therapy is an effective treatment modality for working with the alcohol-dependent individual. However, the authors also note the need for further research into the most effective methods of treating alcohol/drug-addicted clients. Further, the field of family/marital therapy has become a specialized area of expertise, with a vast, evolving literature of its own (Bowen, 1985). It is beyond the scope of this chapter to provide a comprehensive overview of the fields of marital/family therapy in general, or even the specialized application of marital therapy to the treatment of the addictions. The chemical dependency professional should be aware that these are specialized areas of training that seem to offer some promise in substance abuse rehabilitation programs.

Group Therapy Approaches

Group psychotherapy offers some important advantages over individual therapy (Yalom, 1985). First, therapy groups allow one professional to work with several individuals at once. Second, in the therapy group, members learn from each other and offer feedback to each other. Finally, because of the nature of the therapy group, each individual would find his/her family of origin reflected in the group members, allowing the person to work through problems from earlier stages of growth.

These advantages are utilized in chemical dependency treatment programs, where therapy groups are frequently the primary treatment approach offered to clients. While individual sessions may be utilized for special problems too sensitive to discuss in a therapy group situation, clients are usually encouraged to bring their concerns to group, which may meet every other day, daily, or more often than once a day, depending on the pace of the program.

There is limited evidence that group psychotherapy approaches are at all effective in the rehabilitation of substance abusers (Holder et al., 1991). Group therapy formats that utilize cognitive-behavioral approaches to identify and help the client learn how to deal with painful affective states that might contribute to the urge to use chemicals seem to be effective in working with personality-disordered substance abusers (Fisher & Bentley, 1996). In contrast to traditional beliefs about alcohol/drug abusers, however, the harsh, confrontational groups commonly found in therapeutic communities have been found to be ineffective in working with alcohol/drug-abusing clients (Peele, 1989). Peele suggested that therapy groups focus on helping the recovering addict learn effective coping skills such as behavioral response training and stress management techniques.

McCrady (1993) pointed out that women who have substance use problems seem to be somewhat inhibited in group settings. In such cases, the woman seems to do better in an individual therapy setting than in a group, possibly because of shame-based issues. Further, the author suggested, the elderly might feel overwhelmed by the complex pattern of interactions within the group setting and perhaps would respond more favorably if seen on an individual basis. Thus, while group therapy approaches are a common treatment modality, there is limited evidence at best as to its effectiveness.

Assertiveness/Social Skills Training

Lewis et al. (1988) identified special training groups for assertiveness as being useful in building self-esteem and self-confidence in interpersonal relationships. Individuals who are addicted to chemicals often lack the ability to assert themselves (Lewis et al.) and could benefit from training in this interpersonal skill. In addition to assertiveness training, many other social skills may be taught to the recovering addict.

Surprisingly, there is good evidence that assertiveness/social skills training is effective in the rehabilitation of alcoholics (Holder et al., 1991).

Thus, programs that emphasize helping alcohol-addicted individuals learn how to assert themselves appropriately seem to enhance recovery.

Self-Help Groups

The best known self-help group is Alcoholics Anonymous, which is discussed in detail in Chapter 35. However, brief mention of self-help groups such as AA should be made at this time. It has been argued that AA is actually a form of treatment (Tobin, 1992). Whether this is true is a philosophical question, the answer to which depends on the individual's beliefs.

Participation in a self-help group such as AA is often a required component of both inpatient and outpatient treatment programs. Many community AA or Narcotics Anonymous (NA) groups have extended an invitation to local treatment programs to allow their clients to participate in scheduled meetings. If the treatment program is large enough, an on-campus AA or NA meeting may also be scheduled, which is limited to clients in treatment.

There are a number of advantages to AA or NA involvement for clients in treatment. Both AA and NA are potentially chemically free support groups for new members. As such, both AA and NA offer opportunities for members to model drug-free interpersonal interactions for clients in treatment. Each group also offers the opportunity for new members to develop a drug-free support system, to use in times of crisis following treatment. Members in the AA or NA group may, in speaking of their problems, offer newcomers insight into their own problems that may suggest possible solutions.

However, Peele (1989) pointed out that many people recover without joining either AA or NA, raising questions about whether the individual *must* participate in such a self-help group. The treatment program should have some provision for self-help group participation, as such groups have been found by many individuals to be quite helpful. But there is no evidence to suggest that mandatory participation in AA/NA is of value (Holder et al., 1991).

Biofeedback Training

A number of treatment plans advocate biofeedback training as an aid to the treatment of addictive disorders. The technique of biofeedback involves monitoring select body functions, such as skin temperature or muscle tension, and relaying this information to the individual. Depending on the parameter selected (e.g., muscle tension of a certain muscle group, skin temperature, brain wave patterns) and the training provided, the individual is thought to be able to learn how to modify body functions at will. This skill, in turn, is thought to allow the individual to learn how to change these body functions in a desired direction, such as to relax without drugs.

Peniston and Kulkosky (1990) attempted to teach a small number of patients in an alcoholic treatment program to change the frequency with which their brain could produce two specific electrical patterns, known as *Alpha* and *Theta* waves. These patterns of electrical activity in the brain are thought to reflect the individual's relaxation and stress-coping responses. The authors found that their sample had significant changes on standard psychological tests used to measure the personality pattern of the respondent and that these changes continued over an extended follow-up period. It was suggested by the authors that biofeedback training, especially Alpha and Theta brain wave training, might offer a new, possibly more effective, treatment approach for working with the chronic alcoholic.

Ochs (1992) examined the application of biofeedback training techniques to the treatment of addictive disorders. The author concluded that the term "biofeedback training" for the addictions was a bit misleading in that different clinicians employed a wide range of techniques and a wide range of body functions for biofeedback training. Yet, despite the variations in treatment techniques, the author found that biofeedback training for the treatment of addictive disorders did seem to have value, especially when biofeedback was integrated into a larger treatment format designed to address social, economic, vocational, psychological, and familial problems. Thus, evidence suggests that biofeedback training may be a treatment method that will play an increasing role in the treatment of addictive disorders.

Harm Reduction Model

The *Harm Reduction* (HR) model of substance abuse rehabilitation is quite different from the Minnesota Model or the other models of treatment discussed in this chapter. Most other treatment models are based on a "zero tolerance" of chemical use (Marlatt, 1994). This is to say, they do not accept the possibility of *any* chemical use by the individual.

However, the HR model has a different focus: limiting the amount of damage caused by chemical(s), until the individual can achieve total abstinence. Nicotine skin patches and nicotine gum are viewed by Marlatt (1994) as examples of the HR philosophy, in that they reduce the individual's risk of negative consequences from cigarette smoking. From this perspective, formal detoxification from chemicals in a medical setting could also be viewed as a form of harm reduction, in that the individual is protected from many of the dangers of withdrawal during the detoxification program.

The "needle exchange" programs in place in several cities around the country provide another example of the HR philosophy. Because the virus that causes AIDS is often transmitted through contaminated intravenous needles (see Chapter 33), some cities allow addicts to exchange "dirty" needles for new, uncontaminated ones. For example, the mayor of the city of Baltimore, Kurt Schmoke, authorized a needle exchange program in that city to limit the damage done by HIV, on these grounds:

> This program costs $160,000 a year. The cost to the state of Maryland of taking care of just one adult AIDS patient infected through the sharing of a syringe is $102,000 to $120,000. In other words, if just two addicts are protected from HIV through the city's needle exchange, the program will have paid for itself. (Schmoke, 1996, p. 40)

In this way, the transmission of the virus that causes AIDS is slowed, or perhaps even stopped.

While the HR model is somewhat controversial, it offers an alternative to "zero tolerance" approaches.

Aftercare Programs

The *aftercare* program involves those elements of treatment that will be carried out after the individual has been discharged from treatment. If, for example, the person entered into individual psychotherapy to address an issue uncovered in treatment, it is entirely likely that this therapy will continue long after the individual is discharged from the typical 28–35 day inpatient rehabilitation program. Individual therapy on a once-per-week basis with a psychotherapist would then become a part of the aftercare program.

Downing (1990) concluded that an effective aftercare program would: (a) address the chemical dependency issues identified in treatment, (b) address mistaken beliefs and interpersonal conflicts that might contribute to relapse, (c) help the individual establish what Downing termed "the habit of sobriety" (p. 22), (d) help the individual make the necessary changes in lifestyle to maintain sobriety, and (e) "serve as a monitor of sobriety" (p. 22).

Participation in Alcoholics Anonymous or Narcotics Anonymous is often identified as part of an aftercare program, especially those programs that are based on the Minnesota Model of treatment (C. Clark, 1995). A medical problem that requires ongoing medical supervision and support should be a part of the aftercare program, as well as aftercare placement in a transitional living facility such as a halfway house. If the individual presents any special needs, these should also be included as specialized elements of the aftercare program.

The aftercare program is designed and carried out on the assumption that treatment does not end with the individual's discharge from a formal treatment program. Rather, treatment is the first part of a recovery program that (hopefully) continues for the rest of the individual's life. The aftercare component of the treatment plan addresses the issues that require attention following the individual's discharge from the rehabilitation program.

Summary

This chapter reviewed the Minnesota Model of treatment, which is one of the primary treatment models found in this country. The concept of a *comprehensive treatment plan*, which serves as the heart of the treatment process, was also discussed. Pharmacological supports for persons in the early stages of sobriety, and for those going through detoxification from chemicals, were explored.

This chapter also included a discussion of assertiveness training, biofeedback, and marital and family therapy as components of a larger treatment program. The use of blood and urine samples for toxicology screening to verify medication compliance and detect illicit drug use was also reviewed.

CHAPTER TWENTY-NINE

Treatment Formats for Chemical Dependency Rehabilitation

Researchers have long since proven that treatment for substance use problems *is* cost-effective. The current debate centers on the relative merits of rehabilitation programs that utilize an *outpatient* as opposed to an *inpatient* format (Youngstrom, 1990a). This debate has been spirited and has continued for much of the past decade without either side scoring a decisive victory. This chapter focuses on the characteristics of an average outpatient treatment program, the typical inpatient program, and some of the issues that have been raised about the relative advantages and disadvantages of each format.

Outpatient Treatment Programs

Outpatient chemical dependency treatment may best be defined as a formal treatment program (a) that involves one or more professionals who are trained to work with individuals who are addicted to chemicals, (b) that is designed specifically to work with the addicted person to help him/her achieve and maintain sobriety, (c) that utilizes a number of treatment modalities (e.g., psychoeducational approaches; family, marital, individual, and/or group therapies) to help the addicted person come to terms with his/her recreational chemical use problem, and (d) that performs these services on an outpatient basis.

Components of Outpatient Treatment Programs

Outpatient treatment programs use many of the components of treatment discussed in Chapter 28. Such programs usually utilize individual and group therapy formats, as well as possibly marital and family therapy, in working with the addicted person. Most such programs will follow a twelve-step philosophy, usually either Alcoholics Anonymous or Narcotics Anonymous, and the individual is expected to attend regular self-help group meetings as part of the treatment format. The individual's treatment program is usually coordinated by a certified chemical dependency counselor (sometimes called an "addictions" or "substance abuse" counselor). A formal treatment plan is established, review sessions are scheduled on a regular basis, and the client's progress toward the agreed-on goals is monitored by staff.

The general approach of individual and group therapy is to work through the addicted person's system of denial, while providing counseling designed to help the client learn how to face the problems of daily living *without* chemicals. This is accomplished, in part, through psychoeducational lectures that present the individual with factual information about the disease of chemical addiction and its treatment.

Referrals to vocational counseling centers or community mental health centers for individual, family, or marital counseling are made as necessary. Some programs provide a "family night" and encourage family members to participate once a week, or once a month, to discuss their concerns. Other programs feature a "family group" orientation, where couples participate together on a day-to-day basis, as part of the program. In such a format, the spouse of the addicted person will sit in on the group sessions, and participate as an equal with the addicted person in the group therapy.

Whatever the general approach, the goal of any outpatient treatment program is to enhance the highest level of functioning, while providing support for the alcoholic. Some programs require that the detoxification phase of treatment, when the individual is withdrawn from chemicals, is carried out either at a detoxification center or in a general hospital. However, the individual is generally expected to have stopped all chemical use before starting any treatment program.

Abstinence from alcohol/drug use is expected. Many treatment programs require the use of Antabuse (disulfiram) or carry out random urine tests to detect alcohol or drug use by the patient. One advantage of using urine testing is that it allows the staff to check on the individual's compliance with taking Antabuse.

The goal of outpatient treatment is to allow the individual the opportunity to live at home, go to work, and continue family activities, while participating in a rehabilitation program designed to help the client achieve and maintain sobriety (Youngstrom, 1990a). This approach is helpful for some, although research suggests a high dropout rate for outpatient treatment programs.

Varieties of Outpatient Treatment Programs for Substance Abuse Rehabilitation

DWI School

Outpatient rehabilitation programs differ mainly in terms of the frequency with which the individual meets with treatment professionals and the specific methods used by the staff in working with the client. The psychoeducational approach is often the mainstay of the "DWI school" or DWI class. The DWI school is usually limited to first-time offenders, who are assumed to have simply made a mistake by driving under the influence of chemicals. Participants in the DWI school are not addicted to alcohol/drugs in the opinion of the assessor. Participants are exposed to 8 to 12 hours of educational lectures, designed to help them better understand the dangers inherent in driving while under the influence of chemicals. This is done in the hope that they learn from their mistake.

Short-Term Outpatient Programs (STOP)

These are usually time-limited programs. Some STOP-level programs use only individual therapy sessions, while others combine individual and group therapy formats for individuals whose substance use problems is, in the opinion of the assessor, mild to moderate in its severity. These individuals may be required to attend Alcoholics Anonymous (AA) or similar self-help group meetings, in addition to sessions with the therapist that are held at least once a week.

Clients in STOP-level programs are often assigned material to read between sessions with the therapist, and psychoeducational lectures may be used to provide program participants with factual information about the effects of the drugs of abuse. The individual client participates in program activities 1 or 2 nights a week, for a period of time that usually is less than 2 months in duration.

The goal of STOP-level programs is to (a) break through the individual's denial about his/her substance use, (b) achieve a commitment to abstinence from the client, and, (c) make appropriate referrals for those individuals who appear to require more in-depth help.

Intensive Short-Term Outpatient Programs (I-STOP)

Programs at the I-STOP level are aimed at the patient with a moderate to severe substance use problem. Program participants are usually seen in both individual and group therapy sessions, for up to 5 nights a week. Programs at the I-STOP level are time-limited, but in addition to having a level of treatment that is more intense than those on the previous level (1–2 times a week vs. 4–5 times a week), programs at this level usually last longer (up to 6 months). Program participants are often required to attend self-help group meetings, such as AA, in addition to participating in scheduled treatment activities. Additional sessions for family/marital counseling are scheduled outside scheduled treatment hours for those individuals whose recovery requires additional forms of intervention or support.

The goal of I-STOP programs is to (a) break through the individual's denial about his/her substance use, (b) achieve a commitment to abstinence from the client who is unlikely to respond to less intense forms of treatment, and (c) to make appropriate referrals for those individuals who appear to require more in-depth help.

Intensive Long-Term
Outpatient Treatment (ILTOT)

These are usually open-ended programs and are designed for individuals whose substance use problem is moderate to severe in intensity, but for whom less radical treatment would hold little chance of success. ILTOT level programs usually last for a minimum of 6 months, and often for as long as 12 to 18 months. Program participants are involved in a series of individual and group therapy sessions for a specified number of days each week, with the exact timing and sequence of individual and group sessions being determined by the individual's treatment plan.

The goal of ILTOT level programs is to (a) break through the individual's denial about his/her substance use, (b) achieve a commitment to abstinence from the client who either has not been able to benefit from less intense forms of treatment or whose substance use pattern suggests that less intense treatment is likely to fail, (c) support the individual during the early stages of recovery from drug/alcohol use problems, and (d) to make appropriate referrals for those individuals who appear to require more in-depth help.

Advantages of Outpatient
Treatment Programs

Outpatient treatment programs are popular. It has been reported that perhaps as many as 88% of those who are treated for alcohol abuse or addiction, are treated on an outpatient basis (McCaul & Furst, 1994). There is an obvious cost advantage inherent in outpatient treatment compared with inpatient treatment. A 28-day inpatient treatment program might cost between $7,000 and $30,000, depending on the daily fee for each specific treatment setting ("ONDCP," 1990; Turbo, 1989). In contrast, a 6-month outpatient treatment program might cost as little as $1,000 (Turbo).

A major advantage of the outpatient chemical dependency treatment program format is that such treatment avoids the need to remove patients from their environment. Unlike inpatient treatment programs, no community reorientation period is needed after outpatient treatment (Bonstedt, Ulrich, Dolinar, & Johnson, 1984; Youngstrom, 1990a). In addition, outpatient treatment programs tend to last longer than do inpatient rehabilitation programs. Nace (1987) suggested that the ideal outpatient treatment program would last one full year. A treatment program of that duration would offer long-term follow-up for the crucial first year of sobriety, a time when the individual is likely to relapse. The patient who knew he/she would be subjected to random urine toxicology screening as part of a yearlong outpatient program might be less likely to use drugs.

Berg and Dubin (1990) outlined an intensive outpatient treatment program that was divided into four phases. Each of the first three phases, intensive, intermediate, and moderate treatment, was designed to last for two weeks. However, the authors noted, any given individual's placement was determined by "the severity of the patient's addiction, progress in treatment, financial resources, and ability to attend the program" (p. 1175). The final phase of treatment, the extended phase, involved an aftercare meeting once a week for an indefinite period.

Since outpatient treatment programs tend to last longer than do inpatient programs, Lewis et al. (1988) believe that this rehabilitation format offers the counselor a longer period to help clients achieve the goals outlined in their treatment plan. Clients also have an extended period to practice and perfect new behaviors that support sobriety.

Outpatient treatment programs offer yet another advantage over inpatient treatment programs: *flexibility* (Turbo, 1989). Program participation may be through an *outpatient day treatment* program, where treatment activities are scheduled during normal working hours, or through an *outpatient evening treatment* program. As the name implies, an evening program operates during the evening hours to carry out rehabilitation activities. Finally, outpatient treatment programs offer clients the opportunity to practice sobriety while still living in the community. This is a significant advantage over traditional inpatient treatment programs, where clients are removed from their home and community for the duration of treatment.

Disadvantages of Outpatient Treatment Programs

Surprisingly, although inpatient treatment might cost more, because of available insurance coverage, many clients actually pay *less* for inpatient treatment than they would for outpatient treatment. This is because health insurance carriers traditionally do not reimburse outpatient treatment programs at the same rate as the more expensive inpatient substance abuse program by health insurance carriers. This factor often fuels a tendency for health care providers to recommend inpatient over outpatient treatment programs (Berg & Dubin, 1990).

Although statistical research has found no significant difference in the percentage of outpatient treatment program "graduates" who remain sober, as opposed to those who complete inpatient treatment programs for drug addiction, this is not to say that outpatient treatment is as effective as inpatient treatment. Rather, inpatient treatment programs tend to deal more effectively with a different class of client than do outpatient treatment programs, This fact makes it difficult to compare inpatient and outpatient treatment.

The development of an outpatient treatment program for a patient who requires detoxification from chemicals is quite complicated. For example, Dumas (1992) suggested that individuals who smoke cocaine would require inpatient hospitalization, at least at first, to "interrupt the compulsive pattern of drug use, and to treat the ... drug-induced medical and psychiatric problems" (p. 907) caused by cocaine abuse. But in the case of alcohol, it has been suggested that only approximately 10%

of the cases of alcohol withdrawal require hospitalization (Berg & Dubin, 1990). Thus, while the integration of detoxification programs with outpatient treatment is difficult, this is not a problem that will affect the majority of the patients who can benefit from outpatient rehabilitation efforts.

Outpatient treatment programs do not offer the same degree of structure and support found in the inpatient treatment setting. Further, outpatient treatment programs offer less control over the client's environment, since the patient continues to live at home, and thus are of limited value for some patients who require a great deal of support during the early stages of sobriety. While outpatient treatment of substance abuse may work for many clients, it does not seem to be the ultimate answer to the problem of chemical dependency.

Inpatient Treatment Programs

The inpatient treatment program might best be defined as a residential treatment facility, where the client lives while participating in treatment. Such programs usually deal with hard-core, seriously ill, or "difficult" patients. These are individuals for whom outpatient treatment has either not been successful, or for whom outpatient treatment has been ruled out. Residential treatment programs usually have a strong emphasis on a twelve-step philosophy, and use extensive individual and group therapy. The length of stay depends on such factors as the client's motivation and support system, and a range of other variables that the treatment team considers when working with any given individual.

In response to the challenge presented by the client, residential treatment programs have evolved to provide the greatest degree of support and help. Inpatient treatment also is "the most restrictive, structured, and protective of treatment settings" (Klar, 1987, p. 340). It combines the greatest potential for positive change with high financial cost and the possibility of branding the patient for life (Klar). The decision to use inpatient treatment is one that should not be made lightly.

Many general hospitals offer inpatient rehabilitation programs for drug/alcohol use problems. Bell (1995) estimated that 21% of the hospitals surveyed offered inpatient treatment for substance abuse. But there are forms of inpatient treatment that are not hospital-based such as *therapeutic communities* or *halfway houses,* as well as a number of inpatient rehabilitation programs that are not part of a hospital complex.

Varieties of Inpatient Treatment

Hospital/Program Based Inpatient Treatment

Traditional inpatient drug rehabilitation is often carried out either in a center that specializes in chemical dependency treatment, or in a traditional hospital setting as part of a specialized drug treatment unit. Many of these programs follow the Minnesota Model, explored in Chapter 28. There is no standard treatment program under the Minnesota Model, but there is a great deal of flexibility to allow for meeting the needs of different individuals.

Inpatient rehabilitation programs, especially those in a hospital setting, often begin with detoxification. One advantage of having a detoxification component is that a patient can begin treatment in the last stages of withdrawal from chemicals. This blending of withdrawal and treatment might aid in patient retention.

In the treatment program, the individual lives in the treatment setting and follows a daily program of lectures, individual, and group therapy sessions. Each patient is assigned "homework," which might include assignments to read certain material that rehabilitation staff believe would support the individual's recovery. In most programs, they are also expected to begin to follow the Twelve-Step program of AA or a similar self-help group, and attendance in self-help group meetings is required.

Therapeutic Communities

One controversial form of inpatient treatment is the therapeutic community (TC). Surprisingly, there is no generally recognized TC model (DeLeon, 1994; National Academy of Sciences, 1990). Rather, there are a multitude of different programs, which present different recommended lengths of stay, client-to-staff ratios, treatment philosophy, and staff compositions. In general, however, the "traditional" TC might be viewed as a program which operates on the theory that drug abuse is:

a deviant behavior, reflecting impeded personality development or chronic deficits in social, educational, and economic skills . . . . The principal aim of the TC is a global change in life-style: abstinence from illicit substances, elimination of antisocial activity, development of employability, and prosocial attitudes. (DeLeon, 1994, p. 392)

The "traditional" TC programs usually require a commitment of between 1 and 3 years (DeLeon 1989, 1994), although some programs have a minimal commitment of only six months. This extended length of stay is thought to be necessary to change the drug-using behavior. Such long-term residential treatment programs are thought to be effective with those individuals whose addiction is complicated by an antisocial personality disorder, or what "ONDCP," (1990) called "social pathology" (p. 3).

When the TC movement began in the United States, it mainly worked with those individuals who were addicted to opiates. But this is no longer true. The majority of the clients in today's TCs were using chemicals other than opiates prior to their admission to treatment (DeLeon, 1994). Most TC programs follow a single therapeutic model, which is to say that all members of the treatment staff have the same treatment philosophy. This adherence to a single vision seems to contribute to the effectiveness of TCs in working with the drug-dependent individual (Ellis et al., 1988). But the TC model has not been widely accepted in the United States. DeLeon (1989) found that of the estimated 500 drug-free residential treatment programs in the United States, less than a quarter follow the TC model.

A central tenet of the TC model is "its perspective of drug abuse as a *whole person* disorder" (DeLeon, 1989, p. 177, italics in original). Other characteristics of the TC includes social and physical isolation, a structured living environment, a firm system of rewards and punishments, and an emphasis on self-examination and the confession of past wrongdoing. Clients are expected to work, either outside the TC in an approved job, or within the TC itself as part of the housekeeping or kitchen staff. In many TCs, there is some potential mobility from the status of client to that of a paraprofessional staff member (National Academy of Sciences, 1990).

Although many TCs use the services of mental health professionals, there is a tendency for much of the treatment to be carried out by paraprofessional staff members. Often, the paraprofessionals are former residents of the TC itself. This is done on the theory that only a person "who has been there" can understand the addicted person. Such paraprofessional counselors are thought to be effective in breaking through the client's denial and manipulation, since they will have had similar experiences that they can call on in working with the newcomer.

The TC offers an extended family for the individual—a "family" that the recovering addict may be encouraged never to leave. Indeed, the original members of Synanon (one of the early therapeutic communities) were expected to remain there on a permanent basis, as part of that family (Lewis et al., 1988).

Collectively, TCs suffer from significant dropout rates. There is evidence that the first 15 days is an especially difficult period for many clients. It is during this period that the dropout rate is highest ("Therapeutic Community," 1989). DeLeon (1994) suggested that 30% to 40% of those admitted to a TC will drop out in the first 30 days. Further, over the course of treatment, a significant percentage of those who do not leave on their own are asked to leave, or are discharged from treatment for various rule infractions (Gelman, Underwood, King, Hager, & Gordon, 1990). Ultimately, only 15% to 25% of those admitted to TCs actually graduate (DeLeon, 1994; National Academy of Sciences, 1990). The recovery rates of those who drop out of TCs in the earliest phases of treatment "basically cannot be distinguished from those . . . individuals who did not enter any treatment modality" (National Academy of Sciences, 1990, p. 167). Thus, while the TC offers some hope for the addicted person, it also would appear to be a treatment concept that is not for everyone.

There is a great deal of controversy surrounding therapeutic communities. Some (Ausabel, 1983) caution that the therapeutic community might not be a positive step for the individual. Many such programs use methods such as ego stripping and unquestioned submission to the rules of the program. Lewis et al. (1988) point out that the social isolation inherent in the TC prevents the client from going out into the community to try new social skills.

However, others (DeLeon, 1989, 1994; Peele, 1989; Yablonsky, 1967) note that the TC has been effective in some cases where traditional treatment methods have been of limited value. Peele (1989) observed that the TC functions best when it strives to help the individual learn social skills and values inconsistent with drug-using behaviors. The journal *Alcoholism & Drug Abuse Week* ("ONDCP," 1990) concluded in its review of the therapeutic community concept that such programs are quite effective, with upward of 80% *of those who complete the program* remaining drug-free. The National Academy of Sciences (1990) concluded that those who remain in the program the longest were most likely to achieve a sober lifestyle.

Is There a Legitimate Need for Inpatient Treatment?

A decade ago, Miller and Hester (1986) noted that "the relative merits of residential treatment are less than clear" (p. 794). In a similar study, Chick (1993) observed that, for treating alcoholics, "The advantages of inpatient versus outpatient care . . . have been difficult to show" (p. 1374). In an early study that sparked a great deal of controversy, Miller and Hester reviewed 16 different research studies that explored the benefits of inpatient as opposed to outpatient treatment for alcohol-dependent individuals. The authors concluded that there was no significant difference between inpatient and outpatient alcoholism rehabilitation programs on various measures of patient improvement. The authors explored the *length* of inpatient treatment as a possible variable affecting treatment outcome, but found no statistically significant improvement for longer duration alcohol treatment programs compared with shorter inpatient programs.

The authors did admit that their data suggested that inpatient treatment was possibly more advantageous for the long-term addict. But outpatient treatment was thought to be more effective for those clients who had not used chemicals for as long a time, according to the authors. However, posttreatment aftercare programs were found to play a more significant role in posttreatment success/failure than the specific form of treatment utilized (Miller & Hester, 1986).

The team of Miller and Hester do not attempt to hide their criticism of inpatient treatment programs. But they do not:

> advocate the abolition of residential treatment. There may be subpopulations for whom more intensive treatment is justifiable. From the limited matching data available at present, it appears that intensive treatment may be better for severely addicted and socially unstable individuals. (Miller & Hester, 1986, p. 1246)

In response to Miller and Hester's original (1986) work, Adelman and Weiss (1989) conducted their own research into the merits of inpatient treatment. The authors reported that 77% of those alcoholics treated for their alcoholism eventually required some form of inpatient treatment. The authors also found that treatment programs in "medically oriented facilities" (p. 516) had lower dropout rates than did treatment programs in nonmedical centers. The authors also concluded that patients discharged after short inpatient treatment programs tended to relapse more frequently than did those who remained in treatment longer.

There are those who have both advocated for, and challenged the need for, inpatient treatment for chronic cases of alcoholism. In their review of the effectiveness of treatment approaches, the team of Bonstedt et al. (1984) suggested that in most cases "aggressive outpatient treatment" (p. 1039) of alcoholism is more cost-effective than inpatient treatment for alcohol dependence. The authors went on to point out that "the majority of alcoholics do not have to be hospitalized each time they present for treatment" (p. 1039). The issue of whether a prior history of chemical dependency treatment automatically excludes outpatient rehabilitation thus remains one that is disputed by different professionals.

The treatment team of Walsh et al. (1991) randomly assigned 227 workers at a large factory who were known to be abusing alcohol to one of three treatment programs: compulsory attendance of Alcoholics Anonymous, compulsory inpatient treatment, or the patient's choice between these two alternatives. The authors were surprised to find that while the referral to compulsory AA meetings *initially* was more cost-effective, in the long run inpatient treatment resulted in higher abstinence rates.

The team of Moos, King, and Patterson (1996) followed a sample of 2190 men who had been initially treated at a Veterans Administration (VA) medical facility for complications of alcohol abuse/addiction, and who were then discharged to either a hospital-based or residential treatment facility for inpatient treatment of their alcohol use problem. The authors found that for those patients with a coexisting mental health issue, inpatient treatment at a hospital-based program, combined with outpatient mental health care, resulted in lower readmission rates in the first 2 years following admission to treatment.

For those patients who only presented with an alcohol use problem, community-based residential care programs and outpatient mental health counseling seemed to result in longer periods of abstinence, according to the authors. It was concluded that, overall, patients in community-based residential treatment programs were less likely to require readmission to the VA facility over a 2-year follow-up period than those treated in a hospital-based inpatient program. However, those patients who remained in treatment for less than 2 weeks had higher readmission rates than did those patients who remained in treatment for longer than 2 weeks, according to Moos et al. (1996). This finding suggests that there is a "threshold effect" for the treatment process, with stronger results being achieved after 14 days of inpatient treatment.

Inpatient treatment also appears to be a cost-effective approach to the rehabilitation of heroin addicts. Swan (1994) noted that the cost of a 6-month inpatient treatment program for a person addicted to heroin would be about $8,250, while the cost to society for not treating the heroin-addicted person in terms of criminal activity, social support services, and health care services would be approximately $21,500 for the same period. Although a residential treatment program was four times as expensive as simply placing the heroin addict in a methadone maintenance program, it still was only 40% as expensive as not providing any form of treatment for the individual. Thus, one could argue, residential treatment programs appear to be a cost-effective way to deal with individuals who are addicted to heroin.

The Advantages of Inpatient Treatment

Although the case for outpatient treatment programs is a strong one, there are certain advantages to inpatient treatment program as opposed to outpatient rehabilitation programs. Research suggests that inpatient treatment programs have a higher client retention rate than outpatient treatment programs (Bell, Williams, Nelson, & Spence, 1994). The authors found that fully 76% of the clients who were assigned to inpatient treatment completed their program, as opposed to just under 64% of those subjects assigned to an outpatient day treatment program. What are some reasons for this significant difference in retention rates?

One reason a greater percentage of patients who enter inpatient rehabilitation programs actually complete treatment is that such programs offer *more comprehensive treatment programming* than is possible in an outpatient treatment setting (Klar, 1987). This is an advantage in more advanced cases of drug dependency, because these addicted individuals often have centered their life around the chemical for such a long time that they will be unable to use a less restrictive treatment approach. Often, addicted clients live alone or lack close interpersonal support. Because of this lack of close relationships, a medical emergency might go undetected for hours, or days.

In the inpatient treatment setting, medical emergencies are quickly detected, and the appropriate action can be taken by staff to help the client. The close supervision by staff members also helps to discourage further drug use. Clients, especially those with a long-standing drug problem, often are tempted to "help out" the detoxification process, by taking a few additional drugs or drinks during withdrawal. It is not uncommon for opiate-dependent individuals going through withdrawal in a treatment setting to inject illicit chemicals that they brought with them. Alcohol-dependent patients have been known to take a drink or two from a bottle that was thoughtfully hidden away in the suitcase a few days before entering treatment.

Another advantage of the almost total control over the client's environment offered by the inpatient rehabilitation setting is the opportunity for a structured environment with scheduled individual and group therapy sessions, meals, recreational opportunities, self-help group meetings, and spiritual counseling (Berg & Dubin, 1990). For clients who have lived at least the most recent portion of their lives in a drug-centered lifestyle, the concept of a drug-free way of life is often foreign. All too often, clients report that they have not been eating on a regular basis prior to entering treatment. An inpatient rehabilitation setting allows staff to monitor and treat dietary disorders that may have been caused by the individual's addicted lifestyle. Supplementary vitamins, or dietary supplements, have often been found to be of value in such cases, and inpatient treatment allows staff to closely monitor the client's recovery from the physical effects of addiction.

Many clients attend their first AA meeting in an inpatient setting. In some cases, the client will often affirm that he/she would never have attended the meeting of Alcoholics Anonymous, or Narcotics Anonymous, if he/she had not been required to do so by treatment staff. Adelman and Weiss (1989) concluded that participation in Alcoholics Anonymous was an essential component of an effective inpatient treatment program.

Another advantage of inpatient treatment is that it can provide *around-the-clock support during the earliest stages of sobriety.* It is not unusual to find a client sitting up at 2 o'clock in the morning, talking about personal problems with the staff member on duty. Nor is it surprising to find a client still up at 3 o'clock in the morning, pacing through the earliest stages of withdrawal. When such clients are asked what they would do if they were not in treatment, the most common answer is, "I would go out and score some drugs!"[1]

But, because these clients are in treatment, they are able to draw on the support services of the staff on duty, to help them through withdrawal. This support might be in the form of a sympathetic ear when the client needs somebody to talk to, or the administration of previously prescribed medications to help

---

[1] The word *score* usually is interpreted to mean "buy" or "obtain."

the client through the discomfort. Staff members might offer suggestions such as suggesting that the client walk around the ward or have something to eat, and will be able to "be there" for the client during this difficult period.

As Nace (1987) noted, inpatient treatment is of value in cases where outpatient treatment has become a "revolving door" (p. 130) for the individual. Inpatient settings are also of value in cases where the individual has experienced repeated crisis situations while in outpatient treatment, has had several aborted attempts to utilize outpatient treatment, or has been unable to establish an effective therapeutic alliance in a less restrictive setting. Cases where the individual must be treated for multiple problems (physical and psychiatric) while being treated for drug addiction also benefit from inpatient treatment, according to Nace.

Disadvantages of Inpatient Treatment

Residential/inpatient treatment is disruptive to the individual's social, vocational, and family life (Morey, 1996). The individual is forced to leave his/her normal environment, to participate in the rehabilitation program, at the expense of the time necessary to work, participate in family life, or otherwise engage in activities outside the treatment center setting. The economic cost of inpatient treatment is also significantly higher than that of outpatient rehabilitation programs. Finally, the treatment center setting may be isolated, preventing easy contact with the patient and family or friends. All these factors are disadvantages of the inpatient rehabilitation program.

Inpatient or Outpatient Treatment?

The decision whether to use inpatient or outpatient treatment for a client is perhaps one of the most important decisions that a treatment professional will make (Washton et al., 1988). In the past decade, several organizations have published referral guidelines to assist in choosing the proper rehabilitation program. The Group for the Advancement of Psychiatry (1991) identified several criteria that could be used to identify those individuals who would best benefit from inpatient, as opposed to outpatient, treatment programs:

1. Whether the client's condition was associated with significant *medical* or *psychiatric* conditions, or complications.
2. *Severity of actual or anticipated withdrawal* from the drug/s being used.
3. *Multiple failed attempts at outpatient treatment.*
4. The strength of the client's *social support systems.*
5. The *severity of the client's addiction,* and the *possibility of polysubstance abuse.*

Another organization that has produced a list of placement criteria is the American Society of Addiction Medicine (ASAM). Under the ASAM placement criteria system, the patient's strengths and needs in each of six areas, or dimensions, are assessed. Depending on the patient's requirements in each area, placement is made in one of four levels of care. The ASAM placement criteria can be thought of as forming a 4×6 grid for plotting each individual's needs. The ASAM placement grid resembles Table 29-1.

Patient placement guides such as that suggested by ASAM help to guide the rehabilitation professional through an otherwise difficult decision-making process: Which form of treatment is best for the individual client? Both outpatient and inpatient treatment programs offer unique advantages and disadvantages to the individual. It is up to the assessor to determine the best match between the patient's needs and the available treatment options.

In terms of total cost, outpatient treatment programs are usually less expensive than inpatient programs. Outpatient rehabilitation programs are best suited to those clients who have not had an extensive prior treatment history (Nace, 1987). The individual's motivation for treatment and past treatment history offer hints as to whether inpatient or outpatient programs would be most effective. Further, as noted in the ASAM criteria, the patient's need for inpatient detoxification from chemicals should be considered in deciding whether to recommend inpatient or outpatient treatment.

A sad, rarely discussed fact is that restrictions on funding play a role in deciding which treatment options are available for the individual. The person whose insurance will only pay for inpatient chemical dependency treatment has certain financial restrictions placed on his/her treatment options. Thus, availability of funding influences the decision whether to seek inpatient or outpatient treatment for substance abuse. Finally, the individual's psychiatric status, and availability of social support should be evaluated when considering outpatient treatment as an option (Group for the Advancement of Psychiatry, 1991; Nace, 1987). A deeply depressed individual who is recovering from an extended period of cocaine use might benefit from the greater support offered by an inpatient treatment program, at least during the initial recovery period, when the depression is most severe.

Turbo (1989) identified several criteria that suggested an inpatient treatment program might be better for the client than the outpatient setting. These criteria included (a) repeated failure to maintain sobriety in outpatient treatment, (b) the acutely suicidal client, (c) clients with seriously disturbed home environments, (d) clients with serious medical problems, and (e) clients with serious psychiatric problems. In addition, Allen and Phillips (1993) suggested that the patient's legal status be considered in deciding whether to refer the patient to inpatient or outpatient treatment. Those individuals who had been arrested for drug possession charges, or who had been arrested for driving while under the influence of chemicals, might do better in an outpatient treatment program, according to the authors. Court supervision makes relapse less likely. Patients who had achieved periods of sobriety, but who had then relapsed, might be treated briefly on an inpatient basis, according to the authors. But, following a brief stabilization stay in the hospital, these patients could be switched to an outpatient treatment program, according to Allen and Phillips.

TABLE 29-1 ASAM Placement Criteria[2]

Level of care →	*Level I*	*Level II*	*Level III*	*Level IV*
Dimension	*Outpatient treatment*	*Intensive outpatient treatment/partial hospitalization program*	*Medically monitored inpatient treatment (residential treatment)*	*Medically managed inpatient treatment (traditional medical treatment)*
Acute intoxication/ withdrawal potential[1]	None	Minimal	Severe risk, but does not require hospitalization	Severe risk that requires hospitalization
Biomedical conditions or complications[1]	None/stable	Minimal: can be managed in outpatient setting	Serious: requires medical monitoring	Severe: requires inpatient hospitalization
Emotional/behavioral conditions or omplications	None/stable	Mild: but can be managed in outpatient setting	Serious: requires patient to be monitored 24 hours/day	Severe: requires inpatient psychiatric care
Treatment acceptance or resistance	Cooperative: needs guidance and monitoring	Some resistance: intensive treatment needed	Resistance is severe: requires intensive tx	N/A
Relapse potential	Minimal risk of relapse: needs monitoring and guidance only	High risk of relapse without close monitoring and support by staff	Patient is unable to control use without being in inpatient setting	N/A
Recovery environment	Patient has skills and support to abstain on own	Patient lacks environmental support, but has skills to cope with some structure	Environment is dangerous to patient, and s/he must be removed from it	N/A

[1] As determined by licensed physician.
[2] This graph is designed to illustrate the ASAM placement criteria, and should not be utilized as a guide to patient placement.

The final decision whether to suggest an inpatient or an outpatient treatment program ultimately centers around this issue: Given the client's resources and needs, what is the *least restrictive treatment alternative?* (American Psychiatric Association, 1995). The treatment referral criteria advanced by ASAM (Morey, 1996) are useful guides to the selection of the least restrictive alternative that will meet the client's needs. Although there are those who will argue that the inpatient treatment program sounds very similar to a concentration camp experience, the dysfunction caused by drug addiction often requires drastic intervention. Just as drastic intervention is often necessary in the practice of medicine (e.g., emergency surgery where medical treatment of an ulcer has failed), so is the step of inpatient treatment necessary in more advanced cases of addiction to chemicals.

Partial Hospitalization Options

Several new treatment formats have been explored that combine elements of inpatient and outpatient rehabilitation programs. Each of these rehabilitation formats offers advantages and disadvantages, yet each should be considered as a viable treatment option for clients who present themselves for treatment. Depending on the client's needs, some of the new treatment formats may prove to be quite beneficial.

Two-by-Four Programs

One proposed solution to the treatment dilemma of whether to utilize inpatient or outpatient treatment is the so-called two-by-four program. This program format borrows from both inpatient and outpatient treatment programs, to establish a biphasic rehabilitation system that seems to have some promise. Patients are first hospitalized for a short period, usually 2 weeks, to achieve total detoxification from chemicals. Depending on individual needs, the initial period of hospitalization may be somewhat shorter than 2 weeks, or longer than the 2-week time span. However, the goal is to help clients to reach a point as rapidly as possible where they can participate in outpatient treatment. If, as will occasionally happen, a client is unable to function in the less restrictive outpatient rehabilitation program, he/she may be returned to the inpatient treatment format. Later, when additional progress has been made, the

client may again return to an outpatient setting to complete the treatment program there.

Turbo (1989) discussed an interesting variation on the two-by-four program that is carried out through the Schick Shadel chain of hospitals, located in California, Texas, and Washington State. These programs admit the individual for 10 days of inpatient treatment, followed by 2 additional inpatient "reinforcement" days later. The first reinforcement day occurs 1 month after discharge, and another 2 days of inpatient treatment are scheduled for 2 months following the initial admission.

Berg and Dubin (1990) reported, however, that admission to an inpatient treatment program for even short periods resulted in "a lower probability of complying with outpatient after care" (p. 1177) by the client. The authors found a 60% dropout rate for those who were initially hospitalized for a brief period, and then were referred to an intensive outpatient treatment program. It is not known at this time whether these results were specific only to the program with which Berg and Dubin (1990) are affiliated, or if this is a trend that exists in other partial hospitalization programs as well.

Day Hospitalization

The day hospitalization format is also known as *partial-day hospitalization.* Such programs typically provide 3 to 12 hours of treatment a day, for 3 to 7 days of the week. One advantage of partial-day hospitalization programs is that they combine elements of inpatient treatment with the opportunities for growth possible by having the client live at home (Lewis et al., 1988). After detoxification has been achieved, the client lives at home and comes to the treatment center during scheduled treatment hours to participate in the rehabilitation program.

There are a number of advantages to partial hospital programs for substance abuse rehabilitation, including that such programs provide:

> an intensive and structured treatment experience for patients with substance dependence who require more services than those generally available in traditional outpatient settings. (American Psychiatric Association, 1995, p. 23)

Further, day hospitalization programs tend to be less expensive than traditional inpatient treatment programs, with the cost of day treatment being approximately half that of inpatient treatment (French, 1995).

An essential element of day hospitalization is that the client have a supportive, stable family. If the client's spouse (or other family member) also has a chemical abuse problem, day hospitalization may not be a viable treatment option. If the client's spouse is severely codependent and enables the client's continued chemical use, day hospitalization should not be the treatment of choice. But if the client has a stable home environment, day hospitalization offers the opportunity to combine the intensive programming possible through inpatient treatment programs with the opportunities for growth possible by having the client spend the evening hours at home. Such a program is of value for clients who need to rebuild family relationships after a protracted period of chemical use.

Halfway Houses

The halfway house concept emerged in the 1950s, in response to the need for an intermediate step between the inpatient treatment format and independent living (Miller & Hester, 1980). For those clients who lack a stable social support system, the immediate period following treatment is often most difficult. These clients, even if strongly motivated to remain sober, must struggle against the urge to return to chemical use without the social support necessary to aid in this struggle. The halfway house provides a transitional living facility for such clients.

Miller and Hester (1980) identified several common characteristics of halfway houses: (a) small patient population (usually less than 25 individuals), (b) a brief patient stay (less than a few months), (c) emphasis on Alcoholics Anonymous or similar twelve-step philosophy, (d) minimal rules, and (e) small number of professional staff members. As noted, most halfway houses utilize a twelve-step philosophy. Many hold in-house self-help group meetings such as Alcoholics Anonymous, while other halfway houses require a specified number of community self-help group meetings a week. Each individual is expected to find work within a specified period of time (usually 2–3 weeks) or is assigned a job within the halfway house.

The degree of structure in the traditional halfway house setting is somewhere between what is found in an inpatient treatment program setting and what is found in a traditional household. This provides clients with enough support to function during the transitional period between treatment and self-sufficiency, yet allows clients to make choices about their life. As Miller and Hester (1980) pointed out, halfway houses usually have fewer rules than an inpatient treatment center. Halfway house participation is usually time-limited, generally 3 to 6 months, after which clients are ready to assume their responsibilities again.

In their review of treatment modalities, Miller and Hester (1980) concluded that there was little evidence to suggest that the halfway house is a useful adjunct to treatment. They supported this conclusion by pointing to the fact that research had failed to uncover significantly greater improvement from patients admitted to halfway houses following treatment than from patients who were discharged directly into the community following inpatient treatment.

A number of subsequent studies have failed to support this conclusion. Moos and Moos (1995) followed a sample of 1070 subjects who had been treated for substance abuse problems at one of 77 Veterans Administration medical centers across the United States who had been referred to community residential living facilities following completion of their primary treatment program. The authors found that those patients who had remained in the community residential living facility were significantly less likely to have been readmitted for substance use in the 4 years following discharge from the community living unit. In other words, those patients who remained in the halfway house longer were less likely to require additional treatment for substance use problems in the 4 years following discharge from treatment.

These findings were consistent with those of the team of Hitchcock, Stainback, and Roque (1995), who compared the relapse rate of 82 patients who elected not to enter a halfway house setting, against that of 42 patients who were admitted to a halfway house setting. The authors found that patients discharged to a community setting (e.g., home, an apartment, or shared living space with friends/relatives) were significantly more likely to drop out of treatment in the first 60 days following discharge from an inpatient substance abuse rehabilitation program. On the basis of their findings, the authors concluded that halfway house placement can significantly enhance patient retention in aftercare programs, thus improving treatment outcome.

Thus, although the original challenge to the halfway house concept was based on a lack of evidence supporting effectiveness, subsequent research has revealed that halfway houses do indeed seem to be an effective adjunct to the rehabilitation process of chemical abusers.

Summary

There is significant evidence that, at least for some addicted individuals, outpatient treatment is an option that should be considered by treatment professionals. For those with the proper social support, and for whom there is no coexisting psychiatric illness or need for inpatient hospitalization, outpatient therapy for drug addiction may offer the individual the chance to participate in treatment while still living at home. This avoids the need for a reorientation period following treatment, which is often required by patients after discharge from an inpatient rehabilitation facility.

Outpatient treatment also allows for long-term therapeutic support that is often not available from shorter term inpatient programs. Within an outpatient drug addiction program, random urine toxicology screening may be used to check on medication compliance and to identify those individuals who have engaged in illicit drug use. Research evidence suggests that, for many patients, outpatient drug addiction treatment is as effective as inpatient chemical dependency programs. There is a significant dropout rate from outpatient treatment programs, however, and much remains to be learned about how to make outpatient addiction treatment more effective.

Inpatient treatment is often viewed as a drastic step. Yet, for a minority of those who are addicted to chemicals, such a drastic step is necessary if the client is ever to regain control of his/her life. The inpatient rehabilitation program offers many advantages over less restrictive treatment options, including a depth of support services unavailable in outpatient treatment. For many of those in the advanced stages of addiction, inpatient treatment offers the only realistic hope of recovery.

In recent years, questions have been raised concerning the need for inpatient treatment programs or halfway house placement following treatment. It has been suggested that inpatient treatment does not offer any advantage over outpatient treatment, and that a longer length of stay is no more effective than short-term treatment. However, others have concluded that length of stay is inversely related to the probability of relapse following treatment.

CHAPTER THIRTY

Recovery

It is common for substance abuse rehabilitation professionals to speak of the process of recovering from a drug/alcohol use problem as if this were a single step. Even the language of recovery implies that abstinence is a one-time effort. In reality, it is a *process* that, like life itself, has a definite beginning, but no definite end point. In this chapter, the process of recovering from an alcohol/drug use problem is discussed.

The Stages of Recovery

Lichtenstein and Glasgow (1992) presented a model for smoking cessation in which recovery was viewed as a multistage process. Their model was based on the work of Prochaska et al. (1992), who suggested that recovery from drug abuse/addiction is a process involving definite stages (see Figure 30.1). The first stage of recovery is that of *precontemplation* (Lichtenstein & Glasgow, 1992; Prochaska et al., 1992). During the stage of precontemplation, the individual is actively abusing chemicals and has no thought of trying to abstain from chemical use/abuse. This phase can continue for years, or decades. It is during this phase of chemical use that *denial* is most prominent, and the therapeutic challenge for the therapist faced with clients in the precontemplation phase is: (a) to teach them the effects of the drugs of abuse, (b) to teach them the danger(s) associated with continued substance use/abuse, (c) to help awaken within clients a desire for a different lifestyle, (d) to

help clients identify barriers to recovery, and, (e) to help clients identify routes for enhancing their self-esteem.

It is only during the *contemplation* phase that the client begins to entertain vague thoughts about possibly stopping the alcohol/drug use "one of these days." In this phase, the individual remains ambivalent about the possibility of change, but has a growing sense of dissatisfaction with his/her present (alcohol/drug centered) lifestyle. An individual may remain in this phase for months, or even years, while continuing to engage in active chemical use. For the therapist confronted with clients at this stage in the recovery process, the challenge is to (a) enhance the motivation to change, (b) awaken within clients a desire for spiritual growth (see Chapter 35), and (c) help clients learn how the chemical use has affected their life.

In the model of recovery proposed by Prochaska et al. (1992), it is during the contemplation phase that the individual makes a decision to try to quit chemicals within the next 6 months. Brown (1997) suggested that this process takes place during the *determination* phase. In either model, during this phase of recovery, the individual begins to make the cognitive changes necessary to support an attempt at abstinence. It is the therapist's goal to nurture the change process, offering encouragement, support, feedback, gentle confrontation, humor, and external validation for the client's struggles and successes.

In both the Prochaska et al. (1992) model, and the Brown (1997) model, the actual initiation of

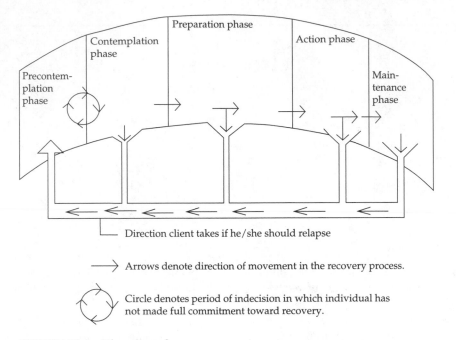

Direction client takes if he/she should relapse

Arrows denote direction of movement in the recovery process.

Circle denotes period of indecision in which individual has not made full commitment toward recovery.

FIGURE 30.1   The stages of recovery.

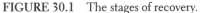

abstinence is the *action* phase of the recovery process. During this period, the individual is actively engaged in the process of change, and taking the first steps toward recovery. The therapist helping clients during this phase must (a) optimize opportunities for growth, (b) be alert to signs that clients are unable to handle the perceived level of stress, (c) encourage clients to begin the process of building a substance-free support system, (d) help clients to handle the emotional roller coaster that they may experience, (e) help clients be realistic about their progress (clients often overestimate their growth and progress), and (f) serve as a parent-substitute, mentor, cheering section, and guide for clients.

Relapse is a real danger during this phase of recovery, and this is a common outcome. In the first 3 to 4 weeks following cessation of cigarette smoking, the individual is especially vulnerable to smoking cues, such as being around other smokers (Bliss et al., 1989). At such times, the individual is less likely to cope effectively with the urge to smoke, and is in danger of a relapse into active cigarette smoking. This is one reason smokers who want to quit typically require an average of 3 to 4 attempts (Prochaska et al., 1992), to perhaps as many as 5 or even 7 "serious attempts"

(Brunton et al., 1994, p. 105; Sherman, 1994) before being able to stop smoking cigarettes. Thus, one task that clients must accomplish during the action phase of recovery is to learn about his/her relapse "triggers" (discussed in Chapter 31).

Finally, after at least 6 months of abstinence the individual will enter the *maintenance* phase. During this phase, the clients work on learning the behaviors that will enable them to continue to abstain from chemical use. During the maintenance phase, clients might have to confront personal issues that contributed to, or at least supported, their use of chemicals. It is during this phase of recovery that they must learn the skills necessary to support an alcohol/drug-free lifestyle, including the need to find/maintain a job and to develop relationships that will support recovery. The maintenance phase has no specific end point, but optimally continues through the client's life. The therapist during this period works to assure the stability of change, to help clients identify issues that might threaten recovery, and finally, to address these issues.

In Figure 30.1, relapse is acknowledged as a possible outcome for the recovery process. There are no guarantees; for example, in the battle against cigarette smoking, the individual's return to the use of tobacco products is so likely that cigarette cessation might best be viewed as a "Dynamic Process" (Cohen et al., 1989, p. 1361), in which periods of abstinence are intermixed with periods of relapse. Indeed, "the return to smoking . . . occurs so frequently that it should be thought of as a part of the process of quitting and not as a failure in quitting (Lee & D'Alonzo, 1993, p. 39).

This is not to say that rehabilitation professionals should *accept* continued chemical use/abuse as being unavoidable. Rather, this is to say that the process of recovery from alcohol/drug addiction is a difficult, ongoing process, in which relapse back to active chemical use is a constant danger.

Surprisingly, the model suggested by Prochaska et al. (1992) seems to apply to those who recover from substance use problems both with, and without, professional intervention. This makes sense, since the majority of those individuals with an alcohol or drug use problem recover without professional treatment (Peele, 1996).

Another model of recovery was suggested by Nowinski (1996). The first stage of recovery from a chemical use problem, according to Nowinski's model, is the stage of *acceptance* (Nowinski). But there appear to be several pathways to recovery: (a) The individual could decide that the consequences of further use of the chemical are not worth the anticipated benefits and cut back/discontinue the use of that chemical (or, possibly, any recreational drug) on his/her own. (b) The individual could turn to a self-help group such as Alcoholics Anonymous (AA) to learn how to abstain from chemical use. (c) The individual could seek outpatient therapy to learn how to abstain from chemical use. (d) Finally, the individual might seek inpatient treatment to learn how to abstain from further chemical use. Figure 30.2 shows a flowchart of the recovery process.

During this stage, the individual struggles to come to understand why willpower alone is not sufficient to guarantee abstinence/recovery. It is only after reaching the second stage, that of *surrender,* that the individual becomes willing to make the changes in lifestyle necessary to support recovery, according to Nowinski (1996). As discussed later in this chapter, the goal of the substance abuse rehabilitation

professional is to facilitate the individual's movement through the different stages of recovery.

In theory, many psychosocial, medical, or legal forces can contribute to the individual's recovery from problematic alcohol/drug use. Humphreys et al. (1995) identified a number of these factors:

- *Interpersonal relationships.* Those individuals who drink more have fewer interpersonal relationships to draw on as sources of support. Those individuals who drink less seem to have stronger interpersonal support systems.

- *Cognitive reappraisals.* Many former drinkers believe it was critical to their recovery that they had reached a point where they realized that their alcohol use was causing physical and emotional damage.

- *Demographic variables.* There is a tendency for those who drink more to come from lower socioeconomic groups.

- *Severity of drinking problems.* Alcohol-related problems such as blackouts, job problems, and legal difficulties may serve as warning signs to some people that their drinking has started to reach problematic levels.

- *Health problems.* Physical ailments may serve as a warning to the individual that his/her alcohol use has started to reach problematic levels.

- *Involvement in AA and/or religious groups.* Membership may help the individual realize that his/her drinking has started to cause problems.

The team of Humphreys et al. (1995) followed a sample of 135 individuals classified as problem drinkers, who either went through an alcohol detoxification program or who contacted an alcoholism information and referral center, to determine what steps these individuals went through in their recovery. The authors found that although their subjects did not enter formal treatment for their alcohol use problems, there were still two pathways away from problem drinking.

The authors discovered that their subjects fell into 3 subgroups at the end of a 3-year period. The first subgroup was made up of individuals who reported that they had achieved stable abstinence and had apparently been able to abstain from further alcohol

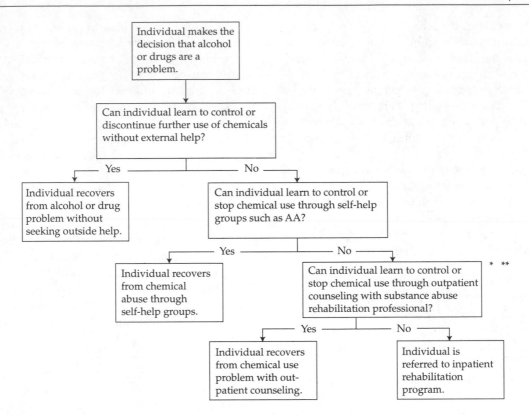

* It is at this point that the individual usually begins the assessment process
  by a substance abuse rehabilitation professional.

** It is only when the individual reaches this point in the rehabilitation process
   if he/she does reach this point, that the individual is likely to be identified as
   having a substance use problem by social scientists.

FIGURE 30.2   The process of recovery.

use during the 3-year follow-up period. The second subgroup was composed of those subjects who had achieved a moderate drinking pattern, consuming no more than five (5) beers/mixed drinks within any given 24-hour time span during the 3-year follow-up period. The final group included those who continued to use alcohol in a problematic manner.

Humphreys et al. (1995) then examined the histories of the individuals in these three groups, to determine what factors seemed relevant to the observed outcome. The authors found that those problem drinkers who became controlled drinkers consumed less alcohol at the start of the study and tended, for the most part, to be members of higher socioeconomic groups. As a group, they also viewed their drinking as being less of a problem than did other drinkers, had higher self-esteem, and were more confident that they could resist the temptation to return to abusive drinking.

Further, the authors found that those individuals who adopted an alcohol-free lifestyle tended to be from lower socioeconomic groups. These individuals tended to have suffered a greater number of lost jobs and economic problems related to their drinking. As a group, the alcohol-free group members were less sure of their ability to control their drinking, and they tended to turn to social support groups such as church and/or AA in their quest for recovery.

Overall, the model that is emerging from clinical experience and research is that recovery from an alcohol/drug use problem is a dynamic process, in which the individual must proceed through a series of specific stages before being able to make any meaningful change(s) in his/her chemical use patterns.

Should Abstinence Be the Goal of Treatment?

One issue that substance abuse rehabilitation professionals fiercely debate is whether the goal of treatment should be to help the individual learn to *control* his/her chemical use or how to abstain from all recreational alcohol/drug use. Although most treatment programs believe that abstinence is the only viable goal of rehabilitation, the truth is that following treatment, the majority of those with alcohol use disorders continue to use alcohol at least occasionally (Peele, 1985; Peele, Brodsky, & Arnold, 1991). In follow-up studies on identified alcohol dependent individuals, George Vaillant (1983, 1996) found that, over the course of their chemical use, they tended to alternate between periods of more and less problematic drinking.

This raises the interesting question of whether treatment centers should advocate that the individual abstain from *all* chemical use, an outcome that is achieved only by a very small minority of those who are treated for alcohol/drug use problems. For example, in the treatment of marijuana addiction, total abstinence from *all* psychoactive drugs is considered essential, if treatment is to be effective (Bloodwortth, 1987). While the ultimate answer to this problem has not been found, it suggests that there is still a great deal to learn about the natural history of alcohol/drug misuse problems and their treatment.

Specific Points to Address with Common Drugs of Abuse

Although the process of recovering from any substance use problem would tend to reflect the steps identified by Prochaska et al. (1992), there are specific issues to consider and address when working with individuals who have been abusing or addicted to different chemicals.

Opiate Addiction: Is Treatment Worthwhile?

Many people seem to believe that, once an opiate addict, always an addict, and they are quite pessimistic about treatment for narcotic addiction. There is some basis for this pessimism, since research has found that 90% of opiate-dependent individuals who are successfully withdrawn from narcotics will return to chemical use within 6 months (Schuckit, 1995a). Another pessimistic view of the evolution of narcotics addiction was provided by Hser et al. (1993). The authors interviewed 581 individuals who were originally identified as being addicted to narcotics by the criminal justice system in the period from 1962 until 1964.

Twenty-four years later, in 1986, the authors found that only 22% of the original sample of 581 narcotics addicts were opiate-free. Some 7% of the original sample was involved in a methadone maintenance program, and 10% reported engaging in only occasional narcotics use. Almost 28% of the original sample had died, with the main causes of death being homicide, suicide, and accidents, in that order.

After reviewing their data, Hser et al. (1993) concluded that if the narcotics addicts in their sample had not stopped chemical use by their late 30s, they were unlikely to do so; the research team then reinterviewed these individuals in 1986. They found that a greater percentage of addicts had died than had achieved abstinence by 1986. This is indeed a rather pessimistic view of the course of narcotics addiction. However, there are also some studies that have concluded that more than a third of all opiate addicts will ultimately be able to achieve and retain sobriety. For those addicts who survive their addiction, abstinence from opiate use is finally achieved in between 6 years (T. Smith, 1994) and 9 years (Jaffe, 1989; Jenike, 1991) after the addiction first developed.

CNS Stimulant Abuse: Withdrawal and Recovery Issues

Although a great deal is known about the manifestations of CNS stimulant abuse/addiction, very little is known about the natural history of dependence on these agents (Jaffe, 1990). A great deal remains to be discovered about the abuse of, and addiction to, cocaine, the amphetamines, and similar drugs. For example, although cocaine has a reputation of being exceptionally addictive, the truth is that not everybody who abuses cocaine will become addicted. Researchers disagree as to the exact percentage of those who use cocaine and then go on to become addicted. The National Institute on Drug Abuse (quoted in Kotulak, 1992) suggested that only about 10% of those who use cocaine actually go on to become heavy users. Restak (1994) gave a higher estimate of 25% to 33% of those who use cocaine going on to become addicted.

The point is that not all cocaine abusers are *addicted* to the drug. The same is true for the other CNS stimulants: not everybody who is abusing a CNS stimulant is addicted to that chemical. It is only through the process of *assessment* (discussed in Chapter 26) that the individual's need for treatment for a cocaine use problem, and the appropriate level of care for that person, is determined. Persons with only CNS stimulant abuse problems rarely require hospital-based detoxification services ("Amphetamines," 1990). This is because withdrawal from the CNS stimulants is rarely life-threatening.

However, hospital-based observation and treatment may be necessary to protect the individual who is depressed as a result of CNS stimulant abuse. Remember that cocaine-induced depression may reach suicidal proportions. The decision to hospitalize/not hospitalize a CNS stimulant abuser should be made on a case-by-case basis by qualified physicians. Some of the factors that must be considered in making the decision to recommend hospitalization for a cocaine abuser include the individual's state of mind, medical status, and whether the person has adequate resources and social support to deal with the withdrawal process on an outpatient basis.

There is very little research into the factors that bring about addiction to the CNS stimulants. In contrast to the research into the genetics of alcoholism, "research on genetic factors in stimulant abuse has not been pursued" (Gawin & Ellinwood, 1988, p. 1177). Thus, there is virtually no information into possible genetic "markers" that might identify the person who is vulnerable to cocaine or amphetamine addiction.

Researchers believe that protracted cocaine abuse may result in a withdrawal syndrome (Satel et al.,

1991). Gawin and Ellinwood (1988) characterized the cocaine-withdrawal syndrome as being "comparable to the acute withdrawal of the alcohol hangover" (p. 1176). Although the cocaine withdrawal syndrome does not include "severe . . . symptoms such as those seen in opiate withdrawal" (Gold & Verebey, 1984, p. 720), research has shown that it is marked by such complaints as paranoia, depression, fatigue, craving for cocaine, agitation, chills, insomnia, nausea, changes in the individual's sleep patterns, ravenous hunger, muscle tremors, headache, and vomiting (DiGregorio, 1990). These symptoms begin 24 to 48 hours after the last dose of cocaine and persist for 7 to 10 days, according to the author.

Stages of Recovery from CNS Stimulant Abuse/Addiction

A triphasic model for the postcocaine binge recovery process has been proposed (Gawin, Khalsa, & Ellinwood, 1994; Gawin & Kleber, 1986). In the early part of the first stage, lasting from 1 to 4 days, the person experienced feelings of agitation, depression, and anorexia (loss of desire to eat), as well as a strong craving for cocaine. As the person progressed through the second half of the first phase, he/she would lose the craving for cocaine, but would experience insomnia and exhaustion, combined with a strong desire for sleep. The second half of the first phase would last from 4 to 7 days, according to the authors.

The second phase of recovery began after 7 days of abstinence; the person would return to a normal sleep pattern and would gradually experience stronger cravings for cocaine and higher levels of anxiety. Conditioned cues would exacerbate the individual's craving for stimulants, drawing the person back to chemical use. If the person was able to withstand the environmental and intrapersonal cues for further drug use, he/she would move into the *extinction* phase and gradually return to a more normal level of function.

The third stage of recovery, extinction, began after 10 weeks of abstinence. If the person could not maintain sobriety and again went on a stimulant binge, the cycle would repeat itself. If the person was able to withstand the craving, there was a good chance of achieving sobriety. Hall et al. (1991) concluded that approximately 80% of those cocaine addicts who were able to abstain from cocaine use for 12 weeks after treatment were still drug-free after 6 months. However, this does not mean that the individual has fully recovered from his/her CNS stimulant addiction. Cocaine and amphetamine addicts might suddenly experience a craving for these drugs "months or years after its last appearance" (Gawin & Ellinwood, 1988, p. 1176), and long after the last period of chemical use.

The research team of Satel et al. (1991) examined the cocaine withdrawal process, and concluded that their data failed to support the model advanced by Gawin and Kleber (1986). The authors found that, for their sample, the cocaine withdrawal process was marked by withdrawal symptoms that declined over the first 3 weeks of inpatient treatment. However, the withdrawal symptoms were much milder than had been anticipated and failed to follow the triphasic model suggested by earlier research.

Thus, researchers have acknowledged that there appears to be a withdrawal syndrome following prolonged cocaine use. But researchers have not reached agreement as to the exact nature of the postcocaine withdrawal syndrome and are exploring various theoretical models to better understand what happens when a cocaine addict stops using chemicals. Further, as part of exploring different ways of working with cocaine addicts, a number of pharmacological agents are being investigated, in the hopes of finding a drug, or combination of drugs, that can control the postcocaine craving that complicates the treatment of cocaine addiction for many of those who are recovering. These agents are discussed in Chapter 32.

The treatment of stimulant addiction involves more than just helping the addicted person stop using the drug. A common complication of stimulant addiction is that the individual has often forgotten what a drug-free life is like (R. K. Siegel, 1982). Further, Gold and Verebey (1984) pointed out that cocaine addiction may lead to vitamin deficiencies, especially of the B complex and C vitamins. Since the stimulant effects of the amphetamines are so similar to that of cocaine, one would expect that the amphetamines would also lead to vitamin deficiencies in a pattern similar to that seen in chronic cocaine abuse.

The authors found that 73% of a sample of cocaine abusers tested had at least one vitamin deficiency. The authors concluded that these vitamin deficiencies reflected the malnutrition found in cocaine abuse, since cocaine may cause anorexia. The authors recommended vitamin replacement therapy as part of the treatment of cocaine addiction.

Total abstinence from drugs of abuse is thought to be essential in the treatment of cocaine or amphetamine use problems. Hall et al. (1991) found that those cocaine-dependent persons who made a commitment to full abstinence following treatment were more likely to avoid further cocaine use than were addicts who did not desire abstinence as a treatment goal. Follow-up treatment should include behavior modification and psychotherapy to help the individual learn the skills to continue abstaining from chemicals (Gold & Verebey, 1984). Social support, and self-help group support in the form of Alcoholics Anonymous, Narcotics Anonymous, or Cocaine Anonymous, is often of great help. As with the other forms of drug addiction, the recovering individual is at risk for cross-addiction to other chemicals, and needs to avoid other drug use for the rest of his/her life.

Issues Surrounding Recovery from Marijuana Use

Although marijuana use has been popular in this country since the Prohibition era, and most certainly after the "hippie" generation "discovered" marijuana in the 1960s, virtually nothing is known about the treatment of marijuana abuse/dependence (Stevens, Roffman, & Simpson, 1994; "Treatment," 1995). It is known that the short-term, acute reaction to marijuana does not require any special intervention (Brophy, 1993). Thus, marijuana-induced feelings of anxiety or panic reactions usually respond to "firm reassurance in a nonthreatening environment" (Mirin et al., 1991, p. 304). However, the patient should be watched to ensure that no harm comes to either the marijuana user, or to others.

There are a number of problems associated with working with marijuana abusers. First, it is rare for a person to be abusing *only* marijuana. Thus, treatment usually must focus on polychemical abuse of a number of chemicals, rather than just marijuana alone. Second, marijuana users usually do not present themselves for treatment, unless there is some form of coercion, in part because they usually do not view themselves as being addicted to a recreational chemical ("Treatment," 1995).

Third, even when the marijuana user *does* enter treatment, the specific therapeutic methods for working with the chronic marijuana user are not well developed (Mirin et al., 1991). It is known that marijuana users often use it as a way to cope with negative feelings, especially anger ("Treatment," 1995). Thus, rehabilitation professionals must help the client identify specific problem areas in his/her life and then help the individual identify non-drug-related coping mechanisms for these trigger situations.

A treatment program that identifies the individual's reason/s for continued drug use and that helps the individual find alternatives to further drug use, is thought to be most effective. Supplemental groups that focus on vocational rehabilitation and socialization skills are also of value in the treatment of the chronic marijuana user (Mirin et al., 1991). Jenike (1991) reported that treatment efforts should focus on understanding the abuser's disturbed psychosocial relationships.

Bloodworth (1987) concluded that "family therapy is almost a necessity" (p. 183). Group therapy as a means of dealing with peer pressure to use chemicals was necessary in this author's opinion and self-help support groups such as Alcoholics Anonymous (AA) or Narcotics Anonymous (NA) "cannot be overemphasized" (Bloodworth, 1987, p. 183).

Issues Surrounding the Treatment of Nicotine Addiction

When one asks cigarette smokers why they continue to smoke despite the dangers associated with this habit, the response is often, "I can't help myself. I'm addicted." It is believed that the addictive power of nicotine is why 90% to 98% of those who attempt to quit smoking in any given year will ultimately fail (Benowitz & Henningfield, 1994; Henningfield, 1995; Sherman, 1994).

Although health care workers have tried for many years to identify which factors contribute to a person's successful attempt to quit smoking, they have met with little success (Kenford et al., 1994).

Thus, cigarette cessation programs are something of a hit-or-miss affair, in which neither the leaders nor the participants have little knowledge of what *really* works. Smoking cessation training programs usually help between 70% to 80% of the participants to stop smoking on a short-term basis. But, of those who attempt to stop smoking, two-thirds may stop for a very few days, but only 2% to 3% will be tobacco-free a year later (Henningfield, 1995). The research team of Hughes et al. (1991) found that 65% of their experimental sample relapsed within the first month of quitting, suggesting that the first month is especially difficult for the recent ex-smoker.

There appears to be a relationship between the frequency with which a given individual smokes, and his/her success in giving up tobacco use. The research team of S. Cohen et al. (1989) reviewed data from 10 different research projects that involved a total of 5000 subjects who were attempting to stop smoking cigarettes.

The authors found that light smokers, who were defined as those who smoked less than 20 cigarettes each day, were significantly more likely to be able to stop smoking on their own than were heavy smokers. S. Cohen et al. (1989) also found that the number of previous attempts to quit smoking was not an indication of hopelessness. Rather, the authors found that the number of unsuccessful previous attempts was unrelated to whether the smoker would be able to quit this time. They concluded that "most people who fail a single attempt [to quit smoking] will try again and again and eventually quit" (p. 1361).

Another factor that seems to be associated with the difficulty smokers experience when attempting to quit is their *expectancies* for the nicotine withdrawal process. The team of Tate et al. (1994) formed 4 subgroups from their research sample of 62 cigarette smokers. Those former smokers who were led to believe that they would not experience any significant distress during the nicotine withdrawal process reported significantly fewer physical or emotional complaints than did the other research groups. It appeared to the authors that the individual's expectations for the nicotine withdrawal process may play a role in how the individual interprets and responds to the symptoms experienced during early abstinence.

There is other evidence to support the theory that the individual's expectations for recovery can influence the experience of abstinence. The team of Kviz et al. (1995) found that for smokers over the age of 50, the perceived degree of difficulty in quitting was negatively associated with the individual's actual attempts to quit smoking. In other words, especially for smokers over the age of 50, the harder the individual expected the task of quitting to be, the less likely he/she was to do so. Thus, the individual's expectations for quitting were found to play a significant role in whether the individual actually did quit smoking cigarettes.

Smokers who want to quit should be warned that the struggle against cigarette smoking is a lifelong one and that their mind-set will play a major role in whether they are successful. Further, former smokers should be warned that they will be vulnerable to relapse for the rest of their life.

Although there has been a great deal of emphasis on formal cigarette cessation treatment programs, perhaps as many as 90% (Brunton et al., 1994; Fiore et al., 1990) to 95% (Hughes, 1992; Kozlowski et al., 1989; Peele, 1989) of cigarette smokers who quit do so without participating in a formal treatment program. Of those smokers who do quit, it would seem that the individual's motivation to quit smoking is most "critical" (Jaffe, 1989, p. 682) to the success of their efforts. These conclusions raise serious questions as to whether extensive treatment programs are necessary for tobacco dependence. But formal treatment programs may be of value to those who are heavy smokers or who are at risk for tobacco-related illness.

Issues Surrounding the Treatment of Anabolic Steroid Abusers

The first step in the treatment of the steroid abuser is identification of those individuals who are indeed abusing anabolic steroids. The physician may, on the basis of clinical history and blood and/or urine tests, be the first person to suspect that a patient is abusing steroids and is in the best position to confront the user. Addictions counselors are not thought to have a significant role to play in the treatment of the anabolic steroid user, at least in the earliest stages.

Once the steroid abuser has been identified, close medical supervision of the patient to identify and treat potential complications of steroid abuse is necessary. The attending physician may need to consider the need for a gradual detoxification program for the steroid abuser. Most medical complications caused by steroid abuse usually clear up after the individual stops the use of steroids (Hough & Kovan, 1990); however, some of the complications caused by steroid abuse (e.g., heart tissue damage) may be permanent. Surgical intervention may be possible to correct some of the side effects of steroid use (Hough & Kovan), but this is not always possible.

Following detoxification from anabolic steroids, staff members should work with the patient to identify why the person started using steroids to begin with. Self-concept issues should be identified, and the proper therapy initiated to help the steroid user learn to avoid artificial crutches in achieving self-acceptance. Proper nutritional counseling may be necessary to help the athlete learn how to enhance body strength without using potentially harmful substances such as anabolic steroids, and individual support programs should be started.

Summary

In this chapter, two models of the recovery process were discussed. The most popular and, apparently, the more widely used model was introduced by Prochaska et al. (1992). This model suggests that clients who want to make behavioral change(s) proceed from a *precontemplation* period, in which no specific change is being contemplated, through a phase in which they are thinking about possibly making some change(s) (*contemplation*), and on to a period in which they actively consider the possibility of change (*determination* phase).

Those clients who proceed enter the *action* phase, in which they attempt to make the desired behavioral change(s), and if successful, they enter the *maintenance* phase, where the new behavior becomes entrenched. Also discussed in this chapter were specific points to address in treating clients who are abusing the popular drugs of abuse.

CHAPTER THIRTY-ONE

Problems in Treating Chemical Dependency

Research has consistently demonstrated that treatment is more effective than criminal justice sanctions in dealing with the problem of drug abuse (Scheer, 1994b). But, no matter which treatment approach therapists choose to use, they may experience problems in working with the recovering addict. In this chapter, we examine some of the more common, and more serious, problems encountered by treatment professionals working with recovering addicts in different settings.

Limit Testing by Clients in Treatment

Clients in therapeutic relationships, including addicted clients in a treatment setting, often "test the limits"—either consciously or unconsciously—to determine whether the professional's treatment will be consistent. The client's limit-testing may assume several forms, from missed appointments to the use of chemicals while in treatment.

The chemical dependency professional should be aware that dependability and consistency also apply to the enforcement of the rules of the program. To counter the problem of chemical use by patients in treatment, McCarthy and Borders (1985) told patients in a methadone maintenance program that their urine would be tested to detect continued chemical abuse. Further, the patients were warned that if their urine tested positive for other drugs four times in the next year, they would be placed on a narcotic withdrawal program in place of the desired methadone maintenance.

It was found that patients in this structured program achieved significantly greater program compliance, and were less likely to use drugs, than were a matched control group of addicts who were not in such a structured program. Thus, enforcement of the rules resulted in a reduced rate of illicit drug use by the patients.

The Counselor and Treatment "Secrets"

A common situation is for the client to ask for an individual conference with the staff member, and then to confess to a rules infraction such as that he/she has used chemicals while in treatment. Often, this admission of guilt is made to a student or intern at the agency, rather than to a regular staff member. Following this admission, the client will ask that the staff member not bring this information to the group, other staff members, or the program director for fear of being discharged from treatment.

The chemical dependency professional who honors a request not to tell other staff members would be entering into a partnership with the addict that makes the professional an enabler. In some situations, to not report this rules violation might make the professional vulnerable to later extortion by the client, who could report the professional to his/her superiors for not passing on the information to staff.

The proper response to this situation is to document the material discussed *immediately*, in writing, through the appropriate channels. This might be a memo, or an entry into the client's progress notes, as well as a discussion of the material revealed by the client with the professional's immediate supervisor. This is done, without malice, to ensure uniform enforcement of the rules for all clients and to protect the professional's reputation.

Treatment Noncompliance

Detractors from treatment for substance use problems often point to the high noncompliance rate as "proof" that rehabilitation is not effective for substance use disorders. Such a position overlooks that the failure of a given patient to follow treatment recommendations, or to benefit from treatment, is not unique to substance abuse rehabilitation programs. "Inadequate response" to treatment because the patient failed to follow the recommendations of the physician is an ongoing problem in many areas of medicine. Lacombe, Vicente, Pages, and Morselli (1996) cited as one example a study in England that found that 14% of the patients who received a prescription failed to have it filled. Patients who fail to have a prescription filled certainly cannot benefit from that treatment intervention. Table 31-1 provides a summary of different medical conditions, and the percentage of patients who do not follow treatment recommendations for that disorder.

As Table 31-1 demonstrates, treatment noncompliance is not limited to substance abuse rehabilitation

TABLE 31-1 Approximate Rates of Treatment Noncompliance

Class of medications	Percentage of patients who fail to follow dosing instructions
Antiepileptics	30–50%
Antihypertensives	30–40
Blood lipid-lowering agents	25–30
Antiarrhythmics	20
Antidepressants	30–40
Immunosuppressive agents	18
Antidiabetics	30–50
Anticoagulants	30
Antiasthmatics	20

Note: Adapted from Lacombe, P. S., Vicente, J. A. G., Pages, J. C., & Morselli, P. L. (1996). "Causes and Problems of Nonresponse or Poor Response to Drugs." *Drugs, 51*, 552–570.

programs. However, only 10% to 30% of those who are deemed to be at risk for an alcohol use disorder actually follow through with recommendations to enter treatment (Cooney et al., 1995). Patient retention is also a problem. More than one addicted person has entered treatment one day and left within a day or two having satisfied the stipulation of parents, judges, or family that they "enter a treatment program." "After all," many seem to reason, "nobody said anything about my *staying* there, did they?"

It is not uncommon for people who are dependent on chemicals to openly admit "I am addicted to chemicals," not because they want to abstain from chemicals, but because in making this admission the individual seems to find an excuse to *continue* using them. Such people follow a circular pattern of logic, almost an elaborate rationalization, by which the word "addicted" comes to mean "hopelessly addicted." Since they are hopelessly addicted, at least in their own mind, they give themselves permission to go on abusing chemicals. This bizarre justification for chemical use overlooks that addiction is a treatable disease. The first part of the "treatment" is often spent convincing people that they are indeed addicted, and need help for the drug dependency that has come to dominate their life. This awareness, and the commitment to enter into treatment, is often achieved through the intervention process.

But, after alcohol/drug dependent individuals enter treatment, they must complete the rehabilitation process. As discussed in Chapter 29, substance abuse treatment programs commonly experience significant levels of patient attrition. For example, McCusker et al. (1996) found that at one publicly funded residential treatment facility in Massachusetts that worked with individuals addicted to chemicals other than alcohol, 50% of the patients admitted to treatment dropped out before the end of 3 months, and two-thirds left treatment before 6 months. Thus, noncompliance is a serious problem for rehabilitation professionals.

Relapse and Relapse Prevention

One of the more destructive forms of treatment noncompliance is for the individual to return to the active use of chemicals. Indeed, "the most common treatment outcome for alcoholics and addicts is relapse" (Dimeff & Marlatt, 1995, p. 176). Thus, entry into treatment should not be seen as a guarantee that the person will actually stop using chemicals. Even patients who complete treatment are likely to return to the use of drugs/alcohol at least briefly, before finally initiating an effective abstinence program.

Since the late 1970s, the focus of treatment has shifted away from simply "getting them sober," to that of arming recovering addicts against the forces that can contribute to relapse. This change in treatment philosophy came about after research revealed that total abstinence from recreational drug use was quite rare after the completion of treatment. Rather than abstaining from all further substance use, most graduates of treatment programs still use chemicals on an episodic basis, "with alternating periods of abstinence and relapse" (DeJong, 1994, p. 682).

Research also revealed that the first 90 days following discharge from treatment is a period of special vulnerability for the individual's potential relapse back to drug use (DeJong, 1994; Dimeff & Marlatt, 1995). Many of those who returned to the use of recreational chemicals did so in the first 90 days following discharge. To some, this is a sign that treatment does not work. However, experienced substance abuse rehabilitation professionals have long known that the disease of addiction is one that can be *arrested*, but can never be *cured*.

If the disease is only arrested, it can spring back into full bloom whenever conditions allow it to reassert itself. Thus, it was not surprising to these professionals to learn that many treatment graduates relapse into the use of chemicals. To combat this tendency for the former patient to return to the use of chemicals, treatment professionals began to place emphasis on *relapse prevention* skills that patients could develop while in treatment, to use after completing the rehabilitation program.

Chiauzzi (1990) found that four elements were common to those who relapsed. First, those individuals who relapsed often demonstrated *personality traits* that interfered with continued sobriety. Such relapse-prone personality traits include a tendency toward compulsive behaviors, since such individuals do not adjust well to even minor changes in routine. Another personality trait that interfered with recovery was a tendency toward dependency, since such individuals had trouble asserting their desire to maintain a recovery program (Chiauzzi).

Passive-aggressive personality traits place the individual at risk for relapse because of a tendency to blame others for one's behavior. The narcissistic traits often found in addicted persons prevents many from admitting to the need for help during a weak moment, while antisocial personality traits underscore a tendency toward impulsiveness and a desire not to follow the road taken by others (Chiauzzi, 1990).

A second factor advanced by Chiauzzi (1990) as contributing to relapse is a tendency for the individual to *substitute addictions*. Often, recovering individuals substitute work, a new relationship, or other chemicals, for the drug that they are no longer using. Caffeine or drug abuse, a relationship where the individual is dependent on the partner, or eating disorders might signal a high-risk situation for relapse.

Third, Chiauzzi (1990) found that the individual's *narrow view of recovery* was often a factor in relapse. All too often, the recovering individual equated abstinence, or simple attendance at a self-help group such as AA as being recovery. Such a view of recovery places individuals at risk for relapse because they are not working to change their personality structure or to solve interpersonal problems that contributed to the development of the addiction in the first place. Such individuals do not develop the self-awareness necessary to be aware of the personal drift toward relapse.

Finally, Chiauzzi (1990) found that what he termed *warning signals* of impending relapse were often overlooked by the individual. Chiauzzi's concept of warning signals is very similar to the concept of the minidecisions first reported by Cummings, Gordon, and Marlatt (1980). Cummings et al. presented a theoretical model of drug relapse in which the relapse was viewed as evolving out of a series of what they called "mini-decisions" (p. 297). The authors found there was no major decision by the individual to return to drug use. Rather, the road to relapse was paved with small decisions that, added together, "begin a chain of behaviors which may set the stage for a relapse to occur" (p. 297).

Examples of such a minidecision might be for the recovering addict to continue a friendship with an active addict, or to go over to the local bar "just to play pool." Chiauzzi (1990) reported that individuals who relapsed failed to notice negative thoughts, a desire to spend time with drug-using friends, or physical illness. Cummings et al. (1980) pointed out that these seemingly innocent minidecisions increase the chance that recovering addicts will encounter a situation where they are likely to relapse.

Often such a minidecision is the individual's choice to stop going to his/her regular AA or NA meetings. The initial decision might be to cut back from five meetings a week to four meetings each week, then the next decision might be to cut back from four meetings each week to perhaps only one or two meetings a week. Eventually, the decision might be to go to meetings only every other week, then once a month, until the individual no longer has any contact with his/her recovery support system.

Another potential threat to the individual's recovery program are those *maladaptive thoughts* that might contribute to the return to active chemical use (Keller, 1996). An example of such a maladaptive thought is the alcohol/drug addicted individual who returns to the old "using" environment, to "see if I could just walk down the same street and not feel the urge to use anymore." Another maladaptive thought is the recovering individual who only "stopped off to pay him some money that I owed him, and I found drugs all over the place!" as if the drug-using behavior of this friend were a revelation. A third example of a maladaptive thought might be the individual who concluded that "I've been doing pretty good . . . one drink surely could not hurt me!". Even after the individual in this hypothetical example has again struggled to reestablish his/her recovery, he/she might not understand how his/her thinking set the stage for the last relapse.

When maladaptive thoughts put the individual "at risk" to use chemicals, the newly recovering individual is at a decision point. He/she must either reaffirm the commitment to personal abstinence, or start back on the path to the active use of chemicals. If the individual has adequate coping skills to support

continued abstinence, her/she will reaffirm the commitment to recovery. However, if the individual's coping skills are inadequate, he/she is in danger of relapsing back to active chemical use.

It is virtually guaranteed that every recovering person will encounter at least one high-risk situation, which is to say a situation where the possibility of dug use is high. Failure to effectively deal with a high-risk situation is a common cause of relapse. For example, Dimeff and Marlatt (1995) reported that fully 75% of all relapses involved the failure to successfully deal with a high-risk situation. Essentially, high-risk situations can be grouped into two categories (Cummings et al., 1980). The first category consists of the acute period of drug withdrawal, when the individual would be motivated to avoid further withdrawal discomfort through the ingestion of chemicals.

The second group of high-risk situations might be viewed as the social, environmental, and emotional states that the individual perceives as stressful, for which drugs were used by the individual as a coping mechanism in the past (Cummings et al., 1980; Keller, 1996). In this second group of high-risk situations, cognitive evaluations of the social, environmental, or emotional stimuli mediate whether the individual considers the possibility of drug use. Such cognitive evaluations may then be interpreted by the individual as an *urge* or *craving* to use a substance.

Many "stimulus factors" (Shiffman, 1992, p. 9) can contribute to lapses in sobriety. Research evidence now suggests that conditioned learning takes place while individuals are using alcohol/drugs. When they are again exposed to the same (or similar) sights, sounds, or emotions that were associated with the chemical use, these persons may again feel a craving for chemicals. For example, it has been found that recovering opiate-dependent individuals can suddenly experience a craving for narcotics even after being drug-free for months, or years, if they return to the neighborhood where they once used chemicals (Galanter, 1993).

To combat the influence of environmental triggers toward chemical use, Shiffman advocated the use of behavioral rehearsals to help the client learn skills for avoiding relapse. A second area of emphasis is the identification of the client's feelings of demoralization and self-blame during the early phases of recovery, according to the author. Such cognitive intervention has been shown to be at least as effective as behavioral training for environmental triggers toward relapse.

Annis and Davis (1991) identified the first step in relapse prevention as being the *identification of potential high-risk situations* for each individual, a step that they termed *anticipating problem situations*. Self-monitoring of internal states by the client and direct observation of the client by treatment center staff were just two of the methods for identifying high-risk situations. The authors also advocated the use of such psychological tests as the Inventory of Drinking Situations (IDS-100), a 100-item questionnaire that their clients took to identify the situations where they were most likely to drink. This test data was then used to develop a hierarchy of drinking situations. Staff would work with the client to identify strengths, resources, and environmental supports for dealing with the potential relapse situation, and help the client develop specific behavioral coping techniques for remaining abstinent. The authors also used rehearsal sessions, where the client practiced useful skills for preventing relapse in high-risk situations.

Niaura et al. (1988) reported that, when the individual is armed with cognitive and behavioral coping mechanisms that counteract feelings of helplessness in the face of cognitive, social, or environmental cues for drug use, that individual is unlikely to relapse. The individual can also carry a reminder card in the wallet or purse with written instructions on the steps to take for limiting the relapse.

DeJong (1994) identified antecedents of relapse:

- Stress.
- Negative emotional states.
- Interpersonal conflict.
- Social pressure.
- Positive emotional states.
- Use of other substances.
- Presence of drug-related cues.

Thus, many potential triggers exist for relapse. Some of the more common triggers are summarized in Table 31-2.

Another potential contributing factor for relapse is for treatment staff to take a short-term view of recovery. Researchers have found that after individuals

TABLE 31-2   Common Relapse Situations

Category of relapse	Description of situation that contributed to or caused relapse	Percentage of cases
Negative emotional states	Patient experiences feelings of frustration, anger, anxiety, depression, boredom, etc.	35%
Peer pressure	Pressure is felt from either a single person (such as a close friend) or group of people (e.g., co-workers) to use chemicals	20
Interpersonal conflict	Conflict arises between patient and a friend, employer, employee, family member, or dating partner	16
Craving for drugs/alcohol	Person becomes preoccupied with use of alcohol and/or drugs, despite abstinence	9
Testing personal control	Person exposes self to high-risk situation, to see if he/she is able to resist urges to use chemicals	5
Negative physical states	Person is experiencing a negative physical state such as illness, postsurgical distress, or injury	3

Note. Adapted from material provided by Dimeff and Marlatt (1995).

who have achieved abstinence for 6 years are unlikely to return to the use of alcohol (Vaillant, 1996). Drawing on a 50-year longitudinal study of white males, Vaillant found that for those men with alcohol use problems, 2, 3, or even 4 years of abstinence was not a sufficiently long period to gauge the individual's prognosis for maintaining abstinence. However, in contrast to the high rate of relapse for those men who were abstinent for less than 5 years, Vaillant found that relatively few men who had been alcohol-free for 6 or more years returned to the use of this chemical. This study suggests that treatment staff must also help recovering patients learn not to let down their guard before abstinence becomes a new lifestyle, a process that seems to take more than 5 years.

The concept of relapse prevention has offered some insight into the forces that can undermine the initial success achieved in treatment. The theoretical models of relapse and its prevention seem to offer some promise in the treatment of chemical dependency, and in the next few years, research should disclose whether current models of relapse prevention are adequate or indicate a need for further study.

Chemical Use—Craving and Urges

The concepts of *craving* and *urges* are often confused by both health care workers, and patients who are recovering from alcohol/drug addiction. Technically, craving is a cognitive state, in which individuals start to think about how they felt while under the influence of alcohol/drugs and how nice it would be to feel that way again (Beck, Wright, Newman, & Liese, 1993). As they begin to think about how they felt, they want to recreate that feeling. The concept of euphoric recall, discussed earlier in this text, is a form of craving.

Individuals who begin to crave chemicals reframe chemical use into positive terms. Since alcohol and/or drugs were needed to experience that feeling before, the individual begins to redefine a return to chemical use as a positive step in the process of recreating the euphoria felt while using chemicals. Vernon Johnson (1980) termed this process *euphoric recall*. As a result of euphoric recall, individuals establish a state of mind where further chemical use not only is acceptable, but is desirable.

Urges, in contrast to craving, are behavioral impulses to find and use alcohol/drugs (Beck et al., 1993). In a sense, chemical use urges reflect the specific actions that the individual might take to use chemicals. Beck et al. identified four different situations that contributed to urges to use chemicals: The first was the individual's learned *response to the discomfort of withdrawal.* As discussed earlier, many recreational chemicals have a characteristic pattern of withdrawal symptoms. Alcohol/drug dependent individuals learn to avoid experiencing these withdrawal symptoms by using more of the chemical that they are addicted to. For example, the nicotine-dependent individual will smoke a cigarette, or the alcohol-dependent individual will have another drink in response to the earliest symptoms of withdrawal.

Next, addicted individuals tend to want to use chemicals when they are unhappy or uncomfortable (Beck et al., 1993). These chemical-use urges are triggered by some of the antecedents of relapse identified by DeJong (1994). These antecedent situations then cause the individual to crave chemicals to cope with the negative situation. Over time, the individual gives in to these cravings by beginning to make specific behavioral plans to use chemicals (the urge to use alcohol/drugs).

The third source of drug-use urges is external drug-use "cues," according to the authors. Such cues might include cleaning out one's apartment, and finding a "stash" of alcohol or drugs. Another cue might be a chance (or intentional) encounter with a former using partner, the return to the same environment where the individual once used chemicals, or a chance encounter with the many sights, sounds, or smells associated with chemical use. For example, some recovering heroin addicts begin to think about using heroin again, if they happen to smell a burning match.

Finally, the fourth source of chemical use urges is the individual's desire to enhance positive experiences (Beck et al., 1993). Many recovering alcohol/drug dependent individuals find that they associated chemical use with feelings of pleasure. When—especially in the early stages of recovery—they find themselves starting to feel good, they begin to fear losing this feeling. The urge is to return to the use of chemicals to extend, or enhance, the positive experience, so that it lasts longer. This category of urge was discussed by DeJong (1994) under the heading "positive emotional states."

It is essential that individuals in the earliest stages of recovery learn about craving and urges, and ways to cope with these experiences. The alternative is that recovery will be threatened, or destroyed, by these urges to return to the use of chemicals.

Controlled Drinking

The concept of helping the alcoholic to return to "social" or "controlled" drinking has been a controversial one for many years (Helzer et al., 1985; Hester, 1995; Schuckit, 1995; Vaillant & Hiller-Sturmhofel, 1996). Ever since the first preliminary reports that it *might* be possible to train a small number of people with alcohol use problems to return to a state of controlled drinking, many alcohol-dependent individuals have seized on this concept to justify their continued drinking.

Research suggests that less than 2% of those alcoholics might safely return to social drinking (Helzer et al., 1985; Vaillant, 1996; Vaillant & Hiller-Sturmhofel, 1996). In contrast to the wishes of those who are alcohol dependent, controlled drinking is a viable goal only for those individuals who are not clearly addicted and who have not experienced significant problems associated with addiction (Hester, 1989). But it is not a goal for the confirmed alcoholic. The authors suggested that it might be possible to teach a large percentage of those who *abuse* alcohol to control their drinking. But, only about 2% of those who are *addicted* may return to social drinking (Helzer et al.).

Researchers have found that individuals who are moderately to severely addicted to alcohol would quickly return to abusive drinking if they attempted to learn how to drink on a social basis. The team of Watson, Hancock, Malovrh, Gearhart, and Raden (1996) tracked a 48-week follow-up study of 102 alcohol-dependent individuals who had been in treatment for substance abuse. Fifty-one of these individuals abstained from alcohol following treatment, while the other 51 attempted to engage in controlled or limited drinking following discharge.

The authors found that those who attempted to use alcohol following treatment were 4 times as likely to return to abusive drinking as were the control subjects. The authors found that the majority of those who tried to drink in a controlled manner returned to total abstinence, following their attempt at limited drinking. These findings lend support to the growing body of evidence that suggests controlled drinking is virtually impossible after physical dependence to alcohol has developed.

Self-control training appears to be most effective only for those individuals with less severe alcohol use problems (Hester, 1995; Meyer, 1989a). *Every* alcoholic, however, wants to believe that he/she is in the 1% to 2% of alcoholics who may be able to return a controlled or social pattern of alcohol use. Given this percentage for successful adaptation, one must question whether controlled drinking should be a viable goal for the person suspected of having an alcohol-use problem.

Those alcohol-dependent individuals who wish to attempt to learn how to drink in a "social" manner be allowed to try to learn to do so. The individual's success/failure at attempting to control his/her drinking will either allow for a successful brief intervention for those clients who do learn how to control their drinking, or set the stage for abstinence-based interventions for those clients who fail this task (Hester, 1995). Thus, a trial of "controlled drinking" may prove of value in helping the individual realize the need for total abstinence (Hester). Further, it is not uncommon for clients to switch from a goal of controlled drinking to abstinence, as they come to more fully understand the consequences of continued alcohol use (Hester). Once individuals fail in this task, they may be more willing to accept that alcoholism is a disease "that can be arrested with abstinence but never cured in a way that will permit the person to drink again" (Brown, 1995, p. 11).

But, the mental health or substance abuse professional needs to weigh the potential benefits from this trial against the potential risks. Confirmed alcoholics who believe they can learn social drinking behaviors once again, *and maintain* a pattern of social drinking for the rest of their lives, are taking a bet where the odds are at best 49:1, if not 99:1, against them. There are few of us who would be willing to chance an operation where the odds were 50 to 1 against us. Few would be willing to consent for a surgical procedure where the person only had a 1% or a 2% chance of recovery. Yet many an alcoholic has voiced the secret wish that he or she could win this bet, and land in what more than one alcoholic has called "the lucky 2%."

Clients Who Appear for Their Appointment while under the Influence of Chemicals

This problem is encountered most often in the outpatient treatment setting, although it does occasionally happen on inpatient treatment units. The client arrives for an appointment, under the influence of chemicals. Perhaps the client slurs words, has an unfocused look, or smells of alcohol, or marijuana. But, for any number of reasons, it appears that the client is under the influence of one or more recreational chemicals.

It is not uncommon for the substance abuse rehabilitation worker to suspect that his/her client is under the influence of chemicals because of the client's behavior. In such cases, the treatment professional may request that the client provide a urine sample under appropriate supervision, so that the appropriate laboratory tests can confirm/rule out possible illicit chemical use. In other cases, simply asking the client whether he/she has been using chemicals will be sufficient to obtain an admission.

The client's use of chemicals prior to a therapy session raises two issues: one a clinical issue, and the second a matter of liability. The client's use of chemicals on his/her therapy can hardly be said to be a minor matter. At the least, it will be impossible to conduct a therapy session when the client is under the influence of recreational chemicals because it is virtually impossible to conduct any form of effective therapy with a client who is intoxicated (Washton, 1995). Thus, such meetings are, essentially, a waste of time and should be rescheduled for a later date.

But the client's use of recreational chemicals prior to a therapy session also raises a number of liability issues for the client and the therapist. Thus, the health care worker's responsibility might not end

with simply rescheduling the appointment. Depending on state law, the therapist might be required to actively intervene, to protect the client and/or others. For example, there is a liability question if the therapist knowingly allows an intoxicated client to drive home. If the client should have an accident on the way home, harming either self or another person, the therapist might be held liable for these injuries, on the grounds that he/she allowed the client to drive while under the influence of chemicals.

The therapist might also be held liable if the client arrives for a session obviously intoxicated, the therapist recommends that the client go home to "sleep it off" and the client then suffers an adverse reaction at home. Thus, depending on the specific state law, mental health workers may be required to intervene in cases of substance use, possibly to the point of initiating an involuntary commitment to a hospital for detoxification. To limit liability, it is recommended that substance abuse rehabilitation professionals be aware of the specific state laws that govern professional responsibility for cases where the therapist should know or suspect that the client is intoxicated during a session.

Toxicology Testing as a Measure of Treatment Compliance and Drug Use

Although it is possible to detect some illicit drugs in blood plasma, the low concentrations at which many recreational chemicals are biologically active does not make blood testing the most efficient way to detect them (Woolf & Shannon, 1995). On the other hand, it is possible to detect metabolites of the recreational chemicals in urine samples for hours, and in some cases days, or even weeks, after the individual stopped using that substance. When properly utilized, urine toxicology testing provides one of the most comprehensive means of monitoring recreational substance use.

But urine toxicology screens are not without their disadvantages. Depending on the circumstances under which the urine sample is obtained, it may be necessary to obtain the patient's consent (Woolf & Shannon, 1995). Obviously, in a medical emergency, a physician would not need to obtain the written consent of a family member of an unconscious patient to test for possible drug use. In such cases, the medical necessity of confirming/ruling out recreational drug use would outweigh the requirement to obtain the written consent of a patient/relative. However, for routine toxicology screening, the patient's written consent is usually required.

Further, urine toxicology testing is not an exact science. It is possible for the test procedure to mistakenly identify a patient as having abused one or more recreational chemicals, when in fact that individual did not do so. Some nonsteroidal antiinflammatory drugs (NSAIDS) such as aspirin, ibuprofen, and Tolmetin may interfere with the tests conducted on urine samples to detect illicit drug use. The nonnarcotic cough suppressant dextromethorphan might register as a metabolite of a narcotic or PCP, on one popular urine toxicology test known as the EMIT, and a number of other over-the-counter or prescription drugs might register as a recreational substance on one or more of the urine toxicology tests currently in use.

Further, commercial testing systems may fail to detect the use of some semisynthetic narcotics such as Dilaudid (hydromorphone) or fentanyl ("Dilandid Users," 1995). Thus, as stated earlier, although it is often a useful adjunct to assessment or treatment, urine toxicology testing is an imperfect procedure.

A further complication of the toxicology testing process is that it is not uncommon for some individuals to attempt to manipulate the results of the urine toxicology test. One small study conducted in England found that 20% of the urine samples tested showed evidence of tampering ("British find 20%," 1995). There are a number of common methods by which drug users attempt to manipulate the results of a urine toxicology test. For example, drug abusers may try either to substitute another person's urine sample for their own or to substitute an old sample of their own urine, for a current urine sample. In the latter case, the person will take care to insure that he/she uses a urine sample from before the time that he/she used chemicals.

A favorite trick is for the client to have a "clean" (i.e., drug-free) urine sample on hand, possibly hidden in a balloon or small bottle. When asked for a urine sample, the client will walk into the toilet stall, then quietly empty the container into the sample bottle. If successful, the client will be able to offer the "clean" urine sample for his/her own, which would show evidence of illicit drug use.

A second method by which clients attempt to tamper with the test results is to "accidentally" dip the bottle into the water in the toilet. This will dilute the urine so much that it is unlikely that the laboratory could detect any *urine*, never mind possible chemical use! One way to avoid this danger is to test the specific gravity and level of acidity of the urine sample, since toilet water has a different specific gravity and acid level than does urine. Another way to avoid this danger is to have the water in the toilet colored with a dye, so that it cannot be substituted for urine.

A third technique that some drug users have tried to avoid having their recreational chemical use detected by urine toxicology testing is to "force" fluids. The intent is to dilute whatever traces of chemicals might be found in the urine sample below the detection value, by providing an unusually large volume of urine. For this reason, many laboratories recommend that the urine sample submitted for testing be drawn from the client's first visit to the toilet in the morning, when urine is most concentrated.

In theory, it *is* possible to dilute one's urine so much that any evidence of illicit drug use would not be detected by current testing techniques. But, according to the "Simple Way," (1994), the person would need to ingest at least *a gallon* of water at once. Even if he/she were able to accomplish this, the specific gravity and creatinine levels of the obtained urine sample would be so low as to alert staff that the urine sample had been altered in some way, according to the authors. Thus, forcing fluids is of limited value to the addict who wants to avoid detection through urine toxicology testing.

A fourth way some clients attempt to defeat the urine toxicology screen is to substitute another substance for the urine sample. For example, some patients have substituted a small sample of a certain unnamed diet soda for the requested urine ("Forum," 1991) . Two ounces of this unnamed diet soda would, after being held under the arm for one hour to simulate the body's warmth, be accepted as a valid urine sample "98 percent of the time" (p. 56). Obviously, this false "urine" sample will not detect *any* drug/alcohol use. However, it would also lack the other characteristics of urine, which would soon be evident if laboratory staff were to test the sample for specific gravity, chemical composition, or acidity.

Finally, some drug users may try to hide evidence of chemical use in a urine sample by adding foreign substances that they believe will defeat the chemical tests conducted on the urine. There are substances that are thought to be able to hide evidence of recent illicit drug use. There are also some commercial products that supposedly will eliminate evidence of illicit drug use from urine samples. For example, depending on the procedure used, Visine eye drops may camouflage any evidence of marijuana use ("Cheaters," 1995; "Forum," 1991). Bleach or table salt added to the urine sample may hide evidence of recent cocaine use ("Forum," 1991; Warner, 1995).

Some drug users have found that adding small amounts of table salt, liquid soap, or Drano drain opener to the urine sample will alter the chemical properties of the fluid enough to avoid detection of chemical use ("Cheaters," 1995; Woolf & Shannon, 1995). On some tests, each of these substances prevents evidence of THC from being detected in a urine sample. But the addition of one or more adulterants to a urine sample is not without its dangers. For example, when Drano was added to a clean urine sample, it tested positive for amphetamine abuse on one test commonly in use ("Cheaters," 1995). While a small amount of the metal salt alum might hide evidence of methamphetamine use, it will also alter the acidity of the urine sample, a characteristic that can easily be detected with a simple test ("Tolmetin," 1995). Thus, there are few adulterants that can safely be added to a urine sample by a drug-using person, without actually increasing the risk of having that urine sample identified as positive for recreational chemicals.

Still, to avoid the risk of a drug user attempting to manipulate the results of a urine toxicology test, *extremely close supervision must be provided for both male and female clients who are giving a urine sample for detection of illicit drug use.* This means that the person supervising the collection of the urine sample *must actually see the urine enter the bottle* and not just stand outside the bathroom or the toilet stall while the client is inside.

If the staff person suspects that the client has substituted another person's urine for his/her own,

several techniques may be utilized to counter this. First, *urine is within 1 or 2 degrees of the core body temperature,* and by immediately taking the temperature of the urine sample, one can determine if it is cooler than a normal human body temperature. The client whose urine sample was 70° is likely to have substituted somebody else's urine sample for his/her own and should be confronted with this fact.

Another technique is for a staff person to wait until he or she sees that the client is about to enter the lavatory, then tell him/her that they have been selected for another urine sample for drug testing. It is unlikely that the client carries around a bottle of substitute urine all the time, on the off chance that he/she will be asked for a urine sample. This procedure is likely to force the client to give a sample of his/her own urine, especially if care is taken to ensure that the client actually provides a sample of his/her own urine.

Still another technique is for the counselor to announce, at the beginning of a group session or other supervised activity, that the client has 2 hours in which to provide a supervised urine sample for toxicology screening. The client will then be unable to leave the group to pick up a urine sample stored in his/her room without staff being aware that he or she has left the group. The client should have access to water, coffee, or soda to stimulate the production of urine, which can be collected for toxicology testing without the client leaving the group room until he/she is escorted to the bathroom for collection of the urine sample.

A major drawback of urine toxicology screening is that the procedure involves an invasion of the patient's right to privacy (Cone, 1993). For this reason, written consent for urine toxicology testing is required. Such written consent states that staff may collect a urine sample at their discretion, as part of the treatment process, and describes the conditions under which a urine toxicology sample is to be obtained.

Depending on the method used, laboratories can detect either the drugs or metabolites produced by the body as the liver breaks down the drugs, for various periods of time. The chemical dependency professional should request a written summary from the laboratory that describes:

1. The *methods* by which the laboratory attempts to detect illicit chemical use.
2. The *accuracy* of this method.
3. *The specific chemicals that can be detected* by that laboratory.
4. *The length of time after the person has used chemicals when the urine test may reveal such drug use.*
5. *Any other drugs* (including over-the-counter medications) that might yield false positive results.

Detection of Marijuana

Surprisingly, there has been little research into the question of how long THC might be detected in the urine of a marijuana user ("Not Enough Data," 1995). Woolf and Shannon (1995) suggested that a urine sample from a person who is a moderate user of marijuana would be positive for THC for 5 days after the last use of this chemical, at a cutoff level of 20 ng/ml of urine. However, chronic marijuana users will, because the body stores THC and gradually releases it back into the blood, test positive at the 20 ng/ml level for 10 to 20 days, according to the authors. D. Roberts (1995) suggested that THC can be detected in the daily user's urine for 3 to 6 weeks following the last use of marijuana, while the *Forensic Drug Abuse Advisor* ("CPPD," 1996) suggested that urine samples will test positive for THC for "at least four days" (p. 42) following the use of a single marijuana cigarette.

Ravel (1989) advocates the testing of new urine samples every 4 or 5 days for chronic users; if there has been no additional marijuana use such serial urine samples should show "a progressive downward trend in the values" (p. 629). The *Forensic Drug Abuse Advisor* ("Secondhand Crack," 1995) suggested daily urine toxicology tests, until the user has tested negative for 3 days in a row, to ensure that any residual THC has been eliminated from the user's body.

Occasionally, a person whose urine tested positive for THC might claim to have passively inhaled marijuana smoke because of being in a room where other people were smoking it. The *Forensic Drug Abuse Advisor* (1995i) did suggest that under special conditions it was possible for a nonusing individual to be exposed to concentrations of secondhand

marijuana smoke high enough to cause his/her urine to test positive for THC. In one study where this was attempted, however, the volunteers had to sit in a chamber so filled with smoke from the marijuana cigarettes that they had to wear special eye protection! Thus, under normal circumstances, it is unlikely that an individual would test positive for THC because of exposure to secondhand smoke from marijuana cigarettes.

Detection of Cocaine

Depending on the route of administration and the amount of cocaine used, it is possible to detect metabolites of cocaine in urine samples for about 24–48 hours after the last drug use (House, 1990; Woolf & Shannon, 1995). However, some authors have suggested that it is possible to detect benzoylecgonine (the major metabolite of cocaine) for up to 96 hours after the person last used the drug (D. Roberts, 1995; Weddington, 1993). The *Forensic Drug Abuse Advisor* ("The Sauna Defense," 1995) suggested that strong evidence suggests that, in extremely heavy users, large amounts of cocaine can be stored in the body tissues, only to be released back into the general circulation days, weeks, or even months after the person last used the drug. The implication of these findings is that a person could continue to test positive for cocaine on a urine toxicology test for many days or weeks after last using the drug ("The Sauna Defense," 1995; "Secondhand Crack," 1995). However, it is doubtful that a client who initially tested negative, or who tested positive at a low level, should suddenly show evidence of high levels of cocaine metabolites in his/her blood. This would suggest recent cocaine use, not the effects of residual cocaine.

As a general rule of thumb, the casual user might show evidence of cocaine use in his/her urine for 2 or 3 days after the episode of drug use using enzyme immunoassay techniques, or up to 7 days if the more sensitive radioimmunoassay technique were utilized. Researchers have found evidence suggesting the possibility for a nonusing individual to absorb some cocaine fumes from secondhand smoke from cocaine smoking. However, the blood levels of cocaine in nonusers was not high enough to cause any physiological reaction, and the concentration of cocaine metabolites in the nonuser's urine would not result in a positive toxicology test at the cutoff levels recommended by the National Institute on Drug Abuse (NIDA).

Detection of PCP Abuse

The hallucinogen PCP or its metabolites can be detected for up to 1 week following its use by a casual user, but for 3 weeks after the chronic user last used this substance (Woolf & Shannon, 1995). As discussed in Chapter 13, the speed at which PCP is excreted from the body depends on the acidity of the urine. Thus, there will be some variation in the speed at which PCP is eliminated from the body. Cone (1993) suggested that PCP can be detected in body fluids for 5 to 8 days in the casual user and for as long as 30 days in the chronic user.

Detection of Amphetamine

The amphetamines, on the other hand, may be detected for only 24 to 48 hours after the last use of this class of drugs (Cone, 1993; D. Roberts, 1995).

Detection of Opiates

The often-abused analgesic Darvon (propoxyphene) may be detected for just 8 hours following its use, although metabolites of propoxyphene may be detected for up to 48 hours following its use (D. Roberts, 1995; Woolf & Shannon, 1995). The "window of detection" for Darvon thus depends on whether the laboratory is testing for the drug itself, or for metabolites of the drug. Other narcotic analgesics such as heroin, morphine, codeine, or Dilaudid (hydromorphone) can be detected for 1 to 2 days following the last use of this class of drugs (Ravel, 1989; Roberts, 1995). Methadone may be detected for a slightly longer period than other narcotic analgesics, according to Roberts. However, even methadone can only be detected for 2 or 3 days following the last dose.

Detection of Rohypno

Although it is possible to test for Rohypnol (flunitrazepam) in urine samples, the drug can be detected only within 60 hours of the time of ingestion (Lively, 1996).

False Positive Test Results, and the Need for Retesting

Urine toxicology testing is an imprecise art, and several factors could cause inaccurate test results. Poppy seeds, for example, are often used in certain kinds of bread. Depending on the method by which the urine sample was tested, a person who ingested some of this bread might then produce a urine sample that tested positive for opioids, even if the person had not used a narcotic (Ravel, 1989). The OTC medication pseudoephedrine hydrochloride (which is sold under a number of different brand names) may cause some urine toxicology tests to be positive for amphetamines (Woolf & Shannon, 1995).

Given these facts, it is unfortunate that on-site testing is becoming increasingly popular at the workplace or other settings where supervisory personnel desire information about possible substance use by another person. On-site tests have a high false positive rate and frequently indicate possible illicit drug use in cases where the individual has not used chemicals ("Why Confirmatory," 1997). On-site test results should *always* be confirmed by independent toxicology testing in a certified laboratory.

Thus, once illicit drug use is detected, it is necessary for the urine sample to be retested by another technique, to rule out a false positive result. Moyer and Ellefson (1987) reported that, when a pure urine specimen is used, the enzyme-mediated immunotechnique (EMIT) is able to detect marijuana use with better than 95% accuracy. When combined with other tests such as gas chromatography/mass spectrometry (GC/MS), it is possible to obtain virtually 100% accuracy when testing urine specimens for evidence of marijuana use.

Because the EMIT procedure has a 3% false positive rate, testing with another technique such as GC/MS is essential to rule out false positive results. Ravel (1989) also advocated the use of additional testing such as mass spectrometry or gas chromatography to confirm/deny the original positive test results for all drugs of abuse. These highly specialized test procedures essentially separate the constituents of a urine sample for identification. Multiple test procedures for all positive urine samples will help to identify those who have truly used illicit chemicals and greatly reduce the danger of false positive test results (Woolf & Shannon, 1995).

Other Uses of Urine Toxicology Tests

A second use of urine toxicology testing is not to detect illicit drug use, but to check medication compliance. Urine toxicology screening help determine whether the client is taking prescribed medications. Obviously, a person being detoxified from narcotics through methadone withdrawal should have evidence of methadone metabolites in his/her urine.

As noted, urine toxicology testing should reveal evidence of methadone for up to 72 hours following the last use of the drug (Woolf & Shannon, 1995). Thus, if, the day after a client supposedly received a dose of methadone, he/she does not test positive for this drug, the staff should consider the possibility that this person has substituted another urine sample for his/her own, and examine why the client should want to do so.

The use of urine for toxicology screens may provide a valuable component to any treatment program. The urine sample must be drawn under closely supervised conditions, however, as clients often try to avoid detection of their alcohol/drug use.

Hair as a Source of Toxicology Test Samples

When a person uses a chemical, molecules of that substance are circulated throughout the body. Some of those drug molecules attach themselves to different tissues in the body, where they may bind to the walls of the cells for extended periods before being released back to the general circulation. But if the cell were to die and be ejected from the body before releasing the drug molecule, it would remain attached to the cell wall. In theory, this characteristic might make it possible to detect evidence of illicit drug use in hair samples of patients. This is because the roots of hair remain alive, but the hair itself is composed of long strands of deal cells pushed outward from the root by the pressure of new hair cells forming at the root.[1] Scientists have developed the technology to detect metabolites of many illicit drugs in the hair of the user, and some people have suggested this as a less intrusive alternative to urine/blood toxicology testing.

It is, however, virtually impossible to determine *when* the user indulged in illicit drug use by hair sample testing. The theory that by measuring the distance that the drug molecules are from the root, and then estimating the time that it would take for hair to grow that distance at a standard rate of growth of 1 centimeter (cm) per month, has not been proven in practice ("Researchers Claim," 1996). Further, questions have been raised as to whether different ethnic groups might not have differing rates of absorbing drug metabolites into the hair itself. Thus, while toxicological testing of hair samples is possible, its value in detecting illicit drug use remains uncertain at best.

Another emerging technology is the use of saliva to test for residual traces of alcohol (Wilson & Kunsman, 1997). Although laboratories have been able to use saliva samples to test for alcohol traces since the 1950s, new techniques are making this procedure attractive for workplace screening programs, according to the authors. The individual will place a cotton swab in his/her mouth, allowing it to become moistened by saliva. The cotton swab is then tested, by exposing it to chemicals that react to the presence of alcohol. The use of saliva allows for a simple, short (less than 20 minute) test that is just as accurate as breath testing, but can be carried out in the workplace. As with any screening procedure, there is a need for follow-up testing to rule out false positive results. But, this procedure allows for on-site testing, making it attractive to employers (Wilson & Kunsman, 1997).

Insurance Reimbursement Policies

As mentioned earlier, there once was a time when the 28-day standard of the Minnesota Model of treatment served as a guide for insurance

---

[1] This is why it is possible to have your hair cut, without feeling pain: the hair is dead, and thus does not have functional nerve endings.

coverage for substance abuse rehabilitation provisions in health insurance policies. Insurance companies that provided health care coverage would use the 28-day standard of the Minnesota Model as a guide, when evaluating the need for reimbursement for inpatient treatment of chemical use problems.

By the early 1990s, health care costs were rising at 2 to 3 times the rate of inflation (Mee-Lee, 1995). To control the rising economic impact of health care, many insurance companies initiated cost containment procedures that included increased accountability on the part of health care providers, a requirement for prior authorization for elective procedures, increased scrutiny of claims for services provided, all in the name of a procedure known as "managed care." In theory, *managed care* (MC) is designed to provide the most appropriate care for the patient at the best possible price to the insurance company. However, many health care providers have come to call managed care by the term "managed profits," because of the way that this process limits the amount of care that an insurance company is liable for under its policy with the individual.

For example, researchers have found that MC companies tend to provide only limited services for substance abuse rehabilitation ("Limits by Managed Care," 1996). An investigation of 50 contracts between MC companies and community mental health/substance abuse rehabilitation programs found that the MC contracts typically provided only a fraction of the range of services available to clients whose health care was covered by insurance programs other than managed care ("Limits by Managed Care," 1996). This finding lends credence to the observation of some professionals that managed care companies tend to be more interested in their profit margin than in providing appropriate levels of care to their clients.

A point often overlooked by health care providers is that insurance companies *do not exist to provide funding for health care procedures.* Rather, insurance companies exist to make money for the owners of the company (stockholders). One way they do this is by selling health insurance. A health insurance policy is, in effect, a gamble by the insurance company that

the policyholder will not become ill while the policy is in effect. The company charges a "premium" that the company will then keep if the policyholder does not become ill with any of the conditions identified by the company as reflecting "illness." If the policyholder *does* become ill, the insurance company is then required to provide a certain level of care, as identified in the policy.

At all times, the company attempts to hold down its costs, to maximize profit. The money that an insurance company spends providing health care coverage for those who purchased such a policy from that company is considered a financial loss to the company. The insurance company thus attempts to maximize the inflow of money while reducing, or eliminating, the need to pay money to policyholders. One way that insurance companies do this is to exclude as many conditions as possible from the health insurance coverage. Another way that insurance companies attempt to limit their losses is to either exclude individuals with known medical problems from participation in the policy, or to charge a higher premium for these individuals to offset the anticipated losses from their care. A third way that insurance companies limit their losses is to adopt a conservative definition of disease.

To this end, it has been charged that insurance companies have come to substitute *symptom reduction* for the "treatment" or "cure" of disease (Kaiser, 1996). In the area of alcohol/drug use problems, insurance companies commonly use a very conservative definition of "recovery" to determine when benefits should be terminated. Thus, research has demonstrated that

> the minimum stay in residential treatment programs needed to yield improvement in long-term outcomes was several months and that improvements in outcomes continue to be manifested for full-time treatment of up to 1 year in length. (McCusker et al., 1996, p. 482)

At best, however, most health insurance companies provide funding for only 2 to 3 weeks of inpatient substance abuse rehabilitation. All too often, funding is even more limited, sometimes to just 5 days of inpatient treatment. Provisions for outpatient treatment are often even more restrictive.

The apparent contradiction is easy to understand if one accepts that insurance companies are able to present *symptom resolution* as a substitute for long-term treatment. Health insurance companies have come to view the stabilization of the immediate crisis as being an acceptable goal for inpatient treatment, in the case of the addictive disorders, *not* long-term rehabilitation. Thus the conflict between insurance companies and health care providers—adequate treatment of the addictive disorders requires time for meaningful change. Few health care providers are willing to accept symptom resolution, which in this case means the immediate cessation of chemical use, as adequate treatment. In contrast, the health care insurance companies, however, interpret "adequate" treatment as just that: the stabilization of the immediate crisis.

A drawback of the managed care concept of health care is that up to half of the fee charged per client goes for administrative fees and company profit (A. Gottlieb, 1997). Further, managed care companies often view substance abuse rehabilitation treatment as being imperfect at best. Among many managed care companies, there is

> a deep suspicion of anything unquantifiable, unprovable, or lingering as probably being poor technique on the therapist's part, self-indulgence on the patient's, and a waste of money by both. (A. Gottlieb, 1997 p. 47)

Yet in this very criticism of psychotherapy is a definition of substance abuse rehabilitation: the treatment methods are unproven, the condition itself may be controlled, but never cured, and the quantification of the condition is virtually impossible. Thus, at many managed care companies, mental health claims in general, and substance abuse rehabilitation claims in specific, are routinely earmarked for administrative review.

Summary

Even after a client has been identified as being in need of substance abuse rehabilitation services, the course of treatment is often a difficult one. Some clients will test the limits imposed by the therapist or the treatment center. Other clients will, with greater or lesser justification, challenge the accuracy of urine toxicology test results. Clients occasionally come to treatment sessions under the influence of chemicals. Virtually every client experiences urges and craving to use chemicals after beginning a recovery program. Some of these individuals relapse and return to active chemical abuse, especially if they fail to respond appropriately to relapse triggers encountered in everyday life. Finally, insurance company policies often place severe constraints on the length of time that a given client can be in either an inpatient or an outpatient rehabilitation program.

While this chapter cannot possibly discuss each and every problem that a client may encounter in a rehabilitation program, it does discuss some of the more common situations that may interfere with a client's recovery from alcohol/drug use problems.

CHAPTER THIRTY-TWO

Pharmacological Intervention Tactics and Substance Abuse[1]

The pharmacological treatment of substance abuse is a logical extension of the medical model. It is based on the premise that through the use of biochemical substances, the individual's substance use can be controlled or totally eliminated. The specific components of treatment may vary from one program to another. For example, a treatment program that specializes in working with alcoholic businesspeople would have little use for a methadone maintenance component. But, whether it is detoxification from alcohol, the prevention of relapse for the chronic drinker, or the control of the craving for cocaine that many addicts report in the early stages of recovery, all forms of pharmacological interventions center on the use of selected chemicals to combat substance abuse.

It is the purpose of this chapter to review these common components of treatment, so that the reader can become familiar with the basic features of chemical dependency programs and better understand how pharmacological treatments are used in the rehabilitation of substance abusers.

The Pharmacological Treatment of Alcohol Abuse and Dependence

Medications Used in the Treatment of the Alcohol Withdrawal Syndrome

As discussed in Chapter 5, the alcohol withdrawal syndrome is a potentially serious condition, which should be treated by a physician. The judicious use of either benzodiazepines such as chlordiazepoxide (20–100 mg either orally or intravenously every 6 hours) or diazepam (5–20 mg either orally or intravenously every 6 hours) has been found to control the tremor, hyperactivity, convulsions, and anxiety associated with alcohol withdrawal (Milhorn, 1992; Miller, Frances, & Holmes, 1989; Yost, 1996).

Not every individual experiencing alcohol withdrawal will require benzodiazepines (Saitz et al., 1994). There is evidence to suggest that following "standing orders" for the administration of benzodiazepines whenever a patient goes into alcohol withdrawal may actually have contributed to excessive hospital stays, according to Saitz et al. Rather than the automatic administration of a predetermined dose of a benzodiazepine whenever a potential alcohol withdrawal situation is encountered, Saitz et al. recommend a "symptom-triggered" (p. 519) approach. The benzodiazepine chlordiazepoxide was administered only if the patient's physical status suggested that the person was going into acute alcohol withdrawal. The authors found that this resulted in fewer doses of medication being administered, and a

[1] The pharmacological support of alcohol or drug withdrawal, or such support as part of the treatment of an ongoing substance abuse problem, should be supervised by a licensed physician who is skilled and experienced in working with substance abuse cases. The information provided in this chapter is not intended to encourage self-treatment of substance abuse problems, nor should it be interpreted as a standard of care for patients addicted to chemicals.

shorter hospital stay, than the standard approach, which placed each patient on a rigid dosing schedule followed by a gradual reduction in the daily dosage level of chlordiazepoxide.

Thus, the approach suggested by Saitz et al. (1994) is an alternative to the standard withdrawal schedule, which suggests that after the withdrawal symptoms have been controlled, the daily dosage level of benzodiazepines should be reduced by 10% to 20% each day, until the medication is finally discontinued (Miller et al., 1989).

In cases where the patient is going through alcohol hallucinosis, Milhorn (1992) advocated the use of low doses of the antipsychotic medication haloperidol, in addition to benzodiazepines, to control the withdrawal symptoms. Usually 1–2 mg of haloperidol every 4 hours, in addition to the benzodiazepines, will control the symptoms of alcohol hallucinosis.

Medications Used in the Treatment of Alcohol Dependence

Frances and Miller (1991) struck a rather pessimistic note when they observed that even after a century of searching for an antidipsotrophic[2] medication:

> At this writing there is no proven biological treatment for alcoholism. Each promising drug that has been tested in the hope it would reduce relapse by intervening in the basic disease process has failed. (p. 13)

However, the authors noted, Antabuse (disulfiram) continues to provide one avenue for the symptomatic treatment of alcoholism.

Antabuse (Disulfiram)

At the 1949 annual meeting of the American Psychiatric Association, Barrera, Osinski, and Davidoff (1949/1994) presented a paper in which they reported the outcome of their research into the possible use of Antabuse as an antidipsotrophic medication. The original theory behind the use of disulfiram was a variation on the process of aversive

conditioning, according to the authors. The combination of alcohol and Antabuse would produce "unpleasant effects" for the drinker, thus reducing the reward value of the alcohol.

In the time since it was first suggested as a way to combat chronic alcoholism, it has been found that disulfiram is a potentially dangerous drug, which should not be used with patients who have serious medical disorders (Schuckit, 1996a). Some of the side effects of disulfiram include skin rash, fatigue, halitosis, a rare, potentially fatal form of hepatitis, peripheral neuropathies, potential damage to the optic nerve, severe depression, and psychosis (Schuckit).

Despite its many dangers, disulfiram has traditionally been viewed by many professionals as a useful tool in the fight against alcohol abuse/addiction. In reality, however, only one large-scale study has shown even a modest positive benefit from disulfiram in the treatment of alcohol dependence (Schuckit, 1996a). But, in theory, for those patients who can use disulfiram, it might provide time for a "second thought" desparately needed by the alcohol-dependent individual who is tempted to drink. Disulfiram *does not decrease the alcoholic's desire to drink*. However, it does interfere with the metabolism of alcohol after it enters the individual's body. The combination of alcohol with disulfiram will cause a number of unpleasant—*potentially fatal*—effects for the individual. This knowledge is then used to help the alcoholic who wants a "second chance" consider the consequences of even one drink in a new light.

The individual is warned about the effects of combining alcohol with disulfiram when the medication is started. Disulfiram interferes with the body's ability to biotransform alcohol, allowing acetaldehyde to build up in the blood. If the individual who has taken disulfiram ingests even small amounts of alcohol, he/she experiences such symptoms as facial flushing, heart palpitations and a rapid heart rate, difficulty in breathing, nausea, vomiting, and possibly a serious drop in blood pressure (Schuckit, 1995a).

Under normal conditions, it takes 3 to 12 hours after the first dose of disulfiram before it can begin to interfere with the metabolism of alcohol. But, when the individual who has been using disulfiram for

---

[2]This term is a carryover from the 19th century, when alcoholics were said to suffer from "dipsomania." A medication that was antidipsotrophic would thus be against dipsomania, or used to treat this disorder.

several days ingests alcohol, he/she will experience the alcohol-disulfiram reaction within about 30 minutes. Typically, the disulfiram-alcohol interaction lasts for 30 to 180 minutes, although there are case reports of it lasting longer than this. The strength of these side effects depends on several factors: (a) how much alcohol has been ingested, (b) the amount of disulfiram being used each day, and (c) the length of time since the last dose of disulfiram was ingested. This time frame is important because the body tends to metabolize disulfiram. Thus, over time, the effects of any given dose become less and less powerful.

To make sure that the user understands the consequences of mixing alcohol with disulfiram, some treatment centers advocate a learning process where patients take disulfiram for a short period (usually a few days) after which they are allowed to drink a small amount of alcohol under controlled conditions. This is done so that the alcoholic can experience the negative consequences of mixing alcohol and dilsulfiram under controlled conditions. When this technique is used, the treatment staff has access to the proper medications and respiratory support equipment, to help the client recover from the alcohol-disulfiram interaction effects. The theory behind this practice is that, by allowing alcoholics to experience the negative consequences after drinking only a small amount of alcohol, they will not be tempted to drink a large amount of alcohol on their own, outside the treatment center.

On occasion, treatment professionals have encountered the situation where a spouse of an alcohol abuser will inquire about the possibility of obtaining disulfiram to "teach him (her) a lesson." Inquiry usually reveals that the spouse wants a sample of disulfiram to place it in the alcoholic's coffee, or "eye opener." The purpose of this exercise is to ensure that the next time that the alcoholic drinks, he or she will experience the alcohol disulfiram interaction, without expecting it. *Disulfiram should never be given to an individual without the user's knowledge and consent* (American Psychiatric Association, 1995). The interaction between disulfiram and alcohol is *potentially serious and may be fatal.*

Disulfiram is not a perfect solution to the problem of alcohol dependence. For example, it is not an effective aversive conditioning agent. Aversive

conditioning programs require *immediate* consequences paired to undesired behavior to be effective. Theoretically, an effective behavior modification program for alcoholism would involve an immediate consequence. In this manner, the person learns to associate drinking behavior with a negative response, and, in theory, will gradually discontinue the undesired behavior. But the 30-minute delay between the ingestion of alcohol and the disulfiram-alcohol reaction is far too long for it to serve as an *immediate* consequence for the drinker. This makes it difficult for the person to associate the use of alcohol with the delayed discomfort caused by the alcohol-disulfiram reaction.

Another disadvantage of disulfiram is that its *full* effects last only about 24 to 48 hours. There have been rare reports of alcohol-disulfiram interactions up to 2 weeks after the last dose of disulfiram. But in most cases, the individual's body ceases to react to alcohol on the 6th or 7th day after his/her last dose of disulfiram. Because of the body's biotransformation of disulfiram, most patients take the drug every day, or perhaps every other day, for optimal effectiveness. Thus, it is up to the individual to take the medication according to the schedule worked out with his/her physician, to ensure that there is an adequate supply of the drug in the body at all times. Obviously, medication compliance is a serious problem for some individuals who use disulfiram.

Further, disulfiram often reacts to the alcohol found in many over-the-counter cough syrups, as well as in aftershaves and a wide range of other products. The individual using disulfiram should be warned by the physician to avoid certain products, to keep from having an unintentional reaction caused by the small amounts of alcohol in these products. Most treatment centers or physicians who utilize disulfiram have lists of such products and foods and will provide a copy to patients taking this drug.

Research has suggested that disulfiram interacts with the neurotransmitter serotonin, to boost brain levels of a by-product of serotonin known as 5-hydrooxy-tryptophol (5-HTOL) (Cowen, 1990). Animal research suggests that increased levels of 5-HTOL result in greater alcohol consumption. While research with human subjects has yet to be completed, preliminary data suggests that there is a need for alcoholics to avoid serotonin-rich foods such as bananas and walnuts, to avoid increasing the craving for alcohol experienced by many recovering alcoholics.

Disulfiram is *not* recommended for individuals who have a history of cardiovascular and cerebrovascular disease, kidney failure, depression, seizure disorders, liver disease, or for women who might be pregnant (Fuller, 1995). It is not recommended for use in elderly patients, because of the potential danger that it might cause/contribute to hypotension, myocardial infarction and stroke in the older individual (Goldstein et al., 1996). This medication has also been implicated as a possible cause of peripheral neuropathies, and has been found to lower the seizure threshold for patients with idiopathic seizure disorders (Fuller, 1995; Schuckit, 1996a). Further, there are reports that suggest disulfiram has caused exacerbation of the symptoms of schizophrenia, in those patients with this disorder (Fuller).

Drug interactions have been reported between disulfiram and phenytoin (sold under the brand name of Dilantin), warfarin, isoniazid (used in the treatment of tuberculosis), diazepam (Valium), chlordiazepoxide (Librium), and several commonly used antidepressants (Fuller, 1989). Patients who are taking the antitubercular drug isoniazid (or, "INH," as it is also called) should not take disulfiram. These drugs may, when used together, bring on a toxic psychosis or cause other neurological problems in the patient (Meyers, 1992).

There are reports that disulfiram may interfere with male sexual performance. Schiavi et al. (1995) noted that one-half of the chronic males in their sample who reported having trouble achieving an erection claimed that this problem only began when they started to take disulfiram. This may prove to be a somewhat frightening side effect for some users, especially if they are not warned of this possibility before starting the medication. Further, patients who use disulfiram should do so only under the supervision of a physician who has a *complete* medication use history on the patient. Because of the danger of disulfiram-medication interactions, the use of multiple prescriptions from different doctors should be most strongly discouraged.

Despite these disadvantages, research has demonstrated a modest benefit from disulfiram. Those alcoholism treatment programs that utilize disulfiram as a part of the overall treatment program have a lower relapse rate than programs that do not (Adelman & Weiss, 1989). What disulfiram does, once the person has taken his/her scheduled dose, is to provide the individual with the knowledge that he or she will be unable to drink for that day, or for perhaps as long as two weeks afterward, at least not without becoming very sick.

Admittedly, some alcoholics will drink despite the disulfiram in their system, which is known as trying to "drink through" the disulfiram. Many alcoholics will stop taking the drug several days before a "spontaneous" relapse, and only about 20% of those individuals who start the drug actually take it for a full year. Further, many alcoholics believe that they know how to neutralize the drug while it is in their body. Nevertheless, for the majority of those who use disulfiram as intended, the drug provides the individual an extra bit of support during a weak moment.

Lithium

In the late 1980s and early 1990s, there was a great deal of interest in the possible use of lithium in the treatment of alcoholism. Lithium has been found to be useful in the treatment of bipolar affective disorders (formerly called manic-depressive disorder). Early research suggested that lithium was also able to reduce the number of relapses that chronic alcoholics experienced, reduce the apparent level of intoxication, and reduce the desire of chronic alcohol users to drink (Judd & Huey, 1984; Miller et al., 1989).

Subsequent research has failed to support the early findings that suggested lithium is a useful agent in the treatment of alcoholism (American Psychiatric Association, 1995; Schuckit, 1996a). A large-scale study suggested that lithium was about as effective as a placebo for patients who took part in the study. Thus, there is little evidence to suggest that lithium would be of value in the treatment of alcohol dependence, although it remains an effective agent in the control of bipolar affective disorders.

Naltrexone Hydrochloride

As discussed in Chapter 4, when an individual consumes alcohol, the person's brain is thought to release endogenous opioids. These are neurotransmitters thought to be involved in the pleasure center of the brain. Researchers have now discovered that drugs that function as antagonists for one of the neurotransmitter binding sites for endogeneous opioids—the receptor site known as the *mu* opioid receptor site—seem to reduce alcohol consumption in both animals and man (Swift, Whelihan, Kuznetsov, Buongiorno, & Hsuing, 1994).

One such drug is naltrexone hydrochloride, which in January 1995 was approved by the Food and Drug Administration (FDA) as a drug for use in the treatment of alcoholics ("FDA Approves," 1995). The research team of Volpicelli, Alterman, Hayashida, and O'Brien (1992) administered 50 mg/day of naltrexone hydrochloride to a sample of diagnosed alcohol-dependent patients. The subjects received the naltrexone hydrochloride following detoxification from alcohol, and their relapse rate was contrasted with that of a matched group of alcoholics who received only a placebo. The authors found that the naltrexone hydrochloride treatment group reported significantly less craving for alcohol than did those individuals who received the placebo. Further, the authors found that 54% of the alcoholics who received the placebo relapsed during the 12 weeks of the study, whereas only 23% of those individuals who received naltrexone hydrochloride relapsed during the study.

The exact mechanism by which naltrexone hydrochloride, a drug normally used in the treatment of narcotics addiction, might block the pleasurable effects of the alcohol is not known at this time. However, naltrexone hydrochloride appears to reduce alcohol's reward value as a drug of abuse as well as the craving for alcohol that so often complicates rehabilitation efforts (American Psychiatric Association, 1995; Holloway, 1991; Swift et al., 1994; Volpicelli et al., 1994).

In addition to its ability to reduce craving for alcohol, clinical evidence suggests that naltrexone is able to make the use of alcohol less rewarding for the individual who has relapsed, so that the individual is less likely to continue drinking (Meza & Kranzler, 1996; Volpicelli et al., 1994). Thus, naltrexone hydrochloride appears to have a role in the fight against alcoholism, although researchers are still not sure which clients might benefit most from its use.

Other Pharmacological Treatments for Chronic Alcoholism

There are other medications, such as Flagyl (or metronidazole), that cause discomfort when mixed with alcohol. Like disulfiram, metronidazole causes nausea, vomiting, flushing, and headache when mixed with alcohol (Graedon, 1980). For this reason, researchers briefly experimented with metronidazole as a possible antidipsotrophic medication in the 1970s. But this research was discontinued when little evidence was found to suggest metronidazole was effective as a possible antidipsotrophic medication (Holder et al., 1991).

However, in the case of one patient who was allergic to disulfiram, the patient's physician elected to use metronidazole as a short-term substitute. This is not currently a recommended use of this medication by the Food and Drug Administration. But, in this case, the physician was able to provide pharmacological support for an alcoholic who needed some external support during his initial period of recovery, when the patient felt most at risk of relapsing. This is not to say that metronidazole should be routinely administered to alcoholics who require pharmacological support. But, when the benefits clearly outweigh the risks presented by this medication, metronidazole might offer an alternative to disulfiram for at least some patients.

European researchers have explored the possible use of Acamprosate (calcium acetylhomotaurinate), a chemical that has a chemical structure similar to that of the neurotransmitter GABA (Whitworth et al., 1996). In a study that used a sample of 455 patients between the ages of 18 and 65, the authors randomly assigned subjects either to a chemical treatment group or a placebo control group. Both groups took their assigned pills each morning. Patients were reassessed at 30, 90, 180, 270, and 360 days following the start of the experiment. Ninety-four of the original 224 members of the medication subgroup completed the yearlong study, while 85 of the 224 control group completed the yearlong treatment period. Equal numbers of both groups relapsed, and similar numbers were either lost to follow-up evaluation, or refused to complete the treatment protocol. At the end of the yearlong study period, the authors found that 18.3% of those patients who received Acamprosate had remained completely abstinent, compared with 7.1% of the placebo control group. Further, the authors found that the Acamprosate treatment group had significantly higher abstinence rate than the placebo control group, with the mean cumulative period of abstinence being 230.8 days for the treatment group, and 183.0 days for the placebo group. The authors interpreted this data to suggest that Acamprosate was a useful tool in treatment programs.

Acamprosate has a different mechanism of action than Antabuse (disulfiram). Rather than interacting with alcohol to cause unpleasant, possibly fatal, physical reactions, Acamprosate stimulates the production of GABA and inhibits the effects of neurotransmitters such as glutamate that stimulate the central nervous system (Whitworth et al., 1996). The apparent effect is that the individual feels less *need* to ingest alcohol, although the exact mechanism of action for Acamprosate is still not known. The drug is not thought to be extensively biotransformed prior to excretion, and its primary route of excretion is thought to be through the kidneys, according to the authors. Although this medication has shown some promise in the treatment of chronic alcohol use/abuse, it still is not available in the United States (Schuckit, 1996a).

Buspirone

Research studies have suggested a possible benefit from the use of buspirone in controlling the symptoms of anxiety and excessive worry associated with protracted abstinence (Meza & Kranzler, 1996; Schuckit, 1996a). Because the first research studies to examine the effectiveness of buspirone in the treatment of alcohol dependence were poorly designed, further research is needed into the possible effectiveness of buspirone as an adjunct to the treatment of alcohol dependence.

Selective Serotonin Reuptake Inhibitors (SSRIs)

In the late 1980s, psychiatrists began to use a new class of medications known as *selective serotonin reuptake inhibitors (SSRIs)* in the treatment of depression. Members of this class of antidepressants include Prozac (fluoxetine). Subsequent research has found that even with those alcohol-dependent individuals who are not depressed, the SSRIs can bring about a modest decrease in alcohol use. However, these initial research studies have involved only small sample groups, and it is still not known whether the SSRIs will prove to be useful with larger groups of alcohol-dependent clients.

Neurotransmitter Precursor Loading

In the 1980s, Blum and Trachtenberg (1988) suggested a different treatment approach to the problem of rehabilitation of the alcoholic. They theorized that alcohol craving might be influenced by the neurochemicals available in the brain. The authors advocated the use of a "neurotransmitter precursor loading" system (Blum & Trachtenberg, 1988, p. 5) to aid in the treatment of alcoholism. According to the authors, proper nutritional supplements would:

> improve brain nutrition, improve the balance of the neurotransmitters, reduce the craving, and help the alcoholic respond more favorably to supportive treatment such as that provided by treatment centers, counselors, and Alcoholics Anonymous. (Blum & Trachtenberg, 1988, p. 35)

This novel treatment was thought to show promise, according to the authors, who offered a patented combination of vitamins, amino acids, and minerals for use in the rehabilitation of alcohol-dependent individuals. An advantage of this approach was that it used the nonaddictive substances for restoring the balance of neurotransmitters found in the otherwise healthy brain. However, subsequent research has failed to find any positive effects from this approach (Peele, 1991).

The Pharmacological Treatment of Narcotics Addiction

Naltrexone hydrochloride is a new tool in the treatment of opioid addiction Depending on the dosage level, it is possible for naltrexone to block the euphoric effects of injected opiates for up to 72 hours. The theory behind the use of naltrexone hydrochloride ("Trexan") is that persons who do not experience any feelings of euphoria from opiates are less likely to try and use opiates again.

This medication should be used *only after the person is completely detoxified from opiates*, to avoid bringing about an undesired withdrawal syndrome in an opiate addict. Callahan (1980) noted that one discovery that has followed the introduction of this narcotic antagonist blocking agent is that few addicts attempt to use narcotics even once while on the blocker. However, when the medication is discontinued, the opiate addict will then begin to reexperience a craving for narcotics. Thus, there is no extinction of the craving for the drug during the period the narcotics addict is usually maintained on a narcotics blocker.

Jenike (1991) reported that a 50-mg dose of naltrexone hydrochloride will block the euphoria of an injection of narcotics for 24 hours, while a 100-mg dose will work for about 48 hours. Further, a 150-mg dose of naltrexone hydrochloride will block the euphoria from injected narcotics for 72 hours. According to Jenike, the usual dosage schedule is three times per week, with 100 mg being administered on Monday and Wednesday, and 150 mg being administered on Friday to provide a longer term dose for the weekend.

To date, there is no research that demonstrates an *unequivocal* benefit from this medication in the treatment of narcotics addiction (Medical Economics Company, 1995). Research has shown that a major drawback of naltrexone hydrochloride is that so many addicts discontinue the drug on their own (Youngstrom, 1990b). One study exploring the application of naltrexone hydrochloride in the treatment of narcotics addiction found that *only 2%* of the original sample continued to take this drug for 9 months (Youngstrom). Thus, naltrexone hydrochloride is not the "magic pill" for the treatment of opiate addiction.

Holloway (1991) suggested that naltrexone hydrochloride was most useful for the narcotics addict who was "motivated to stay drug free" (p. 100). Thus, while this drug seems to offer pharmacological support during the initial period after detoxification, when an addict is most vulnerable to relapse, its applicability in the long-term treatment of narcotics addiction is still unclear.

Other Pharmacological Agents for Treatment of Narcotics Addiction

Ibogaine

An experimental drug under consideration in the rehabilitation of narcotics addicts is an alkaloid obtained from the root bark of the shrub *Tabernanthe iboga*, which grows in some regions of Africa. Some researchers believe that ibogaine might eliminate the individual's craving for narcotics such as heroin in the early phases of recovery ("Ibogaine," 1994).

The mechanism by which ibogaine might accomplish this effect is not known. However, the major metabolite of ibogaine, *noribogaine*, has a biological half-life of several weeks. Researchers are exploring whether this metabolite of ibogaine might account for the report from heroin addicts that their craving for narcotics ended after just one treatment with this chemical. Research into the effectiveness of ibogaine and its relative safety continues at this time. However, some experts in the field have started to question whether ibogaine may be more effective than methadone maintenance or methadone detoxification programs in the rehabilitation of narcotics addicts ("Ibogaine," 1994).

Methadone Maintenance

The concept of methadone maintenance was first advanced by Dole and Nyswander (1965), and has since become the treatment of choice for those individuals addicted to narcotics (especially heroin). Estimates of the number of heroin-addicted individuals in the United States who are involved in a methadone maintenance program range from approximately 99,100 (Strain, Stritzer, Liebson, & Bigelow, 1994) to 120,000 individuals (O'Brien, 1996). Of this number, perhaps 35,000 methadone maintenance patients are in New York City alone (Levy & Rutter, 1992).

The theory behind methadone maintenance is that the use of opiates in certain individuals causes permanent changes in brain function at the cellular level (Booth, 1995; Dole, 1988; Dole & Nyswander, 1965). The early proponents of methadone maintenance programs, Dole and Nyswander postulated that *even a single dose* of narcotics would bring about a change in the structure of the brain of the addict-to-be, forever altering the way the brain functioned. According to this theory, when the narcotics are removed from the body, the individual will crave narcotics for months, or even years afterward. This drug craving then makes it more likely that the individual will ultimately return to the use of narcotics, to feel "normal" again.

According to Dole and Nyswander (1965), structural change formed the basis for narcotics addiction. The authors knew that methadone would, when administered orally in high dosage levels, block the majority of the euphoric effects of injected narcotics. By substituting a sufficiently high dosage of oral methadone to "otherwise intractable" (Dole, 1989, p. 1880) opioid-addicted persons, the authors hoped to eliminate the need for further illegal opiate use. In theory, over time, this was hoped to lead to an extinction of the intravenous narcotics use (National Academy of Sciences, 1990).

Dole (1988), who remains one of the major proponents of the methadone maintenance concept, has observed that this treatment approach is "corrective, but not curative" (p. 3025) for the suspected, but as yet unproven, neurological dysfunction that brings about the compulsive use of narcotics. The usual dosage level used is 40–120 mg of methadone each day, with the most effective dose for most patients being above 90 mg/day (Karch, 1996). The methadone is administered in a single dose, usually in the morning. It is administered to the patient as a liquid, which is often mixed with a fruit juice.

The initial results of the methadone maintenance concept were quite promising (Callahan, 1980), and since the time of its inception methadone maintenance has become *the* treatment of choice for individuals addicted to narcotics. Although the original concept of methadone maintenance was that it would be a part of a larger rehabilitation program, over time, many methadone maintenance clinics became little more than drug distribution centers, with no effort being made at actual rehabilitation (Cohen & Levy, 1992; "Methadone," 1989).

This is unfortunate, because, the methadone maintenance concept originally advanced by Dole and Nyswander (1965) held that when the suspected neurological dysfunction brought on by the use of narcotics "has been normalized, the ex-addict, supported by counseling and social services, can begin the long process of social rehabilitation" (Dole, 1988, p. 3025).

Most certainly, when methadone maintenance is combined with a range of psychosocial support services (e.g., psychotherapy, vocational counseling, social services), significantly larger numbers of narcotics addicts are able to remain drug-free for longer periods than when such services are lacking (McLellan, Arndt, Metzger, Woody, & O'Brien, 1993). The authors concluded that providing such service was "cost effective" (p. 1959) for the severely impaired addicts, and suggested that methadone maintenance programs provide more than simply a steady supply of oral methadone.

Although these results are promising, the concept of methadone maintenance is still not without its critics. Some physicians challenge the concept of methadone maintenance on the grounds that it is only replacing one addictive substance with another, in effect substituting a legal drug for an illegal one (Cornish et al., 1995; "Treatment of Drug Abuse," 1995). This is the view of many European physicians, who accept that such "substitute treatment" (Seivewright & Greenwood, 1996, p. 374) may enable substance abuse treatment professionals to engage the client in long-term rehabilitation programs.

In the United States, many critics of methadone maintenance note that the assumption that narcotics use results in permanent neurological changes has never been proven. The *Harvard Mental Health Letter* ("Treatment of Drug Abuse," 1995) notes that one might take methadone for years, without any apparent toxic effects. This raises serious questions as to whether opiate-addicted individuals really suffer neurological changes as postulated by Dole and Nyswander (1965).

Further, critics argue 50% to 90% of the patients in methadone maintenance programs use other recreational drugs (Glantz & Woods, 1993). It has been found that many of the other recreational drugs, especially alcohol and cocaine, speed up the process of methadone biotransformation, resulting in the patient experiencing earlier withdrawal symptoms and the need to use higher doses of methadone to avoid opiate withdrawal (Karch, 1996). In the eyes of some critics, these drug-seeking behaviors raise serious questions as to the opiate addict's motivation for using methadone.

It is common for patients on methadone to try to obtain prescriptions for the drug propoxyphene (Darvon, Darvocet-N), as this latter chemical enhances the effects of the methadone to produce a sense of euphoria (DeMaria & Weinstein, 1995). Even Dole (1989) acknowledged that methadone is "highly specific for the treatment of opiate addiction" (p. 1880); it will not block the euphoric effects of other drugs of abuse, and there is no similar pharmacological therapy for the other drugs of abuse.

The concept of methadone maintenance has always been controversial, and many problems are inherent in the practice including methadone diversion (Dole, 1995). While the abuse potential of methadone is limited, it still is occasionally abused by opiate-addicted individuals who are unable to obtain other, more desirable, narcotics. Further, methadone maintenance programs suffer from significant dropout rates, which suggests that such programs are not the final answer to the problem of narcotics addiction.

However, there are a number of advantages to the methadone maintenance program concept, not the least of which is cost-effectiveness. After reviewing the literature on methadone maintenance programs, the National Academy of Sciences (1990) concluded that by supplying the addict with methadone so that he/she did not have to use street narcotics to avoid withdrawal symptoms, methadone maintenance programs reduced the participants' level of criminal activity. Swan (1994) reported that the average cost to society, in terms of criminal activity, social support, legal costs, and medical expenses, for a single untreated drug abuser for half a year was $21,500. Yet the cost of methadone maintenance for that same individual for six months was only $1,750 (approximately 8% the cost to society for not treating that individual).

Also, and perhaps most importantly, methadone maintenance programs appear to slow the spread of HIV-1 infection (DeMaria & Weinstein, 1995). Since methadone maintenance programs reduce the tendency for participants to use intravenously administered drugs, these addicts are less likely to be exposed to the virus through contaminated needles. One study from New York City found that less than 10% of those narcotics addicts who were admitted to methadone maintenance programs prior to 1978 were HIV positive, at a time when over 50% of the addicts who were still using narcotics

were infected with this virus (Council on Addiction Psychiatry, 1994).

Thus, while there is little evidence to support Dole and Nyswander's (1965) original theory as to the *cause* of narcotics addiction, methadone maintenance does seem to have a role to play in the treatment of chronic narcotics addiction.

Buprenorphine

In the past decade, researchers have discovered that low doses of orally administered buprenorphine (2–4 mg/day) can actually block the euphoric effects of intravenously administered narcotics (Horgan, 1989; Rosen & Kosten, 1991; Weiss, Greenfield, & Mirin, 1994). For this reason, buprenorphine is being considered as an alternative to methadone, and researchers are attempting to identify the optimum dosage level of buprenorphine for providing relief from opioid craving (Ling, Wesson, Charuvastra, & Klett, 1996).

Like methadone, buprenorphine only needs to be administered once a day. Oral doses of 2–8 mg/day of buprenorphine are thought to be as effective as up to 65 mg of methadone in blocking the euphoric effects of illicit narcotics (Stein & Kosten, 1994; Strain et al., 1994). Unlike methadone, however, buprenorphine provides little incentive for the individual to take more medication than needed. High doses of buprenorphine actually act as a narcotic antagonist, producing effects similar to naltrexone hydrochloride. This means that the medication is, to a significant degree, self-limiting. At high doses, the antagonist effect actually blocks the respiratory depression and euphoria the user might expect to experience from a narcotic analgesic that he/she has intentionally abused (Council on Addiction Psychiatry, 1994).

Another advantage that buprenorphine offers over methadone is that, while withdrawal from methadone may last up to 2 weeks, withdrawal from buprenorphine lasts only a few days (Horgan, 1989). Further, withdrawal from buprenorphine does not seem to make the individual as uncomfortable as methadone withdrawal (Council on Addiction Psychiatry, 1994; Rosen & Kosten, 1991).

Buprenorphine is not a "magic bullet." *Intravenously* administered buprenorphine has a significant abuse potential, which was discussed in Chapter 8. Further, it has been suggested that dosage levels above 8 mg/day might be necessary to suppress illicit opiate use (Fudala & Johnson, 1995). The team of Ling et al. (1996) split a research sample of 225 opiate-dependent individuals into three groups: those who received 30 mg/day of methadone, those who received 80 mg/day of methadone, and those who received 8 mg/day of buprenorphine.

At the end of one year, the authors found that those clients who received 8 mg/day of buprenorphine tended to drop out of treatment or have urine samples that tested positive for illicit opiate use at about the same frequency as those clients who received only 30 mg day of methadone. Thus, because of its abuse potential and uncertainty as to how it should be used most effectively, it is too soon to say how large a role buprenorphine will play in the fight against narcotics addiction.

LAAM

Another chemical that has been approved as a possible agent in treating opiate addicts is L-alpha-acetylmethadol (LAAM), which is sold in this country under the brand name "Orlaam." LAAM can be administered orally. Like methadone, orally administered LAAM is able to prevent the opiate addict from going into withdrawal. But because LAAM has a biological half-life of more than 48 hours (compared with methadone's half-life of 24 hours) the individual must take the drug only once every 2 or 3 days ("Methadone Alternative," 1993). This virtually eliminates the need for the patient to take doses home with him/her, vastly reducing the problem of drug diversion to the illicit market.

Another advantage of LAAM is that research suggests that withdrawal from this drug is possibly easier than withdrawal from methadone ("Methadone Alternative," 1993). However, methadone has been the primary drug used to control narcotics withdrawal symptoms, and it is too early to determine how effective LAAM might be in the treatment of narcotics addiction.

Narcotic Withdrawal

Programs that specialize in the treatment of narcotic addiction often offer controlled withdrawal from opiates. Occasionally, a hospital will offer narcotic withdrawal programs even if that hospital does not attempt to provide long-term treatment for narcotic addicts. The detoxification component in each center is very much the same.

In the United States, methadone is the traditional drug of choice for narcotic withdrawal (Jenike, 1991). The biological half-life of methadone is quite long, and a single dose is usually effective for 24 to 36 hours (Mirin et al., 1991). The authors noted that daily dosage level of 10–40 mg/day of methadone is usually sufficient to prevent withdrawal symptoms in the person addicted to narcotic analgesics. However, Stein and Kosten (1994) challenged this conclusion. It was suggested that opiate-dependent persons who are maintained at low doses of either methadone or buprenorphine may continue to experience a prolonged withdrawal syndrome, after the acute withdrawal symptoms have been controlled. The authors noted that the symptoms of the extended withdrawal syndrome are mild when compared with the acute withdrawal process, but may continue for extended periods. The authors suggested that patients on methadone be maintained at higher dosages, to avoid the protracted withdrawal syndrome, or the temptation to self-medicate these protracted withdrawal symptoms with cocaine.

An initial methadone dosage schedule of 10 mg/hour for the first day is used (Mirin et al., 1991). The individual going through opiate withdrawal receives a dose of 10 mg of methadone each hour, until the withdrawal symptoms are brought under control. Once the withdrawal symptoms have been controlled, the total dose of methadone administered becomes the starting dose for withdrawal. On Day 2 of withdrawal, the narcotics addict receives the same dosage level as was found to terminate withdrawal symptoms on Day 1, but the entire dose is to be administered in the morning, as a single dose. Starting on the Day 3, the daily dose of methadone is reduced by 5 mg/day until the patient is completely detoxified from opiates (Mirin et al., 1991).

The usual detoxification program lasts 3 to 21 days (Mirin et al., 1991), and by law if a detoxification programs lasts longer it must be licensed by the government as a methadone maintenance project (Jenike, 1991). Surprisingly, despite the length of the program, detoxification programs suffer from a significant dropout rate. Mirin et al. noted that as the daily dosage levels drop to the 15 or 20 mg/day range, the individual experiences a return of withdrawal symptoms. At this point, many individuals drop out of detoxification. A timely reminder from the authors is that opiate addicted individuals going through withdrawal should be reminded that they should *not* expect to be symptom-free during withdrawal.

Other programs, however, operate on the philosophy that methadone withdrawal is inappropriate. Some narcotic addicts have reported that methadone withdrawal is, in their opinion, worse than going "cold turkey." As noted in Chapter 11, withdrawal from opiates is not life-threatening, and many addicts have reported that—if the truth be told—withdrawal from narcotics is no more uncomfortable than having a bad cold or the flu.

Some programs offer pharmacological support during the withdrawal phase, such as benzodiazepines to help the person relax and sleep, but do not use narcotics. Other programs use a combination of nonnarcotic drugs to facilitate opiate withdrawal. Stein and Kosten (1992) reviewed a treatment program in which two different drugs, an antihypertensive (clonidine hydrochloride), and an opiate blocker, naltrexone hydrochloride, were used to bring about a 4- to 5-day opiate withdrawal.

The combination of naltrexone hydrochloride and clonidine is not a standard treatment for narcotics withdrawal (Weiss et al., 1994). However, the authors noted that this approach "holds promise" (p. 281) as a method of withdrawal from opiates. When used appropriately, the combination of clonidine and naltrexone hydrochloride hydrochloride appears to be as effective as a 20-day methadone withdrawal program for opiate addicts (Stein & Kosten, 1992). The combined effects of naltrexone hydrochloride hydrochloride (which blocks the opiate receptors in the brain) and the clonidine (which controls the individual's craving for narcotics and the severity of the withdrawal symptoms) thus allow for rapid detoxification from opiates with minimal discomfort.

The authors found that over 95% of their sample were completely withdrawn from narcotics at the end of 5 days. While there is some degree of discomfort for the addict, Stein and Kosten (1992) suggested that addicts reported about the same level of discomfort

from withdrawal using a combination of clonidine and naltrexone hydrochloride as they experienced during a methadone taper. Milhorn (1992) suggested that withdrawal discomfort might be further reduced through the use of transdermal clonidine patches, which would provide a steady supply of the drug while the patch was in place. However, because of the delay in absorption, the author advocated the use of an oral "loading" dose of 0.2 mg of clonidine at the beginning of the withdrawal cycle.

While clonidine would seem to be an effective tool in the control of the discomfort of narcotics withdrawal, some addicts have learned to combine clonidine with methadone, alcohol, benzodiazepines or other drugs to produce a sense of euphoria (Jenike, 1991). Health care professionals must carefully monitor the patient's medication use, to avoid the abuse of clonidine by the addict who is no longer able to use narcotics.

Experimental Methods of Opiate Withdrawal

An exciting, although unproven, method of opiate withdrawal has been advocated by at least some physicians in Israel (Sawicki, 1995). The Center for Investigation and Treatment of Addiction (CITA) in Israel has developed an "ultrarapid" program for opiate detoxification, where the detoxification process is carried out while the patient is in a state of drug-induced sleep. The exact combination of drugs used to induce sleep is a secret; however, detoxification is carried out overnight. Following detoxification, patients receive a 6-month follow-up course of naltrexone, so that if they should try to use opiates again, they would be unable to experience any euphoria from the drug. Proponents of this method of detoxification claim an 80% success rate after 6 months. While it is too soon to determine whether this method of detoxification will become popular, it suggests that there may be alternatives to the traditional methadone withdrawal process for opiate-addicted persons.

Pharmacological Treatment of Cocaine Addiction

Since the last epidemic of cocaine abuse/addiction began, researchers have searched for an agent or agents that will control the craving or hunger for cocaine that many addicts experience in the early stages of recovery. After more than a decade of research, scientists have failed to develop a pharmacological agent(s) that is specific and effective for the treatment of cocaine abuse/dependence (Leshner, 1996; Mendelson & Mellow, 1996).

At one point it was thought that antidepressant medications such as imipramine (Wilbur, 1986) or desipramine hydrochloride (Gawin, Kleber, et al., 1989) would be effective in curbing the postwithdrawal craving for cocaine. It was hoped that, since these antidepressants altered the function of those regions of the brain where cocaine had its main effects, they would prove useful in controlling the individual's urge to return to the use of cocaine.

Although the initial research into the use of antidepressant medication in the treatment of cocaine abuse/addiction was promising, subsequent research failed to support the initial optimistic conclusions by scientists. Meyer (1992) examined the results of the study by Gawin, Kleber, et al. (1989) and challenged the validity of this study on methodological grounds. According to Meyer, the study by Gawin et al. was flawed in that it relied on self-reported levels of cocaine abuse by clients, which were not supported by the results of urine toxicology tests. In other words, the clients *reported* less cocaine use, but the urine toxicology tests did not support these claims, according to Meyer. Thus the conclusions of this early study are suspect.

In another study that challenged the use of pharmacological agents in the treatment of cocaine abuse/addiction, Campbell, Thomas, Gabrielli, Liskow, and Powell (1995) examined the effects of the antidepressant desipramine, the anticonvulsant medication carbamazepine (often used to control the symptoms of epilepsy), and a placebo, on 65 cocaine-dependent patients. In the study, the subject pool was divided into three subgroups. Twenty-one subjects received desipramine, 19 received carbamazepine, and 25 subjects received a placebo, according to the authors. The authors failed to find that the medications had any effect on patient retention or concurrent drug abuse by their subjects, thus casting doubt that these medications are of value in the routine treatment of cocaine dependence.

Desimipramine hydrochloride is thought to be useful only for the subset of cocaine users who either had symptoms of depression prior to their use of cocaine or who became depressed immediately after starting to use cocaine (Mendelson & Mellow, 1996). But, even in this limited number of cocaine users, there still is a possibility that the desimipramine might cause the user to experience cardiac problems (Decker et al., 1987).

To avoid these possible cardiac complications, the research team of Margolin, Kosten, Petrakis, Avants, and Kosten (1991) used a "second generation" antidepressant, *bupropion* (Wellbutrin) in an attempt to control postcocaine craving. The authors reported that five subjects completed the experiment, while one subject was dropped for medical reasons. Of these five individuals, four subjects had stopped cocaine use after a period of 4 weeks, and were still cocaine-free after 3 months.

Their results suggested that bupropion might offer some promise in controlling postcocaine craving. But, the conclusions of this study were marred by the fact that the research sample was made up of only 6 subjects. Subsequent research failed to suggest that bupropion was effective in the treatment of cocaine use/abuse (Mendelson & Mello, 1996). Thus, again, an agent that was initially thought to hold promise in the pharmacological treatment of cocaine abuse/addiction has not lived up to the researchers' expectations.

Another drug that initially demonstrated some promise in controlling cocaine craving, at least in experimental settings, was bromocriptine (sold in this country under the brand name "Parlodel") (DiGregorio, 1990). When administered in a single dose of 1.25 mg, bromocriptine was found to decrease cocaine withdrawal craving, according to DiGregorio, while 0.625 mg given by mouth four times a day was found to reduce psychiatric symptoms associated with cocaine withdrawal.

Bromocriptine's side effects include headaches, sedation, muscle tremor, and dry mouth, which made some users so uncomfortable that they discontinued it. Further, the possibility that bromocriptine is itself addictive was suggested, which raised concern about its use in the treatment of cocaine use problems. Early clinical trials with bromocriptine failed to yield any positive results, and it is now thought that this medication is of little value in the treatment of cocaine addiction (Holloway, 1991; Mendelson & Mello, 1996).

Surprisingly, the drug *flupenthixol* not only has demonstrated some initial promise in the treatment of cocaine use problems, but has also continued to appear effective in controlling cocaine use/abuse (Mendelson & Mello, 1996). Flupenthixol is currently available in Europe, the Far East, and the Caribbean, but not in the United States. This drug seems to be effective in the control of postcocaine craving, according to the authors. Holloway (1991) reported that "some" (p. 100) cocaine addicts on flupenthixol report that their craving for cocaine is "manageable but is not eliminated" (p. 100). Thus, flupenthixol appears to hold promise as a possible pharmacological agent in the treatment of cocaine use problems. But, it remains to be seen whether flupenthixol will live up to its initial promise as a potential agent in the war against cocaine use/abuse.

Another agent that has shown promise in the treatment of cocaine withdrawal craving is buprenorphine. In addition to its effectiveness in laboratory studies with narcotics addicts, buprenorphine has also been shown to have an effect on post-cocaine craving (Holloway, 1991; "Ice Overdose," 1989; Rosen & Kosten, 1991; Youngstrom, 1990b). At low doses, oral buprenorphine seems to reduce the craving for cocaine, although the exact mechanism by which this is accomplished remains unknown (Holloway, 1991; Rosen & Kosten, 1991).

One radical approach to the treatment of cocaine abuse/addiction involves teaching the body to use the immune system against cocaine molecules (Leshner, 1996). There is theoretical evidence to suggest it is possible to target an immune response against certain elements of the cocaine molecule. The body would then form "antibodies" to destroy any molecule that had the same chemical structure. In theory, a vaccine could be developed that would allow the body to develop an immune response to cocaine molecules within the body (Leshner). However, this is still only a theoretical possibility, and there is no such vaccine available for use with humans at this time.

It might be, as Trachtenberg and Blum (1988) suggested, that cocaine brings about its effects, at least in part, by activation of both dopamine and opioid peptide neurotransmitter systems. The authors point out that naloxone, which normally is used to block the effects of narcotics in the brain, actually seems to potentiate the stimulation and euphoria of cocaine. If their theory is true, then the reward mechanism for both cocaine and the narcotics may involve activation of the same neurotransmission systems. It would also seem to make sense that a drug such as buprenorphine might prove of value in controlling the craving to both narcotics and cocaine.

In 1988, a different treatment approach for cocaine addiction was suggested by the authors. Trachtenberg and Blum (1988) suggest a theory that cocaine addiction might be influenced by the neurochemicals available in the brain. The authors, in an extension of the "neurotransmitter precursor loading" system (Blum & Trachtenberg, 1988, p. 5) used in their treatment of alcoholism, advocate the use of a "nutritional neurochemical support" system (Trachtenberg & Blum, 1988, p. 326) to aid in the treatment of cocaine addiction.

The authors suggested using a combination of amino acids, selected minerals, and vitamins to stimulate the formation of the neutransmitters depleated by chronic cocaine use. In one research study, the authors presented claims of a ninefold reduction in dropout rates for patients in an experimental group who received a patented formulation of "nutritional neurochemical support" (p. 326) over those who did not receive such support. But in the past few years, interest in the neuronutrient approach to the treatment of cocaine addiction has waned.

Surprisingly, after conducting an investigation into the cocaine withdrawal process, the research team of Satel et al. (1991) challenged the need for routine pharmacological support of recovering cocaine addicts. The authors concluded that their data "failed to demonstrate the emergence" (p. 1715) of severe withdrawal symptoms following the initiation of abstinence, and that while there were reports of craving for cocaine, their subjects experienced a marked decline in the strength and frequency of such craving over the first 3 weeks of recovery. For these reasons, the authors of this study concluded that there did not seem to be a need for routine pharmacological support of cocaine addicts during the early stages of recovery.

Pharmacological Treatment of Nicotine Dependence

Nicotine Replacement Therapies

Nicotine-Containing Gum

To help smokers in their struggle to quit, health care workers have turned to a number of different pharmacological tools, in the hopes that one or more would prove of value in the battle against cigarette smoking. A form of chewing gum that contains nicotine was introduced as an aid to cigarette cessation in 1984. Originally, nicotine-containing gum was available only with a physician's prescription. However, in 1996 the Food and Drug Administration approved the sale of nicotine-containing gum without a prescription as an aid to cigarette cessation.

The nicotine in the gum is released when it is chewed, and is slowly absorbed through the soft tissues in the mouth. However, the manner in which nicotine-containing gum is chewed differs from that normally used for traditional "chewing gum." With nicotine-containing gum, the individual must adopt a "chew-park-chew-park" (Fiore et al., 1992, p. 2691) system of chewing the gum. When used properly, about 90% of the nicotine in the gum is released in the first 30 minutes that the gum is chewed.

Use of nicotine-containing gum results in a lower blood level of nicotine than that achieved by cigarette smoking. Nicotine-containing gum with 2 mg of nicotine will bring about a blood level of nicotine only about one-third as high as that achieved through cigarette use; likewise, gum with 4 mg of nicotine will produce a blood level only about two-thirds of that reached through smoking (American Psychiatric Association, 1996). Further, nicotine-containing gum may cause such side effects as sore gums, excessive salivation, nausea, anorexia, headache, and the formation of ulcers on the gums (Lee & D'Alonzo, 1993). Also, beverages with a high acid content, such as orange juice or coffee, block the absorption of the nicotine from the gum. Thus, users must monitor their beverage intake to avoid such acidic compounds while using nicotine-containing gum.

Researchers disagree as to the value of nicotine-containing gum in smoking cessation programs.

Some researchers believe that nicotine-containing gum is helpful (although not totally effective) in controlling both the craving for cigarettes and the irritability associated with withdrawal (Hughes et al., 1991). Other researchers have concluded that the success rate of nicotine-containing gum is about the same as that of a placebo, suggesting that this product is of little value in cigarette cessation programs (Fiore et al., 1992).

One reason researchers have reached different conclusions as to the effectiveness of nicotine-containing gum in cigarette cessation programs is that some research studies have paired the use of the gum with intensive individual or group counseling, while other programs have used the gum alone. Research has shown that the effectiveness of nicotine-containing gum varies with the intensity of the supportive counseling that the individual receives (Fiore, Smith, Jorenby, & Baker, 1994). Thus, those studies that utilized nicotine-containing gum alone, or with minimal counseling support, would be less likely to find any significant effect than those programs that included an intensive counseling program for those individuals who wished to stop smoking.

An interesting question surrounding the use of nicotine gum is the role of individual expectations on the observed effects of the gum. Gottlieb et al. (1987) found that when subjects were led to expect nicotine-containing gum, they reported fewer withdrawal symptoms from cigarette withdrawal. However, only some of the subjects in this study actually received nicotine-containing gum. The other subjects received a placebo. The authors found that the individual's expectations as to whether they had received nicotine gum seemed to play a large role in moderating their withdrawal symptoms from cigarettes. This study raises serious questions as to the actual effectiveness of nicotine-containing gum in cigarette cessation.

Transdermal Nicotine Patches

In 1991, several companies introduced transdermal patches containing nicotine, designed to supply a constant blood level of nicotine without the need for the user to smoke cigarettes. The theory behind this treatment technique is that smokers might find it easier to break the habit if they did not actually have to smoke to obtain a moderately high blood level of nicotine. Later (usually 2–8 weeks) after the individual no longer engages in the physical motions of smoking, the dosage levels of nicotine in the patches may be reduced, providing a gradual taper in blood nicotine levels.

Researchers have found that transdermal nicotine patches are an effective adjunct to a cigarette cessation program (Fiore et al., 1992; Fiore, Smith, et al., 1994). The authors found that, of those individuals who had used the patch, approximately 22% to 42% were still smoke-free 6 months after treatment, while only 5% to 28% of those individuals who used a placebo transdermal patch were still smoke-free 6 months after treatment. Thus, the transdermal nicotine patch seems to result in approximately twice as many successful abstainers as a placebo patch system. Further, transdermal nicotine replacement systems reduce some of the more troublesome side effects of cigarette cessation, such as the insomnia that many people experience when they try to quit (Wetter, Fiore, Baker, & Young, 1995).

The transdermal nicotine patch is not without its drawbacks. Individuals who smoke while using the patch run the risk of nicotine toxicity, and even possible cardiovascular problems. Also, while the patch has been shown to reduce the level of nicotine craving, it does not totally eliminate it. Further, many of those who have used a transdermal patch have reported some degree of skin irritation under the patch. Other reported problems associated with the patch include abnormal or disturbing dreams, insomnia, diarrhea, and a burning sensation near where the patch is resting on the skin.

Even with the transdermal nicotine patch, a significant number of smokers will return to the practice of cigarette smoking. The research team of Kenford et al. (1994) attempted to identify factors that would predict which individuals would, and would not, succeed in giving up cigarette smoking while using a patch. Study participants also received group counseling. The authors found that those individuals who were able to abstain from cigarette smoking during the first 2 weeks of treatment, especially during the 2nd week, were most likely to give up their cigarette use. However, 90% of those individuals who smoked during the 2nd week of treatment while using a trans-

dermal nicotine patch were still smoking cigarettes 6 months later, according to the authors.

The results of the study by Kenford et al. (1994) are consistent with earlier studies that suggest the first month of cigarette cessation is especially difficult for the ex-smoker. Further, the results of this study suggest that the transdermal nicotine patch, while useful as an adjunct to cigarette cessation programs, still is not totally effective in helping smokers quit. There is evidence that some former smokers may require transdermal nicotine patches for years to abstain from cigarette use (Sherman, 1994). While these individuals will still be obtaining nicotine in their systems, they will, at least, not be exposing themselves to the multitude of known or suspected toxins contained in cigarette smoke.

A major drawback of the transdermal nicotine patch is that the user can achieve only a relatively low blood level of nicotine (Henningfield, 1995). Thus, the nicotine transdermal patch might not prevent the user from craving more nicotine. To try to eliminate this problem, the American Psychiatric Association (1996) recommended that the user try supplementary doses of nicotine-containing gum if the transdermal skin patch does not provide sufficiently high levels of nicotine to block craving.

Nasal Spray

A nasal spray that contains nicotine has been developed for use in the control of tobacco craving following smoking cessation. In March 1996, the Food and Drug Administration approved the short-term use of a nasal spray in the United States, as an aid to smoking cessation. One provision imposed in the use of nicotine-containing sprays by the Food and Drug administration is that it be used for less than 4 to 6 months. Sutherland et al. (1992) tested the effectiveness of the nasal spray, giving one group of volunteers a supply of nasal spray containing nicotine, while another group of volunteers received a placebo. Both groups participated in group counseling designed to help them remain smoke-free. The authors reported that two advantages of a nicotine-containing nasal spray are that the nicotine is rapidly absorbed through the nasal membranes and that, with the exception of some sinus irritation, there are no serious side effects from this method of nicotine administration. According to the authors, only two subjects had to discontinue use of the nicotine nasal spray because of adverse side effects, which is a reflection of the safety of this method of nicotine replacement.

The authors found that heavy smokers were most likely to benefit from the nasal spray. Further, smokers who used the spray had less weight gain than subjects who received a placebo nasal spray. It was found that 26% of the smokers who had received the nicotine-containing nasal spray had remained smoke-free for a full year, while only 10% of the group that received the placebo remained smoke-free for a year.

But, the nicotine nasal spray also presents its own unique set of dangers. Blood plasma levels of nicotine obtained from this nasal spray approach those achieved from smoking. Because of this characteristic, there is concern that users might become as dependent on the nasal spray as they were on cigarettes (Benowitz, 1992). Sutherland et al. (1992) found that, after 6 months, the nicotine concentrations were three-quarters of those found in active smokers. While the authors concluded that the "systemic nicotine replacement" (p. 328) that the individuals in their research sample achieved with the nasal spray was responsible for lower levels of nicotine craving, one must wonder if their sample was not simply replacing their dependence on tobacco with the nasal spray.

Other Pharmacological Treatments for Nicotine Addiction

Clonidine

A number of researchers have attempted to utilize clonidine, an antihypertensive drug, to control the craving for nicotine often reported by former cigarette smokers. Clonidine has been found to be an effective agent in withdrawal from opioids. Glassman et al. (1988) explored the utility of clonidine to help cigarette smokers stop using tobacco products. The authors found that twice as many of the subjects who received clonidine were able to stop smoking and remain abstinent over a 4-week span than subjects who received a placebo. On the basis of this

study, the authors concluded that clonidine was an effective adjunct in a cigarette cessation program.

The research team of Franks, Harp, and Bell (1989) challenged this conclusion, however. The authors found that "no statistically significant effects on quitting" (p. 3013) existed between those subjects who received clonidine and those subjects who received a placebo. The authors suggested that earlier research studies exploring the application of clonidine to nicotine withdrawal utilized small samples made up of highly motivated subjects. These individuals would be more likely to report success to the researchers than would a general practice population encountered by most physicians, if only because they were highly motivated to quit smoking.

To settle the matter, Gourlay and Benowitz (1995) examined the possibility that clonidine was an effective agent in cigarette cessation programs. After an extensive review of the pharmacology of clonidine, and the findings of earlier research studies, the authors suggested that, for those smokers who had encountered agitation and anxiety in previous attempts to stop smoking, clonidine in addition to nicotine replacement therapies might be an alternative to the use of nicotine replacement techniques alone. However, the authors concluded, clonidine's side effect profile made it a poor first choice for smoking cessation programs. The American Psychiatric Association (1996) recommended that clonidine be used with those individuals who have attempted nicotine replacement therapy, without success.

Silver Acetate

This chemical, when used by a cigarette smoker, will produce a disulfiram-like reaction for the smoker (Hymowitz, Feuerman, Hollander, & Frances, 1993). Chewing gum and lozenges have been used in Europe for the purpose of smoking cessation for more than a decade now, although this medication is not available in the United States. When the individual has recently used the gum or lozenge, and then attempts to smoke, a "noxious metallic taste" (Hymowitz et al., 1993, p. 113) results. This obnoxious taste then causes the smoker to discard the cigarette and replaces the nicotine-based pharmacological reward with an aversive experience.

Silver acetate is dangerous, and overuse may result in *permanent* discoloration of the skin and body organs (Hymowitz et al., 1993). However, the authors point out that this side effect of silver acetate is rare, and is usually seen only after "massive overuse and abuse" (p. 113). Another drawback of silver acetate is that its effectiveness in smoking cessation has not been fully tested. However, preliminary research has suggested a possible role for silver acetate lozenges and gum as an aid in smoking cessation.

Buspar

Buspirone (discussed in Chapter 7) has been found to be of value in the cigarette cessation. The subjects who received buspirone in therapeutic dosage levels reported less fatigue and anxiety while going through nicotine withdrawal. Further, there was no evidence of weight gain in the subjects who received buspirone for nicotine withdrawal. The biochemical mechanism through which buspirone might counter the effects of nicotine withdrawal is not known at this time (Sussman, 1994), but this medication shows promise in cigarette cessation programs.

Other agents that have been utilized in the treatment of nicotine withdrawal over the years include the tricyclic antidepressants and lobeline (a drug derived from a variety of tobacco) (Lee & D'Alonzo, 1993). Despite extensive research, however, no single substance has proven effective in treating the symptoms of nicotine withdrawal beyond any reasonable doubt.

Summary

The pharmacological treatment of substance abuse involves the use of selected chemicals to aid recovering addicts in their attempts to maintain sobriety. To this end, a number of different chemicals have been tried as experimental agents, in the hopes that one or more would prove useful in controlling either the withdrawal symptoms experienced by a recovering addict in the early stages of sobriety or in controlling the craving that many addicts have reported after they stopped using chemicals.

CHAPTER THIRTY-THREE

Infections Frequently Caused by Recreational Substance Abuse[1]

One of the most serious complications of recreational drug use is the development of a viral, bacterial, or fungal infection on the part of the user. There are many ways that infectious agents can gain admission into the individual's body as a direct result of recreational drug use. Among some of the infections commonly found in intravenous drug addicts are peripheral cellulitis, skin abscesses, pneumonia, lung abscesses, and tetanus. Infectious diseases are, collectively, one of the most serious medical complications of intravenous drug abuse (Mathew et al., 1995). These infections might also be indirectly caused by the use of a recreational chemical, such as pneumonia that develops in an alcoholic patient whose resistance has been sapped by years of chronic malnutrition. In this chapter, we discuss some of the more common infections that may be acquired by the recreational chemical abuser.

Why Is Infectious Disease Such a Common Complication of Alcohol/Drug Abuse?

Often, intravenous drug users are malnourished, a condition that may lower their resistance to infection. Chronic alcohol users also tend to be malnourished, both because the individual's body comes to substitute the calories in the alcoholic beverage for those that his/her body should normally obtain from food, and because of vitamin malabsorption syndromes. However, there is another reason intravenous drug abusers are prone to develop infections: the conditions under which they inject their drug(s) of choice make infection almost a guaranteed complication.

Sterile Technique

It is rare for intravenous drug users to use proper "sterile technique" when injecting the chemicals into their bodies. In a hospital setting, staff will sterilize the injection site either with alcohol, or with an antiseptic solution, and then inject a sterile solution containing the pharmaceutical into the patient's body. In contrast, however, intravenous drug addicts usually simply find a vein and then insert the needle directly into that vein, without even attempting to wash the injection site with any kind of an antiseptic. In so doing, addicts will push microscopic organisms found on the surface of the skin directly into their body, bypassing the protective layers of skin that usually keep such microorganisms from the blood-rich tissues within the body.

Another reason IV drug users are prone to infections is that intravenous drug addicts inject illicit compounds, and not pharmaceutical quality products, into their bodies. These street drugs are often contaminated with various microscopic pathogens. Thus, when users inject the compound into their

[1] The author would like to express his appreciation to John P. Doweiko, M.D., for his kindness in reviewing this chapter for technical accuracy.

bodies, they inject whatever microscopic pathogens are in the mixture directly into their bodies as well.

Finally, another common characteristic of intravenous drug users is that they often share needles with other intravenous drug abusers. In some parts of the United States, it is not uncommon for several people to use the same needle and syringe in turn, without stopping to sterilize the intravenous "rig."[2] This practice exposes each subsequent user of that needle to infectious agents in the blood of previous users (Garrett, 1994). Admittedly, some intravenous drug users try to clean the needle before use, perhaps by engaging in such practices as licking the needle clean before use. This transfers microorganisms such as *Neisseria sicca* and *Streptococcus viridans*, bacteria normally limited to the mouth, to the intravenous needle that is about to be inserted under his/her skin, contributing to infection (Dewitt & Paauw, 1996). Other intravenous drug users may wash the needle with water. But ordinary tap water can also contain microorganisms that are harmless to the user when the water is ingested, but that will contaminate an intravenous needle about to be inserted into a person's body (Dewitt & Paauw, 1996).

Among the infections that can be transmitted from one person to another through contaminated needles include several viruses that attack the liver such as those that cause hepatitis types "B" and "C" (discussed later in this chapter). Occasionally, malaria is transmitted from one person to another through contaminated intravenous needles (Cherubin & Sapira, 1993; Garrett, 1994). Any of a large number of other organisms capable of infecting the individual, such as syphilis, may also be transmitted from one person to another through the use of contaminated needles. Some of the more common forms of infection are discussed in this chapter.

Indirect Sources of Infection

Endocarditis

Intravenous drug use might also indirectly contribute to the development of an infection in another way. The chronic use of irritating chemicals such as those often used to adulterate illicit narcotics is thought to contribute to the development of bacterial infections of the heart valves (a condition known as endocarditis) (Mathew et al., 1995). Bacterial endocarditis can arise in individuals who have other medical conditions, but it is also a common complication of intravenous drug use. Researchers believe that 7% to 38% of *all* cases of infectious endocarditis are found in intravenous drug abusers (Abolnik & Corey, 1995; Dewitt & Paauw, 1996). This infection may prove fatal to the individual.

Necrotizing Fascitis

This is an infection in which subcutaneous tissues are attacked by bacteria normally found on the surface of the skin (Karch, 1996). There are clinical indications that suggest cocaine users are more prone to this infection, but it can develop in any intravenous drug abuser who fails to use the proper antiseptic procedures to prepare the skin before injection. The bacteria found on the surface of the skin gain entry to the subcutaneous tissues and spread throughout the body. As the bacteria destroy the tissues under the skin, the infection may spread to internal organs or deeper tissues. The surface of the skin appears normal, until late in the course of the infection, making diagnosis difficult. This condition can result in the death of the patient.

Skin Abscesses

These are a common complication of intravenous drug abuse. It is thought that adulterants mixed with heroin or cocaine cause, or at least contribute, to skin abscesses. Because the adulterants are usually not water soluble, they cause the body to react to their presence at the injection site. Further, most intravenous drug abusers do not use proper antiseptic techniques, setting the stage for bacterial infection. As a result, abscesses form under the surface of the skin, which may become life-threatening.

Fungal Pneumonia

Although a common complication of HIV-1 infection (discussed later in this chapter), pneumonia caused by fungi is also a common complication of heroin abuse/addiction (Karch, 1996). There are two primary reasons for the association between heroin abuse and fungal infections. First, chronic

---

[2] A "rig" is a term applied to the intravenous needle and syringe.

heroin abuse causes the immune system to become less efficient. But, second, many samples of street heroin are contaminated by fungi. Users who then inject the heroin inject the fungi directly into their circulation. Often, the fungi settle in the lungs, causing pneumonia.

Community Acquired Pneumonia

Intravenous heroin abusers and alcohol-dependent persons are known to be at increased risk for a condition known as community-acquired pneumonia (CAP) (Karch, 1996).[3] CAP affects an estimated 2 to 4 million people in the United States each year. While mild cases can be treated on an outpatient basis, fully 20% of those individuals with CAP eventually require hospitalization (G. Campbell, 1994). A quarter of those who are hospitalized with CAP die, despite the best medical care. This means that there are between 100,000 and 200,000 CAP-related deaths each year in the United States.

Several factors determine vulnerability to CAP, including age, general health status, the speed with which the patient begins to be treated for the infection, and the effectiveness of the immune system (G. Campbell, 1994; Leeper & Torres, 1995). Either directly or indirectly, chronic alcohol use and heroin abuse/addiction are known to reduce the effectiveness of the immune system, placing the individual at increased risk for CAP.

As early as the 1890s, pneumonia was recognized as a significant cause of death for alcohol-dependent individuals (Leeper & Torres, 1995). Since then, researchers have found that chronic alcohol use interferes with the defensive ability of the lungs against infectious microorganisms, thus making it a risk factor for CAP (Nelson, Mason, Kolls, & Summer, 1995). With the advent of intravenous drug abuse on a large scale, it has been found that IV drug use is also a risk factor for CAP because this practice can indirectly impair the effectiveness of the immune system. Finally, cigarette smoking, which reduces the effectiveness of the lung's defenses, is also a risk factor for CAP (Leeper & Torres, 1995).

---

[3] As opposed to pneumonia acquired in a hospital setting, or secondary to some form of lung trauma.

Acquired Immune Deficiency Syndrome (AIDS)

In the past generation, the *human immunodeficiency virus type 1* (HIV-1) has spread from its still unknown point of origin, around the globe (King, 1994; Kruger & Jerrells, 1992; Terwilliger, 1995). HIV-1 is the virus that causes AIDS, and infection with this deadly virus is often a complication of alcohol/drug use.

History of AIDS in the United States

In 1981, it became clear to medical researchers that a previously unknown disease had started to spread through the population of the United States. Initially, the disease seemed to be isolated to the homosexual male population, but researchers were not sure what was causing the disorder. About all that was known was that the immune system in certain people would rapidly fail, leaving the victim open to any of a range of rare "opportunistic infections." Medical researchers termed this process the *acquired immune deficiency syndrome* (AIDS).

As physicians studied this disorder, it was discovered that AIDS also developed in some intravenous drug abusers and in individuals whose only apparent risk factor for the infection was that they had received a blood transfusion in the past. These facts suggested to researchers that some kind of blood-borne infection was involved in the development of AIDS. Further studies quickly revealed that the infectious agent was most likely a virus, rather than a new species of bacteria. Within a short period, researchers had isolated a virus that has since been called the *human immunodeficiency virus* (HIV) (King, 1994; McCutchan, 1990). As different, related members of the same virus family have been identified, it has become necessary to identify each by a number. The virus that is thought to cause AIDS is now known to medicine as HIV-1.

What Is AIDS?

It is surprising how many people speak of AIDS as if it were a disease in itself. Technically, AIDS is not a disease, but a *constellation* of symptoms, the most important of which is the destruction of the individual's immune system. AIDS is the end stage of a viral infection caused by HIV-1. As the HIV-1 infection progresses, the patient eventually will die from an infection, neoplasm, or other condition that the immune system was once able to easily control.

Where did HIV-1 come from?   Since it was discovered, a number of stories have been advanced as to how HIV-1 came into being. One of the most provocative myths to emerge is that HIV-1 was a "designer virus" made in a "germ warfare" laboratory that was either accidentally or intentionally released into the population (Weiss, 1994). In reality, HIV-1 is now viewed as one of the multitude of infections that "jump" from one species to another, as the causal microbe adapts to human beings as a new host species.[4] This theory is supported by genetic evidence such as the similarity between HIV-1 and certain other retroviruses that are known to infect only primates (Barre-Sinoussi, 1996; Terwilliger, 1995).

The genetic similarities between HIV-1 and viruses that infect certain monkeys are so strong that researchers believe that HIV-1 and those viruses that infect primates shared a common ancestor as recently as only 600 to 1200 years ago (Barre-Sinoussi, 1996). Then, sometime around the middle of the 20th century, it appears that HIV-1 managed to shift from its original host to humans (Karlen, 1995; Weiss, 1994).

Before the development of modern methods of transportation, Africa's geographic isolation provided an effective barrier to the spread of many infectious diseases. Depending on the form of infection, the infected person might live long enough to travel for a few hours, or a few days. However, for the most part, outbreaks of infectious diseases in Africa tended to be limited to small geographic regions by the barriers that the disease would have to cross, to reach new hosts. It is an unfortunate consequence of modern travel that it is now possible for numerous "new" diseases to move rapidly across the globe.

This is how HIV-1 is thought to have spread. First, as geographic barriers became less and less of a problem for travel, HIV-1 moved out of the backwaters of Africa to the major cities of that continent. Within a few months or, at most, a few years, the virus is thought to have spread around the globe as one infected person after another unknowingly passed the new virus on to new victims. While this theory is consistent with the known facts, it remains only a theory. Scientists have not discovered how HIV-1 evolved into its present form, or, what the history of HIV-1 was like prior to its discovery as the cause of AIDS. There is little, if any, creditable evidence that HIV-1 was intentionally released into the population to target homosexual males or other minority group members, or that it is divine retribution for past sins (Karlen, 1995). It is thought to be just one of many viral infections that has swept through the human population in the past 10,000 years or so.

How Does AIDS Kill?

The process through which HIV-1 is able to infect, and ultimately kill, the victim is based on a remarkable chain of events involving the individual's immune system and the way that HIV-1 replicates in the human host. Every species of bacteria, virus, or fungus has a characteristic pattern of protein molecules in the wall of its cells. When the human body is invaded by a bacterium, fungus, or virus, the immune system learns to recognize the specific pattern of proteins that make up the cell wall of the invader. The body also learns how to tell the difference between the protein pattern of an invading organism from that of the body's own cells. The immune system learns to protect the body from invading organisms by building antibodies that recognize foreign cells and attack them.

The body "tailor-makes" some antibodies for each species of microorganism that it encounters over the years. These pathogen-specific antibodies are designed to recognize the individual protein pattern on the surface of a single species of bacteria, fungus, or virus. These disease-specific antibodies then drift in the individual's blood, spending their entire life searching for just one specific species of virus, or fungus, or bacteria. This is the mechanism through which a person who once had an infection becomes immune to that disease. After recovering from the infection, the individual will have a number of white

---

[4]This is a common occurrence. Karlen (1995) identified almost 300 infectious diseases in humans that were acquired when the microbe that causes that specific disease jumped from the original host to human beings sometime in the past.

blood cells from the previous exposure to the invader in reserve, patiently waiting until the next time that the same microorganism might try to enter his/her body. The person is now immune to that disease.

But the first time that the body is exposed to a new organism, the process of producing the specific antibody necessary to fight off a specific bacteria or virus may take hours, days, weeks, or in some cases, years. Until the body can begin to produce disease-specific antibodies, it must rely on more generalized disease-fighting cells, which are not pathogen-specific. These generalists roam through the body and seek out *any* invader with a foreign protein pattern in the cell wall. These generalist antibodies are the ones that mount the initial attack against a new invader, before the body learns to produce pathogen-specific antibodies.

In the case of an HIV-1 infection, it may require up to 9 months after the virus invades the body, before the immune system begins to produce HIV-1 specific antibodies (McCutchan, 1990). This is one characteristic of the HIV-1 disease process that has contributed to its rapid spread in this country. During this "latency" period between the initial infection and when his/her body has started to produce antibodies against HIV-1, the infected person will not test positive for the infection. This is because current blood tests for HIV-1 test not for the virus itself, but for the *antibodies* that the body produces to try to fight off the infection.

One characteristic of HIV-1 infection is that it is able to work its way into different body tissues (Radetsky, 1990; Terwilliger, 1995). This allows the virus to hide from the body's defenses while it reproduces. HIV-1 demonstrates a preference for the cells of the immune system, especially the type of antibodies known as "T-helper" cells (Branson, 1995). Thus, in the infected individual, one will often find the virus hiding in the cells of the individual's body.

Remember that many of the antibodies are tailor-made to a specific species of virus, bacteria, or fungus. Yet, another characteristic of HIV-1 is that, each time it replicates, it makes slightly different copies of itself. The specific mechanism is quite technical, and well beyond the scope of a text such as this. However, in brief, the virus tends to be "sloppy" in replication, allowing subtle "mistakes" to slip into the genetic code of each new generation of virus particles. These variations in the basic genetic code of HIV-1 then are released back into the general circulation. Because of the differences in their genetic code, these new HIV-1 virus particles are, in effect, "new" viruses, at least as far as the body's defenses are concerned (Nowak & McMichael, 1995; Terwilliger, 1995). As a result, by the later stages of HIV-1 infection a single individual might have as many as *one billion* different forms of the HIV-1 virus in his/her body (Richardson, 1995). At this point in the infectious process, it is not unreasonable to say that the individual's body is host to a "swarm" of viruses (Barre-Sinoussi, 1996, p. 32).

Ultimately, this flood of similar, but distinctly different, HIV-1 cells will overwhelm the body's cellular immune system (Beardsley, 1994; Terwilliger, 1995). The exact means by which HIV-1 destroys the body's immune system is not clear at this time (King, 1994; J. Moore, 1993). But it is known that as the immune system becomes weaker, various "opportunistic infections" begin to develop. Such infections are usually caused by microorganisms that were once easily controlled by the immune system. In some cases, patients have developed opportunistic infections very early in the HIV disease process, when there is a limited degree of immune system impairment (Branson, 1995). Eventually, the body's weakened defenses are overwhelmed by the invading microbes. As the patient enters the final stages of AIDS, death becomes inevitable.

The Chain of HIV-1 Infection

HIV-1 is a fragile virus, which is not easily transmitted (Langone, 1989). The virus must be passed *directly* from one person to another. The apparent modes of HIV-1 transmission are the direct mixing of one's blood with infected body fluids (as when using a contaminated intravenous needle), having received a transfusion of a blood product contaminated with the virus, the passage of the virus from the mother to the fetus, or transmission through the mother's milk to the suckling baby (King, 1994; Kruger & Jerrells, 1992; Quinn, 1995). Sexual contact between an infected and noninfected individual is also a major means by which HIV-1 is transmitted between individuals (M. Cohen, 1995).

Since it is a blood-borne infection, HIV-1 can be transmitted through blood transfusions if the donor is infected with the virus. This fact has resulted in the development of new blood tests to screen out blood donors who have anti-HIV-1 antibodies in their blood. These antibodies suggest that the individual has been exposed to the virus, and thus should not be used for a blood transfusion. This procedure has resulted in a drastic reduction in the level of HIV-1 transfusion in the United States through contaminated blood. Researchers believe that the incidence of HIV-1 infection through blood transfusions in the United States is about 1 case in every 450,000–660,000 units of blood transfused (Lackritz et al., 1995). Schreiber, Busch, Kleinman, and Korelitz (1996) arrived at an estimate of one case of HIV-1 transmission for every 493,000 units of blood used for transfusion in the United States. Thus, blood transfusions are thought to be a rare means by which HIV-1 is transmitted from one person to another in the United States.

One of the most common means by which HIV-1 is transmitted from one person to another in the United States is the practice of sharing drug paraphernalia by intravenous drug abusers. In 1994, more than half of the new cases of HIV-1 infection were drug-related (Swan, 1995b). Overall, 3% to 9% of intravenous drug abusers become infected with HIV-1 each year. To underscore the risk associated with sharing intravenous needles, consider that in some communities blood tests show that up to 80% (Michelson, Carroll, McLane, & Robin, 1988) of intravenous drug users tested are "seropositive." This means that blood samples from these individuals contain antibodies against HIV-1.

The HIV-1 virus can be found in many different body fluids, including the semen of all infected men. Persons involved in sexual relationships with infected partners are thus at risk for contracting HIV-1. Globally, 75% to 85% of all cases of HIV-1 infection are thought to have been acquired when the victim had sex with an infected partner (Royce, Sena, Cates, & Cohen, 1997). For this reason, HIV-1 is increasingly classified as a sexually transmitted disease (STD). As with any other STD, the greater the number of sexual partners that one individual has had, the greater his/her chance of being exposed to somebody who is infected with an STD. In the United States, there is a high probability that

intraveneous drug abusers, those who are sexually promiscuous, prostitutes, and bisexual/homosexual males are infected with HIV-1. Because sexual contact with persons in these catagories can result in the individual contracting HIV-1, it is recommended that sexual relations with such persons be avoided.

In addition to the role that intravenous drug use has in the transmission of HIV-1, recreational drug use may also *indirectly* contribute to HIV-1 infection. Because alcohol lowers inhibitions, it may indirectly contribute to promiscuous behavior, exposing the individual to a partner infected with HIV-1. Further, the use of alcohol by the individual who is infected with HIV-1 may lower the individual's resistance, speeding up the progression of the infection (Kruger & Jerrells, 1992).

The pattern of HIV-1 infection in the United States is unlike that found in other regions of the world. In the United States, homosexual males and intravenous drug users are the groups at highest risk for HIV-1 infection. Slightly over half (52%) of those people in the United States who are infected with HIV-1 contracted the virus through homosexual or bisexual partners. Another 23% of those who are infected with HIV-1 contracted the disease through contaminated needles (Grigg, 1992). Heterosexual transmission of HIV-1 in the United States, while common, is not the primary method by which the virus is passed from one partner to another.

This may be because some subtypes of HIV-1 are able to infect the mucous membranes of the vagina more easily than other subtypes of the same virus. There are at least 10 different subtypes of HIV-1, which have been classified as types "A," "B," and so on (Barre-Sinoussi, 1996). The "E" subtype, which is found mainly in Asia and Africa, is a subtype that is able to more easily pass from an infected male to his female partner. It is thought that this is why heterosexual transmission of HIV-1 is *the* most common means by which the virus is passed on from one person to another in Asia and Africa. But the B subtype of the HIV-1 virus, which is the prevalent strain in the United States, is not able to easily pass into the mucous membranes of the woman, thus making heterosexual transmission of that subtype more difficult (R. Anderson, 1993).

The Scope of the Problem

Since the time that HIV-1 was first identified by medical science in the early 1980s, the face of AIDS has changed. According to current theory, less than 30 years ago HIV-1 was an obscure virus, thought to be found only in geographically isolated parts of Africa. In that span of less than 30 years, AIDS went from being a totally unknown disease, to being the most common cause of death for American men between the ages of 18 and 44, and the 4th most common cause of death for women in the United States between 18 and 44 years old (Anastos, Denenberg, & Solomon, 1997; Branson, 1995; Quinn, 1995).

Globally, an estimated 28 million people around the world are thought to be infected with HIV-1 (Royce et al., 1997). By the year 2000, possibly as many as 100 million people around the world will be infected with the HIV virus (Monteith, 1997). In the United States, an estimated 2 million people are currently infected with HIV-1 ("AIDS and Mental Health," 1994), with 40,000 new cases developing each year in this country. It has been estimated that 1 in every 100 males, and 1 in every 600 females, in the United States is infected with HIV-1 (Grigg, 1992). The World Health Organization (WHO) gave an even higher estimate of 1 in 75 for males in North America, but a lower estimate of 1 in 700 women in North America being infected with HIV-1 ("Update on Global AIDS," 1992).

AIDS is, at this time, predominately a male disease, at least in the United States. More than 88% of the reported cases of AIDS in this country have involved males (Dumas, 1992). Because of this, virtually all the research on the manifestations and treatment of AIDS has involved *male* victims (Amaro, 1995). Very little is known about the evolution of AIDS in women, or whether current treatment programs need to be modified for women (Anastos et al., 1997). This is most unfortunate, since the number of women in the United States who are infected with HIV-1 doubles every 1 to 2 years (Clay, 1996).

Amaro (1995) suggested that the manner in which HIV-1 infection is acquired differs for men and women. The authors reported that only 3% of the men who are infected with HIV-1 acquired the infection through heterosexual contacts. In contrast, 36% of the women who are infected with HIV-1 reportedly acquired the infection from a male partner. This difference in transmission rate reflects that it is estimated to be 12 times as difficult for the woman with HIV-1 to infect the male, as it is for the HIV-1 positive male to infect his female partner, according to the author. As is the case with male AIDS victims, approximately 48% of the women infected with HIV-1 acquired the infection through contaminated intravenous needles (Amaro).

One treatment recommendation for HIV-1 positive women is that they have a Papanicolaou ("Pap") smear immediately after being diagnosed as having been infected (Branson, 1995; Kocurek, 1996). If no abnormalities are found at the time of the first test, a second test should be carried out six months later. The physician should also carry out the appropriate tests to rule out concurrent infection with gonorrhea and chlamydia, according to the author, since the woman who contracts HIV-1 is often exposed to these other STDs at the same time.

How HIV-1 Infection Is Diagnosed

There is a long latency period between the initial exposure to the virus, and the development of the full AIDS syndrome. The median period between infection with HIV-1 and the development of AIDS is 11 years (Quinn, 1995). During this time, HIV-1 infection may be detected only through a series of blood tests. Pope and Morin (1990) outlined the stages necessary to identify whether a person is (or is not) infected with HIV-1 in the following manner:

> Generally, the initial tests screen blood samples of antibodies to the virus; such tests are termed ELISA (enzyme-linked immunosorbent assay). If the individual reacts positively to ELISA tests, a more difficult, expensive, and supposedly accurate test such as the Western Blot (which searches for antibodies against specific protein molecules) or radioimmunoprecipitation or radioimmunoflourescence assay [is carried out]. (p. 47)

The Classification of the Stages of HIV-1 Infection

The HIV-1 infection progresses through three distinct stages, according to Atkinson and Grant (1994). The three stages of HIV-1 are:

1. Seroconversion (the point where antibodies to HIV-1 are detected in the individual's blood for the first time, indicating that he/she has been infected with the virus.
2. A period in which the individual is infected, but during which the individual is essentially asymptomatic.
3. The period during which symptomatic disease and the progression to AIDS begins.

Other Classification Systems

In addition to the classification system offered by Atkinson and Grant (1994), there are numerous other classification systems for the stages of the HIV-1 infectious process. For example, many researchers use the "viral load" measure to determine the number of HIV-1 particles in the blood. However, the most commonly used classification system for HIV-1 infection in the United States was developed by the Center for Disease Control (CDC). This classification system uses approximately the same three stages outlined previously, combined with the number of one form of antibodies in the patient's blood. As researchers have come to understand more about the progression of the HIV-1 infection in the body, they have discovered that the virus seems to have a special affinity for one component of the body's immune system, the CD4+ lymphocyte cells[5] (also known as the CD4+ T-helper cells) (Hollander & Katz, 1993).

The individual who, upon testing, does not have antibodies for the AIDS virus, who does not test positive on the ELISA tests, would be classified as being "seronegative." There are two possible explanations for a "negative" finding: (a) the individual in question has never been exposed to the HIV-1, or (b) the person has been exposed to the virus, but has not had sufficient time to develop antibodies to the HIV-1. In either case, the individual should be tested again at a later date, usually 6 to 10 months after the initial blood test or last high-risk behavior, to rule out the second possibility.[6]

Being seronegative does not mean that the person is not possibly infected, just that the original test did not reveal an immune response to HIV-1. An infected person who still tests seronegative is capable of passing HIV-1 on to others. Evidence now suggests that one time when the virus is most easily transmitted to a new victim is while the first infected person is still seronegative (M. Cohen, 1995). It is only after two blood tests 6 to 10 months apart have been negative that a person can be reasonably assured that his/her last episode of high-risk behavior did not result in contracting the virus.

But, for the person who *is* infected, the disease will proceed. At first, the recently infected person may not have any specific symptom of HIV-1 infection. About 50% of the cases the individual may experience flulike symptoms after being exposed to the virus (Quinn, 1995; Terwilliger, 1995). Then, in the first few months following the transmission of the HIV-1 infection, the individual's body will begin to develop antibodies in an attempt to fight the virus. When this happens, the individual becomes seropositive because there are now antibodies fighting against the HIV-1 virus in the individual's blood. The person may remain seropositive, but essentially asymptomatic, for a number of years. During this phase of the HIV-1 infection process, the virus can be detected only through appropriate blood tests.

The current CDC classification criteria combines the 3 distinct stages of the HIV-1 infectious process outlined earlier, with a second measure that involves the number of certain specialized cells of the immune system, those with the CD4+ protein complex in the cell walls. These cells, which are also known as T-helper cells, are often referred to as "CD4+ T" cells. The CD4+ T cell count is itself broken down into three levels by the CDC classification system (Rubin, 1993):

Category 1	500 or more CD4+ T cells per cubic millimeter of blood.
Category 2	200–499 CD4+ T cells per cubic millimeter of blood.
Category 3	fewer than 200 CD4+ T cells per cubic millimeter of blood.

[5] The name of this cell is based on a pattern of proteins found in the cell wall.

[6] It should be noted that the blood test to detect exposure to HIV-1 is not perfect. The most common blood test for HIV-1 has a false positive rate of less than 1% and a false negative rate of about 3% (Rubin, 1993).

These two sets of criteria are then combined, providing a 3 × 3 classification grid that looks like Table 33-1.

As discussed earlier, because HIV-1 selectively destroys the individual's immune system, the CD4+ T cell count will fall. To avoid problems caused by normal variation in the body's CD4+ T cell count over the course of the day, the individual's blood should be tested at the same time each day (Kocurek, 1996). Further, the same laboratory should conduct the CD4+ T cell count, wherever possible, to ensure that the same procedures are followed each time the same individual is tested.

When the number of CD4+ T cells falls below 200 per cubic millimeter (mm^3) of blood, the individual will usually become vulnerable to any of a range of opportunistic infections rarely seen except in those patients whose immune system has been compromised in some manner. Such disorders include *Pneumocystis carinii pneumonia* (*P. carinii*, or

"*PCP*"), various tumors, and tuberculosis (TB). Thus, if the physician were to encounter a patient whose pneumonia is caused by *P. carinii*, that physician would almost automatically suspect that the patient has AIDS, or that his/her immune system is compromised in some manner.

At one point, physicians spoke of a stage of the HIV-1 infection process known as "Aids Related Complex," or ARC. During this phase, the individual was thought to have an impaired, but still functional, immune system. Further, the patient with ARC did not have the full spectrum of opportunistic infections seen in AIDS. In the past decade, this term has been replaced by the more accurate CD4+ T cell count method of determining the current stage of the HIV-1 infectious process.

Over time, the individual's body will become weakened by any of a range of opportunistic infections that his/her immune system once could easily control. Death is usually caused by one or

TABLE 33-1 Modified Center for Disease Control HIV/AIDS Classification Chart

*Number of CD4+ T-helper cells per mm³ of blood**	*Asymptomatic*	*Symptomatic but not full-blown AIDS*	*Full-blown AIDS*
Greater than or equal to 500 cells	A1	B1	C1
Between 499 and 200 T-helper cells	A2	B2	C2
< 200 T-helper cells	A3	B3	C3

Patients in this column would have developed infections such as bacterial endocarditis, meningitis, pneumonia, or sepsis, which are not specific to AIDS patients alone. For example, it is not uncommon for individuals with normal immune systems to develop bacterial pneumonia. Contrast this with the defining criteria for column "C."

Patients in this column have developed one or more infection(s) rarely seen except in patients who have AIDS. For example, the patient might have a Candidiasis infection of the esophagus or AIDS-induced diarrhea that lasts longer than one month.

Note. Chart based on "Acquired immunodeficiency syndrome" by R. H. Rubin, 1993, in *Scientific American Medicine,* E. Rubenstein & D. D. Federman (Eds.), New York: Scientific American Press.

*The normal person has 800–1200 CD4+ T-helper cells per cubic mm of blood.

more of these infections. Thus, in a technical sense, the acquired immune deficiency syndrome (AIDS) is only one stage, in this case the final stage, of the infection caused by HIV-1 (Glasner & Kaslow, 1990).

AIDS and Suicide

Researchers disagree as to the possibility that a diagnosis of AIDS contributes to suicidal thoughts. In an early study, Pope and Morin (1990) concluded that individuals who knew that they were infected with HIV-1 had a suicide rate *more than 30 times higher* than for individuals who were not infected. Searight and McLaren (1997) identified a confounding variable that raises questions as to this conclusion, however. The authors pointed out that many individuals who are likely to contract HIV-1 often have concurrent forms of psychopathology (personality disorders, etc.) that also might predispose them to suicide attempts. Thus, it is difficult to determine the degree to which the individual's knowledge of being infected with HIV-1 contributes to possible suicidal thoughts. Still, the authors acknowledged that the suicide rate in HIV-1 infected men was seven times that of noninfected men of the same age. Most certainly, there is a need for counseling of individuals who are/ might be infected with HIV-1, to reduce the potential risk of self-harm ("AIDS and Mental Health," 1994).

AIDS and Kaposi's Sarcoma

There was a time when a rare form of cancer known as *Kaposi's sarcoma* was thought to be one of the opportunistic infections that denoted the individual had AIDS. Recent research, however, has suggested that Kaposi's sarcoma may be caused by a different infectious agent, possibly also a virus. By coincidence, this virus seems to have been introduced into the United States at about the same time as the AIDS virus (Oliwenstein, 1990). By the early 1990s, researchers concluded that Kaposi's sarcoma is an entirely separate disease. Because of the similarities in the mode of transmission, both infections are commonly found in homosexual or bisexual males. This led to the mistaken conclusion that Kaposi's sarcoma is a manifestation of AIDS.

The Progression of HIV-1 Infection

Currently, researchers believe that 42% to 62% of those individuals who are infected with HIV-1 will progress to AIDS within 12 years of the time that they were infected (Branson, 1995). However, there is a great deal of variability in this figure, as some people are known to have progressed on to full AIDS within 2 or 3 years of initial infection with HIV-1, while others have not developed AIDS for as long as 15 years after becoming infected with the virus (Nowak & McMichael, 1995). Statistically, it is thought that about 10% of HIV-1 infected individuals progress to AIDS within 2 or 3 years of being infected, while 10% to 15% remain AIDS-free even 10 years after contracting HIV-1 (Haynes, 1996). Each year, 5% to 10% of HIV-1 infected persons progress to the stage of AIDS (Searight & McLaren, 1997).

The Treatment of HIV/AIDS

In order to determine the impact of the latest antiviral treatment methods on AIDS-induced mortality, the team of Palella, Delaney, Moorman, Loveless, Fuhrer, Satten, Aschman, and Holmberg, (1998) examined the data from 1,255 patients who were infected with HIV-1, with a CD4+ cell count of less than 100 per cubic millimeter of blood. The authors concluded that there was a significant reduction in mortality following the introduction of the protease inhibitors, with AIDS-related deaths dropping from 29.4 per 100 patient-years[7] in 1995 to just 8.8 per 100 patient-years in 1997. While these figures are impressive, it still means that almost 9 of every patients whose HIV-1 infection had progressed to AIDS died each year in spite of the most aggressive treatment with the most advanced medications available at this time.

It is for this reason that researchers are hard at work, attempting to develop treatment methods that will *totally arrest* the progression of the disease once the individual has been infected (Gallo & Montagner, 1988; Heaton, 1990). Unfortunately, this goal

---

[7] This is a statistical concept. One hundred patient years means 100 patients, all of whom have a certain condition, who are followed for one year.

remains elusive, current treatment methods are expensive, cause significant side effects for the individual being treated, and are not totally effective in arresting HIV-1 infection in the patient.

If researchers are successful in finding a drug or drugs to completely arrest the progression of AIDS, it will be a significant step forward. Now, however, it would seem that "almost all those currently infected will progress to terminal-stage illness and death" (Monteith, 1997, p. 97). Thus, the outlook remains bleak, although there are hints of treatment methods that *may* offer some hope to those who are infected. For example, since shortly after HIV-1 was isolated, researchers have attempted to identify compounds that might be useful in treating the infection. In the mid-1980s, researchers developed a class of medications known as *nucleoside analogues,* compounds that include agents such as AZT, ddI, ddC, d4T, and 3TC. These chemicals block the action of the enzyme *reverse transcriptase,* which is essential for the reproduction of the virus (Freiberg, 1996).

While somewhat effective in slowing the reproduction of HIV-1, the nucleoside analogues have not been totally effective in the treatment of this infection. Research has demonstrated that some strains of HIV-1 are resistant to the action of nucleoside analogues and that these medications can, at best, only slow the progression of the HIV-1 infection. Thus, the search has continued for other medications that might be useful in the fight against HIV-1 infection. This led to the development of a new class of medications, known as *protease inhibitors* as possible treatments for HIV-1 infection. Like the nucleoside analogues, the protease inhibitors block the viral reproduction process. Unlike AZT and similar antiviral drugs, protease inhibitors block the action of the protease enzyme that is essential in the replication process of HIV-1 (Freiberg, 1996). The first of these agents, Saquinavir, was approved for use in the treatment of HIV-1 in 1996. Unfortunately, the virus HIV-1 also can develop resistance to protease inhibitors (Goldschmidt & Moy, 1996). Because of the rapid development of drug resistance, most specialists in the area of HIV-1 infection now recommend the use of multiple antiviral agents simultaneously

(Goldschmidt & Moy).[8] Such polypharmacy offers hope for slowing the progression of the HIV-1 infection.[9]

But researchers have yet to prove that any single medication, or combination of medications, will permanently suppress HIV-1 (Goldschmidt & Moy, 1996). Ultimately, HIV-1 infection is still expected to progress to AIDS. Before the introduction of the protease inhibitors and nucleoside analogues, once AIDS developed, the average survival period was only 2 to 4 years (Hellinger, 1993). However, the introduction of new drugs that are effective against HIV-1 makes it difficult to estimate long-term survival for those who are infected. Such progress is expensive, however, and it has been estimated that the yearly cost of anti-HIV-1 drugs is $25,000–$35,000/year for each person being treated.

As the 20th century draws to a close, researchers are hopeful that they can eventually develop a treatment program that will completely arrest the progression of HIV-1. Yet, this will not be a cure for AIDS, anymore than insulin can cure diabetes mellitus. The injections of insulin serve as a substitute for the body's own insulin, slowing or even in some cases arresting the progression of the diabetes mellitus. However, the insulin is not a cure for the diabetes.

The ultimate treatment for AIDS at this time lies in prevention. Intravenous drug abusers, however, continue to share contaminated needles, often simply be-cause they do not want to wait until a clean needle or syringe is available. Although rinsing the needle and syringe with bleach will often destroy the AIDS virus, many intravenous drug abusers simply do not engage in this practice, because it takes too much time. Other intravenous drug users have been known to wait in line to use another person's needle and syringe although they had a new needle and syringe at home, because they do not want to wait until then to inject the drug into their body.

---

[8] A point that should be made is that it is possible for a person being treated for HIV-1 infection to *still* pass the infection on to others, although he/she is taking antiviral drugs.

[9] Another group of agents that have shown promise as possible drugs to treat HIV-1 are known as the *integrase inhibitors.* Researchers are exploring the possibility that one or more of these drugs will prove useful in the fight against AIDS by helping to stop HIV-1 replication in the host's body.

There are those who continue to engage in high-risk behavior, although it is not known how representative this group is of national trends. Individuals continue to engage in promiscuous sexual behavior, either heterosexual or homosexual, despite the known association between AIDS and sexual promiscuity. It is thus important for the chemical dependency professional to have a working knowledge of infections such as AIDS and hepatitis B, in order to help their clients understand, and come to terms with, these diseases.

Tuberculosis (TB)

Both directly and indirectly, chronic chemical abuse contributes to the spread of a wide range of infectious diseases. An example of how chronic substance abuse can indirectly contribute to the spread of disease is seen in the return of tuberculosis (TB) (Cherubin & Sapira, 1993). The bacteria that cause TB are common, and it is estimated that 50% of the world's population has been exposed to TB sometime in their lives (Garrett, 1994). However, for the most part, the individual's immune system is able to fight off the danger of infection, and the individual shows no outward sign of having been exposed to TB. But each year, 7 to 8 million new cases of TB develop around the globe, and 2 to 3 million people die from this disease (Hopewell, 1996; Seymour, 1997).

Tuberculosis itself is an opportunistic disease: it preys mainly on those individuals whose immune system has been weakened by illness or malnutrition. Because malnutrition is a common side effect of chronic chemical abuse, alcohol- and drug-dependent individuals are high-risk groups for contracting TB. Further, individuals whose immune systems are compromised, such as individuals with HIV-1, are also at high risk for becoming infected with TB (Garrett, 1994). Indeed, the first outward sign that a person is infected with HIV-1 might be when he/she develops TB (Karlen, 1995).

Tuberculosis was once easily cured by antibiotic medications that were cheap, easily administered, and highly effective. But, to achieve a cure, it was necessary for the infected individual to take the medications daily, for weeks, or even months. The lifestyle of the typical alcohol/drug-dependent person often makes treatment compliance for TB difficult.

This characteristic has contributed to the rise of strains of antibiotic-resistant TB, although there are other reasons why TB no longer responds to antibiotic medications as it once did.

A major reason for physicians' concern about TB is that, in the past, it was a common cause of death. This fact, plus the resistence of many strains of TB to existing antibiotics, has made it a growing threat to some segments of the population in the United States and abroad. The team of Friedman, Williams, Singh, and Frieden (1996) found that alcohol/drug abusing welfare recipients in New York City had rates of TB infection that were 70 times as high as those found across the United States as a whole. The authors did not speculate as to the reasons for these figures, but it is known that several elements of the lifestyle of addicted individuals lend themselves to the transmission of TB.

What Is Tuberculosis?

Tuberculosis (TB) is an infectious disease, caused by the bacteria *Mycobacterium tuberculosis* (Karlen, 1995). Physicians have struggled against TB for hundreds of generations. But, up until recently, the treatment of TB was a long, complicated affair, which did not guarantee success. Then, in the 1950s, antibiotic medications were introduced that offered the hope of completely curing the patient of the disease in just a few months. By the mid-1980s, physicians had concluded that TB was no longer a major threat to the public. Physicians became somewhat complacent about the disease.

By the early 1990s, however, it had become apparent that new strains of TB had evolved that were resistant to many of the medications used to treat it. The complacency of the 1970s was replaced by a sense of alarm, as physicians became aware of strains of TB that were resistant to many of the drugs that had once been effective in treating it (Hopewell, 1996). Within the span of a single decade, TB again emerged as a threat to the health of the world's population.

How Does TB Kill?

TB most often invades the pulmonary system, although it is possible for TB to infect virtually every organ system in the body. The bacteria seem to prefer oxygen-rich body tissues, such as those found in the lungs, central nervous system, and the kidneys (Boutotte, 1993). Since the most common site of infection in this country is the lungs, we will focus our attention on this form of TB.

Tuberculosis is transmitted when the individual inhales a small droplet of body fluid that contains the bacteria. Whenever a person sings, talks, coughs, or sneezes, he/she will release microscopic droplets of moisture from the lungs, which will remain suspended in the air for extended periods. If that person has active TB in the respiratory system, then these moisture droplets will carry bacteria into the surrounding air, where another person might breathe them in (Boutotte, 1993). Once TB gains admission to the individual's body, the individual's immune system attacks the invading bacteria. The initial response by a part of the immune system known as *macrophages* is to engulf the invading bacteria, surround them, and wall them inside little pockets known as granulomas. This then prevents the infection from proceeding further. However, *Mycobacterium tuberculosis* is difficult for the body to destroy, and the bacteria might continue to survive in a dormant stage within the granulomas for years, or decades.

But, if the individual's immune system becomes weakened by another infection, disease, or malnutrition, the body no longer is able to isolate the bacteria in the granulomas. Eventually, the TB bacteria might burst out, and again invade the surrounding body tissue. This is known as "reactivation TB," which accounts for about 85% of all cases of TB in the United States (Boutotte, 1993). At this point, the body attempts a different approach to the invading bacteria. Another part of the immune system, the lymphocytes, attempt to destroy the bacteria that cause TB, but during this process, they release a toxin that destroys surrounding lung tissue. Eventually, as less and less of the lung is able to properly function, the patient dies of pulmonary failure.

Another way that TB might kill is seen in those patients who have been infected with the HIV-1 virus. Concurrent infection with TB and HIV-1 seems to result in shortened life expectancy, since the person's body is not fully able to resist the TB (Fineberg & Wilson, 1996).

The Treatment of TB

Although a great deal has been written about "treatment resistant" TB in the past few years, physicians still have a wide range of medications that they can call on to treat this infection. However, the treatment process may take as long as 6 to 9 months, and the patient needs to take the proper medications on a daily basis for that period (Boutotte, 1993). Failure to follow the established treatment program will result in the patient retaining some active TB germs in his/her body which (because they have survived the patient's initial use of the medication) will be more resistant to these same medications in the future. Over time, new strains of TB emerge, which are totally resistant to medications that once could eradicate the infection.

Viral Hepatitis

There are at least seven different viral infections of the liver. Each virus can cause inflammation of the liver, a condition known as *hepatitis*. Physicians often refer to each virus simply by a letter, such as hepatitis "A," or "B." At least four different forms of viral hepatitis are known to affect alcohol/drug users.

Hepatitis type A (HVA) infections are the most common, with HVA accounting for up to 61% of the new cases of viral hepatitis (Bondesson & Saperston, 1996). The causal agent of HVA was identified as a virus that is transmitted through food or water that has become contaminated with fecal matter. But for many years, physicians were aware that some patients who had received blood transfusions developed symptoms of liver disease suggestive of a viral infection other than HVA. These patients were said to have developed "serum hepatitis." Eventually, a different virus, which they classified as hepatitis type B (HVB), was identified in the blood of these patients, and scientists began to study the virus that caused this disorder, to learn more about how it was transmitted.

Over time, scientists found that HVB was a common disease, accounting for 28% of the new cases of viral hepatitis (Bondesson & Saperston, 1996) and for 5% to 10% of the cases of cirrhosis of the liver in the United States (Hoffnagle & Di Bisceglie, 1997). But, even after HVB was isolated, some patients who had received blood transfusions continued to develop a liver disorder that was suggestive of viral hepatitis, without showing evidence of having been exposed to either HVA or HVB. These patients were said to have "non-A, non-B" hepatitis, and scientists began to search for additional viruses that might account for this disorder. Eventually, four additional viruses were isolated, which have been classified as hepatitis virus type C (HVC), type D (HVD), type E (HVE), type F (HVF), and type G (HVG) (Sjogren, 1996).

Relationship between Viral Hepatitis and Intravenous Drug Abuse

It is uncommon for HVA to be contracted as a result of alcohol/drug abuse. But the sharing of intravenous needles by drug abusers does account for about 2% of the new cases of HVA (Bondesson & Saperston, 1996). Thus, while the most common route of HVA infection is through exposure to food or water that has been contaminated by feces, it is still possible for intravenous drug abusers to pass the infection on to others when they share needles. Because HVA infection is only rarely passed on by intravenous drug abuse, it will not be discussed further.

Unlike HVA, the viruses that cause HVB, HVC, and HVD are all transmitted from one person to another only through exposure to body fluids (Becherer, 1995). A common source of exposure to hepatitis types B, C, and D is through the use of contaminated intravenous needles.

Prevalence

Prevalence of HVB

Globally, 5% of the world's population, or about 300 million (W. Clark 1995) to 400 or 500 million people (Bondesson & Saperston, 1996) are thought to be infected with HVB. In the United States, there are 300,000 new cases of HVB each year (Karlen, 1995).

Prevalence of HVC

Around the world, some 3% of the population is thought to be infected with one of the six subtypes of HVC (Flynn, 1996; Seymour, 1997). But the prevalence of HVC infection varies; 4% to 6% of the population in some regions of the world, such as Africa, have been exposed to the virus, while other regions

have much lower rates of infection (Sharara, Hunt, & Hamilton, 1996). There are an estimated 2 to 4 million people in the United States who have been infected with this virus, and an estimated 150,000 new cases of HVC infection occur each year in this country alone (Flynn).

Transmission

Routes of Transmission for HVB

Both HVB and HVC are *extremely* contagious. By comparison, HVB is perhaps on the order of 100 times as contagious as HIV-1. For example, the virus that causes HIV-1 is fragile and cannot survive for any length of time in the open air. Transmission of HIV-1 requires *direct* exposure to the infected person's body fluids. In contrast, there have been cases where people have contracted HVB by sharing either a toothbrush, or a razor, or simply by kissing an infected person (Brody, 1991). Thus, HVB is easily transmitted by exposure to an infected person's body fluids.

Like HIV-1, the virus that causes HVB may be transmitted through blood transfusions. This fact has resulted in the development of new blood tests, to screen out blood donors who might carry the virus. Two decades ago, the rate of infection with the hepatitis B virus was 1 per 100 units of blood transfused (Edelson, 1993). However, new blood tests for screening potential blood donors (and ways of storing blood prior to use) have reduced the rate of hepatitis B infection to about 1 in 63,000 units of blood used for transfusion in the United States (Schreiber et al., 1996).

In the United States, a common means of transmitting hepatitis B from one person to another is through contaminated drug paraphernalia shared by intravenous drug abusers. Blood tests from intravenous drug abusers reveal that 75% to 98% of intravenous drug users have been exposed to HVB virus sometime in their lives (Michelson et al., 1988). Thus, exposure to contaminated needles or blood products can result in the virus being transmitted to a new victim. Another common source of HVB infection is sexual contact, through which the virus is passed from an infected individual to a noninfected partner. HVB is also found in the semen of most infected men. Thus, like HIV-1, HVB may be passed on to another person through the semen, and it is now classified as a *sexually transmitted disease* (STD). In some communities in the United States, HVB makes up 30% of all new STD cases (Garrett, 1994).

Because HVB may be transmitted through sexual contact with an infected person, anybody involved in a sexual relationship with a person who is infected with HVB is also at risk for contracting HVB. Individuals who are likely to have been exposed to HVB include sexually promiscuous persons, prostitutes, and bisexual and/or homosexual males. Sexual contact with persons in these catagories should be avoided.

Routes of Transmission for HVC

With the advent of new blood tests designed to detect HVC infection, the risk of HVC transmission during blood transfusion is 1 case for each 103,000 units of blood transfused (Schreiber et al., 1996). Thus, while blood transfusions remain a means by which HVC might be transmitted, the rate of transfusion-related infection has been greatly reduced through the use of new screening tests for blood donors. Currently, intravenous drug abusers are thought to make up 40% of the total number of people who are infected with HVC (Najm, 1997). Another 15% of the cases of HVC are thought to have been transmitted sexually (Bondesson & Saperston, 1996; Sharara et al., 1996). Other possible routes of HVC transmission include tattooing, organ transplant procedures where the donor had been infected with HVC, and hemodialysis (Sharara et al., 1996). However, it should be pointed out that 40% to 50% of those known to have been exposed to HVC have no apparent history of having engaged in these high-risk behaviors, suggesting that there are other, as yet unidentified, routes of HVC transmission.

Routes of Transmission for HVD

Little is known about the transmission of HVD. It is known that HVD is a blood-borne virus. Surprisingly, the virus that causes HVD is an "incomplete" or "defective" (Sjogren, 1996, p. 948) virus, which requires prior exposure to HVB in order for an individual to become infected. This accounts for why approximately 10% of those individuals with chronic HVB infections also test positive for exposure to HVD (Di Bisceglie, 1995). Thus, it is thought that for a person to be infected with HVD, he/she must (a) have a preexisting HVB infection, and (b) be exposed to the blood of another person who also is infected with HVD. In the United States, only some 70,000 individuals are thought to have the HVD virus in their bodies (Najm, 1997).

Consequences

What Are the Consequences of HVB Infection?

HVB is potentially fatal; it actually kills more people than AIDS (Karlen, 1995). There are several mechanisms through which the hepatitis B virus may either directly, or indirectly, kill the infected person. First, the virus infects the liver, causing damage to that organ. The body's immune response to HVB infection may cause even more damage to the liver (W. Clark, 1995). If the liver damage is great enough, HVB may kill the infected person through HVB-induced cirrhosis of the liver. It is estimated that 5,000 Americans die each year as a result of HVB-induced cirrhosis (Karlen, 1995).

However, hepatitis B may kill in another way. For reasons that are not known at this time, the person who has been infected with the hepatitis B virus is *10 to 390 times* as likely to develop liver cancer as is a noninfected person (Bondesson & Saperston, 1996). Liver cancer is quite difficult to detect, or treat, and is usually fatal. Each year, there are an estimated 1200 cases of HVB-related liver cancer in the United States (Karlen, 1995).

What Are the Consequences of HVC Infection?

Seventy-five percent of the cases of HVC are asymptomatic and may only be detected by blood tests (Najm, 1997). HVC infection can result in a chronic infection in about 80% of those individuals who are exposed to the virus (Sharara et al., 1996; van der Poel, Cuypers, & Reesink, 1994). Approximately 60% to 80% of those who are infected with HVC will develop chronic hepatitis, and in 20% to 30% of these cases the individual will develop cirrhosis of the liver (Flynn, 1996; Najm, 1997; van der Poel et al., 1994). It usually requires usually 20 to 30 years after the person was infected for cirrhosis to develop (Najm). Another potential complication of HVC infection is the development of liver cancer, possibly as a consequence of the chronic liver inflammation, and HVC-induced necrosis of liver tissue (Flynn).

What Are the Consequences of HVD Infection?

Early evidence suggests that the combination of HVB and HBD infections results in a more severe syndrome than seen in HVB alone (Najm, 1997). Approximately 60% to 70% of those individuals who are infected with HVD will develop cirrhosis of the liver, usually in 2 to 15 years after being infected (Najm, 1997).

Treatment

The Treatment of HVB

The most effective treatment for HVB is prevention. It is possible to immunize against HVB, and immunization is recommended for individuals who are likely to be exposed to the body fluids of an infected individual. Examples of individuals who should be immunized against HVB include children, health care workers, and the spouse of an individual who is infected. Daily injections of the medication interferon alfa for 4 to 6 months have been shown to be effective in only 25% to 40% of the patients who are infected with HVB (Hoffnagle & Di Bisceglie, 1997).

The Treatment of HVC

Injections of interferon is the treatment of choice for patients with HVC infection (Flynn, 1996). After an appropriate period of treatment, approximately half of the patients treated with interferon will not show further evidence of ongoing liver damage when their blood is tested. But, for half of those who initially respond to interferon treatment, the infection seems to redevelop in 6 to 36 months after the cessation of treatment (Flynn). Thus, interferon treatment seems to be effective for only about 25% of the patients who receive this medication. Further, there is little evidence to suggest that liver transplantation will result

in enhanced survival for patients whose natural liver has been destroyed by the HVC infection, according to the author. Thus, like HVB, the most effective treatment for HVC is prevention.

The Treatment of HVD

Preliminary evidence suggests that 9–10 million units of the chemical known as *interferon alfa-2b* injected subcutaneously three times a week for a year might be able to inhibit replication of HVD in infected persons (Najm, 1997). However, the long-term effectiveness of this treatment approach has not been determined. Indeed, it would appear that the disease reasserts itself when interferon therapy is discontinued (Najm). Immunization against HVB blocks the chain of infection, preventing HVD coinfection if an individual should be exposed to this virus (Najm).

The Treatment of HVE, HVF, and HVG

Very little is known about how these viral infections might be treated. Like HVB, the most effective "treatment" for these viral infections is prevention, by avoiding exposure to body fluids of other individuals who are known or suspected to have a form of viral hepatitis.

Summary

It is impossible to identify, in advance, every potential infectious disease that substance abusers are exposed to, as a result of their chemical use. In this chapter, a few of the more common forms of infection that may result from alcohol/drug abuse have been reviewed. Although this chapter is not intended to serve as a guide for the treatment of these infections, it is important that substance abuse rehabilitation professionals understand some of the risk factors associated with such infectious diseases as the hepatitis family of viral infections, HIV-1, and tuberculosis (TB), both to better understand the needs of their patients, and their own potential for being exposed to these disorders as a result of their work with infected individuals.

CHAPTER THIRTY-FOUR

Crime and Drug Use

In the past century, the face of illicit drug use has changed several times. In the middle to late 1800s, a significant percentage of the women in the middle class were addicted to narcotics that had originally been prescribed for the treatment of a wide range of disorders (Jonnes, 1995). The introduction of pharmacologically pure cocaine and heroin in the late 1800s, combined with the development of the intravenous needle, made it possible for illicit drug users to introduce relatively pure concentrations of recreational chemicals directly into the bloodstream.

By the first years of the 20th century, several different forces combined to bring about a wave of opiate and cocaine abuse. First, heroin, opium, and cocaine were available without a prescription. Second, the practice of smoking opium had been introduced in the United States from Asia, where it was common. Finally, there were large numbers of working-class boys who had no hope of advancement, but who had access to recreational chemicals.

At the start of the 20th century, recreational substance use/abuse had become a social concern. By the year 1913, lawmakers were sufficiently alarmed by these social trends to pass a series of local and federal laws in an attempt to control the use of recreational chemicals. The most important of the new federal antidrug laws was the Harrison Narcotics Act of 1914. However, illicit drug use continued to be a major social problem throughout the 1920s and 1930s. It was only with the start of World War II, with the naval blockades instituted by all parties, that the wave of illicit drug use in the United States virtually ended, at least for the duration of the war.

The debate over whether drug abuse/addiction is a medical problem (addiction as illness), or a legal problem (addiction as illegal behavior) is ongoing. In the first half of the 1900s, illicit chemical use was transformed from a medical problem into a legal problem. Ever since then, the problems of illicit drug use and criminal activity have been intertwined in the United States. In the minds of many people, these two social problems are essentially one and the same. From this perspective, illicit drug use is the major cause of criminal activity. There are people who believe that if the problem of recreational drug use were to magically end tomorrow, the problem of criminal activity would also disappear.

This is a rather simplistic view of the relationship between illegal drug use and crime. In reality, illicit chemical abuse and criminal activity are essentially two separate social problems. Crime has been a serious social concern for hundreds of years. But in the past century or so, the social problems of illicit chemical abuse and criminal activity have come to be interrelated in many ways. In this chapter, we explore some of these relationships.

Scope of the Problem of Drug-Related Criminal Behavior

If the truth be told, after more than a century of study, researchers still do not have a clear picture of the incidence of drug-related criminal behavior (Bradford, Greenberg, & Motayne, 1992). It is known that recreational chemical use is one of the most significant factors associated with violent crime (R. Lewis, 1989). It is estimated that fully a quarter of all property crimes (car theft, burglary, etc.) can be traced to recreational drug use (National Academy of Sciences, 1990). But, after more than a century's effort, it remains difficult to determine the degree to which chemical abuse is a causal factor in criminal behavior.

This is because social scientists who try to explore the interrelationship between criminal behavior and substance abuse often use police investigation reports as at least part of their database. While such police reports are helpful, they do not provide a comprehensive overview of the role substance abuse plays in the commission of criminal activity. Some crimes never are solved, and the possible impact of substance use in these cases can never be determined. An excellent example might be an unsolved murder, where the possible relationship between recreational drug use and the crime cannot be determined.

Other crimes are solved only after extended periods. In such cases, it is not clear what role (if any) chemical use might have played in the commission of these crimes. Consider the armed robbery that takes place in a subway system of a large city. The robber might not be identified and arrested until weeks, months, or possibly even years after the robbery. How could researchers determine whether or not substance use/abuse was a factor in a crime that the individual might not even remember committing?

Another factor that complicates the study of the interrelationship between chemical use and criminal activity is that some crimes are ignored by law enforcement authorities because of inadequate evidence, poor witnesses, or other reasons (Bradford et al., 1992). The role of chemical use/abuse in the commission of these crimes will obviously never be investigated. Even when an arrest is made shortly after the commission of a crime, it is unusual for law enforcement officials to carry out urine or blood toxicology tests to determine whether the offender was actually under the influence of alcohol or drugs. In some cases, social scientists have been reduced to simply asking criminals whether they

had been under the influence of chemicals at the time they committed the crime! Such a research technique assumes that the respondent is going to tell the truth, a dubious assumption at best when dealing with a criminal population.

Three Theoretical Perspectives

A little secret researchers rarely discuss is that the theoretical bias of the researcher may influence the outcome of the study. Although one goal of scientific research is to control for the influence of the researcher's personal bias, this is not always possible. The researcher's personal bias, expectations, and possibly his/her political beliefs will shape the design of a research study—what "facts" the researcher considers in the formulation of this study and the conclusions the researcher reaches when evaluating the data.[1]

Many researchers assume that *any* crime committed under the influence of chemicals, or in the service of one's addiction, is automatically drug related. There is the often-repeated example of how heroin addicts are forced to resort to crime to support their habit. Their criminal activity is thus assumed to be caused by their addiction to heroin. The theoretical bias of this research is apparent from the few studies that discuss the relationship between heroin addiction and criminal activity. These studies report that *more than 50%* of heroin addicts in this country have a legal history *prior to their first use of narcotics* (Jaffe, 1989, 1995c).

A second perspective is that individuals who are predisposed to crime may also be predisposed to use alcohol and/or drugs (M. Moore, 1991). From this perspective, it is possible to argue that drug abuse/addiction does not force the individual to resort to crime. Instead, proponents of this school of thought believe that people who engage in the abusive use of chemicals also tend to engage in criminal activity.

In other words, drug users might "commit crimes more frequently than non-users not because they use . . . but because they happen to be the kinds of people who would be expected to have a higher

---

[1] For a discussion of this phenomenon, the reader is referred to Stephen Jay Gould's book *The Mismeasure of Man* (New York: W. W. Norton, 1981).

crime rate" (*National Commission on Marihuana and Drug Abuse*, 1972, p. 77).

According to this line of reasoning, drugs do not so much *cause* criminal activity, as attract those who are predisposed to commit crimes. The fact that the crimes may now be committed to support an addiction to a chemical(s) only serves to obscure that these same individuals often committed crimes before their addiction developed, as well as after they began to use chemicals.

A third perspective on the relationship between criminal activity and chemical abuse was offered by Elliott (1992). The author suggested that chemical abuse and criminal activity both reflect the "decline in the power of cultural restraints" (p. 599) taking place in this country. Thus, to Elliott, drug use and criminal activity are two expressions of a more pervasive sociological phenomenon: a breakdown of traditional restraints and guidelines. The author supported his argument with the observation that Europe experienced "tidal waves of crime" (Elliott, 1992, p. 599) every few decades since the 14th century. According to Elliott, a similar pattern has emerged here in the United States over the past 200 years. A common thread connecting these waves of crime, according to the author, is that in each successive period of social unrest, one could observe "an erosion of personal integrity, widespread dehumanization, a contempt for life, material greed, corruption in high places, sexual promiscuity, *and increased recourse to drugs and alcohol*" (p. 599, italics added for emphasis).

Thus, it is Elliott's (1992) contention that the relationship between drug abuse and criminal activity might be found in the more general breakdown in cultural constraints against antisocial behavior. Rather than a simplistic "drug use causes crime" equation, the author offers a theory that suggests that *both* drug abuse and criminal activity are a reflection of, or perhaps even a reaction to, the more inclusive breakdown in existing social constraints and mores.

Thus, social scientists are unable to identify the exact relationship between recreational chemical use and criminal activity. There does appear to be a relationship between chemical use and crime. However, its exact nature remains unclear, even after more than a century of intense research. Ultimately, the determination of whether the substance use is

causal, one of a number of factors associated with drug use, or totally unrelated to the drug use, must be made on a case-by-case basis.

Criminal Activity and Personal Responsibility

The issue of the limits of personal responsibility in cases where the individual might have been under the influence of chemicals when committing the offense is a difficult one for society. In many cases, this issue is neatly sidestepped through the social fiction that the drugs somehow interfered with the individual's ability to think coherently. Thus, any "perceived correlation between the use of a drug and the unwanted consequences is attributed to the drug, removing the individual from any and all responsibility" (National Commission on Marihuana and Drug Abuse, 1973, p. 4).

The view that crimes committed under the influence of chemicals were caused by the drugs is an extension of the "demon rum" philosophy of the late 1800s (Peele, 1989). According to the belief, once the person ingests even one drink, the alcohol totally overwhelms self-control. From that point on, the person has no control over his/her behavior; it is controlled by the demon hidden within the bottle of alcohol.

The modern version of this belief is that, when a crime is committed by a person who is under the influence of chemicals, the responsibility for that crime is attributed not to the person, but to the chemical used. The individual's role in the commission of that crime is overlooked, or at least minimized, and the person is viewed as a helpless victim of the drug's effects. The outcome is that while drug use in itself is not an excuse for criminal behavior, *extreme* drug use often derails the legal system.

The courts have ruled that the use of recreational chemicals involves some element of choice (Kermani & Castaneda, 1996). Thus, in the eyes of the legal system the individual is still held responsible for the acts committed while under the influence of chemicals. The criminal justice system is often unable to determine whether the individual actually *intended* to commit a crime while under the influence of chemicals. In such cases, the criminal justice system often simply accepts the compromise that the individual suffered a "diminished capacity" as a result of his/her use of chemicals as a way of clearing a difficult case from the court schedule. So popular has this compromise become that "as of 1986, 15 states had . . . created a 'diminished capacity' defense as a legal way station between innocence and full criminal responsibility" (M. Graham, 1989, p. 21).

As a result of this social and legal fiction, it is not unusual for defense attorneys to negotiate a reduced sentence, based on the claim that the defendant was under the influence of chemicals at the time of the offense (M. Graham, 1989). Because of the individual's diminished capacity, a reduced sentence is offered in place of the criminal sanctions usually imposed when the individual was fully aware of his/her actions.

Thus, the demon rum philosophy has actually influenced the workings of the criminal justice system. This defense is quite unlike the "insanity" defense, which is often viewed as a desperation move on the part of the defense attorney in all but extreme cases. Because of the social fiction that the person is a helpless victim of the drug's effects, crimes committed "under the influence, are the only crimes we can generally elude punishment for by utilizing an escape into the recovery process established by our medical society" (Newland, 1989, p. 18).

By invoking the demon rum defense, questions are raised as to the individual's responsibility for the commission of the crime. In extreme cases, substance abuse "treatment" may actually be substituted for the criminal sanctions that normally would be imposed for the individual's behavior.

The Drug Underworld and Crime

In a very real sense, the problem of organized crime can be viewed as a result of society's attempt to deal with the use of illicit chemical use through the criminal justice system. With the exception of alcohol and tobacco, drugs of abuse are not sold in a free market economy. Rather, because these substances are illegal, their production, distribution, and sale are carried out through illegal channels. To meet the demand for the chemicals that society has deemed illegal, a black market has evolved.

This black market generates a significant profit for those who are willing to run the risk of criminal prosecution. Currently, it is estimated that the traffic in illicit chemicals generates an estimated $50 billion to $60 billion a year in *profits* for those who supply the drugs to users (Nadelmann & Wenner, 1994). On a more individual level, some "pushers" have been known to earn upward of $400 or $500 *a day* (above $180,000 a year) (Collier, 1989).[2] Such profits have helped the drug distribution and sales infrastructure become quite resilient in the face of law enforcement attempts to interdict illegal drugs ("Your Heroin, Sir," 1991). There is always somebody willing to risk arrest for the chance to participate in such a highly profitable trade. Thus, law enforcement attempts to control the distribution of illegal drugs may have contributed to the development of an industry so resilient that it is able to defeat any attempt to control it through legislation or criminal sanctions.

Because most recreational drugs are illegal, the price charged for these chemicals is not set by market demand, but, by those who control the distribution monopoly. The high cost of the drugs is justified by their illegality, which means the dealer runs a risk in providing the chemical to those who purchase it. The addict must then find some way to obtain the money necessary to buy drug(s) at inflated prices.

All too often, the addict obtains the money to support chemical purchases through criminal activity. Addicts have been known to steal and to engage in burglary, armed robbery, or prostitution (heterosexual and homosexual) as well as car theft, forgery, and other crimes, to obtain the money that one needs to support their drug habit. Engaging in drug sales (itself a criminal act) to support one's own addiction is also not uncommon.

The person who supports drug use through theft receives only a fraction of the stolen material's worth. As a result, the addict must steal more and more so that the pittance received for the stolen property will meet his/her drug needs. It has been estimated that the typical heroin addict in an average city needs to

---

[2] This money is, essentially, tax-free income, since few illicit drug dealers pay income tax on the money they earn through their illegal activities.

steal some $200,000 worth of goods annually, to support a drug habit (Thomason & Dilts, 1991).

The Illicit Drug Production/Distribution System

Most recreational chemicals are illegal and are not manufactured by legitimate pharmaceutical companies. They must either be produced in clandestine laboratories or be imported into this country through illegal means. The illicit drug network must be viewed as a monopoly, not as a free market economy. The price charged to the consumer is usually the result of an inflationary process where, at each step in the production/distribution system, every person involved will charge a profit. For example, for $75 worth of chemicals, a street "chemist" could manufacture PCP that might ultimately sell for as much as $20,000 on the illicit market (Shepherd & Jagoda, 1990). Heroin or cocaine that might be worth $500 in the country of origin will sell for upward of $100,000 on the streets of a city in the United States (McNamara, 1996).

Another example of the profit margin of the illegal drug distribution system is the amphetamine distribution system that has evolved in the United States. Amphetamine tablets are relatively easy and inexpensive to manufacture. The chemicals needed to produce one of the amphetamines can be legally purchased at virtually any chemical supply store. An investment of $1,000 for the necessary chemicals might eventually yield a return of as much as $40,000 for methamphetamine (Peluso & Peluso, 1988; "Raw Data," 1990). Nationally, the illicit manufacture of amphetamines—an industry mainly centered in Texas and California—is thought to be worth *three billion dollars a year* (Cho, 1990).

At least some of the heroin imported into the United States is obtained from illicit opium poppies grown in Mexico. A native farmer on an illicit opium farm would be paid approximately $100 for the opium gum he obtained from the poppies. For each seven kilograms of opium gum, illicit laboratories would be able to manufacture one kilogram of heroin. Later, when shipped to the United States by various means, this single kilogram of heroin would sell for as much as $500,000 (Shoumatoff, 1995).

The Role of Adulterants

Drugs are not sold on the street in their pure form, but are often mixed with an adulterant(s). Some adulterants are found in illicit drugs as a result of the process of producing the drugs. But drug dealers have also been known to mix the drug with adulterants to increase their profits. For example, a pound of cocaine, when cut and mixed with adulterants so that it is now only 50% pure, becomes *two pounds* of "cocaine" that can be sold.

At each stage of the drug manufacture/distribution process, the price of the chemical being produced is inflated, providing a profit to those involved in obtaining and supplying the drug. For example, in the mid-1980s, raw cocaine leaves were sold by farmers in South America for $2 a kilogram (2.4 pounds). The coca paste produced from the leaves was then sold for $200 a kilogram, while the cocaine base isolated from the coca paste sold for about $1,500 a kilogram. The cocaine hydrochloride obtained from the base was sold for up to $3,000 a kilogram. At this point, the drug was transported to the United States, where it sold at wholesale for upward of $20,000 a kilogram. When packaged for sale on the streets in one-gram lots, this same kilogram ultimately sold for $80,000 to $192,000 (Byrne, 1989b).

At each step in the distribution process, the cocaine is mixed with adulterants, reducing the purity of the resulting mixture, while increasing the amount of the product to be sold. Cocaine and narcotics are adulterated to increase the profit from their sale. Illicit opiates are often "cut" (adulterated) before being sold. At each stage, the potency of the heroin may be reduced by half, or even more. When it is finally sold on the street, a single kilogram of heroin will be sold in powder form in small bags or, occasionally, condoms. These bags sell for between $5 (a "nickel bag") and $10 (a "dime bag") each. A typical bag of heroin contains only between 20% ("Fighting Drug Abuse," 1992) and 73% (Sabbag, 1994) pure heroin. The rest of the contents consists of adulterants that have been added along the way.[3]

---

[3] The adulterants add health risks to the user of illicit chemicals. For example, the intraveneous injection of quinine (frequently used as an adulterant in street heroin) may result in toxic reactions

In 1995 (the last year for which figures are available), chemical analysis of street cocaine revealed that the purity averaged about 61%. This means that, on the average, *approximately 40% of each gram of cocaine purchased* on the street is actually something other than cocaine. These foreign substances, or adulterants, fall into one of five categories, according to the authors (Scarlos, Westra, & Barone, 1990): sugar, stimulants, local anesthetics, toxins, and inert compounds. Cocaine, according to the authors, is frequently adulterated with many different substances.

Various forms of sugar are the most commonly encountered adulterants. As a group, the CNS stimulants:

> are the second most common adulterants, and include caffeine, ephedrine, phenylpropanolamine, amphetamine, or methamphetamine. . . . The local anesthetics are the third most frequent adulterants, and include lidocaine, benzocaine, procaine, and tetracaine. . . . The two most common (lethal toxins used as adulterants) . . . are quinine and strychnine. (p. 24)

Many of the compounds used to adulterate cocaine are also used by drug distributors to cut illicit opiates. Adulterants found in narcotics include food coloring, talcum powder, starch, powdered milk, baking soda, brown sugar, or on occasion, even dog excreta (Scaros et al., 1990). Researchers have found that such compounds as aspirin, amphetamine compounds, belladonna, caffeine, instant coffee, lactose, LSD, magnesium sulfate, meprobamate, pentobarbital, pepper, powdered milk, secobarbital, starch, and warfarin have all been used to cut illicit opiates sold on the streets of the United States (Schauben, 1990).

Marijuana purchased on the street is also frequently adulterated. It is not uncommon for up to half of the "marijuana" purchased on the street to be seeds and woody stems, which must be removed before the marijuana can be smoked. Further, the marijuana may be laced with other compounds ranging from PCP, cocaine paste, or opium, on to toxic compounds such as "Raid" insect spray (Scaros

et al., 1990). Marijuana samples have also been found to have been adulterated with dried shredded cow manure (which may expose the user to salmonella bacteria), as well as herbicide sprays such as paraquat (Jenike, 1991).

Schauben (1990) identified a long list of compounds that have either been mixed in with, or substituted for, marijuana sold on the street at one time or another. Some of these compounds have included alfalfa, apple leaves, catnip, cigarette tobacco, hay, licorice, mescaline, methamphetamine, opium, pipe tobacco, straw, wax, and wood shavings. All of these compounds also gain admission into the user's body when the adulterated marijuana is smoked.

Medical researchers have little understanding of the effects on the human body of compounds that are used to adulterate or are substituted for illicit drugs. The adulterants gain admission to the body, and medical research is hard pressed to predict their impact. In an emergency situation, such as when the user has had a toxic reaction to one or more chemicals that he/she has used, the physician must try to anticipate the effects not only the drug(s) of abuse, but, literally, the effects of any of several score of possible adulterants.

One reason that pharmaceuticals (drugs produced by legal pharmaceutical manufacturers that have been diverted to the streets) are so highly prized among addicts is that these legitimately produced chemicals are of a known quality and potency. Pharmaceuticals are also unlikely to be contaminated. However, pharmaceuticals are also usually difficult to obtain, and the majority of illicit drug users must resort to chemicals produced in illegal laboratories.

Nor are pharmaceuticals without their own dangers. Addicts often attempt to use them in ways that were not intended by the manufacturer. For example, many addicts will attempt to inject tablets or the contents of capsules that were intended for oral use. The contents of the tablet or capsule will often irritate the blood vessel walls, or even totally block that blood vessel (D. Taylor, 1993). This may result in an infection, the development of gangrene, blood clot formation, strokes, and in many cases, the need to amputate the afflicted limb (D. Taylor). In other cases, such as when users crush Ritalin (methylphenidate) tablets and use

---

in the sensitive nerve tissues of the visual system, according to Michelson et al. (1988). Talcum powder, which is also a frequent adulterant for street heroin and cocaine, may cause retinopathy (damage to the retina of the eye).

them for intravenous injection, the talc may block blood vessels in the lungs, causing a form of emphysema (S. Walker, 1996).

The problem of chemical adulterants has existed for generations. It might be argued that the very fact that the drug market is illegal makes chemical adulterants inevitable. In a later section of this chapter, we look at another danger inherent in the drug world today—mistakes that are made in manufacturing chemicals that are then sold on the street to unsuspecting drug users.

The Dilemma of Drug-Related Criminal Activity

Some critics believe it is not drugs that bring about the criminal activity associated with substance abuse, but the legal sanctions *against* drug use that have helped create the combination of a drug underworld and a high crime rate (McWilliams, 1993; Nadelmann, 1989; Nadelmann & Wenner, 1994).

Proponents of this position argue that crime is not a natural consequence of drug use/abuse; it is the attempt to control access and distribution of chemicals through the legal justice system that breeds criminal behavior. In effect, by making chemical use/abuse a criminal justice matter, society has created a whole new group of criminals (Buckley, 1996; Nadelmann, 1989; Nadelmann & Wenner, 1994). The criminal activities of the pre-Prohibition era need only be contrasted with the criminal activities of the Prohibition era to prove this point.

In discussing the relationship between narcotics abuse and crime, Jaffe (1989) concluded:

> The association between opioid use and crime emerges primarily in countries such as the United States, that have tried to restrict the use of opioids to legitimate medical indications, but have been unable to eliminate illicit opioid traffic. (p. 656)

It has even been argued that personal, recreational drug use (as opposed to distribution of illicit chemicals to others) is essentially a consensual crime, in the sense that the individual who is using the chemicals is making a choice to do so (McWilliams, 1993; Royko, 1990). Many individuals have demonstrated a remarkable persistence in obtaining illicit chemicals, despite all that society has done to block their use. By

making drugs legal, they would at least be available to anyone who wanted to "sniff away his nose or addle his brain" (Royko, 1990, p. 46).

One advantage of this system, according to Royko (1990) is that it would avoid the "gun battles, the corruption and the wasted money and effort trying to save the brains and noses of those who don't want them saved" (p. 46) to begin with. Through the legalization of drugs, Royko suggested that some measure of control could be gained over who has access to drugs and at what age they might be allowed to use them, in much the manner that access to alcohol is restricted by law.

The "War On Drugs": Is It Time to Declare a Winner?

For some time, questions have been raised as to whether the efforts of law enforcement agencies to interdict the flow of illegal chemicals has really been very effective. For example, in 1955 there were only an estimated 55,000 heroin addicts in the United States (Garrett, 1994). In the late 1960s, in response to rising rates of illegal substance abuse, Congress approved money for a "full scale attack" (Garrett, 1994, p. 276) on heroin abuse. By 1987, after more than a generation of the war on drugs estimates of the number of heroin addicts in the United States were as high as 1.5 *million* people (Garrett).

These figures argue that the application of law enforcement forces to the problem of illicit drug use has not been effective. It has been suggested that the interdiction efforts against marijuana in the early to mid-1970s may have caused international drug smugglers to switch from transporting marijuana to smuggling cocaine into the United States (Scheer, 1994a). This theory is based on the fact that, pound for pound, cocaine is "less bulky, less smelly, more compact, and more lucrative" (Nadelmann, Kleinman, & Earls, 1990, p. 45) to smuggle, than is marijuana. Thus, smugglers would run less of a risk in attempting to smuggle cocaine into this country than they would if they tried to smuggle marijuana across the borders.

If this theory is true, then the efforts of law enforcement officials to deal with the marijuana problem through interdiction may actually have contributed to the subsequent development of the wave of cocaine abuse that began to sweep this country in the late 1970s and early 1980s.

The prohibition against recreational cocaine use has also contributed to the violence that spread across the United States in the late 1980s, according to Hatsukami and Fischman (1996). The authors suggested that the legal sanctions against drug dealers led them to recruit juveniles to sell cocaine, since juveniles are not punished as severely as adults when caught selling cocaine. Many of these juveniles began to carry firearms, with the result that impulsive adolescents with firearms were introduced to the drug trade, sparking a wave of violence that has yet to peak.

One consequence to the prohibition against chemical use is that the individual must use drug(s) under hazardous conditions. For example, it has been suggested that narcotics addicts utilize injected narcotics only because it is the most efficient method to administer the limited amount of the drug available. When allowed access to unlimited supplies of relatively pure narcotics, the preferred method of administration is by smoking, as was found in the turn-of-the-century opium dens. It is only when supplies become scarce that addicts begin to inject the drug into their bodies and to share needles. In a very real sense, the prohibition against narcotics use can be said to be one contributing factor to the spread of HIV in this country.

The two-pronged policy of prohibition and interdiction of illicit chemicals has been the watchword in this country for almost a century, now. Each year, an estimated *$75 billion* is spent on the war on drugs (Buckley, 1996). Yet, despite the investment of all this time, energy, and money, there is strong evidence that "the . . . 'War on Drugs' has failed as a strategy to decrease the level of drug use in the United States" (Selwyn, 1993, p. 1044). In fact, there is evidence that there are *more* drugs on the street now, and these drugs are of greater purity in many cases, than was the case *before* the war on drugs started (Sabbag, 1994; Scheer, 1994a).

Still, one must wonder, how committed the U.S. government has been to winning this war. For, despite the investment of federal financial and legal resources, one agency of the U.S. government, the Central Intelligence Agency (CIA) was busy *smuggling more than a ton of cocaine into this country* for

sale by drug dealers, at the very time when the United States was deeply involved in the so-called war on drugs (*60 Minutes*, 1993). Given these facts, is it any wonder that some people are openly calling the war a failure, and are looking for alternatives for this social policy?

Should Drugs Be Legalized?

In the early 1980s, the U.S. government initiated a "zero tolerance" program, in its war against drug use. Legal sanctions and incarceration were immediately imposed on those who were convicted of a drug-related criminal offense through mandatory sentencing provisions in the law. Although political support for mandatory sentencing was almost universal, its success has recently been criticized by many social scientists, physicians, and several lawmakers.

As we near the year 2000, it is all too easy to forget that in the 1950s, Congress passed a series of similar mandatory minimum-sentence laws in the fight against narcotics use/abuse in this country (Schlosser, 1994). These laws were loosely termed the "Boggs Act," which defined minimum prison sentences that Congress thought should be imposed for the illicit use of narcotics in this country. While support for the Boggs Act was almost universal, the then director of the United States Bureau of Prisons, James V. Bennett, expressed strong reservations about the effectiveness of the Boggs Act. Although he had not personally broken any laws in doing so, Mr. Bennett, himself a federal employee, was subsequently followed by agents of the Federal Bureau of Narcotics, who submitted regular reports to their superiors as to the content of speeches that he gave (Schlosser, 1994).

By the late 1960s, it was clear that Mr. Bennett was right—mandatory sentencing did little to reduce the scope of narcotics use/abuse in this country. In 1970, the Boggs Act was replaced by a more appropriate series of sentencing guidelines, through which a judge could assign appropriate sentences to defendants based on the merits of each case. However, in one of the great reversals of all time, just 14 years later Congress again imposed mandatory prison sentences for drug-related offenses. The lessons of past decades were forgotten. Through the Sentencing Reform Act of 1984,

Congress took away the judges' power to determine appropriate prison sentences through the application of mandated minimum prison terms. Even first-time offenders were sent to prison for extended periods, without the hope of parole.

One result of the Sentencing Reform Act of 1984 is that the prison system soon became filled with individuals serving lengthy mandatory sentences. Whereas in 1970, only 16% of all federal prisoners were incarcerated because of drug-related convictions, currently 62% of those incarcerated in federal penitentiaries are there because of drug-related convictions ("The Drug Index," 1995b; Nadelmann & Wenner, 1994; Schlosser, 1994). By the year 2001, it is possible that *more than three-quarters* of all federal inmates might be incarcerated for drug-related mandatory minimum prison terms.

To underscore the cost of incarcerating individuals who are incarcerated for drug-use related offenses, consider the following statistics: In 1972, there were an estimated 200,000 jail and prison cells in the entire United States. By the year 1998, the state of California alone was projected to have at least this number of cells in its prison system (Ryglewicz & Pepper, 1996). The vast majority of these new jail/prison cells are necessary to house individuals convicted of drug-related crimes. In 1981, the state of California spent six times as much on higher education as it did on corrections. By 1995, the annual corrections budget exceeded that of higher education in California and accounted for 10% of the entire state budget. At the present rate of growth, the annual budget for the California Department of Corrections will leave just 1% of the entire state budget available to fund higher education by the year 2001 ("New Law," 1996).

It is expensive to keep a person in prison. For example, Nadelmann and Wenner (1994) reported that there are 300,000 individuals incarcerated for drug-related convictions. It costs $40,000 *per inmate per year* to keep a person incarcerated (D. Smith, 1997). This means that more than *$12 billion per year* is being spent just to keep already convicted drug offenders incarcerated. The "war on drugs" initiated by President Ronald Reagan, and reaffirmed by every President elected since then, costs each man, woman, and child in the United States $133 each year (Buckley, 1997). In return for

this investment, the past 16 years have seen an erosion of traditional constitutional rights, and we are yet to become drug-free (Elders, 1997).

A significant number of those individuals incarcerated are first-time offenders, who have never had a prior conviction for *any* offense. Yet, because of mandatory sentencing guidelines, they are sentenced to lengthy prison terms without the hope of parole. Some critics of mandatory sentencing for possession of illegal chemicals believe it results in prison terms that are not proportional to the offense. For example, although the offender who is convicted of intentional homicide is usually sentenced to life in prison:

> The average sentence *served* for murder in the U.S. is six and a half years, while eight years with no possibility of parole is *mandatory* for the possession of 700 marijuana plants. (Potterton, 1992, p. 47, italics added for emphasis)

To put the mandatory sentencing laws into a different perspective, a first-time offender convicted of stealing $80,000,000 would face a mandatory sentence of 4 years in a federal correctional facility and could apply for early release from prison under the parole provisions of the law. Yet a first-time offender convicted of possession of $1500 worth of LSD would be sentenced to a mandatory 10 years in prison under the Sentencing Reform Act of 1984, without benefit of parole ("Raw Data," 1993).

The impact of mandatory prison sentences for those convicted of drug-related offenses has reached the point where habitual and violent prisoners are being released from prison, to make room for *first-time* offenders convicted and sentenced under mandatory drug-enforcement laws (Asseo, 1993; Potterton, 1992). If the existing federal laws against drug possession/use were to be fully implemented, it would be necessary for the U.S. government to build a new 650-bed prison *every month* just to house those convicted of violating just the federal antidrug laws ("Ibogaine," 1994).

Other critics of the mandatory sentencing laws for possession of illegal substances point out that the small-time user is usually the victim of lengthy mandatory prison terms (N. Steinberg, 1994). The author points out that, despite the intent of the law (which was to punish those involved in drug distribution), mid-level and upper-level suppliers are frequently able to bargain their knowledge of who is buying drugs from them for lighter prison sentences. As a result of the plea bargains offered to these drug dealers in return for "cooperation":

> The former hippie with 1,000 marijuana plants growing in his basement and no drug ring to rat on gets the full decade in prison, while the savvy dealer bringing in boatloads of pot from south of the border can finger a few friends and be out in half the time. (p. 33)

An excellent example of the unfair application of this principle is in the case (reported in Schlosser, 1994) where a major drug dealer was caught with 20,000 kilograms (44,092 pounds) of cocaine. He was able to trade his knowledge of the drug distribution system for a reduced sentence of less than 4 years in prison. Yet, as noted, a person growing 1000 marijuana plants in his basement for personal use would go to prison for a full decade.

Another outgrowth of the war on drugs is that a number of employers have started to carry out random, mandatory urine toxicology testing to detect illicit drug use. Some employers require that job applicants submit to urine toxicology testing, as a precondition of employment. This process has been termed "a chemical loyalty oath" (Grinspoon & Bakalar, 1993, p. 000), similar to the "loyalty oaths" seen in the United States during the McCarthy era of the 1950s, especially since the ability of urine toxicology tests to deter recreational chemical use has been challenged by the authors.

The question of whether drugs should/should not be legalized has sparked fierce debate in this country. Advocates of drug legalization point out that through legalization an important source of revenue for what is loosely called "organized crime" would be removed. Currently, the illegal drug trade supports organized crime not only in this country, but around the world ("Bring Drugs," 1993). For example, the weekly supply of illicit drugs that might cost the user $1000 in today's "market" might have a free-market value of only $20 (Buckley, 1996). The rest of this amount of money is profit for the illicit drug distributors. Through legalization, an important source of revenue for organized crime would be eliminated.

On the other hand, Frances (1991) argued against the legalization of drugs, in part because the increased availability of drugs would result in higher levels of chemical use. The author suggested that the number of cocaine users would triple, for example, if cocaine were ever to be legalized. Drawing on the pattern of chemical use that emerged in the 1800s, when drugs were legal, Frances argued that society would be swept by a wave of addiction the likes of which has never been seen before. If drugs were to be legalized now, the black market would be destroyed, but the price of chemicals of abuse would fall so drastically that prices would come ". . . within reach of lunch money for elementary school children" (p. 120), according to the author.

This is a frightening prediction. But, it is difficult to be certain it is accurate. For example, in New Zealand, there are no laws that prohibit minors from buying or consuming alcohol in public, if they are with their parents. In England and Austria, alcohol can be purchased by adolescents as young as 16 years of age, while in Portugal and Belgium there are no minimum age restrictions for the purchase of alcohol (Peele, 1996). In these countries, it is felt that adolescents should learn to drink within the context of their families in order to learn moderate, social drinking skills. Thus, although young adolescents may purchase alcohol in many European countries, they do so only in the company of their parents. Yet despite this rather liberal pattern of alcohol use, these countries do not suffer from rates of childhood/adolescent alcohol abuse problems that are much higher than those seen here in the United States.

One alternative to the free-market legalization program so fearfully envisioned by Frances (1991) would be that recreational drugs be made available through a physician's prescription (Lessard, 1989; Schmoke, 1997). This is a very similar approach to that adopted by England, where physicians who hold a special license may prescribe heroin to individuals proven to be addicts (*60 minutes*, 1992). The medical journal *The Lancet* ("Deglamorising Cannabis," 1995) went so far as to call for the legalization of marijuana, with controls similar to those on the sale of cigarettes put in place, on the grounds that the criminal sanctions currently in place against marijuana only add a degree of glamour to its use.

Admittedly, chemical users might experience health problems. However, Curley (1995) suggested that insurance companies might be permitted to charge higher health insurance premiums for drug users, as they do now for cigarette smokers. These higher health care premiums would be to cover the expense of providing health care to people who engage in such high-risk behaviors as abusing chemicals. In this way, access to the drugs could be limited, while the profit incentive for criminals would be removed. Lessard (1989) suggested, in other words, that the problem of drug abuse be approached from a health perspective, as it is in Holland and England.

The Dutch Experience

The social experiment that has been underway in Holland for the past two decades has yielded conflicting evidence as to which approach to the problem of drug abuse is the best one. In 1976, the Dutch revised their antidrug laws, making possession of less than one ounce of marijuana only a misdemeanor. Further revisions of the antidrug statutes, or the ways that they were interpreted, resulted in a policy decision being made not to enforce the strict antidrug laws already on the books. To do so, government officials reasoned, would be to drive what was essentially a health problem underground, turning it into a legal problem.

Dutch authorities would rather tolerate the use of "soft" drugs, to protect young adults from the temptations of "hard" drugs such as cocaine or heroin. To this end, small amounts of marijuana and hashish are sold openly in Dutch coffeehouses, and users are allowed to purchase up to 30 grams of marijuana legally. The coffeehouses are not permitted to advertise or to sell cannabis to adolescents under the age of 16 ("Deglamorising Cannabis," 1995). Surprisingly, even the possession of "hard" drugs is tolerated by authorities, as long as the drug is for personal use, and the individual has not engaged in other illegal behaviors such as burglary (R. Lewis, 1989; "War by Other Means," 1990).

Despite this open toleration for marijuana use, the number of heroin addicts dropped by approximately one-third after this change in national philosophy took place. Holland has continued to enjoy extremely low rates of hard drug use. Currently, the percentage of the population classified as heavy users of heroin or cocaine is about 1.6 per 1000 inhabitants, a rate that is half that of other European countries, and one-sixth that found in the United States (*Washington Post*, 1995).

However, the rather liberal philosophy of Dutch authorities has caused some friction with its European neighbors (*Washington Post*, 1995). French authorities have complained that Dutch coffeehouses are little more than transshipment points for drugs that are then exported to other European countries, and have threatened to close their boarders with Holland (*Washington Post*). In response to a wave of drug-related crime, Dutch authorities have also started to clamp down on drug use. Much of this crime apparently is caused by individuals who are either visiting or have moved to Holland to take advantage of the permissive attitudes toward drug use in that country. Relatively little of the drug-related crime is caused by native Dutch drug users. Further, the Health Minister of Holland, Els-Borst-Eilers, and the Justice Minister, Winniee Sorgdrager, suggested that even heroin should be freely distributed to Dutch addicts, although the heroin addict would have to obtain a prescription for the drug from a physician ("European Drug Dealings," 1994).

Under their proposed plan, physicians would be required to keep strict records, and the number of physicians who would be licensed to prescribe heroin to addicts would be limited. However, it was suggested, this approach would limit or eliminate the incentive for organized crime to become involved in heroin distribution in Holland. Thus, again, Dutch authorities suggest a public health response to what seems to be an evolving drug use problem in that country.

It is not clear how the Dutch experiment will end, or, how the population will react to a wave of nonnative drug users moving to their country. Some Dutch officials have suggested mandatory treatment of drug addicts, in an attempt to deal with addiction in their country (Kleber, 1994). This may signal a change in the guiding philosophy of the "Dutch government."

The English Experience

England followed a drug interdiction and incarceration model that was similar to that used in the United States throughout much of the 1980s. Drug addiction in England tripled during this decade-long experiment (60 Minutes, 1992). At that point, questions were asked as to whether it was time to reconsider their national approach to the problem of drug abuse. The policymakers in England concluded that "as the sole or major player in a drug-control system, the law is at best a blunt instrument" (Berridge, 1996, p. 304). Control and treatment of drug addicts was turned over to physicians, as it had been in the 1920s through the 1970s. A limited number of physicians could prescribe the drugs that the addicts needed to supply their "habit."

The physician who prescribes the drugs for the addict must hold a special license (60 Minutes, 1992). At the same time, the addict must have proven that he/she is unwilling, or unable, to give up drugs. The goal of this system is to help the addicted individual avoid the dangers inherent in the drug-using lifestyle, at least until he/she is able to "mature out" of the need to use drugs. One measure of the success of this approach is that, whereas more than 50% of the intravenous drug abusers in cities such as New York have been found to carry HIV-1, only 1% of the addicts in Liverpool, England, have been found to have this virus in their blood (60 Minutes, 1992).

Given this different approach to the problem of illicit drug use, it is surprising to observe a rise in child/adolescent recreational chemical use in England, similar to that observed in the United States in the mid-1990s (Webb, Ashton, & Kamali, 1996). It is not known why there are simultaneous increases in the rates of child/adolescent recreational chemical abuse in both the United States and England. However, both the Dutch and the English responses to the drug "crisis" have been unlike the American approach. The success of each alternative approach suggests that there might be room for improvement in the traditional American approach to the problem of alcohol/drug addiction.

Drug Use and Violence: The Unseen Connection

Researchers have recently discovered what police officers have long known: there is a relationship between substance abuse and violence. Although research has established that, as a group, the mentally ill are 5 times as likely to become violent as the general population, as a group substance abusers are 12 to 16 times as likely to resort to violence (Marzuk, 1996).

Some recreational drugs such as the amphetamines and cocaine tend to predispose the user toward violence. One study found that 31% of homicide victims in New York City had cocaine in their bodies at the time of their death (Swan, 1995a). Overall, cocaine users are 10 to 50 times as likely to be murdered than are nonusers, according to the author. There are several reasons for this: cocaine users tend to associate with people who are more likely to respond with violence and are less likely to avoid situations where violence might occur. Further, individuals under the influence of cocaine may behave in ways that trigger others to respond violently to them, resulting in what is known as a "victim-precipitated homicide."

The disinhibition effects of many recreational drugs may also account for some of the observed tendency toward violence among alcohol/drug abusers. As discussed in Chapter 4, alcohol is a common factor in violent behaviors. For example, "more than half" (Kermani & Castaneda, 1996, p. 2) of those who commit homicide were actively using chemicals at the time of the commission of the murder. But a significant percentage of those homicides were planned in advance, and the murderer then drank to bolster his/her courage before committing the act. Thus, the relationship between alcohol and interpersonal violence is more complex than a simple cause and effect.

The world of illicit drug use/abuse is a violent one. Jaffe (1989) reported that one study in St. Louis found that 35% of the addicts surveyed reported having been shot or wounded with a knife at some point during their drug-using careers. Drug pushers have been known to attack customers in order to steal their money, armed with the knowledge that the drug user is unlikely to press charges. After all, when one engages in illegal acts (such as the use of illicit chemicals) or has obtained money through illegal channels (such as burglary), one is unlikely to call the police to report being victimized by another criminal.

Drug pushers have been known to kill their customers in retaliation for unpaid drug debts, and as a warning to others who might be behind in their payments. For example, Goldstein (1990) concluded that fully 18% of all the homicides committed in New York State in 1986 were the result of drug-related debts. On occasion, drug pushers themselves are shot, then dropped in front of the hospital emergency room, or simply left to die where they fall. Sometimes, this is done by other drug pushers, to scare off competition over "territory" (i.e., an area where one drug dealer will sell drugs). On other occasions, the murder is carried out by others associated with the drug trade, mainly because of unpaid drug debts. Although the drug dealer might earn profits of several hundred to several thousand dollars per day, few dealers carry health insurance. When a drug user/dealer is beaten, shot, or stabbed as a result of involvement in the drug underworld, his/her medical care can cost tens or hundreds of thousands of dollars. If, as is often the case, the drug user/dealer is uninsured, these expenses are passed on to the government, or to patients with insurance, through a financial process known as "cost shifting" (Headden, 1996).

The violent world in which the opiate-dependent person lives increases the risk of premature death through drug overdose, infections, malnutrition, accidents, and violence. It has been estimated that 2% of all active heroin-addicted persons die each year (Anthony et al., 1995). For those heroin-addicted persons who are infected with HIV, the annual death rate is 4% per year, according to the authors. There does not appear to be any end to the drug-related violence. There are those who argue that the prohibition against chemical abuse has contributed to the rise of violence among those who use chemicals. If this is true, then the logical conclusion would be that if drug use were legalized, then there would be a significant *decrease* in the level of violence in this country. However, this is only a theory, and it is not known whether this would happen in reality.

Unseen Victims of Street Drug Chemistry

As discussed earlier, many of the illicit chemicals used in this country are produced in illicit laboratories.

Product reliability is hardly a strong component of clandestine, illegal drug laboratories. This is not a new phenomenon. During Prohibition, a constant danger was that the "bathtub gin" or "home brew" (beverages containing alcohol) might have accidentally produced methanol (a form of alcohol that could blind or even kill a person) instead of the desired ethanol. The number of victims of methanol poisoning during Prohibition was thought to number in the "tens of thousands" (Nadelmann et al., 1990, p. 46). One reason smuggling alcohol was so popular during Prohibition is that people could trust a legitimate imported alcoholic beverage would not blind or kill them.

Nor were the problems associated with illegally manufactured alcohol limited to the Prohibition era. Even today, whiskey produced by illegal stills, known in many parts of the country as "moonshine" (or, "shine"), is frequently contaminated with high levels of lead (Pegues, Hughes, & Woernie, 1993). The lead contamination is caused by the tendency of many producers to filter the brew through old automobile radiators, according to the authors, where it comes into contact with lead from soldered joints. So common is this problem that the authors concluded that illegal whiskey is "an important and unappreciated source of lead poisoning" (p. 1501) in some parts of this country.

In today's world, contaminants are commonly found in the drugs sold on the street. If the drug was manufactured in an illegal laboratory, a simple mistake in the production process might produce a dangerous, or even a lethal, chemical combination. For example, although the illicit production of methamphetamine requires only a few common chemicals, and only a basic knowledge of chemistry, mistakes made in the production process can contaminate the drug with high levels of lead (Norton, Burton, & McGirr, 1996).

In the mid-1970s, heroin addicts in California were sold a compound that was, they were told, "synthetic heroin." These addicts injected the drug and quickly developed a drug-induced condition very similar to advanced cases of Parkinson's disease (Kirsch, 1986). Chemists discovered that, as a result of a mistake in the production process, what had been produced was not 1-methyl-4–4-phenyl-4-pro-pionoxy-piperidine (a synthetic narcotic known as MPPP), but the chemical 1-methyl-4-phenyl-1,2,3,6-tetrahydropyridine (known as MPTP).[4] Once in the body, the enzyme monoamine oxidase biotransforms MPTP into a neurotoxin known as 1-methyl-4-phenylpyridinium (MPP+), which is a neurotoxin that kills the dopamine-producing brain cells in the nigrostriatal region of the brain (Langston & Palfreman, 1995; Lopez & Jeste, 1997).

Subsequent research revealed that the loss of these same neurons is implicated in the development of Parkinson's disease. Thus, indirectly, this mistake in the manufacture of illicit narcotics allowed researchers to make an important discovery into the cause of Parkinson's disease. Because MPTP was sold on the street, however, many opiate abusers died as a result of this mistake. Others developed a lifelong drug-induced disorder very similar to Parkinson's disease, as a result of a simple mistake in the process of making illicit synthetic heroin.

There is no way to determine how many people have suffered, or died, because of other impurities in illicit drugs. But, it is known that addicts have been, and still are, being poisoned because of mistakes made in the production of street drugs. In the late 1980s, a heroin addict was found to have developed lead poisoning, as a result of the use of lead-contaminated heroin (Parras et al., 1988). Cases have been reported where the users of amphetamines have also been exposed to toxic levels of lead or other possibly carcinogenic compounds, as a result of impure street drugs (Centers for Disease Control, 1990; Evanko, 1991). In France, some samples of heroin were found to be contaminated with the heavy metal thallium, which killed at least one individual ("Bald Is Not Beautiful," 1996).

Lombard, Levin, and Weiner (1989) reviewed a case where a cocaine abuser was found to have had developed arsenic poisoning, a rather rare condition. Physicians concluded that the arsenic was contained in the cocaine that this patient was using. When they told him that the cause of his nausea, vomiting, and diarrhea was a contaminant in the cocaine that he was using, the patient was reportedly quite unimpressed. The addict informed the physicians that it

was "common knowledge" (p. 869) that cocaine might be mixed with compounds that contained arsenic. The authors warned that similar cases might be encountered by other physicians.

Nor is the problem of contaminated drugs limited to narcotics or cocaine alone. Most of the drugs

> intended for popular recreational use are most often produced in clandestine laboratories with little or no quality control, so generally speaking users cannot be sure of the purity of what they are ingesting. (Hayner & McKinney, 1986, p. 341)

Where illicit drugs are concerned, "misrepresentation is the rule" (Brown & Braden, 1987, p. 341). A capsule might be sold on the street as "THC," but actually contain PCP, a far different chemical. The buyer cannot, without a detailed chemical analysis, be sure what the substance purchased actually is, whether it is contaminated, or how potent it might be.

Toward the end of the 1980s, one study revealed that only 60% of the samples of "amphetamines" purchased on the street actually contained amphetamines (Scaros et al., 1990). It is not uncommon for "amphetamine tablets" sold on the street to actually be nothing more than caffeine tablets. In some cases, police chemists have found that what was sold as the hallucinogen MDMA actually contained "anything from MDA, LSD and amphetamine to fish-tank oxygenating tablets and cold cure powders" (Abbott & Concar, 1992, p. 33).

Thus, one should not assume that any illicit drug is actually what it was reported to be. One should not even accept that the chemical is safe for human consumption, without a chemical analysis of that substance. In the world of illicit drug use, it is indeed a case of "let the buyer beware."

Drug Analogs: The "Designer" Drugs

When a pharmaceutical company develops a new drug for use in the fight against disease, that drug is patented. To apply for a patent, the pharmaceutical company must identify the chemical structure of the new drug molecule; and the exact location of each atom in relation to every other atom in the chemical chain of that drug molecule is identified

---

[4]The very names of these chemicals gives the reader some idea as to how easy it would be for chemists to make mistakes in their manufacture.

and recorded. After review by the Food and Drug Administration, the pharmaceutical company is then granted a patent on that drug molecule for a specific period.

When law enforcement agencies want to classify a drug as an illicit substance, they must go through much the same process. Chemists must identify the chemical structure of the new drug molecule; and the exact location of each atom in relation to every other atom in the chemical chain of that drug molecule must be identified, and recorded. This process can take several months, but will yield a chemical formula that can then be used to identify that specific compound as an illicit substance.

Because drug molecules are very complex, it is often possible to add, rearrange, or remove some atoms from the "parent" drug molecule, without having much of an impact on the original drug's psychoactive effect. Depending on the exact chemical structure of the parent drug, it is possible to develop dozens, or even hundreds, of variations of the original drug molecule. For example, there are 184 known potential variations of the parent drug from which the hallucinogen MDMA is developed ("Market Update," 1993). These variations on the original drug molecule are called "analog" drugs, or "analogs." Many of the drug analogs have no psychoactive effect, and thus are of little interest to the illicit chemists who produce chemicals for sale on the street. But some drug analogs are abusable, and thus would be of interest to illicit drug producers. A drug analog might be less potent than the parent compound, equally potent or even, in some cases, more potent than the original chemical. As discussed later in this chapter, some analogs of the pharmaceutical fentanyl are more powerful than the original drug.

The main point to keep in mind is that, even if the difference is just one atom that has been added, or moved around on the chemical chain, the chemical structure of the drug analog will be different from that of the parent drug. If the parent drug has been classified as an illegal substance, it is possible that by removing just one atom from the chemical chain of the original drug, to create a "new" drug that has not yet been outlawed. For the sake of discussion, assume that the simplified drug "molecule"

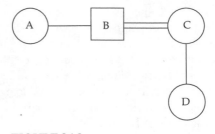

FIGURE 34.1

shown in Figure 34.1 has been outlawed as an illegal hallucinogen.[5]

In this example, the parent drug "molecule" only has four atoms, not the hundreds of atoms found in some actual chemical molecules. However, a drug with the chemical structure shown in Figure 34.2 would technically be a "different" drug, since its molecular structure is not *exactly* the same as the first chemical.

This chemical would be a drug analog of the parent drug. There is an obvious difference in the chemical structure of the first and the second drug. The new atom that was added to the chemical structure might not make the analog more potent than the parent compound. But, it will change the chemical structure of that drug just enough so that it is not covered by the law that made the original parent drug illegal. For this analog to be declared illegal, researchers would have to identify the location of every atom in the second compound, and the nature of the chemical bond that held that atom in place. Then, law enforcement officials would have to present their findings to the appropriate agency for the drug analog to be outlawed. This process might take months, or even longer. When this happens, it would be a simple matter to again change the chemical structure a little bit, build a new analog, and start the whole cycle over again. For example, the new analog might look like the structure shown in Figure 34.3.

Notice that there is a subtle difference in the chemical structure of the last two hypothetical drug molecules. In each case, however, in the eyes of the

---

[5] For the sake of illustration, I have not used real drug molecules.

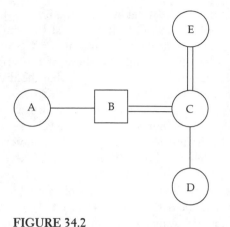

FIGURE 34.2

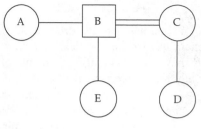

FIGURE 34.4

law, they are "different" drugs. Technically, this is a new "drug," which is not covered by the law that prohibited the parent drug. If this drug molecule *were* to be outlawed, the street chemist might again change the drug into something like the structure shown in Figure 34.4.

The drug molecule in this example is a very simple one, with only five atoms. However, even with this simplistic example, it has been possible to produce several different analogs of the parent molecule. When you stop to consider that many of the psychoactive drugs have drug molecules that contain many hundreds, or even thousands, of atoms, the number of potential combinations is rather impressive.

Some Existing Drug Analogs

It should be no surprise that street chemists have been manipulating the chemical structure of known drugs of abuse, in the hopes of coming up with a

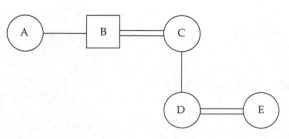

FIGURE 34.3

new drug that has not yet been outlawed. Some of the following drug analogs have been outlawed by government agencies, while action against some of the other compounds is still pending.

Analogs of the Amphetamines

The amphetamine molecule lends itself to experimentation, and several analogs of the original amphetamine molecule have been identified by law enforcement agencies. Some known analogs of the amphetamines include 2,5-dimethoxy-4-methylamphetamine, or the hallucinogenic DOM (Scaros et al., 1990). MDMA, also known as "ecstacy," is itself a drug analog of the amphetamine family of chemicals. There are, in turn, 184 known analogs of the parent drug of MDMA, some of which are known to have a psychoactive effect on the user.

The drug 3,4-methylenedioxyamphetamine, or MDEA, is another drug analog of the amphetamine family. When the hallucinogen ecstacy (MDMA) was classified as a controlled substance in 1985, many street chemists simply started to produce MDEA. The chemical structure of MDEA is very similar to that of MDMA, and its effects are reported to be very similar to those of MDMA (Mirin et al., 1991). This substance is often sold under the name of "Eve." There have been isolated reports of death associated with MDEA use, and it is not known what role, if any, MDEA had in these deaths. Further, the long-term effects of MDEA are still unknown.

A recent addition to the list of illicit stimulants being produced by street chemists in this country is methcathinone, or "Kat." This compound was discussed in Chapter 8. However, the reader should be aware that Kat is also a "designer" drug.

Analogs of PCP

PCP is a popular parent drug molecule with illicit chemists. To date, at least 30 drug analogs of PCP have been identified, many of which are actually more potent than PCP itself (Crowley, 1995b; Weiss et al., 1994). These are the drugs N-ethyl-1-phenylcyclohexylamine (also known as PCE), [1-(1–2-thienylcyclohexyl) piperidine] (TCP), [1-(1-phenylcyclohexyl)-pyrrolidine] (PHP), [1-piperidinocyclohexanecarbonitrile] (PCC), and Eu⁴ia (pronounced "euphoria"), an amphetamine-like drug synthesized from legally purchased, over-the-counter chemicals (Scaros et al., 1990).

Ketamine

Another street analog of PCP that is occasionally produced by illicit laboratories includes [2-o-chorophenyl-2-methylamine cyclohexanone] (or Ketamine). Ketamine, surprisingly, is a legitimate pharmaceutical agent, which is used as a surgical anesthetic for both humans and animals (Bushnell & Justins, 1993). When used as a surgical anesthetic, Ketamine may be introduced into the body by way of intraveneous injection, intramuscular injection, or in oral form, according to the authors. Further, since Ketamine does not cause respiratory or cardiac depression, it is of value in situations where opioid-based anesthetics cannot be used.

When abused, Ketamine is said to have effects similar to those of heroin ("Ice Overdose," 1989). In addition to causing a short-lived sense of euphoria, Some of the side effects of Ketamine abuse include a sense of psychological dissociation, panic states, and hallucinations (Jansen, 1993). Long-term use, especially at high doses may result in drug-induced memory problems, according to the author. This effect has reportedly made Ketamine popular as a "date rape" drug.

Aminorex

For a number of years, the drug analog 2-amino-4-methyl-5-phenyl-2-oxazoline has appeared on the streets, from time to time. This compound is derived from a diet pill sold in Europe under the brand name of "Aminorex" in the 1980s, and it is easily synthesized (Karch, 1996). The effects of this drug, often sold on the street by the name of "U-4-E-UH" or "EU4EA" are not well known at this time, but available evidence suggests that it is a CNS stimulant, with effects similar to those of the amphetamines (Karch). There are reports that the drug has been sold on both the East and West Coasts.

Following a single oral dose of the pharmaceutical compound Aminorex, peak blood levels are seen in about 2 hours, and the half-life of Aminorex is approximately 7.7 hours (Karch, 1996). There is no clinical research into the effect of illicit forms of 2-amino-4-methyl-5-phenyl-2-oxazoline on the human body, and the potential for harm from Aminorex-like compounds available on the street remains unknown.

GHB

Another illicit drug that has appeared on the streets in recent years is the CNS depressant known as Gamma hydroxybutyrate (GHB). This drug is a metabolite of the neurotransmitter GABA, discussed in earlier chapters. It is relatively easy to make, and information on how to make GHB is available on the Internet ("Introduction to GHB," 1997). Thus, there is little to keep illicit chemists from attempting to make this compound. At doses of 10 mg per kilogram of body weight, the drug can produce a sense of euphoria. Doses of 50 mg/kg of body weight can produce anesthesia, coma, respiratory depression, and possible death. The drug was once used as an experimental anesthetic, but it was found that it had only a narrow therapeutic window, and even when used by physicians it could cause seizures ("Introduction to GHB," 1997). This compound was outlawed by the Food and Drug Administration in 1990, but has been growing in popularity in the United States.

Fentanyl: The Best Known Designer Drug?

Street chemists must like fentanyl. The drug molecule is easy to manipulate, and it may be synthesized from a few ordinary industrial chemicals (Langston & Palfreman, 1995). By making just a minor change in the drug molecule, by adding a few atoms to the right portion of the fentanyl molecule, it is possible to produce a fentanyl analog that will extend the drug's effects from the normal 30 to 90 minutes up to 4 or 5 hours or, with the right modifications to the parent drug, even 4 or 5 *days*, according to the authors. Thus, it is a popular drug for illicit drug manufacturers to produce.

In the early 1980s, there was a series of fatal narcotic overdoses in California, as street chemists started to produce various designer drugs that were similar to the analgesic fentanyl (discussed in the chapter on narcotic analgesics) (Hibbs, Perper, & Winek, 1991). Kirsch (1986) identified nine different drug analogs to fentanyl that are known, or suspected, to have been sold on the streets. These drug analogs range in potency from one-tenth that of morphine for the fentanyl analog benzylfentanyl, to 1000 times (Hibbs et al., 1991) to 3000 times (Kirsch) more potent than morphine for 3-methyl fentanyl.

The drug 3-methyl fentanyl is also known to chemists as "TMF." This analog of fentanyl has been identified as the cause of narcotics overdoses in the area around Pittsburgh, Pennsylvania (Hibbs et al., 1991), and also in New York City ("A New Market," 1991). Hibbs et al. conducted a retrospective analysis to determine how serious a problem TMF-induced overdoses were for the Allegheny County region, which surrounds Pittsburgh. Surprisingly, the authors found that in the year 1988, fully 27% of the drug overdose deaths in Allegheny County were caused by TMF. This would suggest that designer narcotics are a significant part of the narcotics problem in this country.

The chemical structure of fentanyl makes it possible for the drug molecule to be snorted, much like cocaine. When used intranasally, the drug is deposited on the blood-rich tissues of the sinuses, where it is absorbed into the general circulation. Fentanyl can also be smoked. Like cocaine, when fentanyl is smoked, the molecules easily cross into the general circulation through the lungs. So rapidly is fentanyl absorbed through the lungs that it is possible for the user to overdose on the medication after just one inhalation ("Take Time to Smell," 1994).

Given the characteristics of fentanyl, it is safe to assume that analogs of this chemical present similar abuse profiles. Law enforcement officials have struggled to deal with the problem of diversion of fentanyl products to illicit users almost from the moment that the drug was introduced. But the drug is so powerful that even small amounts have a value to illicit drug users. For example, some opiate abusers scrape the residual medication from transdermal fentanyl patches, to obtain small amounts of fentanyl that can then be smoked.

Fentanyl is so potent a drug that extremely small doses are effective in humans. To be detected in a blood or urine sample, a special test procedure must be carried out (Evanko, 1991). Routine drug toxicology screens easily miss the presence of such small amounts of fentanyl in the blood or urine of a suspected drug user ("Take Time to Smell," 1994). Thus, even a clean urine or blood drug screen might not rule out fentanyl use on the part of an addict.

Some opiate abusers have been known to die so rapidly after using fentanyl that they were found with the needle still in their arms (Evanko, 1991). This phenomenon is well documented in cases of narcotic overdoses, but is not understood by medicine. Some researchers attribute the rapid death to the narcotic itself, while others have suggested that the user's death is caused by chemicals added to the drug to "cut" or dilute it on the street. Fentanyl is so potent that some samples of the drug sold on the street are made up of 0.01% fentanyl, and 99.9% filler (Langston & Palfreman, 1995).

It is difficult to understand the addictive potential of fentanyl. Dr. William Spiegelman (quoted in Gallagher, 1986) observed, "it can take years to become addicted to alcohol, months for cocaine, and one shot for fentanyl" (p. 26). To further complicate matters, street chemists are manipulating the chemical structure of fentanyl, adding a few atoms to the basic fentanyl chain here, snipping a few atoms there, to produce drug analogs. In the past 20 years, fentanyl and its analogs have become a significant part of the drug abuse problem in the United States, and there is no end in sight.

Summary

The relationship between criminal activity and substance use/abuse is exceptionally complex, and in this chapter the relationship between alcohol/drug use and crime were briefly explored. Although some criminal activity *does* seem to result from the use/abuse of recreational chemicals, it also has been suggested that many of those who engage in criminal activity and substance use are the types of people who are prone to engage in illegal activities. In such cases, the apparent relationship between substance use and criminal behavior is not a causal one, but a complex interaction between the individual's personality, his/her use of chemicals, and his/her tendency to engage in illegal behaviors.

There is strong evidence that at least some of the criminal behavior associated with drug abuse is caused by the legal status of the chemicals in society, and proponents have used this information to call for the legalization of recreational drugs. The sanctions against chemical use have resulted in overburdened courts, overcrowded jails/prisons, and no apparent reduction in the level of illicit drug use in this country. In this chapter, alternatives to the legalistic approach used in the United States were reviewed, including the public health approach utilized in England and Holland.

The fact that illicit drug producers are motivated to find new "designer" drugs in part because of the way that drugs are identified/regulated in the United States, and the rewards for finding unregulated drug molecules for sale by consumers of recreational drugs was discussed. The role that adulterants play in the production/distribution of illicit drugs was discussed, and many of the more common adulterants were identified. The relationship between the individual's use of recreational chemicals and his/her responsibility for that person's behavior was discussed. The fact that many drug distributors trade their knowledge about who is involved in the drug trade for reduced sentences, and the history of the present "war" on drugs were briefly reviewed.

CHAPTER THIRTY-FIVE

Self-Help Groups

The Twelve Steps of Alcoholics Anonymous[1]

Step One: We admitted that we were powerless over alcohol—that our lives had become unmanageable.

Step Two: Came to believe that a Power greater than ourselves could restore us to sanity.

Step Three: Made a decision to turn our will and our lives over to the care of God *as we understood Him.*

Step Four: Made a searching and fearless moral inventory of ourselves.

Step Five: Admitted to God, to ourselves, and to another human being the exact nature of our wrongs.

Step Six: Were entirely ready to have God remove all these defects of character.

Step Seven: Humbly asked Him to remove our shortcomings.

Step Eight: Made a list of all persons we had harmed, and became willing to make amends to them all.

Step Nine: Made direct amends to such people wherever possible, except when to do so would injure them or others.

Step Ten: Continued to take personal inventory and when we were wrong, promptly admitted it.

[1] The Twelve Steps are reprinted by permission of Alcoholics Anonymous World Services, Inc.

Step Eleven: Sought through prayer and meditation to improve our conscious contact with God *as we understood Him,* praying only for knowledge of His will for us, and the power to carry that out.

Step Twelve: Having had a spiritual awakening as the result of these steps, we tried to carry this message to alcoholics, and to practice these principles in all our affairs.

Alcoholics Anonymous (AA) is the "most frequently consulted source of help for drinking problems" (Miller & McCrady, 1993, p. 3). Approximately 1 in every 10 adults in the United States has attended AA at least once (Miller & McCrady, 1993; Zweben, 1995). This is not to say that all these people had alcohol use problems of their own, however. Perhaps two-thirds of those who have attended at least one AA meeting, have done so out of a concern for another person's drinking (Zweben). However, this still means that one-third of those who have attended AA, or 3.1% of the adults in the United States, have done so because they thought that they might have an alcohol use problem (Godlaski, Leukefeld, & Cloud, 1997).

Despite its popularity, however, AA is perhaps the least rigorously studied element in the spectrum of rehabilitation programs (Meza & Kranzler, 1996). Even after having existed for close to 60 years, "the empirical research on the efficacy of Alcoholics Anonymous is sparse and inconclusive" (Watson et al., 1997, p. 209). AA remains something of a mystery not only to nonmembers, but, all too often, even to active members. Further, AA or similar self-help groups are controversial. Supporters claim that AA is the most effective means of treating alcoholism. Critics of AA, or similar programs, challenge this claim. In this chapter, the self-help group phenomenon patterned after the Alcoholics Anonymous program is examined.

The History of AA

The diverse forces that were to blend together to form Alcoholics Anonymous (AA) include the American temperance movement of the late 1800s (Peele, 1984, 1989), a nondenominational religious group known as the Oxford Group, which was popular in the 1930s (Nace, 1987), and the psychoanalysis of an American alcoholic by Carl Jung in the year 1931 (Edmeades, 1987). Over the years, many early members of Alcoholics Anonymous were hospitalized, mistakes were made, questions were asked, and the early pioneers of AA embarked on a struggle for sobriety that transcended individual members.

Historically, AA was thought to have been founded on June 10, 1935, the day that an alcoholic physician had his last drink (Nace, 1987). Earlier, following a meeting between a stockbroker, William Griffith Wilson, and the surgeon, Dr. Robert Holbrook Smith, the foundation to AA was set down. William Wilson was struggling to protect his newfound sobriety while on a business trip in a strange city. After making several telephone calls to try to find support in his struggle, Wilson was asked to talk to Dr. Smith, who was drinking at the time that Wilson called.

Rather than looking out for his own needs, Wilson chose a different approach. He carried a message of sobriety to another alcoholic. The self-help philosophy of AA was born from this moment. In the half century since then, it has grown to a fellowship of 87,000 "clubs" or AA groups including chapters in 150 countries, with a total membership estimated at more than 2 million persons (Humphreys & Moos, 1996). Of this number, 1.2 million members are from either the United States or Canada (Marvel, 1995). Thus, 68% of the entire world membership of AA is found just in North America.

During its early years, AA struggled to find a method that would support its members in their struggle to both achieve and maintain sobriety.

Within three years of its founding, three AA groups were in existence, but even with three groups "it was hard to find two score of sure recoveries" (*Twelve Steps and Twelve Traditions*, 1981, p. 17). But, the fledgling organization slowly grew, until, by the fourth year following its inception, there were about 100 members in isolated AA groups (Nace, 1987). Despite this limited beginning, the early members decided to write about their struggle to achieve sobriety, in order to share their discoveries with others. The book that was published in 1939 as a result of this process was the first edition of the book *Alcoholics Anonymous*. The organization took its name from the title of this book, which has since come to be known as the "Big Book" of AA (*Twelve Steps and Twelve Traditions*, 1981).

Elements of AA

In their exploration of why certain self-help groups are so effective, Roots and Aanes (1992) identified eight characteristics that seem to contribute to a group's success:

1. Members have *shared experience*, in this case their inability to control their drug or alcohol use.
2. *Education*, not psychotherapy, is the primary goal of AA membership.
3. Self-help groups are *self-governing*.
4. The group places emphasis on *accepting responsibility for one's behavior*.
5. There is but a *single purpose* to the group.
6. Membership is *voluntary*.
7. The individual member must make a *commitment to personal change*.
8. The group places emphasis on *anonymity and confidentiality*.

The core characteristics of AA are very much a product of society in the United States in the late 1930s. Culturally, Americans have always had a strong belief in the process of public confession, contrition, and salvation through spirituality, all of which are elements in the AA program. Further, as the *Twelve Steps and Twelve Traditions* (1981) acknowledged, the early members of AA also freely borrowed from the fields of medicine and religion to establish a program that worked for them. The program that emerged is the famous "Twelve Steps" of AA. The Twelve Steps serve as the core of the recovery program that AA offers.

A Breakdown of the Twelve Steps

The book *Al-Anon's Twelve Steps and Twelve Traditions*, which has borrowed the Twelve Steps of AA for use with families, divides the Twelve Steps into three groups. The first three steps are viewed as necessary for the acceptance of one's limitations. Through these first three steps, the individual is able to come to accept that his/her own resources are not sufficient to solve life's problems, especially the problems inherent in living with an addicted person. In the AA Step program, these steps help the individual accept that his/her resources are insufficient for dealing with the problems of life, especially one's addiction to alcohol.

Steps Four through Nine are a series of change-oriented activities. These steps are designed to help the individual identify, confront, and ultimately overcome character shortcomings that were integral to the individual's addicted lifestyle. Through these steps, one may work through the guilt associated with past behaviors, and learn to recognize the limits of personal responsibility. These steps allow the person to learn the tools of non-drug-centered living, something which at first is often alien to both the alcohol-dependent person, and his/her family.

Finally, Steps Ten through Twelve challenge the individual to continue to build on the foundation established in Steps Four through Nine. The individual is asked to continue to search out personal shortcomings and to confront them. The person also is challenged to continue the spiritual growth initiated during the earlier steps, and to carry the message of hope to others.

In a sense, AA might be viewed as functioning as a form of psychotherapy (Alibrandi, 1978; Peck, 1993; Tobin, 1992). From this perspective, the AA program consists of five phases (Alibrandi, 1978). The first stage starts on the first day of membership in AA, and lasts for the next week. During this phase, the individual's goal is simply to stay away from his/her first drink (or, episode of chemical use).

The second phase of recovery starts at the end of the 1st week, and lasts until the end of the 2nd month of AA membership (Alibrandi, 1978). Major steps during this part of the recovery process include the recovering addict's acceptance of the disease concept of addiction, and learning the willingness to accept help with his/her addiction. During this phase, the individual struggles to replace old drug-centered behavioral habits with new, sobriety-oriented habits. The third stage of recovery spans the interval from the 2nd through to the 6th month of recovery, according to Alibrandi. During this stage, the individual is to use the Twelve Steps as a guide, and to try letting go of old ideas. Guilt feelings about past chemical use are to be replaced with gratitude for sobriety, wherever possible, and the member is to stand available for service to other addicts.

The fourth stage begins at around the sixth month of sobriety, and lasts until after the first year of sobriety (Alibrandi, 1978). During the fourth stage, the addict is encouraged to take a searching and fearless moral inventory of "self," and to share this with another person. At the same time, if the individual is still "shaky," he/she is encouraged to work with another member. Emphasis during this phase of recovery is on acceptance of responsibility, and the resolution of the anger and resentments that so often underlie addiction. Finally, after the first year of sobriety, the recovery process has reached what Brown (1985) termed "ongoing sobriety." Alibrandi identified the goal during this phase of recovery as being the maintenance of a "spiritual condition." The person is warned not to dwell on the shortcomings of others, to suspend judgment of self and others, and to beware of the false pride that could bring one back to chemical use again.

The Twelve Steps essentially provide a program for spiritual growth (Peck, 1993). The core of the AA program is the correction of the spiritual defects that form the foundation of the alcoholism. Although W. Dyer (1989) did not address AA specifically when he explored the issue of spiritual growth, his observations could also be applied to the process of spiritual growth that is a central component of the AA program when he said:

> Once you start to make the transformational awakening journey, there is no going back. You develop

a knowledge that is so powerful that you will wonder how you could have lived any other way. The awakened life begins to own you, and then you simply know within that you are on the right path. (p. 17)

Whether the Twelve Steps are effective, or why they are effective, is often disputed. But, within the AA community, there are those who believe that the Twelve Steps offer a program within which personality transformation can be accomplished (DiClemente, 1993). Others believe that the Twelve Steps represent a series of successive approximations toward the goal of sobriety (McCrady & Delaney, 1995). Surprisingly, the Steps are not required for AA membership. But, they are viewed within AA as a proven method of behavioral change that offers the addict a chance to rebuild his/her life. There are many who believe that these Steps were instrumental in saving their lives.

AA and Religion

Alcoholics Anonymous makes a distinction between spirituality and religion (Berenson, 1987; Wallace, 1996), and it identifies with no single religious group or doctrine (*Twelve Steps and Twelve Traditions*, 1981). But, as a spiritual growth program, AA embraces the tenet that the individual's distorted self-perception of being the center of the universe helps to make the individual vulnerable to alcoholism (McCrady, 1994). To counter this narcissistic perception, AA places emphasis on establishing a relationship with a Higher Power, without endorsing a specific religious doctrine for its members.

An example of this process is Step Three of the AA twelve-step program. This step "doesn't demand an immediate conversion experience . . . but . . . does call for a decision" (Jensen, 1987b, p. 22) by the alcohol-dependent person to turn his/her will over to God. The concept of a Higher Power, which is not incorporated into formal religious doctrine is, perhaps, best reflected by the Lakota Wisdomkeeper Mathew King:

You can call Wakan-Tanka by any name you like. In English I call Him God or the Great Spirit.

He's the Great Mystery, the Great Mysterious. That's what Wakan-Tanka really means—the Great Mysterious.

You can't define Him. He's not actually a "He" or a "She," a "Him" or a "Her." We have to use those kinds of words because you can't just say "It." God's never an "It." (Arden, 1994, pp. 4–5)

The Third Step of the AA program "simply assumes that there is a God to understand and that we each have a God of our own understanding" (Jensen, 1987b, p. 23). In this manner, AA sidesteps the question of religion, while still addressing the spiritual disease that it views as forming the foundation for the addiction. In turning one's will over to a Higher Power, the individual comes to accept that his/her own will is not enough to maintain recovery. Thus, AA offers a spiritual program that ties the individual's will into that of a "higher power," without offering a specific religious dogma that might offend members. Still the heavy emphasis on a Higher Power has resulted in criticism of AA by some former members (Marvel, 1995; Wallace, 1996).

One "A" Is for Anonymous

Anonymity is central to the AA program (*Understanding Anonymity*, 1981). This is a major reason for most meetings being "closed." There are three types of closed meetings. In the first, where there is a designated speaker, one individual will talk at length about his/her life, substance use and how he/she came to join AA and benefit from the program (Nowinski, 1996). In the second form of closed AA meeting, the "discussion" meeting, a theme or problem of interest to the members of the AA group is identified, and each member of the group is offered the chance to talk about how this problem affects him/her. Finally, in the last type of closed meeting, the "Step" meeting, the group will focus on one of the Twelve Steps for a month at a time, with each member being offered the chance to talk about his/her understanding of the step and how he/she attempts to put that step into practice in his/her recovery program. Closed meetings are limited to members of AA. In contrast to the closed meetings, there are also "open" AA meetings. In the open meeting, which is open to any interested person, one or two volunteers will speak, and visitors are encouraged to ask questions about AA and how it works.

Anonymity is a central concept of AA. For this reason, many AA members believe that court-ordered or employer-mandated attendance of AA runs counter to the central philosophy of anonymity; to verify attendance, the individual must ask a member of AA to break anonymity and to confirm that the person was present at the meeting(s) he/she was ordered to attend. The AA program places emphasis on anonymity to protect the identities of members and to ensure that no identified spokesperson emerges who claims to "speak" for AA (*Understanding Anonymity*, 1981). Through this policy, the members of AA strive for humility, each knowing that he/she is equal to the other members. The concept of anonymity is so important that it is said to serve "as the spiritual foundation of the Fellowship" (*Understanding Anonymity*, 1981, p. 5) of AA.

The concept of equality of the members underlies the AA tradition that no "directors" are nominated or voted upon. Rather, "service boards" or special committees are created from the membership as needed. These boards always remain responsible to the group *as a whole*, and must answer to the entire AA group. As is noted in Tradition Two of AA, "our leaders are but trusted servants; they do not govern" (*Twelve Steps and Twelve Traditions*, 1981, p. 10). Because of this emphasis on equality, the structure of AA has evolved into one that minimizes if not almost totally avoids the "interpersonal conflicts and the petty jealousy, greed or self-importance that could create havoc among fellowship members" (DiClemente, 1993, p. 85).

AA and Outside Organizations

Each Alcoholics Anonymous group is both self-supporting and not-for-profit. Individual groups are autonomous and must support themselves only through the contributions of the members. Further, each individual member is prohibited from contributing more than $1,000 per year to AA. Outside donations are discouraged, to avoid the problem of having to decide how to deal with these gifts. Outside commitments are also discouraged for AA groups. As is stated in the text *Twelve Steps and Twelve Traditions* (1981), AA groups will not "endorse, finance, or lend the AA name to any related facility or outside enterprise, least problems of money, property and prestige divert us from our primary purpose" (p. 11).

The relationships between different autonomous AA groups, and between different AA groups and other organizations, are governed by the Twelve Traditions of AA. The Traditions are a set of guidelines or a framework within which different groups may interact, and through which AA as a whole may work together. They will not be reviewed in this chapter; however, interested readers might wish to read *The Twelve Steps and Twelve Traditions* (1981) to learn more about the Traditions.

The Primary Purpose of AA

Carrying the Message

This "primary purpose" of AA is twofold. First, the members of AA strive to "carry the message to the addict who still suffers" (*Group*, 1976, p. 1). Second, AA seeks to provide for its members a program for living without chemicals. This is done not by preaching at the alcohol/drug addicted individual. Rather, this is accomplished by presenting to the individual a simple, truthful, realistic picture of the disease of addiction. This is accomplished by confronting the alcohol/ drug addicted person in language that he/she can understand. This confrontation is carried out in a somewhat different manner than the usual methods of confrontation. In AA, speakers share their own life stories, a public confession of sorts where each individual tells of the lies, the distortions, the self-deceptions, and the denial that supported his/her own chemical use. In so doing, the speaker hopes to break through the defensiveness of the alcohol-addicted person, by showing that others have walked the same road and yet found a way to recovery.

Helping others is a central theme of AA, in part because:

> Even the newest of newcomers finds undreamed rewards as he tries to help his brother alcoholic, the one who is even blinder than he. . . . And then he discovers that by the divine paradox of this kind of giving he has found his own reward, whether his brother has yet received anything or not. (*Twelve Steps and Twelve Traditions*, 1981, p. 109)

In this, one finds a therapeutic paradox (not the only one!) in AA. For the speaker seeks first of all to help him-/herself through the public admission of his/ her powerlessness over chemicals. Through the public admission of weakness, the speaker seeks to gain strength from the group. It is almost as if, by owning the reality of his/her own addiction, the speaker says "This is what *my* life was like, and by having shared it with you, I am reminded again of the reason why I will not return to alcohol again."

This is the method pioneered by Bill Wilson, in his first meeting with Bob Smith. In that meeting, Bill Wilson spoke at length of his own addiction to alcohol, of the pain and suffering that he had caused others, and that he had suffered, in the service of his addiction. He did not preach, but simply shared with Dr. Smith the history of his own alcoholism. Bill Wilson concluded with the statement: "So thanks a lot for hearing me out. I know now that I'm not going to take a drink, and I'm grateful to you" (Kurtz, 1979, p. 29).

As noted earlier, the methods of AA present a paradox, in that it is by helping others that the speaker receives help for his/her own addiction to alcohol/drugs. At the same time, he/she confronts the defenses of the new member by saying, in effect, "I am a mirror of yourself, and just as you cannot look into a mirror without seeing your own image, you cannot look at me without seeing a part of yourself."

A New Lifestyle

As mentioned, Alcoholics Anonymous is a spiritual program that is at the same time not religious. The second part of AAs basic purpose is to offer members the promise of a new lifestyle and the tools to accomplish this goal. Within the AA program, alcoholism is viewed as a

> spiritual illness, and drinking as a symptom of that illness. The central spiritual "defect" of alcoholics is described as an excessive preoccupation with self . . . . Treatment of the preoccupation with self is at the core of AA's approach. (McCrady & Irvine, 1989, p. 153)

From the theoretical model of AA, alcoholism is viewed as the end product of a process that begins when the individual loses his/her spirituality (McCrady, 1994; Miller & Hester, 1995). To combat the excessive preoccupation with self, AA offers the Twelve Steps as a guide for spiritual growth, and for living. But the individual is not *required* to follow the Steps to participate in AA. Rather, "*the program* does not issue orders; it merely *suggests* Twelve Steps to recovery" (Jensen, 1987a; p. 15, italics in original). Thus, the individual is offered a choice between the way of life that preceded AA, or acceptance of a program that others have used to achieve and maintain their sobriety. But, the individual does not simply *passively* accept the Twelve Steps. Rather, the emphasis is on *working* the Steps, a process that requires "the active participation and intentional engagement of each individual who desires to change their drinking and become sober" (DiClemente, 1993, p. 80).

The Twelve Steps offer the promise and the tools necessary for daily abstinence. One of these tools is that the member of AA is not encouraged to look for the "cause" of his/her addiction to alcohol. Rather, the individual's alcoholism is accepted as a given fact. "It is not so much *how* you came to this place, as what you are going to do now that you are here," as one member said to a newcomer. Neither is the member admonished for being unable to live without chemicals. Members of AA know from bitter experience that relapse is possible and common (McCrady & Irvine, 1989). Chemical addiction is assumed in membership: "If chemicals were not a problem for you, you would not be here!" In place of the chemical-centered lifestyle, the new member is offered a step-by-step program for living that allows the person to achieve, and maintain, recovery.

To take advantage of this opportunity, the member need only accept the *program*. Admittedly, in doing so the individual is asked to accept yet another therapeutic paradox, known as Step One. The First Step, which is the only one that specifically mentions alcohol by name, asks that the individual accept that s/he is powerless over this chemical. The individual is asked to do so not on the most superficial of levels necessary to speak the words "I am powerless over chemicals," but on the deepest level of his/her being. This is a difficult step, which often must be carried out time and time again, as this lesson is learned and relearned, over and over again. The essence of the First Step is the acceptance in the deepest level of the individual's soul, that he/she is *addicted to and totally powerless over* alcohol.

It is not uncommon for new members to continue to believe that alcohol alone was the problem. When they finally confront the rationalization that they are helpless victims of the disease of addiction, they will be forced to accept that

> it is we ourselves, not the pills or alcohol, who cause most of our problems. Chemicals will not bring destruction upon a person until that person learns how to justify continual use and abuse of those chemicals. (Springborn, 1987, p. 8)

Members are helped to see that while they are not responsible for having the bio/psycho/spiritual/genetic predisposition for alcoholism, they are responsible for working toward their recovery (Wallace, 1996).

Hitting Bottom

The process of learning how completely alcohol/drugs have come to dominate a person's life is often called "hitting bottom." This is a moment of painful self-discovery, when the person accepts the bitter, frightening reality that his/her life is being spent in the service of the addiction. The person then comes to understand that he/she can do *nothing* to control the chemical use, for he/she is *addicted.*

In this moment of extreme despair, the addicted person may turn to another and say, "I need help." According to the AA model, it is at this moment in time that the alcohol/drug dependent individual takes the First Step (the ultimate admission of powerlessness) and becomes receptive to learning how to face problems without the continued use of alcohol or other chemicals.

Of AA and Recovery

Alcoholics Anonymous does not refer to a "cure" for the disease of alcoholism. The members of AA do not speak of themselves as having "recovered." For while the members of AA believe that addiction is a disease whose progress may be arrested, it is acknowledged that alcoholism can never be cured. Thus, a person may speak of themselves as *recovering,* but never as having *recovered.* An excellent example of this is that there is often a time lapse of several months between the time when new members begin to attend AA, and when they stop drinking. New members may attend AA for 20 months before they even will admit to

being a member of AA, and 8 more months before they stop drinking (Zweben, 1995). Thus, it takes the average person slightly over two years to stop drinking after joining AA.

Alcoholics Anonymous also does not speak of itself as an ultimate cure for alcoholism because it views the recovering person as being only a moment away from the next slip. The 25-year veteran may, in a weak moment, relapse back into active drinking. Simple affiliation with AA does not guarantee abstinence from alcohol/drugs (McCrady & Irvine, 1989). Each member engages in a personal struggle to abstain from alcohol/drugs that must be faced "one day at a time." If "today" is too long a period to think about, the individual is encouraged to think about abstaining for the next hour, or the next minute, or just the next second.

Once addicted persons accept the program, they find a way of living that provides support for recovery 24 hours a day, for the rest of their life (DiClemente, 1993). In accepting the program, addicted persons may discover a second chance that they thought was forever lost.

Sponsorship

To help individuals on the spiritual odyssey that leads to sobriety, new members of AA are encouraged to find a "sponsor." Sponsorship is seen as a key element to the AA program (McCrady & Delaney, 1995; Zweben, 1995). Sponsors are persons who have worked their way through the step program and who have achieved a basic understanding of their own addiction. Sponsors act as spiritual (but not religious) guides, offering confrontation, insight, and support, in equal amounts to new members.

It is the duty of the sponsor to take an interest in the newcomer's progress, but *not to take responsibility for it* (Alibrandi, 1978; McCrady & Irvine, 1989). Each new AA member is expected to have daily contact with his/her sponsor either by telephone, or in person, at least at first (Nowinski, 1996). Despite frequent communications between the new member and his/her sponsor, the responsibility for recovery remains with the individual. In a sense, the sponsor says to the client: "I can be concerned for you, but I am not responsible for you." In today's terminology, the sponsor is a living example of what might be called "tough love." In a sense, the sponsor's role is similar to that of a skilled folk psychotherapist (Peck, 1993).

The sponsor should not try to control the newcomer's life, ideally should recognize his/her personal limitations, and should be the same sex as the new AA member being sponsored (McCrady & Delaney, 1995). The sponsor should also possess many, if not all, of the same characteristics of the healthy human services professional identified by Rogers (1961).

The sponsor, acting as an extension of AA, is a tool. But, while the sponsor is a tool, it is up to the newcomer to grasp and use this tool to achieve sobriety. There are no guarantees, and the sponsor often struggles with many of the same issues facing the newcomer. The newcomer must assume the responsibility for reaching out and using the tools that are offered. Sponsorship is, in essence, an expression of the mission of AA to "carry the message" to other addicts, who are still actively using chemicals. This is a reflection of Step Twelve, and one often hears a sponsor speak of having participated in a Twelfth Step visit, or of having been involved in Twelfth Step work. The sponsor is, in a sense, a guide, friend, peer counselor, fellow traveler, conscience, and devil's advocate, all rolled into one.

AA and Psychological Theory

The psychiatrist and popular writer M. Scott Peck (1993) advanced the theory that AA offers a form of folk psychology. But, the AA/ NA step programs are different from other therapeutic programs that the addict may have been exposed to, in the sense that the steps are "reports of action taken rather than rules not to be broken . . ." (Alibrandi, 1978, p. 166). Each step then is a public (or private) demonstration of action taken in the struggle to achieve and maintain sobriety, rather than a rule that might be broken.

Brown (1985) speaks of the Twelve Steps as also serving to keep recovering addicts focused on their addiction. For, just as the alcohol was an axis around which these individuals centered their lives while drinking, through the Twelve Steps addicts continue to center their lives around alcohol in a different

way: a lifestyle without chemicals. During the period of active chemical use, life centered around the drug of choice (Brown). To avoid the danger of being deceived, individuals need to learn a new way to openly relate to addiction that allows them to achieve and maintain sobriety. According to Brown, the Twelve Steps accomplish this with a structured program through which members can relate to their addiction while being able to draw on the group for support and strength.

How Does AA Work?

Although AA has been a social force in the United States for more than half a century, there has been surprisingly little research into what elements of the program are effective (Emrick, Tonigan, Montgomery, & Little, 1993). Charles Bufe (1988) offered three reasons he thought AA was effective "at least for some people" (p. 55). First, AA provides a social outlet for its members. "Loneliness," as Bufe observed, "is a terrible problem in our society, and people will flock to almost *anything* that relieves it—even AA meetings" (p. 55, italics in original).

Second, AA allows its members to recognize that their problems are not unique (Alibrandi, 1978; Bufe, 1988). Nace (1987) noted that AA participation helps the individual member to restore identity and self-esteem through the unconditional acceptance of its members, all of whom suffer from the same disease. In this way, each member of AA is able to discover a relatedness to others. Finally, AA can offer a proven path to follow, which can "look awfully attractive when your world has turned upside down and you no longer have your best friend—alcohol—to lean on" (Bufe, 1988, p. 55). Thus, the AA program offers the individual *hope* at a time when there seems to be nobody to turn to (Bean-Bayog, 1993). Although hope is an essential part of recovery, one must wonder if, as Bufe concluded, "These things, especially the first two, are all that is really needed" (p. 55). Bufe's view, while perhaps accurate, also appears to be rather limited. For AA seems to offer more than just a way to deal with loneliness, or a way of relating to others.

Herman (1988) observed that twelve-step programs such as AA offer at least one more feature to the recovering addict: *predictability*. Consistency was identified by Rogers (1961) as being a valuable characteristic in the helping relationship, and the predictability of AA may be one of the curative forces of this self-help group. However, this remains only a hypothesis.

The AA twelve-step program provides a format for "a planned spontaneous remission" (Berenson, 1987, p. 29) that is "designed so that a person can stop drinking by either education, therapeutic change, or transformation" (p. 30). As part of the therapeutic transformation inherent in AA participation, Berenson (1987) speculated that people would "bond to the group and use it as a social support and as a refuge to explore and release their suppressed and repressed feelings" (p. 30).

Alcoholics Anonymous meetings, as noted by Nace (1987) "are generally characterized by warmth, openness, honesty, and humor" (p. 242), attributes that may promote personal growth. AA is thought to be "the treatment of choice" (Berenson, 1987, p. 27) for active alcoholics, although Brodsky (1993) challenged this claim. Indeed, Brodsky noted that the twelve-step program advocated by AA is potentially "damaging, violative and ineffective" (p. 21) for many individuals. The author bases his criticism of the program on the assumption that, while it might be a useful tool for some, it is based on "a 19th century fundamentalist tradition" (p. 21) that is essentially conservative Protestant in nature. Such a program might, when forced on many people, prove more destructive than helpful, according to Brodsky.

Outcome Studies: The Effectiveness of AA

Many substance abuse rehabilitation professionals view AA as being the single most important component of a person's recovery program. At least one study found that AA participation was the *only* significant predictor of long-term recovery (McCaul & Furst, 1994). Nevertheless, AA is not without its critics (Brodsky, 1993; Marvel, 1995; Ogborne & Glaser, 1985; Uva, 1991). Virtually everything about AA has been challenged and/or defended. There are those who suggest that AA "should be used only as a supportive adjunct to treatment" (Lewis et al., 1988,

p. 151) and should not be considered as "treatment" of alcoholism by itself. At the same time, there are those who argue that AA and similar twelve-step programs have many similarities to a therapeutic program of change and thus should be viewed as a form of treatment (Tobin, 1992).

In light of the controversy that surrounds AA, there has been surprisingly little empirical research into its effectiveness (Watson et al., 1997), or for what types of people it might be most useful (Galanter, Castaneda, & Franco, 1991; George & Tucker, 1996; McCaul & Furst, 1994; Tonigan & Hiller-Sturmhofel, 1994). Questions have even been raised as to whether AA is necessary for every individual with an alcohol/drug use problem (Peele, 1989; Peele et al., 1991). However, even critics of AA seem to accept that it may be helpful at least to some, but not necessarily all, of those who have a problem with chemicals (Brodsky, 1993; Ogborne & Glaser, 1985).

It has been pointed out that those people who join and remain in AA are not a representative sample of alcoholics (Galanter et al., 1991). This is true because only certain people elect to join and remain in AA of their own free will. Thus, the membership of AA is different from those alcohol-dependent individuals who choose not to join AA, or those who join, but do not remain active members.[2]

As stated earlier, simple membership in AA is not a guarantee of recovery. *At least half* of newcomers to AA stop going to meetings within 3 months, and at the end of 1 year 95% of the new members will have dropped out (Dorsman, 1996). Even of those who remain in AA, there is a significant relapse rate. Only 70% of those who abstain from alcohol for 1 year will still be alcohol-free at the end of their 2nd year, while 90% of those who abstained from alcohol for 2 full years were still alcohol-free at the end of their 3rd year of AA participation. Thus, statistically, only 2% of those individuals who initially join AA will be alcohol-free at the end of 2 years (Dorsman).

In the past few years, a small number of studies have attempted to answer the question of whether AA is effective. Humphreys and Moos (1996) followed a

---

[2]Yet, as the reader will recall, it was on data obtained from members of AA that Jellinek (1960) based his model of alcoholism.

sample of 201 alcohol-dependent individuals, of whom 135 elected to join AA while the remainder chose professional outpatient counseling for their alcoholism. There were no significant differences between these two subgroups in terms of age, sex, or socioeconomic status, according to the authors. Research subjects were interviewed at the start of the research project and at the end of 1 and 3 years. The authors found that at the end of 3 years' time, the group that had entered into outpatient counseling had the same percentage of abstinent members as did those subjects who elected to join AA. The authors cautioned that their sample was self-selected, in that the clients themselves elected to either enter AA or professional outpatient counseling for their alcohol use problems. Thus, this study did not utilize a randomized assignment to treatment groups. However, despite this limitation, the authors concluded that "alcohol self-help organizations may promote positive outcomes in alcohol-dependent individuals and may also take a significant burden off the public and private health care sectors" (p. 712).

The team of Watson et al. (1997) followed a sample of 150 men, who had been treated on an inpatient basis at a Veterans Administration hospital for chemical dependency for 48 weeks. Subjects were grouped according to whether they had attended AA Frequently (9+ meetings), Moderately (5–8 meetings), Occasionally (1–4 meetings), or were Nonattenders (0 meetings) in the first 4 weeks since their discharge from treatment. The authors found a positive relationship between the number of meetings attended in the time following discharge from inpatient treatment and the abstinence rate from chemicals. The Frequent, Moderate, or Occasional AA participants were statistically more likely to remain abstinent from alcohol than Nonattenders. The findings of this study suggested that AA was of value in the rehabilitation of alcohol-dependent individuals.

One popular belief is that life stressors trigger increased alcohol use. In a study designed to identify the role of life stressors on alcohol use and abstinence, Humphreys, Moos, and Finney (1996) followed 439 problem drinkers for a 3-year period. The authors found that there was little evidence to suggest that stress *initiated* problem drinking among their sample. Rather, the authors found that alcohol use *predated the development of many stressors,*

which then set the stage for even more alcohol use by the individual. An unexpected finding of their study, however, was that the one factor that was most consistently involved in a reduction in alcohol intake was the individual's involvement in AA. The authors suggested that friendships made through AA would almost automatically be supportive of the individual's abstinence since members of AA are themselves working toward their own recovery. Further, AA provides its members with a range of social activities (dances, conventions, etc.) that are recovery oriented. Thus, AA involvement was the one factor that the authors found consistently predicted a reduction in alcohol use by the problem drinker.

While the results of these studies are suggestive, there still is insufficient evidence to conclude that AA is effective in the treatment of alcoholism (Hester, 1994; Holder et al., 1991). Even if future research proves that AA is an effective tool in the rehabilitation of the problem drinker, the majority of alcohol-dependent individuals never join an AA group (Bean-Bayog, 1993). This may be because AA "is not effective for *all* kinds of persons with alcohol problems" (Ogborne & Glaser, 1985, p. 188). At best, it would appear that AA is most effective with a subset of problem drinkers: those socially stable white males, over 40 years of age, who are physically dependent on alcohol, prone to guilt, and the firstborn or only child.

But this picture of the person who is most likely to benefit from AA membership is only the first preliminary effort to identify the "typical" AA member. The research data "is not currently developed enough to provide us with a composite profile of the most likely AA affiliates" (Emrick et al., 1993, p. 53). There are many members of AA who do not demonstrate the same characteristics of a successful member outlined by Ogborne and Glaser (1985). In 1991 it was estimated that fully 35% of the membership of AA was composed of women ("AA Survey," 1991). This is in direct contrast to the conclusion reached by Ogborne and Glaser that the person for whom AA was most effective was male. These conflicting studies underscore the need for more research in this area.

Although some would dispute this observation, AA does not seem to be effective with those who are coerced into attending AA by the courts (C. Clark, 1995; Glaser & Ogborne, 1982; Humphreys & Moos, 1996; Peele, 1989; Peele et al., 1991). Humphreys and Moos (1996) noted that the members of AA, and the very nature of the AA movement itself, might be adversely affected by the influx of large numbers of involuntary members who seek admission only because of marital, legal, and/or employment pressure. Further, there is evidence to suggest that those individuals who face legal consequences as a result of driving while intoxicated (i.e., were sent to jail or were placed on probation) seem to have better subsequent driving records (i.e., fewer accidents or further arrests) than those "sentenced" to treatment (Peele, 1989; Peele et al., 1991). For these reasons, it is suggested that clients not be coerced into attending AA.

Peele (1989) is critical of AA as it exists today, in part because there is so little research data that supports AA as an appropriate method of treatment for alcohol-addicted individuals. Many of the basic tenets of AA are not supported by research data. For example, consider the twin beliefs that: (a) alcoholism will *always* grow worse without treatment, and (b) that the individual cannot cut back or quit drinking on his/her own. Research (Peele, 1989; Vaillant, 1983) has shown just the opposite of this belief: alcoholics rarely follow the downward spiral thought to be inescapable by AA. Further, individuals with alcohol-use problems often control or discontinue drinking without formal intervention.

It has been suggested that the question of whether AA is effective is far too complex to be measured by a single research study (Glaser & Ogborne, 1982; Ogborne, 1993). The composition of AA ensures that there will be vast differences between different AA groups. Although they all share the same name, different AA groups do not offer a fixed form of treatment (Ogborne). There is a need for a series of well-controlled research studies to identify all the variables that might influence the outcome of AA participation (McCrady & Irvine, 1989).

It is likely that the very nature of the question "Is AA effective?" makes it unanswerable. For example, would the chronic alcoholic who, as a result of participation in AA, stopped drinking on a daily basis, but then began a pattern of binge drinking, be measured as a successful outcome or as a failure? Would the chronic alcoholic who entered AA, stopped drinking, but who died of alcohol-induced liver disease 6 weeks later, be a successful or unsuccessful outcome? These examples illustrate how difficult it is to generate a meaningful answer (Ogborne & Glaser, 1985). A more meaningful approach would be to attempt to identify which types of people are most likely to benefit from a twelve-step program such as that offered by AA.

Narcotics Anonymous

In 1953, a self-help group patterned after AA was founded that called itself "Narcotics Anonymous" (NA). Although this group honors its debt to Alcoholics Anonymous, the members of Narcotics Anonymous feel that:

> We follow the same path with only a single exception. Our identification as addicts is all-inclusive in respect to any mood-changing, mind-altering substance. "Alcoholism" is too limited a term for us; our problem is not a specific substance, it is a disease called "addiction." (*Narcotics Anonymous*, 1982, p. x)

To the members of NA, it is not the specific chemical that is the problem, but the common disease of addiction. Narcotics Anonymous emerged as a self-help group to help those whose only "common denominator is that we failed to come to terms with our addiction" (*Narcotics Anonymous*, 1982, p. x). On the other hand, many outsiders view the major difference between AA and NA as being one of emphasis. Alcoholics Anonymous addresses only alcoholism, while NA addresses addiction to chemicals in addition to alcohol.

The growth of NA has been phenomenal, with there being a 600% increase in the number of NA groups from 1983–1988 (P. Coleman, 1989), and there are more than 25,000 chapters of NA meetings in the United States (Humphreys, 1997). Alcoholics Anonymous and Narcotics Anonymous are not affiliated with each other, although there is an element of cooperation between AA and NA (M. Jordan, Personal Communication, February 27, 1989). Each follows essentially the same twelve-step program, which offers the addict a day-by-day program for recovery. This is understandable, since NA is essentially an outgrowth of

AA. The language of AA speaks of alcoholism, whereas NA speaks of "addiction" or "chemicals." Each offers the same program, with minor variations, to help the addicted person struggle to achieve sobriety.

The most important point is this: which group works best for the individual? Some people feel quite comfortable going to AA for their addiction to alcohol. Other people feel that NA offers them what they need to deal with their addiction. In the final analysis, the name of the group does not matter as much as its ability to offer the recovering person the support and understanding necessary to remain sober for today.

Al-Anon and Alateen

The book *Al-Anon's Twelve Steps and Twelve Traditions* provides a short history of Al-Anon in its introduction. According to this history, wives would often wait while their husbands were at the early AA meetings. As they waited, they would often talk over their problems. At some point, the decision was made to try applying the same Twelve Steps that their husbands had found so helpful to their own lives, and the group known as *Al-Anon* was born.

In the beginning, each isolated group made whatever changes it felt necessary in the Twelve Steps. By 1948, however, the wife of one of the cofounders of AA became involved in the growing organization, and in time a uniform family support program emerged. This program, known as the Al-Anon Family Group, borrowed and modified the AA Twelve Steps and Twelve Traditions to make them applicable to the needs of families of alcoholics. Although joining Al-Anon is the most common recommendation for spouses of alcohol-abusing individuals, there is limited research into its effectiveness (O'Farrell, 1995). Little is known about the characteristics of an effective Al-Anon group or the successful Al-Anon member. Thus, although Al-Anon is viewed as a resource for the spouse of the alcohol-abusing individual, its effectiveness is still not proven.

By 1957, in response to the recognition that teenagers presented special needs and concerns, Al-Anon itself gave birth to a modified group for teens known as *Alateen*. Alateen members follow the same Twelve Steps outlined in the Al-Anon program. The goal of the Alateen program, however, is to provide the opportunity for teenagers to come together to share their experiences, discuss current problems, learn how to cope more effectively with their various concerns, and to provide encouragement to each other (*Facts about Alateen*, 1969).

Through Alateen, teenagers learn that alcoholism is a disease and are helped to detach emotionally from the alcoholic's behavior, while still loving the individual. The goal of Alateen is also to help the individual learn that he/she did not "cause" the alcoholic to drink and to see that they can build a rewarding life despite the alcoholic's continued drinking (*Facts about Alateen*, 1969).

Support Groups Other than AA

Criticism has been aimed against the AA program for its emphasis on spiritual growth, its failure to empower women, or for its basic philosophy. Several new self-help groups have emerged since 1986 that offer alternatives to AA.

Rational Recovery (RR)

Rational Recovery was founded in 1986 ("Groups Offer Self-Help," 1991). Currently, it is estimated that RR has 600 groups around the United States (McCrady & Delaney, 1995). The program draws heavily on the cognitive-behavioral school of psychotherapy, and views alcoholism as reflecting negative, self-defeating thought patterns (Ouimette et al., 1997). Members are encouraged to stop drinking as a sign of self-respect, as opposed to drinking to feel good about themselves. Groups are advised by mental health professionals and strive to help the individual addict identify and correct self-defeating ways of viewing self and the world.

Gorski (1993) identified two general irrational thought groups that contribute to substance use. The first of these, termed *addictive thinking* (p. 26), was defined as the individual's use of irrational thoughts to support a claim that he/she has a "right" to use chemicals, and, that chemical use is not the cause of the problems facing the person. The second group of irrational thoughts used to support substance use were *relapse justifications* (p. 26), according to the author. These were specific thoughts used to justify the person's return to chemical use. "I can't cope with the stress without having a drink!" is an example of this kind of thinking. From a Rational Recovery perspective, the task of the group, and the individual, would be to learn more rational ways of looking at the individual's behavior, so that he/she would not continue to support substance use through such self-defeating thoughts.

In a comparison of the effectiveness of traditional twelve-step programs, and cognitive-behavioral (CB) treatment approaches, the team of Ouimette et al. (1997) discussed the results of a multicenter experiment involving 3018 patients who were being treated for substance use problems at one of 15 selected Veterans Administration hospitals in the United States. The subjects in this study were assigned to one of three treatment conditions: pure twelve-step treatment, pure CB treatment, or a mixed CB/twelve-step format. Participants in this study were interviewed after one year's time, to determine their employment and substance use status. The authors concluded that pure cognitive-behavioral and twelve-step programs were equally effective in helping people address substance use problems. This study thus supported treatment approaches such as RR for persons with substance use problems.

Secular Organizations of Sobriety (SOS)

This program was also founded in 1986 and currently it is estimated that there are approximately 1200 SOS groups meeting each week (Dorsman, 1996), with in excess of 100,000 members around the world (Marvel, 1995). SOS is a self-help group that emerged as a reaction to the heavy emphasis on spirituality found in AA and NA ("Groups Offer Self-Help," 1991). The guiding philosophy of SOS stresses personal responsibility and the role of critical thinking in recovery. Members also struggle to identify their own "cycle of addiction."

Women for Sobriety (WFS)

Women for Sobriety was founded in 1975 ("Groups Offer Self-Help," 1991). Approximately 325 WFS groups meet in the United States (McCrady & Delaney, 1995). It is an organization specifically for women and was founded on the theory that the AA program failed to address the very real differences between the meaning of alcoholism for men and women. There are 13 core statements, or beliefs, aimed at providing the member with a new perspective on herself. There is a great deal of emphasis on self-esteem and on building self-esteem for the member.

Alcoholics Anonymous for Atheists and Agnostics (Quad A)

This is a twelve-step program that draws heavily from traditional AA (Rand, 1995). However, Quad A, as the group is known, tends to downplay the emphasis on religion inherent in traditional AA and thus tends to be attractive to those individuals whose beliefs do not include the possibility of a Supreme Being. The Quad A format tends to place less emphasis on "letting go" of one's personal will and ego, features that make it attractive to many women (Rand). Further, in place of the emphasis on the "Power Greater than Ourselves" found in traditional AA meetings, Quad A tends to place stress on the forces in the individual's life that support recovery (Rand).

Quad A is mainly found in the Chicago area, where it has made a home for itself. There are an estimated 400 to 500 members at this time (Rand, 1995). While traditional AA meetings usually last about an hour, Quad A meetings may last for several hours, especially when members become involved in a heated discussion of a topic of interest to a number of those present. Only time will tell whether the Quad A format will spread across this country or will remain a local phenomenon. However, for those in the Chicago area, it offers an interesting alternative to traditional AA meetings.

Moderation Management (MM)

The Moderation Management program has been controversial since its inception. The program resulted from the frustration of its founder with traditional alcohol rehabilitation programs. The founder of MM is Shirley Kishline. Her addiction to alcohol was apparently never firmly established, and she had trouble using abstinence-based programs such as AA in her struggle against excessive drinking. In time, Ms. Kishline came to accept *moderation* as a more appropriate goal than abstinence (Kishline,

1996). Her justification for this decision is that she was a "problem drinker" (p. 53), as opposed to an alcoholic.

Ms. Kishline defines a "problem drinker" as a person who consumes no more than 35 drinks per week and who has experienced only mild to moderate alcohol-related problems (Kishline, 1996). In contrast, chronic drinkers are viewed by MM as persons who will, in the majority of cases, experience severe withdrawal symptoms when they stop drinking, and whose drinking has resulted in serious social, financial, personal, vocational, legal, or medical consequences.

The goal of MM is to "provide a supportive environment in which people who have made the decision to reduce their drinking can come together to help each other change" (p. 55).

The MM concept rests on a foundation of behavior modification techniques used by professionals to help individuals learn how to change their behavior. While the founder has apparently identified an underserved population, there is a potential danger inherent in the MM concept (Resler, 1994). The danger is that members with actual alcohol dependence problems will use the group as an excuse to continue to try and achieve "controlled" drinking (discussed in Chapter 30).

However, MM group leaders strive to complete an *accurate* assessment of the individual, his/her alcohol use history, emotional resources, and motivation for membership. The individual's progress is monitored, and if he/she should prove unable to return to a moderate pattern of alcohol use, a traditional self-help group such as AA, or a formal treatment program for substance abuse, is recommended for the member.

Summary

The self-help group Alcoholics Anonymous (AA) has emerged as one of the predominant forces in the field of drug abuse treatment. Drawing on the experience and knowledge of its members, AA has developed a program for living that is spiritual without being religious, confrontive without using confrontation in the traditional sense of the word, which relies on no outside support, and which many of its members believe is effective in helping them stay sober on a daily basis.

The program for living established by AA is based on those factors that early members believed were important to their own sobriety. This program for living is known as the Twelve Steps. The Steps are suggested as a guide to new members. Emphasis is placed on the equality of all members, and there is no board of directors within the AA group.

Whether or not AA is effective is a continuing question. Researchers agree that it seems to be effective for some people, but not for all those who join. How to measure the effectiveness of AA is a complex problem. A series of well-designed research projects is required to identify the multitude of variables involved in making AA effective for some people.

Despite these unanswered questions, however, AA has served as a model for many other self-help groups, including Narcotics Anonymous (NA). A central tenet of Narcotics Anonymous is that the alcohol focus of AA is too narrow for persons who have become addicted to other chemicals, either alone or in combination with alcohol. Narcotics Anonymous expounds the belief that addiction is a common disease that may express itself through many different forms of drug dependency. NA has established a twelve-step program based on the Twelve Steps of Alcoholics Anonymous and draws heavily from its parent. But, NA seeks to reach out to those whose addiction involves chemicals other than alcohol.

Other self-help groups that have emerged from the AA experience include Al-Anon and Alateen. Al-Anon emerged from informal encounters between the spouses of early AA members and strives to provide an avenue for helping the families of those who are addicted to alcohol. Alateen emerged from Al-Anon, in response to the recognition that adolescents have special needs. Both groups strive to help members learn how to be supportive, without being dependent on, the alcoholic, and how to detach from the alcoholic and his/her behavior.

Sample Assessment:
Alcohol Abuse Situation[1]

HISTORY AND IDENTIFYING INFORMATION

Mr John D_____ is a 35-year-old married white male, from _____ county, Missouri. He is employed as an electrical engineer for the X X X X company, where he has worked for the past three years. Prior to this, Mr. D_____ was in the United States Navy, where he served for four years. He was discharged under Honorable conditions, and reported that he only had "a few" minor rules infractions. He was never brought before a court-martial, according to Mr. D_____.

CIRCUMSTANCES OF REFERRAL

Mr. D_____ was seen after having been arrested for the charge of driving while under the influence of alcohol. Mr. D_____ reported that he had been drinking with co-workers, to celebrate a promotion at work. His measured blood alcohol level (or BAL) was .150, well above the legal limit necessary for a charge of driving while under the influence. Mr. D_____ reported that he had "seven or eight" mixed drinks in approximately a 2-hour time span. By his report, he was arrested within a quarter hour of the time that he left the bar. After his initial court appearance, Mr. D_____ was referred to this evaluator by the court, to determine whether or not Mr. D_____ has a chemical dependency problem.

1

DRUG AND ALCOHOL USE HISTORY

Mr. D_____ reports that he first began to drink at the age of 15, when he and a friend would steal beer from his father's supply in the basement. He would drink an occasional beer from time to time after that, and first became intoxicated when he was 17, by Mr. D_____'s report.

When he was 18, Mr. D_____ enlisted in the United States Navy, and after basic training he was stationed in the San Diago area. Mr. D_____ reported that he was first exposed to chemicals while he was stationed in San Diago, and that he tried both marijuana and cocaine while on weekend liberty. Mr. D_____ reported that he did not like the effects of cocaine, and that he only used this chemical once or twice. He did like the effects of marijuana and reported that he would smoke one or two marijuana cigarettes obtained from friends perhaps once a month.

During this portion of this life, Mr. D_____ reports that he would drink about twice a weekend, when on liberty. The amount that he would drink ranged from "one or two beers" on through to twelve or eighteen beers. Mr. D_____ reported that he first had an alcohol-related blackout while he was in the Navy, and reported that he "should" have been arrested for driving on base while under the influence of alcohol on several different occasions, but was never stopped by the Shore Patrol.

Following his discharge from the Navy under Honorable Conditions at the age of 22, Mr. D_____ enrolled in college. His chemical use declined to the weekend use of alcohol, usually in moderation, but Mr. D_____ reported that he did drink to the point of an alcohol-related blackout "once or twice" in the 4 years that he was in college. There was no other chemical use following his discharge from the Navy, and Mr. D_____ reports that he has not used other chemicals since the age of 20 or 21.

After graduation, at the age of 26, Mr. D_____ began to work for the X X X X X Company, where he is employed now. He met his wife shortly after he began work for the X X X X X Company, and they were married after a courtship of 1 year. Mr. D_____'s wife, Pat, does not use chemicals other than an "occasional" social drink. Exploration of this revealed that Mrs. D_____ will drink a glass of wine with a meal about twice a month. She denied other chemical use.

Mrs. D_____ reported that her husband does not usually drink more than one or two beers, and that he will drink only on weekends. She reported that the night when he was arrested was "unusual" for him, in the sense that he is not a drinker. His employer was not contacted, but court records failed to reveal any other arrest records for Mr. D_____.

Mr. D_____ admitted to several alcohol-related blackouts, but none since he was in college. He denied seizures, DTs or alcohol-related tremor. There was no evidence of ulcers, gastritis, or cardiac problems noted. His last physical was "normal" according to information provided by his personal physician. There were no abnormal blood chemistry findings, nor did his physician find any evidence suggesting alcoholism. Mr. D_____ denied having ever been hospitalized for an alcohol-related injury, and there was no evidence suggesting that he has been involved in fights.

On the Michigan Alcoholism Screening Test (MAST), Mr. D_____'s score of four (4) points would not suggest alcoholism. This information was reviewed in the presence of his wife, who did not suggest that there was any misrepresentation on his test scores. On this administration of the MMPI, there was no evidence of psychopathology noted. Mr. D_____'s MacAndrew Alcoholism Scale score fell in the normal range, failing to suggest an addictive disorder at this time.

PSYCHIATRIC HISTORY

Mr. D_____ denied psychiatric treatment of any kind. He did admit to having seen a marriage counselor "once" shortly after he married, but reported that overall he and his wife are happy together. Apparently, they had a question about a marital communications issue that was cleared up after one visit, which took place after three or four years of marriage.

SUMMARY AND CONCLUSIONS

There is little evidence to suggest an ongoing alcohol problem. Mr. D_____ would seem to be a well-adjusted young man, who drank to the point of excess after having been offered a long-desired promotion at work. This would seem to be an unusual occurrence for Mr. D_____, who usually limits his drinking to one or two beers on the weekends. There was no evidence of alcohol-related injuries, accidents, or legal problems noted.

RECOMMENDATIONS

Recommend light sentence, possibly a fine, limited probation, with no restrictions on license. It is also recommended that Mr. D_____ attend "DWI School" for 8 weeks, to learn more about the effects of alcohol on driving.

Sample Assessment:
Chemical Dependency Situation[1]

HISTORY AND IDENTIFYING FEATURES

Mr. Michael S_____ is a 35-year-old divorced white male, who is self-employed. He has been a resident of _____ County, Kansas, for the past 3 months. Prior to this, he apparently was living in _____ County, New York, according to information provided by Mr. S_____. On the night of June 6 of this year, Mr. S_____ was arrested for the charge of possession of a Controlled Substance. In specific, Mr. S_____ was found to be in possession of two grams of cocaine, according to police records. This is his first arrest for a drug-related charge in Kansas, although by history he has been arrested on two other occasions for similar charges, in New York State. A copy of his police record is attached to this report.

CIRCUMSTANCES OF REFERRAL

Mr. Michael S_____ was referred to the undersigned for a chemical dependency evaluation, which will be part of his presentence investigation (or, PSI) for the charge of Felony Possession of a Controlled Substance, and the charge of Sale of a Controlled Substance.

DRUG AND ALCOHOL USE HISTORY

Mr. S_____ reported that he began to use alcohol when he was 13 years of age, and that by the age of 14 he was drinking on

1

---

[1] This case is entirely fictitious. Any similarity between the person in this report, and any person living or dead, is entirely coincidental.

a regular basis. Exploration of this revealed that, by the time just prior to his 15th birthday, Mr. S_____ was drinking on "weekends" with friends. He reported that he first became intoxicated on his 15th birthday, but projected responsibility for this on to his friends, who by his report "kept on pouring more and more into the glass until I was drunk."

By the age of 16, Mr. S_____ was using alcohol "four or five nights a week," and was also using marijuana and hallucinogenics perhaps two or three times a week. He projected responsibility for his expanded chemical use onto his environment, noting that "everybody was selling the stuff, you couldn't walk down the street without people stopping you to ask if you wanted to buy some."

Also, by the age of 16, Mr. S_____ was supporting his chemical use through burglaries, which he committed with his friends. He was never caught, but volunteered this information explaining to the undersigned that since the statute of limitations has expired, he does not have to fear being charged for these crimes, anymore.

By the age of 21, Mr. S_____ was using cocaine "once or twice a week." He was arrested for the first time when he was about 22, for possession of cocaine. This was when he was living in the state of _____. After being tried in court, he was convicted of Felony Possession of Cocaine, and placed on probation for five years. When asked if he used chemicals while he was on probation, Mr. S_____ responded that "I don't have to answer that."

Mr. S_____ reported that he first entered treatment for chemical dependency when he was 27 years of age. At that time, he was found to be addicted to a number of drugs, including alcohol, cocaine, and "downers." Although in treatment for two months, at the chemical dependency unit of _____ Hospital, Mr. S_____ reported that "I left as addicted as when I arrived" and reported with some degree of apparent pride that he had found a way to use chemicals even while in treatment. His chemical use apparently was the reason for his ultimate discharge from this program. While Mr. S_____ was somewhat vague about why he was discharged, he did report that "they did not like how I was doing" while he was in treatment.

Since that time, Mr. S_____ has been using cocaine, alcohol, various drugs obtained from a series of physicians, and

2

opiates. Mr. S_____ was quite vague as to how he supported his chemical use, but noted that "there are ways of getting money, if you really want some."

In the past year, Mr. S_____ reported that he has been using cocaine "four or five times a week," although on occasion he did admit to having used cocaine "for a whole week straight." He has been sharing needles with other cocaine users from time to time, but reported that "I am careful." Despite this, however, he was diagnosed as having hepatitis B in the last year, according to Mr. S_____ . He also reported that he has overdosed on cocaine "once or twice," but that he treated this overdose himself with benzodiazepines and alcohol.

In addition to the possible cocaine overdoses noted above, Mr. S_____ admitted to having experienced chest pain while using cocaine on at least two occasions, and has used alcohol or tranquilizers to combat the side effects of cocaine on a regular basis. He has admitted to frequently using tranquilizers or alcohol to help him sleep after using cocaine for extended periods of time. He also admits to having spent money on drugs that was meant for other expenses (loan payments, etc.) and by his report has had at least one automobile repossessed for failure to make payments on the loan.

Mr. S_____ has been unemployed for at least the past 2 years, but is rather vague as to how he supports himself. He apparently was engaged in selling cocaine at the time of his arrest, this being one of the charges brought against him by the police.

Mr. S_____ had not seen a physician for several years, prior to this arrest. During this interview, however, it was noted that he had scars strongly suggestive of intravenous needle use on both arms. When asked about these marks, he referred to them as "tracks," a street term for drug needle scars. This would suggest long-term intravenous drug use on Mr. S_____'s part. He denied the intravenous use of opiates, but a urine toxicology screen detected narcotics. This would suggest that Mr. S_____ has not been very open about his narcotic drug use.

On his administration of the Michigan Alcoholism Screening Test (MAST) Mr. S_____ achieved a score of 17 points, which is strongly suggestive of alcoholism. He reported that "hours" represents the longest period he has been able to go without using chemicals in the past five years. His profile on this administration

3

of the Minnesota Multiphasic Personality Inventory (MMPI) was suggestive of a very impulsive, immature individual, who is likely to have a chemical dependency problem.

PSYCHIATRIC HISTORY

Mr. S_____ reported that he has been hospitalized for psychiatric reasons only "once." This hospitalization took place several years ago, while Mr. S_____ was living in the state of X X X X X. Apparently, he was hospitalized for observation following a suicide attempt in which he slit his wrists with a razor blade. Mr. S_____ was unable to recall whether he had been using cocaine prior to this suicide attempt, but thought that it was "quite possible" that he had experienced a cocaine-induced depression.

MEDICAL HISTORY

As noted, Mr. S_____ had not seen a physician for several years prior to his arrest. Since the time of his arrest, however, he has been examined by a physician for a cough that he has had for some time. The physician (report enclosed) concluded that Mr. S_____ is "seropositive" for HIV, and classified Mr. S_____ as falling into category CDC_1. While it is not possible to determine whether Mr. S_____ contracted HIV through sharing needles, this is at least a possibility.

SUMMARY AND CONCLUSIONS

Overall, it is apparent that Mr. S_____ has a long-standing chemical dependency problem. Despite his evasiveness and denial, there was strong evidence of significant chemical dependency problems. Mr. S_____ seems to support his drug and alcohol use through criminal activity, although he is rather vague about this. He has been convicted of drug-related charges in the state of XXXXX, and was on probation following this conviction. One might suspect that Mr. S_____'s motivation for treatment is quite low at this time, as he has expressed the belief that his attorney will "make a deal for me" where he will not have to spend time in prison.

RECOMMENDATIONS

1. Given the fact that Mr. S_____ has contracted HIV and hepatitis B from infected needles, it is strongly recommended

that he be referred to the appropriate medical facility for treatment.

    2. It is the opinion of this reviewer that Mr. S_____'s motivation for treatment is low at this time. If he is referred to treatment, it is recommended that this be made part of his sentencing agreement with the court. If he is incarcerated, chemical dependency treatment might be made part of his treatment plan in prison.

    3. Referral to a therapeutic community should be considered for Mr. S_____, for long-term residential treatment.

Signed /s/

References

AASE, J. M. (1994). Clinical recognition of FAS. *Alcohol Health & Research World, 18*(1), 5–9.

AASE, J. M., JONES, K. L., & CLARREN, S. K. (1995). Do we need the term "FAE"? *Pediatrics, 95,* 428–430.

AA SURVEY FINDINGS RELEASED. (1991). *The Alcoholism Report, 19*(7), 8–10.

ABBOTT, A., & CONCAR, D. (1992). A trip into the unknown. *New Scientist, 135,* 30–34.

ABBOTT, P. J., QUINN, D., & KNOX, L. (1995). Ambulatory medical detoxification for alcohol. *American Journal of Drug and Alcohol Abuse, 21,* 549–564.

ABEL, E. L. (1982). *Drugs and behavior: A primer in neuropsychopharmacology.* Malabar, FL: Krieger.

ABOLNIK, I. Z., & COREY, G. R. (1995). Pinning down infectious endocarditis. *Emergency Physician, 27*(8), 85–90.

ABOOD, M. E., & MARTIN, B. R. (1992). Neurobiology of marijuana abuse. *Trends in Pharmacological Sciences, 13*(5), 201–206.

ABRAMS, R. C., & ALEXOPOULOS, G. (1987). Substance abuse in the elderly: Alcohol and prescription drugs. *Hospital and Community Psychiatry, 38,* 1285–1288.

ABT ASSOCIATES, INC. (1995a). *What America's user's spend on illegal drugs, 1988–1993.* Washington, DC: Office of National Drug Control Policy.

ABT ASSOCIATES, INC. (1995b). *Pulse check.* Washington, DC: Office of National Drug Control Policy.

A CALL FOR NEW CURBS ON TEENS. (1993). *U.S. News & World Report, 114*(10), 15.

ACHORD, J. L. (1995). Alcohol and the liver. *Scientific American Science & Medicine, 2*(2), 16–27.

ACKERMAN, R. J. (1983). *Children of alcoholics: A guidebook for educators, therapists, and parents.* Holmes Beach, FL: Learning Publications.

ADAMS, J. K. (1988). Setting free chemical dependency. *Alcoholism & Addiction, 8*(4), 20–21.

ADAMS, W. L., YUAN, Z., BARBORIAK, J. J., & RIMM, A. A. (1993). Alcohol-related hospitalizations of elderly people. *Journal of the American Medical Association, 270,* 1222–1225.

ADDICTION—PART I. (1992a). *The Harvard Mental Health Letter, 9*(4), 1–4.

ADDICTION—PART II. (1992b). *The Harvard Mental Health Letter, 9*(5), 1–4.

ADELMAN, S. A., & WEISS, R. D. (1989). What is therapeutic about inpatient alcoholism treatment? *Hospital and Community Psychiatry, 40*(5), 515–519.

ADGER, H., & WERNER, M. J. (1994). The pediatrician. *Alcohol Health & Research World, 18,* 121–126.

AIDS AND MENTAL HEALTH—PART I. (1994). *The Harvard Mental Health Letter, 10*(7), 1–4.

AL-ANON'S TWELVE STEPS & TWELVE TRADITIONS. (1985). New York: Al-Anon Family Group Headquarters.

ALBERTSON, T. E., WALBY, W. F., & DERLET, R. (1995). Stimulant-induced pulmonary toxicity. *Chest, 108,* 1140–1150.

ALCOHOL ALERT. (1993a). Alcohol and the liver. Washington, DC: National Institute on Alcohol Abuse and Alcoholism.

ALCOHOL ALERT. (1993b). Alcohol and cancer. Washington, DC: National Institute on Alcohol Abuse and Alcoholism.

ALCOHOL ALERT. (1993c). Alcohol and nutrition. Washington, DC: National Institute on Alcohol Abuse and Alcoholism.

ALCOHOL ALERT. (1994a). Alcohol-related Impairment. Washington, DC: National Institute on Alcohol Abuse and Alcoholism.

ALCOHOL ALERT. (1994b). Alcohol and hormones. Washington, DC: National Institute on Alcohol Abuse and Alcoholism.

ALCOHOL ALERT. (1995). Alcohol-medication interactions. Washington, DC: National Institute on Alcohol Abuse and Alcoholism.

ALCOHOL ALERT. (1996). Drinking and Driving. Washington, DC: National Institute on Alcohol Abuse and Alcoholism.

ALCOHOLICS ANONYMOUS. (1976). New York: Alcoholics Anonymous Worlds Services.

ALEMI, F., STEPHENS, R. C., LLORENS, S., & ORRIS, B. (1995). A review of factors affecting treatment outcomes: Expected treatment outcome scale. *American Journal of Drug and Alcohol Abuse, 21,* 483–510.

ALEXANDER, B. (1991). Alcohol abuse in adolescents. *American Family Physician, 43*(2), 527–532.

ALEXANDER, D. E., & GWYTHER, R. E. (1995). Alcoholism in adolescents and their families. *Pediatric Clinics of North America, 42,* 217–234.

ALEXANDER, M. J. (1996). Women with occurring addictive and mental disorders. *American Journal of Orthopsychiatry, 66,* 61–70.

ALIBRANDI, L. A. (1978). The folk psychotherapy of Alcoholics Anonymous. In S. Zimberg, J. Wallace, & S. Blume (Eds.), *Practical approaches to alcoholism psychotherapy.* New York: Plenum Press.

ALLEN, M. G., & PHILLIPS, K. L. (1993). Utilization review of treatment for chemical dependence. *Hospital and Community Psychiatry, 44,* 752–756.

ALLISON, M. C., HOWATSON, A. G., TORRANCE, C. J., LEE, F. D., & RUSSELL, R. I. (1992). Gastrointestinal damage associated with the use of nonsteroidal anti-inflammatory drugs. *New England Journal of Medicine, 327,* 749–754.

ALTERMAN, A. I., ERDLEN, D. I., LaPORTE, D. J., & ERDLEN, F. R. (1982). Effects of illicit drug use in an inpatient psychiatric population. *Addictive Behaviors, 7,* 231–242.

ALUM MAY MASK METHAMPHETAMINE ABUSE. (1996). *Forensic Drug Abuse Advisor, 8*(3), 27.

AMARO, H. (1995). Love, sex and power. *American Psychologist, 50,* 437–447.

AMERICAN ACADEMY OF FAMILY PHYSICIANS. (1989). Screening for alcohol and other drug abuse. *American Family Physician, 40*(1), 137–147.

AMERICAN ACADEMY OF FAMILY PHYSICIANS. (1990a). Marijuana use and memory loss. *American Family Physician, 41*(3), 930–932.

AMERICAN ACADEMY OF FAMILY PHYSICIANS. (1990b). Effects of fetal exposure to cocaine and heroin. *American Family Physician, 41*(5), 1595–1597.

AMERICAN CANCER SOCIETY. (1990). Data bank. *Breakthroughs, 1*(2), 12.

AMERICAN MEDICAL ASSOCIATION. (1992). Costs from drug abuse doubled since 1986. *American Medical News, 35*(30). 37.

AMERICAN MEDICAL ASSOCIATION. (1993a). *Factors contributing to the health care cost problem.* Chicago: American Medical Association.

AMERICAN MEDICAL ASSOCIATION. (1993b). Injury prevention must be part of nation's plan to reduce health costs, say control experts. *Journal of the American Medical Association, 270,* 19–20.

AMERICAN MEDICAL ASSOCIATION. (1994). *Drug Evaluations Annual 1994.* Washington, DC: Author.

AMERICAN PSYCHIATRIC ASSOCIATION. (1990). *Benzodiazepine dependence, toxicity, and abuse.* Washington, DC: Author.

AMERICAN PSYCHIATRIC ASSOCIATION. (1994). *Diagnostic and statistical manual of mental disorders* (4th ed.). Washington, DC: Author.

AMERICAN PSYCHIATRIC ASSOCIATION. (1995). Practice guidelines for the treatment of patients with substance use disorders: Alcohol, cocaine, opioids. *American Journal of Psychiatry, 152*(11) (Suppl.).

AMERICAN PSYCHIATRIC ASSOCIATION. (1996). Practice guidelines for the treatment of patients with nicotine dependence. *American Journal of Psychiatry, 153*(10) (Suppl.).

AMERICAN SOCIETY OF HOSPITAL PHARMACISTS. (1994). *AHFS drug information.* Bethesda, MD: Author.

AMES, D., WIRSHING, W. C., & FRIEDMAN, R. (1993). Ecstasy, the serotonin syndrome, and neuroleptic malignant syndrome—a possible link? *Journal of the American Medical Association, 269,* 869–870.

AMPHETAMINES. (1990). *The Harvard Medical School Mental Health Letter, 6*(10), 1–4.

ANAND, K. J. S., & ARNOLD, J. H. (1994). Opioid tolerance and dependence in infants and children. *Critical Care Medicine, 22,* 334–342.

ANANTH, J., VANDEWATER, S., KAMAL, M., BRODSKY, A., GAMAL, R., & MILLER, M. (1989).Missed diagnosis of substance abuse in psychiatric patients. *Hospital & Community Psychiatry, 40,* 297–299.

ANASTOS, K., DENENBERG, R., & SOLOMON, L. (1997). Human immunodeficiency virus infection in women. *Medical Clinics of North America, 81,* 533–553.

ANDERSON, D. J. (1989a). Inhalant abusers risk death, permanent injury. *Minneapolis Star-Tribune, VIII*(165), 4EX.

ANDERSON, D. J. (1989b). An alcoholic is never too old for treatment. *Minneapolis Star-Tribune, VIII*(200), 7EX.

ANDERSON, D. J. (1991). Alcohol abuse takes a toll in head injuries. *Minneapolis Star-Tribune, X*(152), 7E.

ANDERSON, D. J. (1993). Chemically dependent women still face barriers. *Minneapolis Star-Tribune, XII*(65), 8E.

ANDERSON, D. J. (1995). Adult children of alcoholics must deal with anger. *Minneapolis Star-Tribune, XIII*(274), 4EX.

ANDERSON, R. (1993). AIDS: Trends, predictions, controversy. *Nature, 363,* 393–394.

ANDERSON, R. M., & MAY, R. M. (1992). Understanding the AIDS pandemic. *Scientific American, 266*(5), 58–66.

A NEW MARKET FOR A LETHAL DRUG. (1991). *Newsweek, CXVII*(7), 58.

ANGELL, M., & KASSIRER, J. P. (1994). Alcohol and other drugs—toward a more rational and consistent policy. *The New England Journal of Medicine, 331*, 537–539.

ANGIER, N. (1990). Storming the wall. *Discover, 11*(5), 67–72.

ANKER, A. L., & SMILKSTEIN, M. J. (1994). Acetaminophen. *Emergency Medical Clinics of North America, 12*, 335–349.

ANNIS, H. M., & DAVIS, C. S. (1991). Relapse prevention. *Alcohol Health & Research World, 15*(3), 204–212.

ANSEVICS, N. L., & DOWEIKO, H. E. (1983). A conceptual framework for intervention with the antisocial personality. *Psychotherapy in Private Practice, 1*(3), 43–52.

ANTHONY, J. C., ARRIA, A. M., & JOHNSON, E. O. (1995). Epidemiological and public health issues for tobacco, alcohol, and other drugs. In J. M. Oldham & M. B. Riba (Eds.), *Review of psychiatry* (Vol. 14). Washington: American Psychiatric Press.

ANTON, R. F. (1994). Medications for treating alcoholism. *Alcohol Health & Research World, 18*, 265–271.

APPELBAUM, P. S. (1992). Controlling prescription of benzodiazepines. *Hospital & Community Psychiatry, 43*, 12–13.

ARDEN, H. (1994). *Noble red man.* Hillsboro, OR: Beyond Words.

ARONOFF, G. M., WAGNER, J. M., & SPANGLER, A. S. (1986). Chemical interventions for pain. *Journal of Consulting and Clinical Psychology, 54*, 769–775.

ASHTON, H. (1992). *Brain function and psychotropic drugs.* New York: Oxford University Press.

ASHTON, H. (1994). Guidelines for the rational use of benzodiazepines. *Drugs, 48*(1), 25–40.

ASIATIC AMPHETAMINE ABUSE: STROKES, INFARCTS, AGITATED DELIRIUM, AND POSTMORTEM LEVELS. (1994). *Forensic Drug Abuse Advisor, 6*(8), 60–62.

ASPIRIN FOR PREVENTION OF MYOCARDIAL INFARCTION AND STROKE. (1989). *The Medical Letter, 31*(799), 77–79.

ASPIRIN IN THE PREVENTION OF CARDIOVASCULAR DISEASE. (1989). *Psychiatry Drug Alerts, III*(8), 64.

ASPIRIN REDUCES THE RISK OF HEART ATTACK—THE PHYSICIAN'S HEALTH STUDY DATA. (1989). *Internal Medicine Alert, 11* (15), 57–58.

ASSEO, L. (1993). Drug war clogs system, ABA says. *St. Paul Pioneer Press, 144*(287), 2A

ASSOCIATED PRESS. (1992). Women smoker deaths are expected to double. *St. Paul Pioneer Press, 143*(341), 12A.

ASSOCIATED PRESS. (1993). Drug dealers find new prey—the deaf. *San Francisco Examiner, 128*(21), B-7.

ASSOCIATED PRESS. (1994a). About 2.2 million children smoke, heart group says. *Minneapolis Star-Tribune, XII*(212), 2A

ASSOCIATED PRESS. (1994b). Spraying away the cigarette craving? *Minneapolis Star-Tribune, XIII*(120), 5A, 6A.

ASTHMA DEATHS BLAMED ON COCAINE USE. (1997). *Forensic Drug Abuse Advisor, 9*(2), 14.

ASTRACHAN, B. M., & TISCHLER, G. L. (1984). Normality from a health systems perspective. In D. Offer & M. Sabshin (Eds.), *Normality and the life cycle.* New York: Basic Books.

ATKINSON, I. H., & GRANT, I. (1994). Natural history of neuropsychiatric manifestations of HIV disease. *Psychiatric Clinics of North America, 17*, 17–33.

AUSABEL, D. P. (1983). Methadone maintenance treatment: The other side of the coin. *International Journal of the Addictions, 18*, 851–862.

AVANTS, S. K., MARGOLIN, P., CHANG, T. R., & BIRCH, S. (1995). Acupuncture for the treatment of cocaine addiction: Investigation of a needle puncture control. *Journal of Substance Abuse Treatment, 12*, 195–205.

AYD, F. J. (1994). Prescribing anxiolytics and hypnotics for the elderly. *Psychiatric Annals, 24*(2), 91–97.

AYD, F. J., JANICAK, P. G., DAVIS, J. M., & PRESKORN, S. H. (1996). Advances in the pharmacotherapy of anxiety and sleep disorders. *Principles and Practice of Psychopharmacotherapy, 1*(4), 1–22.

AZUMA, S. D., & CHASNOFF, I. J. (1993). Outcome of children prenatally exposed to cocaine and other drugs: A path analysis of three year data. *Pediatrics, 92*, 396–402.

BABERG, H. T., NELESEN, R. A., & DIMSDALE, J. E. (1996). Amphetamine use: Return of an old scourge in a consultation psychiatry setting. *American Journal of Psychiatry, 153*, 789–793.

BAGATELL, C. J., & BREMNER, W. J. (1996). Androgens in men—uses and abuses. *New England Journal of Medicine, 334*, 707–714.

BAHRKE, M. S. (1990). *Psychological research, methodological problems, and relevant issues.* Paper presented at the 1990 meeting of the American Psychological Association, Boston.

BALD IS NOT BEAUTIFUL, THALLIUM FOUND IN FRENCH HEROIN. (1996). *Forensic Drug Abuse Advisor, 8*(5), 35–36.

BALES, J. (1988). Legalized drugs: Idea flawed, debate healthy. *APA Monitor, 19*(8), 22.

BALLENGER, J. C. (1995). Benzodiazepines. In A. F. Schatzberg & C. B. Nemeroff (Eds.), *Textbook of psychopharmacology.* Washington, DC: American Psychiatric Association.

BANERJEE, S. (1990). Newest wrinkle for smokers is on their faces. *Minneapolis Star-Tribune, VIII* (341), 1EX, 5EX.

BARDEN, J. C. (1991). In depth. *Minneapolis Star-Tribune, X*(153), 4A, 6A.

BARKER, D. (1994). Reasons for tobacco use and symptoms of nicotine withdrawal among adolescent and young adult tobacco users—United States, 1993. *Journal of the American Medical Association, 272*, 1648–1649.

BARNHILL, J. G., CIRAULO, A. M., CIRAULO, D. A., & GREENE, J. A. (1995). Interactions of importance in chemical dependence. In D. A. Ciraulo, R. I. Shader, D. J. Greenblatt, & W. Creelman (Eds.), *Drug interactions in psychiatry* (2nd ed.). New York: Williams & Wilkins.

BARR, W. G., & MERCHUT, M. P. (1992). Systemic lupus erythematosus with central nervous system involvement. *The Psychiatric Clinics of North America, 15,* 439–454.

BARRERA, S. E., OSINSKI, W. A., & DAVIDOFF, E. (1949/1994). The use of Antabuse (tetraethylthiuramdisulphide) in chronic alcoholics. *American Journal of Psychiatry, 151,* 263–267.

BARRE-SINOUSSI, F. (1996). HIV as the cause of AIDS. *Lancet, 348,* 31–35.

BARTECCHI, C. E., MacKENZIE, T. D., & SCHRIER, R. W. (1994). The human costs of tobacco use. *New England Journal of Medicine, 330,* 907–912.

BAUGHAN, D. M. (1995). Barriers to diagnosing anxiety disorder in family practice. *American Family Physician, 52*(2), 447–450.

BAUGHMAN, R. D. (1993). Psoriasis and cigarettes. *Archives of Dermatology, 129,*1329–1330.

BAUMAN, J. L. (1988). Acute heroin withdrawal. *Hospital Therapy, 13,* 60–66.

BAUMAN, K. E., & ENNETT, S. T. (1994). Peer influence on adolescent drug use. *American Psychologist, 63,* 820–822.

BAYS, J. (1990). Substance abuse and child abuse. *Pediatric Clinics of North America, 37,* 881–903.

BAYS, J. (1992). The care of alcohol and drug-affected infants. *Pediatric Annals, 21*(8), 485–495.

BEAN-BAYOG, M. (1988). Alcohol and drug abuse: Alcoholism as a cause of psychopathology. *Hospital and Community Psychiatry, 39,* 352–354.

BEAN-BAYOG, M. (1993). AA processes and change: How does it work? In B. S. McCrady & W. R. Miller (Eds.), *Research on Alcoholics Anonymous.* New Brunswick, NJ: Rutgers Center of Alcohol Studies.

BEARDSLEY, T. (1994). The lucky ones. *Scientific American, 270*(5), 20, 24, 28.

BEASLEY, J. D. (1987). *Wrong diagnosis, wrong treatment: The plight of the alcoholic in America.* New York: Creative Infomatics.

BEATTIE, M. (1987). *Codependent no more.* New York: Harper & Row.

BEATTIE, M. (1989). *Beyond codependency.* New York: Harper & Row.

BEAUVAIS, F., & OETTING, E. R. (1988). Inhalant abuse by young children. In *Epidemiology of inhalant abuse: An update.* Washington, DC: National Institute on Drug Abuse.

BECHERER, P. R. (1995). Viral hepatitis. *Postgraduate Medicine, 98,* 65–74.

BECK, A. T., WRIGHT, F. D., NEWMAN, C. F., & LIESE, B. S. (1993). *Cognitive therapy of substance abuse.* New York: Guilford Press.

BECKMAN, L. J. (1993). Alcoholics Anonymous and gender issues. In B. S. McCrady & W. R. Miller (Eds.), *Research on Alcoholics Anonymous.* New Brunswick, NJ: Rutgers Center of Alcohol Studies.

BECKMAN, L. J. (1994). Treatment needs of women with alcohol problems. *Alcohol Health & Research World, 18,* 206–211.

BEEBE, D. K., & WALLEY, E. (1991). Substance abuse: The designer drugs. *American Family Physician, 43,* 1689–1698.

BEEBE, D. K., & WALLEY, E. (1995). Smokable methamphetamine ("Ice"): An old drug in a different form. *American Family Physician, 51,* 449–454.

BEEDER, A. B., & MILLMAN, R. B. (1995). Treatment strategies for comorbid disorders: Psychopathology and substance abuse. In A. M. Washton (Ed.), *Psychotherapy and substance abuse.* New York: Guilford Press.

BEHNKE, M., & EYLER, F. D. (1993). The consequences of prenatal substance use for the developing fetus, newborn and young child. *International Journal of the Addictions, 28,* 1341–1391.

BEITNER-JOHNSON, D., & NESTLER, E. J. (1992). Basic neurobiology of cocaine: Actions within the mesolimbic dopamine system. In T. R. Kosten & H. D. Kleber (Eds.), *Clinician's guide to cocaine addiction.* New York: Guilford Press.

BELL, D. C., MONTOYA, I. D., & ATKINSON, J. S. (1997). Therapeutic connection and client progress in drug abuse treatment. *Journal of Clinical Psychology, 53,* 215–224.

BELL, D. C., WILLIAMS, M. L., NELSON, R., & SPENCE, R. T. (1994). An experimental test on retention in residential and outpatient program. *American Journal of Drug and Alcohol Abuse, 20*(3), 331–341.

BELL, G. L., & LAU, K. (1995). Perinatal and neonatal issues of substance abuse. *Pediatric Clinics of North America, 42,* 261–281.

BELL, R. (1995). Determinants of hospital-based substance abuse treatment programs. *Hospital & Health Services Administration, 39*(1), 93–102.

BENET, L. Z., KROETZ, D. L., & SHEINER, L. B. (1995). Pharmacokinetics: The dynamics of drug absorption, distribution and elimination. In J. G. Hardman, & L. E. Limbird (Editors-in-Chief),*The pharmacological basis of therapeutics* (9th ed.). New York: McGraw-Hill.

BENOWITZ, N. L. (1992). Cigarette smoking and nicotine addiction. *Medical Clinics of North America, 76,* 415–437.

BENOWITZ, N. L., & HENNINGFIELD, J. E. (1994). Establishing a nicotine threshold for addiction. *New England Journal of Medicine, 331,* 123–126.

BENOWITZ, N. L., & JACOB, P. (1993). Nicotine and cotinine elimination pharmacokinetics in smokers and nonsmokers. *Clinical Pharmacology & Therapeutics, 53,* 316–323.

BENZER, D. G. (1995). *Use and abuse of benzodiazepines.* Paper presented at the 1995 annual Frank P. Furlano, M. D. memorial lecture: Gunderson-Lutheran Medical Center, La Crosse, WI.

BERENSON, D. (1987). Alcoholics Anonymous: From surrender to transformation. *The Family Therapy Networker, 11*(4), 25–31.

BERG, B. J., & DUBIN, W. R. (1990). Economic grand rounds: Why 28 days? An alternative approach to alcoholism treatment. *Hospital and Community Psychiatry, 41*, 1175–1178.

BERG, I. K., & MILLER, S. D. (1992). *Working with the problem drinker.* New York: Norton.

BERG, R., FRANZEN, M. M., & WEDDING, D. (1994). *Screening for brain impairment: A manual for mental health practice* (2nd ed.). New York: Springer.

BERGER, P. A., & DUNN, M. J. (1982). Substance induced and substance use disorders. In J. H. Griest, J. W. Jefferson, & R. L. Spitzer (Eds.), *Treatment of mental disorders.* New York: Oxford University Press.

BERKOWITZ, A., & PERKINS, H. W. (1988). Personality characteristics of children of alcoholics. *Journal of Consulting and Clinical Psychology, 56*, 206–209.

BERNSTEIN, E., TRACEY, A., BERNSTEIN, J., & WILLIAMS, C. (1996). Emergency department detection and referral rates for patients with problem drinking. *Substance Abuse, 17*, 69–76.

BERRIDGE, V. (1996). Drug policy: Should the law take a back seat? *Lancet, 347*, 301–305.

BETTER THAN WELL: SOCIETY'S MORAL CONFUSION OVER DRUGS IS NEATLY ILLUSTRATED BY ITS DIFFERING REACTIONS TO PROZAC AND ECSTACY. (1996). *The Economist, 339*(7960), 87–89.

BHANDARI, M., SYLVESTER, S. L., & RIGOTTI, N. A. (1996). Nicotine and cigarette smoking. In L. Friedman, N. F. Fleming, D. H. Roberts, & S. E. Hyman (Eds.), *Source book of substance abuse and addiction.* New York: Williams & Wilkins.

BLACK, C. (1982). *It will never happen to me.* Denver, CO: M.A.C. Printing.

BLACK, C. (1987). How different is recovery for a COA? *Alcoholism & Addiction, 8*(6).

BLAIR, D. T., & RAMONES, V. A. (1996). The undertreatment of anxiety: Overcoming the confusion and stigma. *Journal of Psychosocial Nursing, 34*(6), 9–17.

BLAKE, R. (1990). Mental health counseling and older problem drinkers. *Journal of Mental Health Counseling, 12*(3), 354–367.

BLANSJAAR, B. A., & ZWINDERMAN, A. H. (1992). The course of alcohol amnesic disorder: A three-year follow up study of clinical signs. *Acta Psychiatricia Scandinavica, 86*, 240–246.

BLAU, M. (1990). Toxic parents, perennial kids: Is it time for adult children to grow up? *Utne Reader, 42*, 60–65.

BLEIDT, B. A., & MOSS, J. T. (1989). Age-related changes in drug distribution. *U.S. Pharmacist, 14*(8), 24–32.

BLISS, R. E., GARVEY, A. J., HEINOLD, J. W., & HITCHCOCK, J. L. (1989). The influence of situation and coping on relapse crisis outcomes after smoking cessation. *Journal of Consulting and Clinical Psychology, 57*, 443–449.

BLONDELL, R. D., FRIERSON, R. L., & LIPPMANN, S. B. (1996). Alcoholism. *Postgraduate Medicine, 100*, 69–72, 78–80.

BLOODWORTH, R. C. (1987). Major problems associated with marijuana abuse. *Psychiatric Medicine, 3*(3), 173–184.

BLOOMER, S. (1994). Caffeine abuse widespread, researchers show. *APA Monitor, 25*(2), 17.

BLUM, K. (1984). *Handbook of abusable drugs.* New York: Gardner Press.

BLUM, K. (1988). The disease process in alcoholism. *Alcoholism & Addiction, 8*(5), 5–8.

BLUM, K., NOBLE, E. P., SHERIDAN, P. J., MONTGOMERY, A., RITCHIE, T., JAGADEESWARAN, P., NOGAMI, H., BRIGGS, A. H., & COHN, J. B. (1990). Allelic association of human dopamine D_2 receptor gene in alcoholism. *Journal of the American Medical Association, 263*(15), 2055–2060.

BLUM, K., & PAYNE, J. E. (1991). *Alcohol and the addictive brain.* New York: Free Press.

BLUM, K., & TRACHTENBERG, M. C. (1988). Neurochemistry and alcohol craving. *California Society for the Treatment of Alcoholism and Other Drug Dependencies News, 13*(2), 1–7.

BLUME, S. B. (1994). Gender differences in alcohol-related disorders. *Harvard Review of Psychiatry, 2*, 7–14.

BLUNTS AND CRUDE: TWO NEW MARIJUANA PRODUCTS ARE ON THE STREETS. (1993a). *The Addiction Letter, 9*(11), 1, 7.

BOARD OF TRUSTEES. (1991). Drug abuse in the United States. *Journal of the American Medical Association, 256*, 2102–2107.

BOBO, J. K., SLADE, J., & HOFFMAN, A. L. (1995). Nicotine addiction counseling for chemically dependent patients. *Psychiatric Services, 46*, 945–947.

BODE, C., MAUTE, G., & BODE, J. C. (1996). Prostaglandin E_2 and prostaglandin F_{2a} biosynthesis in human gastric mucosa: Effect of chronic alcohol misuse. *Gut, 39*, 348–352.

BODENHAM, A. R., & MALLICK, A. (1996). New dimensions in toxicology: Hyperthermic syndrome following amphetamine derivatives. *Intensive Care Medicine, 22*, 622–624.

BOHN, M. J. (1993). Alcoholism. *Psychiatric Clinics of North America, 16*, 679–692.

BOLOS, A. M., DEAN, M., LUCAS-DERSE, S., RAMSBURG, M., BROWN, G. L., & GOLDMAN, D. (1991). Population and pedigree studies reveal a lack of association between the dopamine D_2 receptor gene and alcoholism. *Journal of the American Medical Association, 264*, 3156–3160.

BOND, W. S. (1989). Smoking's effects on medications. *American Druggist, 200*(1), 24–25.

BONDESSON, J. D., & SAPERSTON, A. R. (1996). Hepatitis. *Emergency Medical Clinics of North America, 14,* 695–718.

BONSTEDT, T., ULRICH, D. A., DOLINAR, L. J., & JOHNSON, J. J. (1984). When and where should we hospitalize alcoholics? *Hospital & Community Psychiatry, 35,* 1038–1040.

BOOTH, M. (1995). The quiet addiction. *The Denver Post Magazine, 103*(353), 12–15, 18.

BOUTOTTE, J. (1993). T.B. The second time around . . . *Nursing 93, 23*(5), 42–49.

BOWDEN, S. J. (1994). Neuropsychology of alcohol and drug dependence. In S. Touyz, D. Byrne, & A. Gilandas (Eds.), *Neuropsychology in clinical practice.* New York: Academic Press.

BOWEN, M. (1985). *Family therapy in clinical practice.* Northvale, NJ: Jason Aronson.

BOWER, B. (1991). Pumped up and strung out. *Science News, 140*(2), 30–31.

BOYD, C. (1992). Self-help sickness? *St. Paul Pioneer Press, 143*(346), 1C, 4C.

BOYD, L. M. (1995). Moved by the spirit. *San Francisco Chronicle, 130*(16), 10.

BRADFORD, J. M. W., GREENBERG, D. M., & MOTAYNE, G. G. (1992). Substance abuse and criminal behavior. *Psychiatric Clinics of North America, 15,* 605–622.

BRADLEY, B. P., GOSSOP, M., BREWIN, C. R., PHILLIPS, G., & GREEN, L. (1992). Attributions and relapse in opiate addicts. *Journal of Consulting and Clinical Psychology, 60,*470–472.

BRADSHAW, J. (1988a). Compulsivity: The black plague of our day. *Lear's Magazine, 42,* 89–90.

BRADSHAW, J. (1988b). *Bradshaw on: The family.* Deerfield Beach, FL: Health Communications.

BRADY, K. T., GRICE, D. E., DUSTAN, L., & RANDALL, C. (1993). Gender differences in substance use disorders. *American Journal of Psychiatry, 150,* 1707–1711.

BRANDT, J., & BUTTERS, N. (1986). The alcoholic Wernicke-Korsakoff syndrome and its relationship to long term alcohol use. In I. Grant & K. M. Adams (Eds.), *Neuropsychological assessment of neuropsychiatric disorders.* New York: Oxford University Press.

BRANSON, B. M. (1995). Early intervention for persons infected with human immunodeficiency virus. *Clinical Infectious Diseases, 20*(Suppl. 1), S3–S22.

BRECHER, E. M. (1972). *Licit and illicit drugs.* Boston: Little, Brown.

BRENDEL, D., WEST, H., & HYMAN, S. E. (1996). Hallucinogens and phencyclidine. In L. Friedman, N. F. Fleming, D. H. Roberts, & S. E. Hyman (Eds.), *Source book of substance abuse and addiction.* New York: Williams & Wilkins.

BRENNAN, D. F., BETZELOS, S., REED, R., & FALK, J. L. (1995). Ethanol elimination rates in an ED population. *American Journal of Emergency Medicine, 13,* 276–280.

BRENNAN, P. L., & MOOS, R. H. (1996). Late-life drinking behavior: The influence of personal characteristics, life context, and treatment. *Alcohol Health & Research World, 20,* 197–204.

BRENNER, D. E., KUKULL, W. A., VAN BELLE, G., BOWEN, J. D., MCCORMICK, W. C., TERI, L., & LARSON, E. B. (1993). Relationship between cigarette smoking and Alzheimer's disease in a population-based case-control study. *Neurology, 43,* 293–300.

BRENT, D. A., KUPFER, D. J., BROMET, E. J., & DEW, M. A. (1988). The assessment and treatment of patients at risk for suicide. In A. J. Frances & R. E. Hales (Eds.), *American psychiatric association annual review* (Vol. 7). Washington, DC: American Psychiatric Association Press.

BRENT, J. A. (1995). Drugs of abuse: An update. *Emergency Medicine, 27*(7), 56–70.

BREO, D. L. (1990). Of MD's and muscles—lessons from two "retired steroid doctors." *Journal of the American Medical Association, 263,* 1697–1705.

BRESLAU, N., KILBEY, M., & ANDRESKI, P. (1993). Vulnerability to psychopathology in nicotine-dependent smokers: An epidemiologic study of young adults. *American Journal of Psychiatry, 150,* 941–946.

BRESLIN, J. (1988). Crack. *Playboy, 35*(12), 109–110, 210, 212–213, 215.

BRIGGS, G. G., FREEMAN, R. K., & YAFFE, S. J. (1986). *Drugs in pregnancy and lactation* (2nd ed). Baltimore: Williams & Wilkins.

BRING DRUGS WITHIN THE LAW. (1993). *The Economist, 327*(7811), 13–14.

BRITISH FIND 20% OF URINE SAMPLES ADULTERATED. (1995). *Forensic Drug Abuse Advisor, 7*(8), 59.

BRODSKY, A. (1993). The 12 steps are not for everyone—or even for most. *Addiction& Recovery, 13*(2), 21.

BRODY, J. (1991). Hepatitis B still spreading. *Minneapolis Star-Tribune, X*(269), 4E.

BRODY, J. (1993). To drink or not to drink? For women its benefit to heart vs. cancer risk. *Minneapolis Star-Tribune, XII*(168), 12EX.

BROOKOFF, D., COOK, C. S., WILLIAMS, C., & MANN, C. S. (1994). Testing reckless drivers for cocaine and marijuana. *New England Journal of Medicine, 331,* 528–522.

BROOKS, J. T., LEUNG, G., & SHANNON, M. (1996). Inhalants. In L. Friedman, N. F. Fleming, D. H. Roberts, & S. E. Hyman (Eds.), *Source book of substance abuse and addiction.* New York: Williams & Wilkins.

BROPHY, J. J. (1993). Psychiatric disorders. In L. M. Tierney, S. J. McPhee, M. A. Papadakis, & S. A. Schroeder (Eds.), *Current medical diagnosis and treatment.* Norwalk, CT: Appleton & Lange.

BROWER, K. J. (1993). Anabolic steroids. *Psychiatric Clinics of North America, 16,* 97 103.

BROWER, K. J., BLOW, F. C., YOUNG, J. P., & HILL, E. M. (1991). Symptoms and correlates of anabolic-androgenic steroid dependence. *British Journal of Addiction, 86,* 759–768.

BROWER, K. J., CATLIN, D. H., BLOW, F. C., ELIOPULOS, G. A., & BERESFORD, T. P. (1991). Clinical assessment and urine testing for anabolic-androgenic steroid abuse and dependence. *American Journal of Drug and Alcohol Abuse, 17*(2), 161–172.

BROWN, R. L. (1997, May 2). *Stages of change.* Paper presented at symposium, Still Getting High, a 30 year perspective on drug abuse, Gundersen Lutheran Medical Center, La Crosse, WI.

BROWN, R. L., LEONARD, T., SAUNDERS, L. A., & PAPASOULIOUTIS, O. (1997). A two-item screening test for alcohol and other drug problems. *Journal of Family Practice, 44,* 151–160.

BROWN, R. T., & BRADEN, N. J. (1987). Hallucinogens. *Pediatric Clinics of North America, 34*(2), 341–347.

BROWN, S. (1985). *Treating the alcoholic: A developmental model of recovery.* New York: Wiley.

BROWN, S., & LEWIS, V. (1995). The alcoholic family: A developmental model of recovery. In S. Brown (Ed.), *Treating alcoholism.* New York: Jossey-Bass.

BROWN, S. A. (1990). Adolescent alcohol expectancies and risk for alcohol abuse. *Addiction & Recovery, 10*(5/6), 16–19.

BROWN, S. A. (1995). Introduction. In S. A. Brown (Ed.), *Treating alcoholism.* New York: Jossey-Bass.

BROWN, S. A., CREAMER, V. A., & STETSON, B. A. (1987). Adolescent alcohol expectancies in relation to personal and parental drinking patterns. *Journal of Abnormal Psychology, 96,* 117–121.

BROWN, S. A., GOLDMAN, M. S., INN, A., & ANDERSON, L. R. (1980). Expectations of reinforcement from alcohol: Their domain and relation to drinking patterns. *Journal of Abnormal Psychology, 96,* 117–121.

BROWN, V. B., RIDGELY, M. S., PEPPER, B., LEVINE, I. S., & RYGLEWICZ, H. (1989). The dual crisis: Mental illness and substance abuse. *American Psychologist, 44,* 565–569.

BROWNING, M., HOFFER, B. J., & DUNWIDDIE, T. V. (1993). Alcohol, memory and molecules. *Alcohol Health & Research World, 16*(4), 280–284.

BROWNLEE, S., ROBERTS, S. V., COOPER, M., GOODE, E., HETTER, K., & WRIGHT, A. (1994). "Should cigarettes be outlawed?" *U.S. News and World Report, 116*(15), 32–36, 38.

BROWNSON, R. C., NOVOTNY, T. E., & PERRY, M. C. (1993). Cigarette smoking and adult leukemia. *Archives of Internal Medicine, 153,* 469–475.

BRUNSWICK, M. (1989). More kids turning to inhalant abuse. *Minneapolis Star-Tribune, VII*(356), 1A, 6A.

BRUNTON, S. A., HENNINGFIELD, J. E., & SOLBERG, L. I. (1994). Smoking cessation: What works best? *Patient Care, 25*(11), 89–115.

BRUST, J. C. M. (1993). Other agents: Phencyclidine, marijuana, hallucinogens, inhalants, and anticholinergics. *Neurologic Clinics, 11,* 555–561.

BUBER, M. (1970). *I and thou.* New York: Charles Scribner's Sons.

BUCKLEY, N. A., DAWSON, A. H., WHYTE, I. M., & O'CONNELL, D. L. (1995). Relative toxicity of benzodiazepines in overdose. *British Medical Journal, 310*(6974), 219–222.

BUCKLEY, W. F. (1996). The war on drugs is lost. *National Review, XLVIII*(2), 35–38.

BUCKLEY, W. F. (1997). Save money, cut crime, get real. *Playboy, 44*(1), 129, 192–193.

BUDIANSKY, S., GOODE, E. E., & GEST, T. (1994). The cold war experiments. *U.S. News & World Report, 116*(3), 32–38.

BUFE, C. (1988). AA: Guilt and god for the gullible. *Utne Reader, 30,* 54–55.

BUGLIOSI, V. T. (1996). *The Phoenix solution.* Beverly Hills, CA: Dove.

BUKSTEIN, O. G. (1994). Treatment of adolescent alcohol abuse and dependence. *Alcohol Health and Research World, 18,* 297–301.

BUKSTEIN, O. G. (1995). *Adolescent substance abuse.* New York: Wiley Interscience.

BUKSTEIN, O. G., BRENT, D. A., PERPER, J. A., MORITZ, G., BAUGHER, M., SCHWEERS, J., ROTH, C., & BALACH, L. (1993). Risk factors for completed suicide among adolescents with a lifetime history of substance abuse: A case controlled study. *Acta Psychiatrica Scandinavica, 88,* 403–408.

BURKE, J. D., BURKE, K. C., & RAE, D. S. (1994). Increased rates of drug abuse and dependence after onset of mood or anxiety disorders in adolescence. *Hospital and Community Psychiatry, 45,* 451–455.

BURKETT, G., YASIN, S. Y., PALOW, D., LAVOIE, L. & MARTINEZ, M. (1994). Patterns of cocaine binging: Effects on pregnancy. *American Journal of Obstetrics and Gynecology, 171*(2), 372–379.

BURNAM, M. A., STEIN, J. A., GOLDING, J. M., SIEGEL, J. M., SORENSEN, S. B., FORSYTHE, A. B., & TELLES, C. A. (1989). Sexual assault and mental disorders in a community population. *Journal of Consulting and Clinical Psychology, 56*(6), 843–850.

BURNS, D. M. (1991). Cigarettes and cigarette smoking. *Clinics in Chest Medicine, 12,* 631–642.

BUSHNELL, T. G., & JUSTINS, D. M. (1993). Choosing the right analgesic. *Drugs, 46,* 394–408.

BUTCHER, J. N. (1988). Introduction to the special series. *Journal of Consulting and Clinical Psychology, 56,* 171.

BUTTERWORTH, R. F. (1995). The role of liver disease in alcohol-induced cognitive defects. *Alcohol Health & Research World, 19,* 123–129.

BYCK, R. (1987). Cocaine use and research: Three histories. In S. Fisher, A. Rashkin, & E. H. Unlenhuth

(Eds.), *Cocaine: Clinical and behavioral aspects.* New York: Oxford University Press.

BYRD, R. C., & HOWARD, C. R. (1995). Children's passive and prenatal exposure to cigarette smoke. *Pediatric Annals, 24,* 640–645.

BYRNE, C. (1989a). Pregnancy and crack: Trying to heal horror. *Minneapolis Star-Tribune, VIII*(89), 1, 4A.

BYRNE, C. (1989b). Cocaine alley. *Minneapolis Star-Tribune, VIII*(215), 29a–32a.

CAINE, S. B., & KOOB, G. F. (1993). Modulation of cocaine self-administration in the rat through D-3 dopamine receptors. *Science, 260,* 1814–1817.

CALABRESI, M., FOWLER, D., SCALA, T., THOMPSON, D., & WILLWERTH, J. (1994). The butt stops here. *Time, 143*(16), 58–64,

CALLAHAN, E. J. (1980). Alternative strategies in the treatment of narcotic addiction: A review. In W. R. Miller (Ed.), *The addictive behaviors.* New York: Pergamon Press.

CALLAHAN, J. (1993). Blueprint for an adolescent suicidal crisis. *Psychiatric Annals, 23*(5), 263–270.

CAMPBELL, G. D. (1994). Overview of community-acquired pneumonia. *Medical Clinics of North American, 78,* 1035–1048.

CAMPBELL, J. (1995). Making sense of . . . the effects of alcohol. *Nursing Times, 91*(3), 38–39.

CAMPBELL, J. L., THOMAS, H. M., GABRIELLI, W., LISDOW, B. I., & POWELL, B. J. (1995). Impact of desipramine or carbamazepine on patient retention in outpatient cocaine treatment: Preliminary findings. *Journal of Addictive Diseases, 13*(4), 191–199.

CAMPBELL, J. W. (1992). Alcoholism. In R. J. Ham & P. D. Sloane (Eds.), *Primary care geriatrics* (2nd ed.). Boston: Mosby.

CARDIEUZ, R. J. (1996). Azapirones: An alternative to benzodiazepines for anxiety. *American Family Physician, 53,* 2349–2353.

CARDONI, A. A. (1990). Focus on *adinazolam:* A benzodiazepine with antidepressant activity. *Hospital Formulary, 25,* 155–158.

CAREY, K. B. (1989). Emerging treatment guidelines for mentally ill chemical abusers. *Hospital and Community Psychiatry, 40,* 341–342, 349.

CAREY, K. B., COCCO, K. M., & SIMONS, J. S. (1996). Concurrent validity of clinicians' ratings of substance abuse among psychiatric outpatients. *Psychiatric Services, 47,* 842–847.

CARLSON, J. L., STROM, B. L., MORSE, L., WEST, S. L., SOPER, K. A., STOLLEY, P. D., & JONES, J. K. (1987). The relative gastrointestinal toxicity of the nonsteroidal anti-inflammatory drugs. *Archives of Internal Medicine, 147,* 1054–1059.

CARROLL, K. M., & ROUNSAVILLE, B. J. (1992). Contrast of treatment-seeking and untreated cocaine abusers. *Archives of General Psychiatry, 49,* 464–471.

CASTLEMAN, M. (1994). Aspirin: Not just for your heart. *Reader's Digest, 144*(864), 85–89.

CATANZARITE, V. A., & STEIN, D. A. (1995). "Crystal" and pregnancy methamphetamine associated maternal deaths. *Western Journal of Medicine, 162,* 545–547.

CATON, C. L. M., GRALNICK, A., BENDER, S., & SIMON, R. (1989). Young chronic patients and substance abuse. *Hospital and Community Psychiatry, 40,* 1037–1040.

"CAT" POSES NATIONAL THREAT, EXPERTS SAY (methcathione). (1993). *Alcoholism & Drug Abuse Week, 5*(47), 5–6.

CATTARELLO, A. M., CLAYTON, R. R., & LEUKEFELD, C. G. (1995). Adolescent alcoholl and drug abuse. In J. M. Oldham & M. B. Riba (Eds.), *Review of Psychiatry* (Vol. 14). Washington, DC: American Psychiatric Press.

CAVALIERE, F. (1995). Substance abuse in the deaf community. *APA Monitor, 26*(10), 49.

CENTERS FOR DISEASE CONTROL. (1990). Lead poisoning associated with intravenous methamphetamine use—Oregon, 1988. *Journal of the American Medical Association, 263,* 797.

CETARUK, E. W., DART, E. C., HOROWITZ, R. S., & HURIBUT, K. M. (1996). Extended-release acetaminophen overdose. *Journal of the American Medical Association, 275,* 686.

CHAN, P., CHEN, J. H., LEE, M. H., & DENG, J. F. (1994). Fatal and nonfatal methamphetamine intoxication in the intensive care unit. *Journal of Toxicology: Clinical Toxicology, 32,* 147–156.

CHARNESS, M. E., SIMON, R. P., & GREENBERG, D. A. (1989). Ethanol and the nervous system. *New England Journal of Medicine, 321*(7), 442–454.

CHASNOFF, I. J. (1988). Drug use in pregnancy: Parameters of risk. *Pediatric Clinics of North America, 35*(6), 1403–1412.

CHASNOFF, I. J. (1991a). Cocaine and pregnancy: Clinical and methadologic issues. *Clinics in Perinatology, 18,* 113–123.

CHASNOFF, I. J. (1991b). Drugs, alcohol, pregnancy, and the neonate. *Journal of the American Medical Association, 266,* 1567–1568.

CHASNOFF, I. J., & SCHNOLL, S. H. (1987). Consequences of cocaine and other drug use in pregnancy. In A. M. Washton & M. S. Gold (Eds.), *Cocaine: A clinician's handbook.* New York: Guilford Press.

CHASSIN, L., CURRAN, P. J., HUSSONG, A. M., & COLDER, C. R. (1996). The relation of parent alcoholism to adolescent substance use: A longitudinal follow-up study. *Journal of Abnormal Psychology, 105,* 70–80.

CHASSIN, L., & DELUCIA, C. (1996). Drinking during adolescence. *Alcohol Health & Research World, 20,* 175–180.

CHATLOS, J. C. (1996). Recent developments and a developmental approach to substance abuse in adolescents.

Child and Adolescent Psychiatric Clinics of North America, 5, 1–27.

CHAVEZ, G. F., MULINARE, J., & CORDERO, J. F. (1989). Maternal cocaine use during early pregnancy as a risk factor for congenital urogenital anomalies. *Journal of the American Medical Association, 262*(6), 795–798.

CHEATERS ADVISED TO AVOID USING DRANO. (1995). *Forensic Drug Abuse Advisor, 7*(1), 3–4.

CHERNY, N. I., & FOLEY, K. M. (1996). Nonopioid and opioid analgesic pharmacology of cancer pain. *Hematology/Oncology Clinics of North American, 10*, 79–102.

CHERUBIN, C. E., & SAPIRA, J. D. (1993). The medical complications of drug addiction and the medical assessment of the intraveneous drug user: 25 years later. *Annals of Internal Medicine, 119*, 1017–1028.

CHIAUZZI, E. (1990). Breaking the patterns that lead to relapse. *Psychology Today, 23*(12), 18–19.

CHICK, J. (1993). Brief interventions for alcohol misuse. *British Medical Journal, 307*, 1374.

CHO, A. K. (1990). Ice: A new dosage form of an old drug. *Science, 249*, 631–634.

CHRISTENSEN, W. G., MANSON, J. E., SEDDON, J. M., GLYNN, R. J., BURING, J. E., ROSNER, B., & HENNEKENS, C. H. (1992). A prospective study of cigarette smoking and risk of cataract in men. *Journal of the American Medical Association, 268*, 989–993.

CHUCK, R. S., WILLIAMS, J. M., GOLDBERG, M. A., & LUBNIEWSKI, A. J. (1996). Recurrent corneal ulcerations associated with smokable methamphetamine abuse. *American Journal of Ophthalmology, 121*, 571–573.

CIANCIO, S. G., & BOURGAULT, P. C. (1989). *Clinical pharmacology for dental professionals* (3rd ed.). Chicago: Year Book Medical.

CIRAULO, D. A., CREELMAN, W., SHADER, R. I., & O'SULLIVAN, R. O. (1995). Antidepressants. In D. A. Ciraulo, R. I. Shader, D. J. Greenblatt, & W. Creelman (Eds.), *Drug interactions in psychiatry* (2nd ed.). Baltimore: Williams & Wilkins.

CIRAULO, D. A., SARID-SEGAL, O., KNAPP, C., CIRAULO, A. M., GREENBLATT, D. J., & SHADER, R. I. (1996). Liability to alprazolam abuse in daughters of alcoholics. *American Journal of Psychiatry, 153*, 956–958.

CIRAULO, D. A., SHADER, R. I., CIRAULO, A., GREENBLATT, D. J., & VON MOLTKE, L. L. (1994a). Alcoholism and its treatment. In R. I. Shader (Ed.), *Manual of psychiatric therapeutics* (2nd ed.). Boston: Little, Brown.

CIRAULO, D. A., SHADER, R. I., CIRAULO, A., GREENBLATT, D. J., & VON MOLTKE, L. L. (1994b). Treatment of alcohol withdrawal. In R. I. Shader (Ed.), *Manual of psychiatric therapeutics* (2nd ed.). Boston: Little, Brown.

CIRAULO, D. A., SHADER, R. I., GREENBLATT, D. J., & BARNHILL, J. G. (1995). Basic concepts. In D. A. Ciraulo, R. I. Shader, D. J. Greenblatt, & W. Creelman (Eds.), *Drug interactions in psychiatry* (2nd ed.). Baltimore: Williams & Wilkins.

CLARK, C. M. (1995). Alcoholics Anonymous. *The Addictions Newsletter, 2*(3), 9, 22.

CLARK, D. C., GIVVONS, R. D., HAVILAND, M. G., & HENDRYX, M. S. (1993). Assessing the severity of depressive states in recently detoxified alcoholics. *Journal of Studies on Alcohol, 54*, 107–114.

CLARK, R. E. (1994). Family costs associated with severe mental illness and substance abuse. *Hospital and Community Psychiatry, 45*, 808–813.

CLARK, W. G., BRATLER, D. C., & JOHNSON, A. R. (1991). *Goth's medical pharmacology* (13th ed.). Boston: Mosby.

CLARK, W. R. (1995). *At war within.* New York: Oxford University Press.

CLAUNCH, L. (1994). Intervention can be used as a tool or as a weapon against clients. *The Addiction Letter, 10*(4), 1–2.

CLAY, R. A. (1996). Targeted interventions curb the spread of HIV. *APA Monitor, 27*(6), 29.

CLIMKO, R. P., ROEHRICH, H., SWEENEY, D. R., & AL-RAZI, J. (1987). Ecstacy: A review of MDMA and MDA. *International Journal of Psychiatry in Medicine, 16*(4), 359–372.

CLONINGER, C. R., GOHMAN, M., & SIGVARDSSON, S. (1981). Inheritance of alcohol abuse: Cross fostering analysis of adopted men. *Archives of General Psychiatry, 38*, 861–868.

CLONINGER, C. R., SIGVARDSSON, S., & BOHMAN, M. (1996). Type I and Type II alcoholism: An update. *Alcohol Health & Research World, 20*(1), 18–23.

COCAINE IN THE BRAIN. (1994). *Forensic Drug Abuse Advisor, 6*(9), 67.

COCAINE USE . . . BY THE TON. (1994). *USA Today, 12*(235), 1A.

COCAINE USE DANGEROUS FOR MOTHERS, TOO. (1995). *Forensic Drug Abuse Advisor, 7*(6), 44.

COHEN, D. A., RICHARDSON, J., & LaBREE, L. (1994). Parenting behaviors and the onset of smoking and alcohol use: A longitudinal study. *Pediatrics, 94*, 368–375.

COHEN, G., FLEMING, N. S., GLATTER, K. A., HAGHIGI, D. B., HALBERSTADT, J., McHIGH, K. M.,& WOOLF, A. (1996). Epidemiology of substance use. In L. Friedman, N. F. Fleming, D. H. Roberts, & S. E. Hyman (Eds.), *Source book of substance abuse and addiction.* New York: Williams & Wilkins.

COHEN, J., & LEVY, S. J. (1992). *The mentally ill chemical abuser: Whose client?* New York: Lexington Books.

COHEN, L. S. (1989). Psychotropic drug use in pregnancy. *Hospital and Community Psychiatry, 40*(6), 566–567.

COHEN, M. S. (1995). HIV and sexually transmitted diseases. *Postgraduate Medicine, 98*(3), 52–64.

COHEN, N. L., & MARCOS, L. R. (1989). The bad-mad dilemma for public psychiatry. *Hospital and Community Psychiatry, 40*, 677.

COHEN, S. (1977). Inhalant abuse: An overview of the problem. In C. W. Sharp, & M. L. Brehm (Eds.), *Review of inhalants: Euphoria to dysfunction*. Washington, DC: U.S. Government Printing Office.

COHEN, S., LICHTENSTEIN, E., PROCHASKA, J. O., ROSSI, J. S., GRITZ, E. R., CARR, C. R., ORLEANS, C. T., SCHOENBACH, V. J., BIENER, L., ABRAMS, D., DiCLEMENTE, C., CURRY, S., MARLATT, G. A., CUMMINGS, K. M., EMONT, S. L., GIOVINO, G., & OSSIP-KLEIN, D. (1989). Debunking myths about self-quitting. *American Psychologist, 44*, 1355–1365.

COHEN, S. I. (1995). Overdiagnosis of schizophrenia: Role of alcohol and drug misuse. *Lancet, 346*, 1541–1542.

COHN, J. B., WILCOX, C. S., BOWDEN, C. L., FISHER, J. G., & RODOS, J. J. (1992). Double-blind clorazepate in anxious outpatients with and without depressive symptoms. *Psychopathology, 25*(Suppl. 1), 10–21.

COLBURN, N., MEYER, R. D., WRIGLEY, M., & BRADLEY, E. L. (1993). Should motorcycles be operated within the legal alcohol limits for automobiles? *The Journal of Trauma, 34*(1), 183–186.

COLE, J. O., & KANDO, J. C. (1993). Adverse behavioral events reported in patients taking alprazolam and other benzodiazepines. *Journal of Clinical Psychiatry, 54*(10)(Suppl.), 49–61.

COLE, J. O., & YONKERS, K. A. (1995). Nonbenzodiazepine anxiolytics. In A. F. Schatzberg & C. B. Nemeroff (Eds.), *Textbook of psychopharmacology*. Washington,DC: American Psychiatric Association Press.

COLEMAN, E. (1988). Chemical dependency and intimacy dysfunction: Inextricably bound. In E. Coleman (Ed.), *Chemical dependency and intimacy dysfunction*. New York: Haworth Press.

COLEMAN, P. (1989). Letter to the editor. *Journal of the American Medical Association, 261*(13), 1879–1880.

COLLETTE, L. (1988). Step by step: A skeptic's encounter. *Utne Reader, 30*, 69–76.

COLLETTE, L. (1990). After the anger, what then? *Networker, 14*(1), 22–31.

COLLIER, A. (1989). To deal and die in LA *Ebony, 44*(10), 106–108.

COLLINS, J. J., & ALLISON, M. (1983). Legal coercion and retention in drug abuse treatment. *Hospital and Community Psychiatry, 34*, 1145–1150.

COLLINS, J. J., & MESSERSCHMIDT, P. M. (1993). Epidemiology of alcohol-related violence. *Alcohol Health & Research World, 17*(2), 93–100.

COMMITTEE ON SUBSTANCE ABUSE. (1995). Alcohol use and abuse: A pediatric concern. *Pediatrics, 95*, 439–442.

COMMITTEE ON SUBSTANCE ABUSE AND COMMITTEE ON CHILDREN WITH DISABILITIES. (1993). Fetal alcohol syndrome and fetal alcohol effects. *Pediatrics, 91*, 1004–1006.

CONE, E. J. (1993). Saliva testing for drugs of abuse. In D. Malamud & L. Tabak(Eds.), *Saliva as a diagnostic fluid*. New York: New York Academy of Sciences.

CONLAN, M. F. (1990). Research and development plan proposed for pharmacotherapy. *Drug Topics, 134* (1), 50.

CONSEQUENCES OF PCP ABUSE ARE UP. (1994). *The Addiction Letter, 10*(3), 3.

CONTROLLING THE WEED IN PUBLIC. (1993). *Lancet, 341*, 525–526.

COOK, A. (1995). Ecstasy (MDMA): Alerting users to the dangers. *Nursing Times, 91*(16), 32–33.

COONEY, N. L., ZWEBEN, A., & FLEMING, M. F. (1995). Screening for alcohol problems and at-risk drinking in health-care settings. In R. K. Hester & W. R. Miller (Eds.), *Handbook of alcoholism treatment approaches* (2nd ed.). New York: Allyn & Bacon.

COOPER, J. R., BLOOM, F. E., & ROTH, R. H. (1986). *The biochemical basis of neuropharmacology* (5th ed.). New York: Oxford University Press.

COOPER, J. R., BLOOM, F. E., & ROTH, R. H. (1996). *The biochemical basis of neuropharmacology* (7th ed.). New York: Oxford University Press.

CORDERO, J. F. (1990). Effect of environmental agents on pregnancy outcomes: Disturbances of prenatal growth and development. *Medical Clinics of North America, 72*(2), 279–290.

CORNELL, W. F. (1996). Capitalism in the consulting room. *Readings, 11*(1), 12–17.

CORNISH, J. W., McNICHOLAS, L. F., & O'BRIEN, C. P. (1995). Treatment of substancerelated disorders. In A. F. Schatzberg & C. B. Nemeroff (Eds.), *Textbook of psychopharmacology*. Washington, DC: American Psychiatric Association.

CORRIGAN, B. (1996). Anabolic steroids and the mind. *Medical Journal of Australia, 165*, 222–226.

CORWIN, J. (1994). Outlook. *U.S. News & World Report, 116*(23), 15–16.

COTTON, P. (1990). Medium isn't accurate "ice age" message. *Journal of the American Medical Association, 263*, 2717.

COTTON, P. (1993). Low-tar cigarettes come under fire. *Journal of the American Medical Association, 270*, 1399.

COTTON, P. (1994). Smoking cigarettes may do developing fetus more harm than ingesting cocaine, some experts say. *Journal of the American Medical Association, 271*, 576–577.

COUNCIL ON ADDICTION PSYCHIATRY. (1994). Position statement on methadone maintenance treatment. *American Journal of Psychiatry, 151*, 792–794.

COUNCIL ON SCIENTIFIC AFFAIRS. (1990a). The worldwide smoking epidemic. *Journal of the American Medical Association, 263*, 3312–3318.

COUNCIL ON SCIENTIFIC AFFAIRS. (1990b). Medical and nonmedical uses of anabolicandrogenic steroids. *Journal of the American Medical Association, 264*, 2923–2927.

COUNCIL ON SCIENTIFIC AFFAIRS. (1996). Alcoholism in the elderly. *Journal of the American Medical Association, 275*, 797–801.

COUSINS, N. (1989). *Head first: The biology of hope.* New York: Dutton.

COVINGTON, S. S. (1987). Alcohol and female sexuality. *Alcoholism & Addiction, 7*(5), 21.

COWEN, R. (1990). Alcoholism treatment under scrutiny. *Science News, 137*, 254.

COWLEY, G. (1992). Halcion takes another hit. *Newsweek, CXIX*(7), 58.

CPPD IN PUERTO RICO, MEETING HIGHLIGHTS. FRENCH HEROIN. (1996). *Forensic Drug Abuse Advisor, 8*(6), 41–44.

CRABBE, J. C., & GOLDMAN, D. (1993). Alcoholism. *Alcohol Health & Research World, 16*(4), 297–303.

CRACK INJECTING IN CHICAGO—FIRST U.S. REPORTS OF DANGEROUS NEW PRACTICE. (1996). *Forensic Drug Abuse Advisor, 8*(8), 60.

CRAFT, N. (1994). WHO denounces health benefits of alcohol. *British Medical Journal, 309*, 1249.

CRAIG, T. J. (1996). Drugs to be used with caution in patients with asthma. *American Family Physician, 54*, 947–953.

CREELMAN, W., SANDS, B. F., CIRAULO, D. A., GREENBLATT, D. J., & SHADER, R. I. (1989). Benzodiazepines. In D. A. Ciraulo, R. I. Shader, D. J. Greenblatt, & W. Creelman (Eds.), *Drug interactions in psychiatry.* Baltimore: Williams & Wilkins.

CREIGHTON, F. J., BLACK, D. L., & HYDE, C. E. (1991). "Ecstacy" psychosis and flashbacks. *British Journal of Psychiatry, 159*, 713–715.

CROWLEY, T. J. (1988). *Substance abuse treatment and policy: Contributions of behavioral pharmacology.* Paper presented at the 1988 meeting of the American Psychological Association, Atlanta, GA.

CROWLEY, T. J. (1995a). Inhalant-related disorders. In H. I. Kaplan & B. J. Sadock (Eds.), *Comprehensive textbook of psychiatry* (6th ed.). Baltimore: Williams & Wilkins.

CROWLEY, T. J. (1995b). Pneycyclidine- (or Phencyclidine-like) related disorders. In H. I. Kaplan & B. J. Sadock (Eds.), *Comprehensive textbook of psychiatry* (6th ed.). Baltimore: Williams & Wilkins.

CUFFEL, B. J., HEITHOFF, K. A., & LAWSON, W. (1993). Correlates of patterns of substance abuse among patients with schizophrenia. *Hospital and Community Psychiatry, 44*, 247–251.

CUMMINGS, C., GORDON, J. R., & MARLATT, G. A. (1980). Relapse: Prevention and prediction. In W. R. Miller (Ed.), *The addictive behaviors.* New York: Pergamon Press.

CUNNIEN, A. J. (1988). Psychiatric and medical syndromes associated with deception. In R. Rogers (Ed.), *Clinical assessment of malingering and deception.* New York: Guilford Press.

CURLEY, B. (1995). Drugs demand distinction between rights and responsibilities. *Alcoholism & Drug Abuse Week, 7*(19), 5.

CYR, M. G., & MOULTON, A. W. (1993). The physician's role in prevention, detection, and treatment of alcohol abuse in women. *Psychiatric Annals, 23*, 454–462.

CZEIZEL, A. E., KODAJ, I., & LENZ, W. (1994). Smoking during pregnancy and congenital limb deficiency. *British Medical Journal, 308*, 1473–1476.

DAGHESTANI, A. N., & SCHNOLL, S. H. (1994). Phencyclidine. In M. Galanter & H. D. Kleber (Eds.), *Textbook of substance abuse treatment.* Washington, DC: American Psychiatric Press.

D'ANDREA, L. M., FISHER, G. L., & HARRISON, T. C. (1994). Cluster analysis of adult children of alcoholics. *International Journal of the Addictions, 29*, 565–582.

DANGEROUS INHALANTS ARE INCREASINGLY POPULAR AMONG ADOLESCENTS. (1993). *The Addiction Letter, 9*(8), 1, 7.

DAVIS, J. M., & BRESNAHAN, D. B. (1987). Psychopharmacology in clinical psychiatry. In *American psychiatric association annual review* (Vol. 6). Washington, DC: American Psychiatric Association Press.

DAWN: EMERGENCY ROOMS SEEING FEWER DRUG CASES. (1991). *Alcoholism & Drug Abuse Week, 3*(6), 1.

DAWN SURVEY: SURGE IN HEROIN-RELATED DEATHS, COCAINE DEATHS RISE. (1995). *Forensic Drug Abuse Advisor, 7*(5), 33–34.

DAY, N. L., & RICHARDSON, G. A. (1991). Prenatal marijuana use: Epidemiology, methodologic issues, and infant outcome. *Clinics in Perinatology, 18*, 77–91.

DAY, N. L., & RICHARDSON, G. A. (1994). Comparative tetragenicity of alcohol and other drugs. *Alcohol Health & Research World, 18*, 42–48.

DEANGELIS, T. (1989). Behavior is included in report on smoking. *APA Monitor, 20*(3), 1, 4.

DEANGELIS, T. (1994a). People's drug of choice offers potent side effects. *APA Monitor, 25*(2), 16.

DEANGELIS, T. (1994b). Perceptions influence student drinking. *APA Monitor, 25*(12), 35.

DECKER, K. P., & RIES, R. K. (1993). Differential diagnosis and psychopharmacology of dual disorders. *Psychiatric Clinics of North America, 16*, 703–718.

DECKER, S., FINS, J., & FRANCES, R. (1987). Cocaine and chest pain. *Hospital & Community Psychiatry, 38*, 464–466.

DEGLAMORISING CANNABIS. (1995). *Lancet, 346*, 1241.

DEJONG, W. (1994). Relapse prevention: An emerging technology for promoting long-term abstinence. *International Journal of the Addictions, 29*, 681–785.

DELBANCO, T. L. (1996). Patients who drink alcohol. *Journal of the American Medical Association, 275*, 803–804.

DEL BOCA, F. K., & HESSELBROCK, M. N. (1996). Gender and alcoholic subtypes. *Alcohol Health & Research World, 20,* 56–62.

DELEON, G. (1989). Psychopathology and substance abuse: What is being learned from research in therapeutic communities. *Journal of Psychoactive Drugs, 21*(2),177–188.

DELEON, G. (1994). Therapeutic Communities. In M. Galanter & H. D. Kleber (Eds.), *Textbook of substance abuse treatment.* Washington, DC: American Psychiatric Press.

DEMARIA, P. A., & WEINSTEIN, S. P. (1995). Methadone maintenance treatment. *Postgraduate Medicine, 97*(3), 83–92.

DERLET, R. W. (1989). Cocaine intoxication. *Postgraduate Medicine, 86*(5), 245–248, 253.

DERLET, R. W., & HEISCHOBER, B. (1990). Methamphetamine: Stimulant of the 1990's? *Western Journal of Medicine, 153,* 625–629.

DERLET, R. W., & HOROWITZ, B. Z. (1995). Cardiotoxic drugs. *Emergency Medicine Clinics of North American, 13,* 771–791.

DEWITT, D. E., & PAAUW, D. S. (1996). Endocarditis in injection drug users. *American Family Physician, 53,* 2045–2049.

DEYKIN, E. Y., BUKA, D. P. H., & ZEENA, B. S. (1992). Depressive illness among chemically dependent adolescents. *American Journal of Psychiatry, 149,* 1341–1347.

DI BISCEGLIE, A. M. (1995). Chronic hepatitis B. *Postgraduate Medicine, 98,* 99–103.

DICLEMENTE, C. C. (1993). Alcoholics Anonymous and the structure of change. In B. S. McCrady & W. R. Miller (Eds.), *Research on Alcoholics Anonymous.* New Brunswick, NJ: Rutgers Center of Alcohol Studies.

DIETCH, J. (1983). The nature and extent of benzodiazepine abuse: An overview of recent literature. *Hospital and Community Psychiatry, 34,* 1139–1144.

DIFRANZA, J. R., RICHARDS, J. W., PAULMAN, P. M., WOLF-GILLESPIE, N., FLETCHER, C., JAFFE, R. D., & MURRAY, D. (1991). RJR Nabisco's cartoon camel promotes Camel cigarettes to children. *Journal of the American Medical Association, 266,* 3149–3153.

DIFRANZA, J. R., & TYE, J. B. (1990). Who profits from tobacco sales to children? *Journal of the American Medical Association, 263,* 2784–2787.

DIGREGORIO, G. J. (1990). Cocaine update: Abuse and therapy. *American Family Physician, 41*(1), 247–251.

DILAUDID USERS MAY BE ESCAPING DETECTION. (1995). *Forensic Drug Abuse Advisor, 7*(3), 26–27.

DIMEFF, L. A., & MARLATT, G. A. (1995). Relapse prevention. In R. K. Hester & W. R. Miller (Eds.), *Handbook of alcoholism treatment approaches* (2nd ed.). New York: Allyn & Bacon.

DIONNE, R. A., & GORDON, S. M. (1994). Nonsteroidal antiinflammatory drugs for acute pain control. *Dental Clinics of North America, 38,* 645–667.

DIRECTOR, L. (1995). Dual diagnosis: Outpatient treatment of substance abusers with coexisting psychiatric disorders. In A. M. Washton (ed.), *Psychotherapy and substance abuse.* New York: Guilford Press.

DOGHRAMJI, K. (1989). Sleep disorders: A selective update. *Hospital and Community Psychiatry, 40,* 29–40.

DO-IT-YOURSELF DRUG DETECTOR. (1995). *Minneapolis Star-Tribune, XIII*(359), 1A.

DOLE, V. P. (1988). Implications of methadone maintenance for theories of narcotic addiction. *Journal of the American Medical Association, 260,* 3025–3029.

DOLE, V. P. (1989). Letter to the editor. *Journal of the American Medical Association, 261*(13), 1880.

DOLE, V. P. (1995). On Federal regulation of methadone treatment. *Journal of the American Medical Association, 274*(16), 1307.

DOLE, V. P., & NYSWANDER, M. A. (1965). Medical treatment for diacetylmorphine (heroin) addiction. *Journal of the American Medical Association, 193,* 645–656.

DOMENICO, D., & WINDLE, M. (1993). Intrapersonal and interpersonal functioning among middle-aged female adult children of alcoholics. *Journal of Consulting and Clinical Psychology, 61,* 659–666.

DOMINGUEZ, R., VILA-CORO, A. A., AGUIRRE, V. C., SLIPIS, J. M., & BOHAN, T. P. (1991). Brain and ocular abnormalities in infants in utero exposure to cocaine and other street drugs. *American Journal of Diseases of Children, 145,* 688–694.

DONOVAN, D. M. (1992). The assessment process in addictive behaviors. *The Behavior Therapist, 15*(1), 18.

DORIA, J. (1990). Alcohol, women and heart disease. *Alcohol Health & Research World, 14*(4), 349–351.

DORLAND'S ILLUSTRATED MEDICAL DICTIONARY (27th ed.). (1988). Philadelphia: Saunders.

DORSMAN, J. (1996). Improving alcoholism treatment: An overview. *Behavioral Health Management, 16*(1), 26–29.

DOWNING, C. (1990). The wounded healers. *Addiction & Recovery, 10*(3), 21–24.

DRAKE, R. E., & MUESER, K. T. (1996). Alcohol abuse disorder and severe mental illness. *Alcohol Health & Research World, 20,* 87–93.

DRAKE, R. E., MUESER, K. T., CLARK, R. E., & WALLACH, M. A. (1996). The course, treatment,and outcome of substance disorder in persons with severe mental illness. *American Journal of Orthopsychiatry, 66,* 42–51.

DRAKE, R. E., OSHER, F. C., & WALLACH, M. A. (1989). Alcohol use and abuse in schizophrenia. *Journal of Nervous and Mental Disease, 177,* 408–414.

DRAKE, R. E., & WALLACH, M. A. (1989). Substance abuse among the chronic mentally ill. *Hospital and Community Psychiatry, 40,* 1041–1046.

DRAKE, R. E., & WALLACH, M. A. (1993). Moderate drinking among people with severe mental illness. *Hospital and Community Psychiatry, 44,* 780–781.

DREGER, R. M. (1986). Does anyone really believe that alcoholism is a disease? *American Psychologist, 37,* 322.

DREHER, M. C., NUGENT, K., & HUDGINS, R. (1994). Prenatal marijuana exposure and neonatal outcomes in Jamaica: An ethnographic study. *Pediatrics, 93,* 254–260.

DREWS, R. C. (1993). Alcohol and cataract. *Archives of Ophthalmology, 111,* 1312.

DREYFUSS, I. (1989). Federal agency to probe anabolic steroid abuse. *The Physician and Sports Medicine, 17*(7), 16.

DRUG PROBLEMS IN PERSPECTIVE. (1990). *Health News, 8*(3), 1–10.

DUBE, C. E., & LEWIS, DC (1994). Medical education in alcohol and other drugs: Curriculum development for primary care. *Alcohol Health & Research World, 18,*146–155.

DUKE, S. B. (1996). The war on drugs is lost. *National Review, XLVIII*(2), 47–48.

DUMAS, L. (1992). Addicted women. *Nursing Clinics of North America, 27,* 901–915.

DUNLOP, J., MANGHELLI, D., & TOLSON, R. (1989). Senior alcohol and drug coalition statement of treatment philosophy for the elderly. *Professional Counselor, 4*(2), 39–42.

DUNN, G. E., PAOLO, A. M., RYAN, J. J., & VAN FLEET, J. (1993). Dissociative symptoms in a substance abuse population. *American Journal of Psychiatry, 150,* 1043–1047.

DUNNE, F. J. (1994). Misuse of alcohol or drugs by elderly people. *British Medical Journal, 308,* 608–609.

DURANT, R. H., ESCOBEDO, L. G., & HEALTH, G. W. (1995). Anabolic-steroid use, strength training, and multiple drug use among adolescents in the United States. *Pediatrics, 96,* 23–29.

DURANT, R. H., RICKERT, V. I., ASHWORTH, C. S., NEWMAN, C., & SLAVENS, G. (1993). Use of multiple drug among adolescents who use anabolic steroids. *New England Journal of Medicine, 328,* 922–926.

DURELL, J., LECHTENBERG, B., CORSE, S., & FRANCES, R. J. (1993). Intensive case management of persons with chronic mental illness who abuse substances. *Hospital and Community Psychiatry, 44,* 415–416, 428.

DYER, C. (1992). Upjohn claims exoneration after FDA's decision. *British Medical Journal, 305,* 1384.

DYER, C. (1993). Halcion edges its way back into Britain in low doses. *British Medical Journal, 306,* 1085.

DYER, W. W. (1989). *You'll see it when you believe it.* New York: Morrow.

DYGERT, S. L., & MINELLI, M. J. (1993). Heroin abuse progression chart. *Addiction & Recovery, 13*(1), 27–31.

ECCLES, J. S., MIDGLEY, C., WIGFIELD, A., BUCHANAN, C. M., REUMAN, D., FLANAGAN, C., & MACIVER, D. (1993). Development during adolescence. *American Psychologist, 48,* 90–101.

EDELSON, E. (1993). Fear of blood. *Popular Science, 242*(6), 108–111, 122.

EDMEADES, B. (1987). Alcoholics Anonymous celebrates its 50th year. In W. B. Rucker & M. E. Rucker (Eds.), *Drugs, society and behavior.* Guilford, CN: Dashkin.

EDWARDS, M. E., & STEINGLASS, P. (1995). Family therapy treatment outcomes for alcoholism. *Journal of Marital and Family Therapy, 21,* 475–509.

EDWARDS, R. W. (1993). Drug use among 8th grade students is increasing. *International Journal of the Addictions, 28,* 1621–1623.

EFRAN, J. S., HEFFNER, K. P., & LUKENS, R. T. (1987). Alcoholism as an opinion. *Family Therapy Networker, 11*(4), 43–46.

EHRENREICH, B. (1992). Stamping out a dread scourge. *Time, 139*(7), 88.

EHRMAN, M. (1995). Heroin chic. *Playboy, 42*(5), 66–68, 144–147.

EIDELBERG, E., NEER, H. M., & MILLER, M. K. (1965). Anticonvulsant properties of some benzodiazepine derivatives. *Neurology, 15,* 223–230.

EISEN, S. A., LYONS, M. J., GOLDBERG, J., & TRUE, W. R. (1993). The impact of cigarette and alcohol consumption on weight and obesity. *Archives of Internal Medicine, 153,* 2457–2463.

EISENHANDLER, J., & DRUCKER, E. (1993). Opiate dependence among the subscribers of a New York area private insurance plan. *Journal of the American Medical Association, 269,* 2890–2891.

EISON, A. S., & TEMPLE, D. L. (1987). Buspirone: Review of its pharmacology and current perspectives on its mechanism of action. *American Journal of Medicine, 80*(Suppl. 3B), 1–9.

ELDERS, M. J. (1997). Save money, cut crime, get real. *Playboy, 44*(1), 129, 191–192.

ELLIOTT, F. A. (1992). Violence. *Archives of Neurology, 49,* 595–603.

ELLIS, A., MCINERNEY, J. F., DIGIUSEPPE, R., & YEAGER, R. J. (1988). *Rational emotive therapy with alcoholics and substance abusers.* New York: Pergamon Press.

EMONSON, D. L., & VANDERBEEK, R. D. (1995). The use of amphetamines in the U.S. Air Force tactical operations during Desert Shield and Storm. *Aviation, Space and Environmental Medicine, 66*(3), 260–263.

EMRICK, C. D., TONIGAN, S., MONTGOMERY, H., & LITTLE, L. (1993). Alcoholics Anonymous: What is currently known? In B. S. McCrady & W. R. Miller (Eds.), *Research on Alcoholics Anonymous.* New Brunswick, NJ: Rutgers Center of Alcohol Studies.

ENGELMAN, R. (1989). Researcher says quest for intoxication is common throughout animal kingdom. *Minneapolis Star-Tribune, VIII*(173), 12E.

ENGLISH, T. J. (1992). Hong Kong outlaws. *Playboy, 39*(6), 94–96; 168–170.

EPHEDRINE IS USED ILLEGALLY AS A PRECURSOR TO STREET DRUGS. (1995). *The Addiction Letter, 11*(2), 5.

ESMAIL, A., MEYER, L., POTTIER, A., & WRIGHT, S. (1993). Deaths from volatile substance abuse in those under 18 years: Results from a national epidemiological study. *Archives of Disease in Childhood, 69,* 356–360.

ESTROFF, T. W. (1987). Medical and biological consequences of cocaine abuse. In A. M. Washton & M. S. Gold (Eds.), *Cocaine: A clinician's handbook.* New York: Guilford Press.

EUROPEAN DRUG DEALINGS. (1994). *Forensic Drug Abuse Advisor, 6*(10), 79.

EVANKO, D. (1991). Designer drugs. *Postgraduate Medicine, 89*(6), 67–71.

EVANS, G. D. (1993). Cigarette smoke = radiation hazard. *Pediatrics, 92,* 464.

EVANS, K., & SULLIVAN, J. M. (1990). *Dual diagnosis.* New York: Guilford Press.

EVANS, S. M., FUNDERBURK, F. R., & GRIFFITHS, R. R. (1990). Zolpidem and triazolam in humans: Behavioral and subjective effects and abuse liability. *Journal of Pharmacology and Experimental Therapeutics, 255,* 1246–1255.

EWING, J. A. (1984). Detecting alcoholism: The CAGE questionnaire. *Journal of the American Medical Association, 252,* 1905–1907.

FACTS ABOUT ALATEEN. (1969). New York: Al-Anon Family Group Headquarters.

FALLS-STEWART, W., & LUCENTE, S. (1994). Treating obsessive-compulsive disorder among substance abusers: A guide. *Psychology of Addictive Behaviors, 8,* 14–23.

FARIELLO, D., & SCHEIDT, S. (1989). Clinical case management of the dually diagnosed patient. *Hospital and Community Psychiatry, 40,* 1065–1067.

FARROW, J. A. (1990). Adolescent chemical dependency. *Medical Clinics of North America, 74,* 1265–1274.

FASSINGER, R. E. (1991). The hidden minority: Issues and challenges in working with lesbian women and gay men. *Counseling Psychologist, 19,* 157–176.

FAWCETT, J., & BUSCH, K. A. (1995). Stimulants in psychiatry. In A. F. Schatzberg & C. B. Nemeroff (Eds.), *Textbook of psychopharmacology.* Washington, DC: American Psychiatric Association Press.

FDA APPROVES NEW ALCOHOLISM TREATMENT. (1995). *Minneapolis Star-Tribune,* XIII(288), 7A.

FEDERAL DRUG PLANS AND STATISTICS. (1996). *Forensic Drug Abuse Advisor, 8*(6), 46–47.

FEDS SAY HEROIN USE UP, COCAINE AND HEROIN PRICES DOWN, AND COCAINE SNORTING BACK IN FASHION. (1994). *Forensic Drug Abuse Advisor, 6*(6), 41–43.

FEIGHNER, J. P. (1987). Impact of anxiety therapy on patients' quality of life. *American Journal of Medicine, 82*(Suppl. A), 14–19.

FERNANDEZ-SOLA, J., ESTRUCH, R., GRAU, J. M., PARE, J. C., RUBIN, E., & URBANO-MARQUEZ, A. (1994). The relation of alcoholic myopathy to cardiomyopathy. *Annuals of Internal Medicine, 120,* 529–536.

FIGHTING DRUG ABUSE: TOUGH DECISIONS FOR OUR NATIONAL STRATEGY. (1992). Washington, DC: Majority staff of the United States Senate Judiciary Committee.

FIGUEREDO, V. M. (1997). The effects of alcohol on the heart. *Postgraduate Medicine, 101,* 165–176.

FINEBERG, H. V., & WILSON, M. E. (1996). Social vulnerability and death by infection. *New England Journal of Medicine, 334,* 859–860.

FINGARETTE, H. (1988). Alcoholism: The mythical disease. *Utne Reader, 30,* 64–69.

FINGER, W. W., LUND, M., & SLAGEL, M. A. (1997). Medications that may contribute to sexual disorders: A guide to assessment and treatment in family practice. *Journal of Family Practice, 44,* 33–44.

FINNEY, J. W., MOOS, R. H., & CHAN, D. A. (1975). Length of stay and program component effects in the treatment of alcoholism. *Journal of Studies on Alcohol, 36,* 88–108.

FIORE, M. C. (1992). Trends in cigarette smoking in the United States. *Medical Clinics of North America, 76,* 289–303.

FIORE, M. C., EPPS, R. P., & MANLEY, M. W. (1994). A missed opportunity. *Journal of American Medical Association, 271,* 624–626.

FIORE, M. C., JORENBY, D. E., BAKER, T. B., & KENFORD, S. L. (1992). Tobacco dependence and the nicotine patch. *Journal of the American Medical Association, 268,* 2687 2694.

FIORE, M. C., NOVOTNY, T. E., PIERCE, J. P., GIOVINO, G. A., HATZIANDREU, E. J., NEWCOMB, P. A., SURAWICZ, T. S., & DAVIS, R. M. (1990). Methods used to quit smoking in the United States. *Journal of the American Medical Association, 263,* 2760–2765.

FIORE, M. C., SMITH, S. S., JORENBY, D. E., & BAKER, T. B. (1994). The effectiveness of the nicotine patch for smoking cessation. *Journal of the American Medical Association, 271,* 1940–1947.

FISCHBACH, G. D. (1992). Mind and brain. *Scientific American, 267*(3), 48–57.

FISCHER, C., HATZIDIMITRIOU, G., WLOS, J., KLATZ, J., & RICAURTE, G. (1995). Reorganization of ascending 5-HT axon projections in animals previously exposed to recreational drug 3,4-methelenedioxymethamphetamine (MDMA, "Ecstasy"). *Journal of Neuroscience, 15,* 5476–5485.

FISCHER, R. G. (1989). Clinical use of nonsteroidal anti-inflammatory drugs. *Pharmacy Times, 55*(8), 31–35.

FISHER, M. S., & BENTLEY, K. J. (1996). Two group therapy models for clients with a dual diagnosis of substance abuse and personality disorder. *Psychiatric Services, 47,* 1244–1250.

FISHMAN, R. H. B. (1996). Normal development after prenatal heroin. *Lancet, 347,* 1397.

FISHMAN, S. M., & CARR, D. B. (1992). Clinical issues in pain management. *Contemporary Medicine, 4*(10), 92–103.

FLAUM, M., & SCHULTZ, S. K. (1996). When does amphetamine-induced psychosis become schizophrenia? *American Journal of Psychiatry, 153,* 812–815.

FLEGAL, K. M., TROIANO, R. P., PAMUK, E. R., KUCZMARSKI, R. J., & CAMPBELL, S. M. (1995). The influence of smoking cessation on the prevalence of overweight in the United States. *New England Journal of Medicine, 333,* 1165–1170.

FLEMING, N. F., POTTER, D., & KETTYLE, C. (1996). What are substance abuse and addiction? In L. Friedman, N. F. Fleming, D. H. Roberts, & S. E. Hyman (Eds.), *Source book of substance abuse and addiction.* New York: Williams & Wilkins.

FLETCHER, J. M., PAGE, J. B., FRANCIS, D. J., COPELAND, K., NAUS, M. J., DAVIS, C. M., MORRIS, R., KRAUSKOPF, D., & SATZ, P. (1996). Cognitive correlates of long-term cannabis use in Costa Rican men. *Archives of General Psychiatry, 53,* 1051–1057.

FLYNN, P. M. (1996). Hepatitis C infections. *Pediatric Annals, 25,* 496–500.

FOA, P. P. (1989). Letters to the editor. *Smithsonian, 20*(6), 18.

FOLEY, K. M. (1993). Opioids. *Neurologic Clinics, 11,* 503–522.

FONTHAM, E. T. H., CORREA, P., REYNOLDS, P., WU-WILLIAMS, A., BUFFLER, P. A., GREENBERG, R. S., CHEN, V., ALTERMAN, T., BOYD, P., AUSTIN, D. F., & LIFF, J. (1994). Environmental tobacco smoke and lung cancer in nonsmoking women. *Journal of the American Medical Association, 271,* 1752–1759.

FORNAZZAZRI, L. (1988). Clinical recognition and management of solvent abusers. *Internal Medicine for the Specialist, 9*(6), 99–108.

FORUM. (1991). *Playboy, 38*(1), 52.

FOULKS, E. F., & PENA, J. M. (1995). Ethnicity and psychotherapy. *Psychiatric Clinics of North America, 18,* 607–620.

FRANCES, R. J. (1991). Should drugs be legalized? Implications of the debate for the mental health field. *Hospital and Community Psychiatry, 42,* 119–120, 125.

FRANCES, R. J., & MILLER, S. I. (1991). Addiction treatment: The widening scope. R. J. In Frances & S. I. Miller (Eds.), *Clinical textbook of addictive disorders.* New York: Guilford Press.

FRANK, D. A., BAUCHNER, H., ZUCKERMAN, B. S., & FRIED, L. (1992). Cocaine and marijuana use during pregnancy by women intending and not intending to breast feed. *Journal of the American Dietetic Association, 92,* 215–217.

FRANKLIN, J. (1987). *Molecules of the mind.* New York: Dell.

FRANKLIN, J. E. (1989). Alcoholism among blacks. *Hospital and Community Psychiatry, 40,* 1120–1122, 1127.

FRANKLIN, J. E. (1994). Addiction medicine. *Journal of the American Medical Association, 271,* 1650–1651.

FRANKS, P., HARP, J., & BELL, B. (1989). Randomized, controlled trial of clonidine for smoking cessation in a primary care setting. *New England Journal of Medicine, 321,* 3011–3013.

FREDERICKSON, P. A., RICHARDSON, J. W., ESTHER, M. S., & LIN, S. (1990). Sleep disorders in psychiatric practice. *Mayo Clinic Procedures, 65,* 861–868.

FREEBORN, D. (1996). By the numbers. *Minneapolis Star-Tribune, XV*(94), D2.

FREIBERG, P. (1991). Panel hears of families victimized by alcoholism. *APA Monitor, 22*(4), 30.

FREIBERG, P. (1996). New drugs give hope to AIDS patients. *APA Monitor, 27*(6), 28.

FRENCH, M. T. (1995). Economic evaluation of drug abuse treatment programs: Methodology and findings. *American Journal of Drug and Alcohol Abuse, 21*(1), 111–135.

FREZZA, M., DI PADOVA, C., POZZATO, G., TERPIN, M., BARAONA, E., & LIEBER, C. S. (1990). High blood alcohol levels in women. *New England Journal of Medicine, 322,* 95–99.

FRIEDMAN, D. (1987) Toxic effects of marijuana. *Alcoholism & Addiction, 7*(6), 47.

FRIEDMAN, L. N., WILLIAMS, W. T., SINGH, T. P., & FRIEDEN, T. R. (1996). Tuberculosis, AIDS, and death among substance abusers on welfare in New York City. *New England Journal of Medicine, 334,* 828–833.

FRIEDMAN, R. C., & DOWNEY, J. I. (1994). Homosexuality. *New England Journal of Medicine, 331,* 923–930.

FROMM, E. (1956). *The art of loving.* New York: Harper & Row.

FROMM, E. (1968). *The revolution of hope.* New York: Harper & Row.

FUDALA, P. J., & JOHNSON, R. E. (1995). Clinical efficacy studies of buprenorphine for the treatment of opioid dependence. In A. Cowan & J. W. Lewis (Eds.), *Buprenorphine.* New York: Wiley-Liss.

FULLER, P. G., & CABANAUGH, R. M. (1995). Basic assessment and screening for substance abuse in the pediatrician's office. *Pediatric Clinics of North America, 42,* 295–307.

FULLER, R. K. (1989). Antidipsotropic medications. In R. K. Hester & W. R. Miller (Eds.), *Handbook of alcoholism treatment approaches.* New York: Pergamon Press.

FULLER, R. K. (1995). Antidipsotropic medications. In R. K. Hester & W. R. Miller (Eds.), *Handbook of alcoholism treatment approaches* (2nd ed.). New York: Allyn & Bacon.

FULTON, J. S., & JOHNSON, G. B. (1993). Using high-dose morphine to relieve cancer pain. *Nursing '93, 23*(2), 35–39.

FULTZ, O. (1991). 'Roid rage. *American Health, X*(4), 60–64.

FURSTENBERG, F. F. (1990). Coming of age in a changing family system. In S. S. Feldman & G. R. Elliott (Eds.),

At the threshold. Cambridge, MA: Harvard University Press.

GABRIEL, T. (1994). Heroin finds a new market along cutting edge of style. *The New York Times, CXLIII*(49,690), 1, 17.

GALANTER, M. (1993). Network therapy for addiction: A model for office practice. *American Journal of Psychiatry, 150*, 28–36.

GALANTER, M., CASTANEDA, R., & FRANCO, H. (1991). Group therapy and self-help groups. In R. J. Frances & S. I. Miller (Eds.), *Clinical textbook of addictive disorders*. New York: Guilford Press.

GALANTER, M., & FRANCES, R. (1992). Addiction psychiatry: Challenges for a new psychiatric subspeciality. *Hospital and Community Psychiatry, 43*, 1067–1068, 1072.

GALLAGHER, W. (1986). The looming menace of designer drugs. *Designer, 7*(8), 24–35.

GALLIC HEARTS. (1994). *Discover, 15*(9), 14–15.

GALLO, R. C., & MONTAGNIER, L. (1988). Aids in 1988. *Scientific American, 259*(4), 41–48.

GANNON, K. (1994). OTC naproxen sodium set to shake OTC analgesics. *Drug Topics, 138*(3), 34.

GARBARINO, J., DUBROW, N., KOSTELNY, K., & PARDO, C. (1992). *Children in danger*. New York: Jossey-Bass.

GARRETT, L. (1994). *The coming plague*. New York: Farrar, Straus and Giroux.

GARRO, A. J., ESPINA, N., & LIEBER, C. S. (1992). Alcohol and cancer. *Alcohol Health & Research World, 16*(1), 81–85.

GARRY, P. (1995). Oh, judge, can't you make them stop picking on me? *Minneapolis Star-Tribune, XIV*(106), 10A.

GAWIN, F. H., ALLEN, D., & HUMBLESTONE, B. (1989). Outpatient treatment of "Crack" cocaine smoking with flupenthixol deconate: A preliminary report. *Archives of General Psychiatry, 46*, 122–126.

GAWIN, F. H., & ELLINWOOD, E. H. (1988). Cocaine and other stimulants: Actions, abuse, and treatment. *New England Journal of Medicine, 318*, 1173–1182.

GAWIN, F. H., KHALSA, M. E., & ELLINWOOD, E. (1994). Stimulants. In M. Galanter & H. D. Kleber (Eds.), *Textbook of substance abuse treatment*. Washington, DC: American Psychiatric Press.

GAWIN, F. H., & KLEBER, H. D. (1986). Abstinence symptomology and psychiatric diagnosis in cocaine abusers. *Achieves of General Psychiatry, 43*, 107–113.

GAWIN, F. H., KLEBER, H. D., BYCK, R., ROUNSAVILLE, B. J., KOSTEN, T. R., JATLOW, P. I., & MORGAN, C. (1989). Desipramine facilitation of initial cocaine abstinence. *Archives of General Psychiatry, 46*, 117–121.

GAY, G. R. (1990). Another side effects of NSAIDs. *Journal of the American Medical Association, 164*, 2677–2678.

GAZZANIGA, M. S. (1988). *Mind matters*. Boston: Houghton Mifflin.

GELERNTER, J., GOLDMAN, D., & RISCH, N. (1993). The A1 allele at the D_2 dopamine receptor gene and alcoholism. *Journal of the American Medical Association, 269*, 1673–1677.

GELLES, R. J., & STRAUS, M. A. (1988). *Intimate violence: The definitive study of the causes and consequences of abuse in the American family*. New York: Simon & Schuster.

GELMAN, D., UNDERWOOD, A., KING, P., HAGER, M., & GORDON, J. (1990). Some things work! *Newsweek, CXVI*(13), 78–81.

GENTILELLO, L. M., DONOVAN, D. M., DUNN, C. W., & RIVARA, F. P. (1995). Alcohol interventions in trauma centers: Current practice and future directions. *Journal of the American Medical Center, 274*, 1043–1048.

GEORGE, A. A., & TUCKER, J. A. (1996). Help-seeking for alcohol-related problems: Social contexts surrounding entry into alcoholism treatment or Alcoholics Anonymous. *Journal of Studies on Alcohol, 57*, 449–457.

GIACONA, N. S., DAHL, S. L., & HARE, B. D. (1987). The role of nonsteroidal antiinflammatory drugs and non-narcotics in analgesia. *Hospital Formulary, 22*, 723–733.

GILBERTSON, P. K., & WEINBERG, J. (1992). Fetal alcohol syndrome and functioning of the immune system. *Alcohol Health & Research World, 16*(1), 29–38.

GILLIN, J. C. (1991). The long and the short of sleeping pills. *New England Journal of Medicine, 324*, 1735–1736.

GILMAN, S. (1992). Advances in neurology. *New England Journal of Medicine, 326*, 1608–1616.

GIOVANNUCCI, E., RIMM, E. B., SAMPFER, M. J., COLDITZ, G. A., ASCHERIO, A., & WILLETT, W. C. (1994). Aspirin use and the risk for colorectal cancer and adenoma in male health professionals. *Annals of Internal Medicine, 121*, 241–246.

GIUNTA, C. T., & COMPAS, B. E. (1994). Adult daughters of alcoholics: Are they unique? *Journal of Studies on Alcohol, 55*, 600–606.

GLANTZ, J. C., & WOODS, J. R. (1993). Cocaine, heroin, and phencyclidine: Obstetric perspectives. *Clinical Obstetrics and Gynecology, 36*, 279–301.

GLANTZ, S., & PARMLEY, W. W. (1995). Passive smoking and heart disease. *Journal of the American Medical Association, 273*, 1047–1053.

GLANTZ, S. A., BARNES, D. E., BEREO, L., HANAUER, P., & SLADE, J. (1995). Looking through a keyhole at the tobacco industry. *Journal of the American Medical Association, 274*, 219–224.

GLANTZ, S. A., SLADE, J., BEREO, L. A., HANAUER, P., & BARNES, D. E. (1996). *The cigarette papers*. Los Angeles: University of California Press.

GLASER, F. B., & OGBORNE, A. C. (1982). Does AA really work? *British Journal of the Addictions, 77*, 88–92.

GLASNER, P. D., & KASLOW, R. A. (1990). The epidemiology of human immunodeficiency virus infection.

Journal of Clinical and Consulting Psychology, 58, 13–21.

GLASS, R. M. (1993). Methadone maintenance. *Journal of the American Medical Association, 269,* 1995–1996.

GLASSMAN, A. H. (1993). Cigarette smoking: Implications for psychiatric illness. *American Journal of Psychiatry, 150,* 546–553.

GLASSMAN, A. H., STETNER, F., WALSH, T., RAIZMAN, P. S., FLEISS, J. L., COOPER, T. B., & COVEY, L. S. (1988). Heavy smokers, smoking cessation and clonidine. *Journal of the American Medical Association, 259,* 2863–2866.

GLEICK, E. (1996). Tobacco blues. *Time, 147*(11), 54–55, 57–58, 60.

GLOWA, J. R. (1986). *Inhalants: The toxic fumes.* New York: Chelsea House.

GODLASKI, T. M., LEUKEFELD, C., & CLOUD, R. (1997). Recovery: With and without selfhelp. *Substance Use & Misuse, 32,* 621–627.

GOLD, D. R., WANG, X., WYPIJ, D., SPEIZER, F. E., WARE, J. E., & DOCKERY, D. W. (1996). Effects of cigarette smoking on lung function in adolescent boys and girls. *New England Journal of Medicine, 335,* 931–937.

GOLD, M. S. (1988). Alcohol, drugs, and sexual dysfunction. *Alcoholism & Addiction, 9*(2), 13.

GOLD, M. S. (1989a). Medical implications of cocaine intoxication. *Alcoholism & Addiction, 9*(3), 16.

GOLD, M. S. (1989b). Opiates. In A. J. Giannini & A. E. Slaby (Eds.), *Drugs of abuse.* Oradell, NJ: Medical Economics Books.

GOLD, M. S. (1990a). Weekend warriors and addicts. *Alcoholism & Addiction, 10*(3), 12.

GOLD, M. S. (1990b). Another Ice age? *Alcoholism & Addiction, 10*(2), 10.

GOLD, M. S. (1993). Opiate addiction and the locus coeruleus. *Psychiatric Clinics of North America, 16,* 61–73.

GOLD, M. S., & PALUMBO, J. M. (1991). The future treatment of cocaine addiction. *Alcohol & Addiction, 11*(3), 35–37.

GOLD, M. S., SCHUCHARD, K., & GLEATON, T. (1994). LSD use among US high school students. *Journal of the American Medical Association, 271,* 426–427.

GOLD, M. S., & VEREBEY, K. (1984). The psychopharmacology of cocaine. *Psychiatric Annuals, 14,* 714–723.

GOLDMAN, B. (1991). How to thwart a drug seeker. *Emergency Medicine, 23*(6), 48–61.

GOLDSCHMIDT, R. D., & MOY, A. (1996). Antiretroviral drug treatment for HIV/AIDS. *American Family Physician, 54,* 574–580.

GOLDSTEIN, M. Z., PATAKI, A., & WEBB, M. T. (1996). Alcoholism among elderly persons. *Psychiatric Services, 47,* 941–943.

GOLDSTEIN, P. (1990). *Drugs and violence.* Paper presented at the 1990 meeting of the American Psychological Association, Boston.

GOLDSTONE, M. S. (1993). "Cat": Methcathinone, a new drug of abuse. *Journal of the American Medical Association, 269,* 2508.

GONDALF, E. W., & FOSTER, R. A. (1991). Wife assault among VA alcohol rehabilitation patients. *Hospital and Community Psychiatry, 42,* 74–79.

GONZALES, J. J., STERN, T. A., EMMERICH, A. D., & RAUCH, S. L. (1992). Recognition and management of benzodiazepine dependence. *American Family Physician, 45,* 2269–2276.

GOODWIN, D. W. (1989). Alcoholism. In H. I. Kaplan & B. J. Sadock (Eds.), *Comprehensive textbook of psychiatry* (Vol. V). Baltimore: Williams & Wilkins.

GOODWIN, D. W. (1991). Inpatient treatment of alcoholism—new life for the Minneapolis plan. *New England Journal of Medicine, 325,* 804–806.

GOODWIN, D. W., & WARNOCK, J. K. (1991). Alcoholism: A family disease. In R. J. Frances & S. I. Miller (Eds.), *Clinical textbook of addictive disorders.* New York: Guilford Press.

GORDIS, E. (1995). The National Institute on Alcohol Abuse and Alcoholism. *Alcohol Health & Research World, 19,* 5–11.

GORDIS, E. (1996a). Alcohol research. *Archives of General Psychiatry, 53,* 199–201.

GORDIS, E. (1996b). Drinking and driving—A commentary by NIAAA director Enoch Gordis, M. D. *Alcohol Alert, 31,* 3.

GORSKI, T. T. (1992). Diagnosing codependence. *Addiction & Recovery, 12*(7), 14–16.

GORSKI, T. T. (1993). Relapse prevention. *Addiction & Recovery, 13*(2), 25–27.

GOSSOP, M., BATTERSBY, M., & STRANG, J. (1991). Self-detoxification by opiate addicts. *British Journal of Psychiatry, 159,* 208–212.

GOTTESMAN, J. (1992). Little is known about effects of steroids on women. *Minneapolis Star-Tribune, XI*(211), 7C.

GOTTLIEB, A., POPE, S., RICKERT, V. I., & HARDIN, B. H. (1993). Patterns of smokeless tobacco use by young adolescents. *Pediatrics, 91,* 75–78.

GOTTLIEB, A. M. (1997). Crisis of consciousness. *Utne Reader, 79,* 45–48.

GOTTLIEB, A. M., KILLEN, J. D., MARLATT, G. A., & TAYLOR, C. B. (1987). Psychological and pharmacological influences in cigarette smoking withdrawal: Effects of nicotine gum and expectancy on smoking withdrawal symptoms and relapse. *Journal of Clinical and Consulting Psychology, 55,* 606–608.

GOTTLIEB, M. I. (1994). Alcohol and pregnancy: A potential for disaster. *Emergency Medicine, 26*(1), 73–79.

GOURLAY, S. G., & BENOWITZ, N. L. (1995). Is clonidine an effective smoking cessation therapy? *Drugs, 50,* 197–207.

GRAEDON, J., & FERGUSON, T. (1993). *The aspirin handbook.* New York: Bantam Books.

GRAEDON, J., & GRAEDON, T. (1991). *Graedons' best medicine.* New York: Bantam Books.

GRAEDON, J., & GRAEDON, T. (1995). *The people's guide to deadly drug interactions.* New York: St. Martin's Press.

GRAEDON, J., & GRAEDON, T. (1996). *The people's pharmacy—revised.* New York: St. Martin's Griffin.

GRAFF, J. L., RIVERA, E., SIMMONS, A. M., & WILLERTH, J. (1996). Kids and pot. *Time, 148*(26), 26–30.

GRAHAM, B. (1988). The abuse of alcohol: Disease or disgrace? *Alcoholism & Addiction, 8*(4), 14–15.

GRAHAM, J. R. (1990). *MMPI-2 assessing personality and psychopathology.* New York: Oxford University Press.

GRAHAM, M. (1989). One toke over the line. *The New Republic, 200*(16), 20–22.

GRAHAM, P. (1996). Alcohol and the young. *Archives of Disease in Childhood, 75,* 361–363.

GRANT, I. (1987). Alcohol and the brain: Neuropsychological correlates. *Journal of Clinical and Consulting Psychology, 55,* 310–324.

GRANT, P. D., & HEATON, R. K. (1990). Human immunodeficiency virus—type 1 (HIV-1) and the brain. *Journal of Clinical and Consulting Psychology, 58,* 22–30.

GREDEN, J. F., & WALTERS, A. (1992). Caffeine. In J. H. Lowinson, P. Ruiz, R. Millman, & J. G. Langrod (Eds.), *Substance abuse: A comprehensive textbook* (2nd ed). New York: Williams & Wilkins.

GREENBAUM, P. E., FOSTER-JOHNSON, L., & PETRILA, A. (1996). Co-occuring addictive and mental disorders among adolescents: Prevalence research and future directions. *American Journal of Orthopsychiatry, 66,* 52–60.

GREENBERG, D. A. (1993). Ethanol and sedatives. *Neurologic Clinics, 11,* 523–534.

GREENE, W. C. (1993). AIDS and the immune system. *Scientific American, 269*(3), 99–105.

GRIFFIN, M. L., WEISS, R. D., MIRIN, S. M., & LANG, U. (1989). A comparison of male and female cocaine abusers. *Archives of General Psychiatry, 46,* 122–126.

GRIFFITHS, H. J., PARANTAINEN, H., & OLSON, P. (1994). Alcohol and bone disorders. *Alcohol Health & Research World, 17,* 299–304.

GRIGG, W. (1992). Don't bet your life on statistics. *Minneapolis Star-Tribune, XI*(106), 23A.

GRINSPOON, L., & BAKALAR, J. B. (1990). What is phencyclidine? *Harvard Medical School Mental Health Letter, 6*(7), 8.

GRINSPOON, L., & BAKALAR, J. B. (1992). Marijuana. In J. H. Lowinson, P. Ruiz, R. B. Millman, & J. G. Langrod (Eds.), *Substance abuse: A comprehensive textbook* (2nd ed.). New York: Williams & Wilkins.

GRINSPOON, L., & BAKALAR, J. B. (1993). *Marijuana: The forgotten medicine.* New Haven, CT: Yale University Press.

GRINSPOON, L., & BAKALAR, J. B. (1995). Marijuana as medicine. *Journal of the American Medical Association, 273,* 1875–1876.

GRINSPOON, L., & BAKALAR, J. B. (1997). Smoke screen. *Playboy, 44*(6), 49–53.

GROB, L. H., BRAVO, G., & WALSH, R. (1990). Second thoughts on 3, 4-methylenedioxymethamphetamine (MDMA) neurotoxicity. *Archives of General Psychiatry, 47,* 288.

GROUP FOR THE ADVANCEMENT OF PSYCHIATRY. (1990). Substance abuse disorders: A psychiatric priority. *American Journal of Psychiatry, 148,* 1291–1300.

GROUP, THE. (1976). Narcotics Anonymous World Service Office, Inc.

GROUPS OFFER SELF-HELP ALTERNATIVES TO AA. (1991). *Alcoholism & Drug Abuse Week, 3*(37), 6.

GROVER, S. A., GRAY-DONALD, K., JOSEPH, L., ABRAHAMOWICZ, M., & COUPAL, L. (1994). Life expectancy following dietary modification or smoking cessation. *Archives of Internal Medicine, 154,* 1697–1704.

GUSLANDI, M. (1997). Gastric toxicity of antiplatelet therapy with low-dose aspirin. *Drugs, 53,* 1–5.

GUTTMAN, M. (1996). The new pot culture. *Minneapolis Star-Tribune, XIV*(318), USA Weekend 4–7.

HALL, S. M., HAVASSY, B. E., & WASSERMAN, D. A. (1991). Effects of commitment to abstinence, positive moods, stress and coping on relapse to cocaine use. *Journal of Consulting and Clinical Psychology, 59,* 526–532.

HALL, W., & SANNIBALE, C. (1996). Are there two types of alcoholism? *Lancet, 348,* 1258.

HALL, W. C., TALBERT, R. L., & ERESHEFSKY, L. (1990). Cocaine abuse and its treatment. *Pharmacotherapy, 10*(1), 47–65.

HAMNER, M. B. (1993). PTSD and cocaine abuse. *Hospital and Community Psychiatry, 44,* 591–592.

HAND, R. P. (1989). Taking another look at triazolam—Is this drug safe? *Focus on pharmacology: Theory and practice, 11*(6), 1–3.

HANDELSMAN, L., ARONSON, M. J., NESS. R., COCHRANE, K. J., & KANOF, P. D. (1992). The dysphoria of heroin addiction. *American Journal of Drug and Alcohol Abuse, 18*(3), 275–287.

HANKINSON, S. E., WILLETT, W. C., COLDITZ, G. A., SEDDON, J. M., ROSNER, B., SPEIZER, F. E., & STAMPFER, M. J. (1992). A prospective study of cigarette smoking and risk of cataract surgery in women. *Journal of the American Medical Association, 268,* 994–998.

HANSEN, W. B., & ROSE, L. A. (1995). Recreational use of inhalant drugs by adolescents: A challenge for family physicians. *Family Medicine, 27,* 383–387.

HARRIS, M., & BACHRACH, L. L. (1990). Perspectives on homeless mentally ill women. *Hospital & Community Psychiatry, 41,* 253–254.

HARTMAN, D. E. (1995). *Neuropsychological toxicology* (2nd ed.). New York: Plenum Press.

HARTMANN, P. M. (1995). Drug treatment of insomnia: Indications and newer agents. *American Family Physician, 51*(1), 191–194.

HATFIELD, A. B. (1989). Patients' accounts of stress and coping in schizophrenia. *Hospital and Community Psychiatry, 40*, 1141–1145.

HATSUKAMI, D. K., & FISCHMAN, M. W. (1996). Crack cocaine and cocaine hydrochloride. *Journal of the American Medical Association, 276*, 1580–1588.

HAVERKOS, H. W., & STEIN, M. D. (1995). Identifying substance abuse in primary care. *American Family Physician, 52*, 2029–2035.

HAWKES, C. H. (1992). Endorphins: The basis of pleasure? *Journal of Neurology, Neurosurgery and Psychiatry, 55*, 247–250.

HAWLEY, T. L., HALLE, T. G., DRASIN, R. E., & THOMAS, N. G. (1995). Children of addicted mothers' effects of the "crack epidemic" on the caregiving environment and the development of preschoolers. *American Journal of Orthopsychiatry, 65*(3), 364–379.

HAYNER, G. N., & McKINNEY, H. (1986). MDMA: The dark side of ecstasy. *Journal of Psychoactive Drugs, 18*(4), 341–347.

HAYNES, B. F. (1996). HIV vaccines: Where we are and were we are going. *Lancet, 348*, 933–937.

HEADDEN, S. (1996). Guns, money and medicine. *U.S. News & World Report, 121*(1), 30–40.

HEALTH SPENDING CRITICIZED. (1996). *Wisconsin State Journal, 157*(260), 1A, 3A.

HEARN, W. (1995). Considering cannabis. *American Medical News, 38*(37), 18–24.

HEATH, D. B. (1994). Inhalant abuse. *Behavioral Health Management, 14*(3), 47–48.

HEATON, R. K. (1990). Introduction to the special series on acquired immune deficiency syndrome (AIDS). *Journal of Consulting and Clinical Psychology, 58*, 3–4.

HEEREMA, D. L. (1990). Drug use in the 1990's. *Business Horizons, 33*(1), 127–132.

HEESCH, C. M., NEGUS, B. H., STEINER, M., SNYDER, R. W., McINTIRE, D. D., GRAYBURN, P. A., ASHCRAFT, J., HERNANDEZ, J. A., & EICHORN, E. J. (1996). Effects of in vivo cocaine administration on human platelet aggregation. *American Journal of Cardiology 78*, 237–239.

HEIMEL, C. (1990). Its now, it's trendy, it's codependency. *Playboy, 37*(5), 43.

HEIMEL, C. (1991). Sickos "R" us. *Playboy, 38*(9), 42.

HEINZ, A., DUFEU, P., KUHN, S., DETTLING, M., GRAF, K., KURTEN, I., ROMMELSPACHER, H., & SCHMIDT, L. G. (1996). Psychopathological and behavioral correlates of dopaminergic sensitivity in alcohol-dependent patients. *Archives of General Psychiatry, 53*, 1123–1128.

HELLINGER, F. J. (1993). The lifetime cost of treating a person with HIV. *Journal of the American Medical Association, 270*, 474–478.

HELLMAN, R. E., STANTON, M., LEE, J., TYTUN, A., & VACHON, R. (1989). Treatment of homosexual alcoholics in government-funded agencies: Provider training and attitudes. *Hospital and Community Psychiatry, 40*, 1163–1168.

HELZER, J. E., ROBINS, L. N., TAYLOR, J. R., CAREY, K., MILLER, R. H., COMBS-ORME, T., & FARMER, A. (1985). The extent of long-term moderate drinking among alcoholics discharged from medical and psychiatric treatment facilities. *New England Journal of Medicine, 312*, 1678–1682.

HENDERSON, L. A. (1994a). About LSD. In L. A. Henderson & W. J. Glass (Eds.), *LSD: Still with us after all these years.* New York: Lexington Books.

HENDERSON, L. A. (1994b). Adverse reactions. In L. A. Henderson & W. J. Glass (Eds.), *LSD: Still with us after all these years.* New York: Lexington Books.

HENNEKENS, C. H., JONAS, M. A., & BURING, J. E. (1994). The benefits of aspirin in acute myocardial infarction. *Archives of Internal Medicine, 154*, 37–39.

HENNESSEY, M. B. (1992). Identifying the woman with alcohol problems. *Nursing Clinics of North America, 27*, 917–924.

HENNINGFIELD, J. E. (1995). Nicotine medications for smoking cessation. *New England Journal of Medicine, 333*, 1196–1203.

HENNINGFIELD, J. E., & NEMETH-COSLETT, R. (1988). Nicotine dependence. *Chest, 93*(2), 37s–55s.

HENRETIG, F. (1996). Inhalant abuse in children and adolescents. *Pediatric Annals, 25*(1), 47–52.

HENRY, J. A. (1996). Management of drug abuse emergencies. *Journal of Accident & Emergency Medicine, 13*, 370–372.

HENRY, J. A., JEFFREYS, J. A., & DAWLING, S. (1992). Toxicity and deaths from 3, 4-methylenedioxymethamphetamine ("ecstasy"). *Lancet, 340*, 384–387.

HERMAN, E. (1988). The twelve step program: Cure or cover? *Utne Reader, 30*, 52–53.

HERMAN, R. (1993). Alcohol debate may drive you to drink. *St. Paul Pioneer Press, 144*(356), 11G.

HEROIN IS BACK, WITH YOUNGER USERS. (1994). *The Addiction Letter, 10*(11), 1–3.

HEROIN SMOKING ANALYZED BY SWISS RESEARCHERS. (1996). *Forensic Drug Abuse Advisor, 8*(10), 78–79.

HERRERA, S. (1997). The morphine myth. *Forbes, 159*, 258–260.

HESTER, R. K. (1994). Outcome research: Alcoholism. In M. Galanter & H. D. Kleber (Eds.), *Textbook of substance abuse treatment.* Washington, DC: American Psychiatric Press.

HESTER, R. K. (1995). Self-control training. In R. K. Hester & W. R. Miller (Eds.), *Handbook of alcoholism treatment approaches.* New York: Allyn & Bacon.

HIBBS, J., PERPER, J., & WINEK, C. L. (1991). An outbreak of designer drug-related deaths in Pennsylvania. *Journal of the American Medical Association, 265*, 1011–1013.

HIGGINS, J. P., WRIGHT, S. W., & WRENN, K. D. (1996). Alcohol, the elderly, and motor vehicle crashes. *American Journal of Emergency Medicine, 14*, 265–267.

HIGH COURT WEIGHS SCHOOL DRUG TESTING. (1995). *Minneapolis Star-Tribune*, XIII(359), 7A.

HILL, S. Y., (1995). Vulnerability to alcoholism in women. In M. Galanter (Ed.), *Recent developments in alcoholism* (Vol. 12). New York: Plenum Press.

HILTS, P. J. (1994). Labeling on cigarettes called a smoke screen. *St. Paul Pioneer Press*, 146(5), 1A, 6A.

HILTS, P. J. (1996). *Smoke screen.* New York: Addison-Wesley.

HINGSON, R. (1996). Prevention of drinking and driving. *Alcohol Health & Research World*, 20, 219–226.

HIRSCH, D., PALEY, J. E., & RENNER, J. A. (1996). Opiates. In L. Friedman, N. F. Fleming, D. H. Roberts, & S. E. Hyman (Eds.), *Source book of substance abuse and addiction.* New York: Williams & Wilkins.

HIRSCHFIELD, R. M. A., & DAVIDSON, L. (1988). Risk factors for suicide. In A. J. Frances & R. E. Hales (Eds.), *Review of psychiatry* (Vol. 7). Washington, DC: American Psychiatric Association Press.

HITCHCOCK, H. C., STAINBACK, R. D., & ROQUE, G. M. (1995). Effects of halfway house placement on retention of patients in substance abuse aftercare. *American Journal of Drug and Alcohol Abuse*, 21, 379–391.

HOBBS, W. R., RALL, T. W., & VERDOORN, T. A. (1995). Hypnotics and sedatives; ethanol. In J. G. Hardman & L. E. Limbird (Editors-in-Chief), *The pharmacological basis of therapeutics* (9th ed.). New York: McGraw-Hill.

HOBERMAN, J. M., & YESALIS, C. E. (1995). The history of synthetic testosterone. *Scientific American*, 272(2), 76–81.

HOBSON, J. A. (1989). Dream theory: A new view of the brain-mind. *Harvard Medical School Mental Health Letter*, 5(8), 3–5.

HOCHBERG, M. C. (1992). NSAIDs: Mechanisms and pathways of actions. *Hospital Practice*, 24(3), 185–198.

HOEGERMAN, G., & SCHNOLL, S. (1991). Narcotic use in pregnancy. *Clinics in Perinatology*, 18, 52–76.

HOEKSEMA, H. L., & DE BOCK, G. H. (1993). The value of laboratory tests for the screening and recognition of alcohol abuse in primary care patients. *Journal of Family Practice*, 37, 268–276.

HOFFMAN, B. B., & LEFKOWITZ, R. J. (1990). Catecholamines and sympathomimetic drugs. In A. G. Gilman, T. W. Rall, A. S. Nies, & P. Taylor (Eds.), *The pharmacological basis of therapeutics* (8th ed.). New York: Pergamon Press.

HOFFMANN, N. G., BELILLE, C. A., & HARRISON, P. A. (1987). Adequate resources for a complex population? *Alcoholism & Addiction*, 7(5), 17.

HOFFNAGLE, J. H., & DI BISCEGLIE, A. M. (1997). The treatment of chronic viral hepatitis. *New England Journal of Medicine*, 336, 347–356.

HOLDER, H., LONGABAUGH, R., MILLER, W. R., & RUBONIS, A. V. (1991). The cost effectiveness of treatment for alcoholism: A first approximation. *Journal of Studies on Alcohol*, 52, 517–540.

HOLLAND, W. W., & FITZSIMONS, B. (1991). Smoking in children. *Archives of Disease in Childhood*, 66, 1269–1270.

HOLLANDER, H., & KATZ, M. H. (1993). HIV Infection. In L. M. Tierney, S. J. McPhee, M. A. Papadakis, & S. A. Schroeder (Eds.), *Current medical diagnosis & treatment.* Norwalk, CT: Appleton & Lange.

HOLLANDER, J. E. (1995). The management of cocaine-associated myocardial ischemia. *New England Journal of Medicine*, 333, 1267–1271.

HOLLANDER, J. E., HOFFMAN, R. S., BURNSTEIN, J. L., SHIH, R. D., & THODE, H. C. (1995). Cocaine-associated myocardial infarction. *Archives of Internal Medicine*, 155,1081–1086.

HOLLANDER, J. E., SHIH, R. D., HOFFMAN, R. S., HARCHELROAD, F. P., PHILLIPS, S., BRENT, J., KULIG, K., & THODE, H. C. (1997). Predictors of coronary artery disease in patients with cocaine-associated myocardial infarction. *American Journal of Medicine*, 102, 159–163.

HOLLANDER, J. E., TODD, K. H., GREEN, G., HEILPERN, K. L., KARRAS, D. J., SINGER, A. J., BROGAN, G. X., FUNK, J. P., & STRAHAN, J. B. (1995). Chest pain associated with cocaine: An assessment of prevalence in suburban and urban emergency departments. *Annals of Emergency Medicine*, 26, 671–676.

HOLLOWAY, M. (1991). Rx for addiction. *Scientific American*, 264(3), 94–103.

HONG, R., MATSUYAMA, E., & NUR, K. (1991). Cardiomyopathy associated with smoking of crystal methamphetamine. *Journal of the American Medical Association*, 265,1152–1154.

HOPEWELL, P. C. (1996). Mycobacterium tuberculosis an emerging pathogen? *Western Journal of Medicine*, 164, 33–35.

HOPFENSPERGER, J. (1995). Babies overcome odds. *Minneapolis Star-Tribune*, XIII(335), 1A, 8A.

HOPPER, J. L., & SEEMAN, E. (1994). The bone density of female twins discordant for tobacco use. *New England Journal of Medicine*, 330, 387–392.

HORGAN, J. (1989). Lukewarm turkey: Drug firms balk at pursuing a heroin-addiction treatment. *Scientific American*, 260(3), 32.

HORNEY, K. (1964). *The neurotic personality of our time.* New York: Norton.

HOUGH, D. O., & KOVAN, J. R. (1990). Is your patient a steroid abuser? *Medical Aspects of Human Sexuality*, 24(11), 24–32.

HOUSE, M. A. (1990). Cocaine. *American Journal of Nursing*, 90(4), 40–45.

HOUSE PANEL CONSIDERS IMPACT OF DRUGS ON EMERGENCY ROOMS. (1990). *Alcoholism & Drug Abuse Week*, 2(38), 4–5.

HOW COCAINE CAUSES SUDDEN DEATH. (1994). *Forensic Drug Abuse Advisor*, 6(10), 76–77.

HOW MUCH MARIJUANA DO AMERICANS REALLY SMOKE? (1995). *Forensic Drug Abuse Advisor*, 7(1), 7–8.

HOWARD, D. L., & MCCAUGHRIN, W. C. (1996). The treatment effectiveness of outpatient substance misuse treatment organizations between court-mandated and voluntary clients. *Substance Use & Misuse*, (31), 895–925.

HOWARD, M. O., KIVLAHAN, D., & WALKER, R. D. (1997). Cloninger's tridimensional theory of personality and psychopathology: Applications to substance use disorders. *Journal of Studies on Alcohol, 58*, 48–67.

HOWLAND, R. H. (1990). Barriers to community treatment of patients with dual diagnoses. *Hospital & Community Psychiatry, 41*, 1136–1138.

HSER, Y., ANGLIN, D., & POWERS, K. (1993). A 24 year follow-up of California narcotics addicts. *Archives of General Psychiatry, 50*, 577–584.

HUGHES, J. R. (1992). Tobacco withdrawal in self-quitters. *Journal of Consulting and Clinical Psychology, 60*, 689–697.

HUGHES, J. R., GUST, S. W., SKOOG, K., KEENAN, R. M., & FENWICK, J. W. (1991). Symptoms of tobacco withdrawal. *Archives of General Psychiatry, 48*, 52–59.

HUGHES, R. (1993). Bitch, bitch, bitch . . . *Psychology Today, 26*(5), 28–30.

HUGHES, T. L., & WILSNACK, S. C. (1997). Use of alcohol among lesbians: Research and clinical implications. *American Journal of Orthopsychiatry, 67*, 20–36.

HUMPHREYS, K. (1997). Clinicians' referral and matching of substance abuse patients to self-help groups after treatment. *Psychiatric Services, 48*, 1445–1449.

HUMPHREYS, K., & MOOS, R. H. (1996). Reduced substance-abuse-related health care costs among voluntary participants in Alcoholics Anonymous. *Psychiatric Services, 47*, 709–713.

HUMPHREYS, K., MOOS, R. H., & FINNEY, J. W. (1995). Two pathways out of drinking problems without professional treatment. *Addictive Behaviors, 20*, 427–441.

HUMPHREYS, K., MOOS, R. H., & FINNEY, J. W. (1996). Life domains, Alcoholics Anonymous, and tole incumbency in the 3 year course of problem drinking. *Journal of Nervous and Mental Disease, 184*, 475–481.

HUMPHREYS, K., & RAPPAPORT, J. (1993). From the community mental health movement to the war on drugs. *American Psychologist, 48*, 892–901.

HUNTER, M., & KELLOGG, T. (1989). Redefining ACA characteristics. *Alcoholism & Addiction, 9*(3), 28–29.

HURT, R. D., FINLAYSON, R. E., MORSE, R. M., & DAVIS, L. J. (1988). Alcoholism in elderly persons: Medical aspects and prognosis of 216 inpatients. *Mayo Clinic Proceedings, 63*, 753–760.

HURT, R. D., OFFORD, K. P., CROGHAN, I. T., GOMEZ-DAHL, L., KOTTKE, T. E., MORSE, R. M., & MELTON, J. (1996). Mortality following inpatient addictions treatment. *Journal of the American Medical Association, 275*, 1097–1103.

HUSSAR, D. A. (1990). Update 90: New drugs. *Nursing 90, 20*(12), 41–51.

HUSTON, C. J. (1996). Ruptured esophageal varicies. *American Journal of Nursing, 96*(4), 43.

HUTCHINSON, B. M., & HOOK, E. W. (1990). Syphilis in adults. *Medical Clinics of North America, 74*, 1389–1416.

HYDE, G. L. (1989). Management of the impaired person in the OR. *Bulletin of the American College of Surgeons, 74*(11), 6–9.

HYMAN, S. E. (1996). Drug abuse and addiction. In E. Rubenstein & D. D. Federman (Eds.), *Scientific American medicine*. New York: Scientific American Press.

HYMAN, S. E., & CASSEM, N. H. (1995). Alcoholism. In E. Rubenstein & D. D. Federman (Eds.), *Scientific American medicine*. New York: Scientific American Press.

HYMAN, S. E., & NESTLER, E. J. (1996). Initiation and adaption: A paradigm for understanding psychotropic drug action. *American Journal of Psychiatry, 153*, 151–162.

HYMOWITZ, N., FEUERMAN, M., HOLLANDER, M., & FRANCES, R. J. (1993). Smoking deterrence using silver acetate. *Hospital and Community Psychiatry, 44*, 113–114, 116.

IBOGAINE AND MINIMUM SENTENCING HOT TOPICS AT DPF MEETING. (1994). *Forensic Drug Abuse Advisor, 6*(10), 78–79.

ICE OVERDOSE. (1989). *The Economist, 313*(7631), 29–31.

IGGERS, J. (1990). The addiction industry. *Minneapolis Star-Tribune, IX*(102), 1E, 4E, 10EX.

IMHOF, J. E. (1995). Overcoming countertransference. In A. M. Washton (Ed.), *Psychotherapy and substance abuse*. New York: Guilford Press.

INTRODUCTION TO GHB. (1997). *Forensic Drug Abuse Advisor, 9*(5), 37–38.

IRWIN, K. (1995). Ideology, pregnancy and drugs: Differences between crack cocaine, heroin and methamphetamine users. *Contemporary Drug Problems, 22*(4), 613–638.

ISENHART, C. E., & SILVERSMITH, D. J. (1996). MMPI-2 response styles: Generalization to alcoholism assessment. *Psychology of Addictive Behaviors, 10*, 115–123.

ISNER, J. M., & CHOKSHI, S. K. (1989). Cocaine and vasospasm. *New England Journal of Medicine, 321*, 1604–1606.

IS THERE AN ADDICTIVE PERSONALITY? (1990). *The Wellness Letter, 6*(9), 1–2.

JACOBSON, J. M. (1992). Alcoholism and tuberculosis. *Alcohol Health & Research World, 16*(1), 39–45.

JAFFE, D. L., CHUNG, R. T., & FRIEDMAN, L. S. (1996). Management of portal hypertension and its complications. *Medical Clinics of North America, 80*, 1021–1034.

JAFFE, J. H. (1986). Opioids. In *American Psychiatric Association Annual Review* (Vol. 5). Washington, DC: American Psychiatric Association.

JAFFE, J. H. (1989). Drug dependence: Opioids, non-narcotics, nicotine (Tobacco) and caffeine. In H. I. Kaplan & B. J. Sadock (Eds.), *Comprehensive textbook of psychiatry* (Vol. V). Baltimore: Williams & Wilkins.

JAFFE, J. H. (1990). Drug addiction and drug abuse. In A. G. Gilman, T. W. Rall, A. S. Nies, & P. Taylor (Eds.), *The pharmacological basis of therapeutics* (8th ed.). New York: Macmillan.

JAFFE, J. H. (1992). Opiates: Clinical aspects. In J. H. Lowinson, P. Ruiz, R. B. Millman, & J. G. Langrod (Eds.), *Substance abuse: A comprehensive textbook* (2nd ed.). New York: Williams & Wilkins.

JAFFE, J. H. (1995a). Amphetamine (or amphetaminelike) disorders. In H. I. Kaplan & B. J. Sadock (Eds.), *Comprehensive textbook of psychiatry* (6th ed.). Baltimore: Williams & Wilkins.

JAFFE, J. H. (1995b). Cocaine-related disorders. In H. I. Kaplan & B. J. Sadock (Eds.), *Comprehensive textbook of psychiatry* (6th ed.). Baltimore: Williams & Wilkins.

JAFFE, J. H. (1995c). Opioid-related disorders. In H. I. Kaplan & B. J. Sadock (Eds.), *Comprehensive textbook of psychiatry* (6th ed.). Baltimore: Williams & Wilkins.

JAFFE, J. H., & MARTIN, W. R. (1990). Opioid analgesics and antagonists. In A. G. Gilman, T. W. Rall, A. S. Nies, & P. Taylor (Eds.), *The pharmacological basis of therapeutics* (8th ed.). New York: Macmillan.

JANSEN, K. L. R. (1993). Non-medical use of ketamine. *Lancet, 306,* 601–602.

JAPENGA, A. (1991). You're tougher than you think! *Self, 13*(4), 174–175, 187.

JARVIK, M. E., & SCHNEIDER, N. G. (1992). Nicotine. In J. H. Lowinson, P. Ruiz, R. B. Millman, & J. G. Langrod (Eds.), *Substance abuse: A comprehensive textbook* (2nd ed.). New York: Williams & Wilkins.

JELLINEK, E. M. (1952). Phases of alcohol addiction. *Quarterly Journal of Studies on Alcohol, 13,* 673–674.

JELLINEK, E. M. (1960). *The disease concept of alcoholism.* New Haven, CT: College and University Press.

JENIKE, M. A. (1991). Drug abuse. In E. Rubenstein & D. D. Federman (Eds.), *Scientific American medicine.* New York: Scientific American Press.

JENSEN, G. B., & PAKKENBERG, B. (1993). Do alcoholics drink their neurons away? *Lancet, 342,* 1201–1204.

JENSEN, J. G. (1987a). Step Two: A promise of hope. In *The twelve steps of Alcoholics Anonymous.* New York: Harper & Row.

JENSEN, J. G. (1987b). Step Three: Turning it over. In *The twelve steps of Alcoholics Anonymous.* New York: Harper & Row.

JOHNSON, M. D. (1990). Anabolic steroid use in adolescent athletes. *Pediatric Clinics of North America, 37,* 1111–1123.

JOHNSON, M. R., & LYDIARD, R. B. (1995). The neurobiology of anxiety disorders. *Psychiatric Clinics of North America, 18,* 681–725.

JOHNSON, V. E. (1980). *I'll quit tomorrow.* San Francisco: Harper & Row.

JOHNSON INSTITUTE. (1987). *The family enablers.* Minneapolis, MN: Author.

JOHNSTON, L. D., O'MALLEY, P. M., & BACHMAN, J. G. (1993). *National survey results on drug use from the monitoring the future study, 1975–1992.* Rockville, MD: U.S. Department of Health and Human Services.

JOHNSTON, L. D., O'MALLEY, P. M., & BACHMAN, J. G. (1994). *National survey results on drug use.* Rockville, MD: U.S. Department of Health and Human Services.

JOHNSTON, L. D., O'MALLEY, P. M., & BACHMAN, J. G. (1996). *National survey results on drug use from the monitoring the future study, 1975–1995.* Rockville, MD: U.S. Department of Health and Human Services.

JONES, A. L., JARVIE, D. R., McDERMID, G., & PROUDFOOT, A. T. (1994). Hepatocellular damage following amphetamine intoxication. *Journal of Toxicology, 32*(4),435–445.

JONES, R. L. (1990). Evaluation of drug use in the adolescent. In L. M. Haddad & J. F. Winchester (Eds.), *Clinical management of poisoning and drug overdoses* (2nd ed.). New York: Saunders.

JONES, R. T. (1987). Psychopharmacology of cocaine. In A. G. Washton & M. S. Gold (Eds.), *Cocaine: A clinician's handbook.* New York: Guilford Press.

JONNES, J. (1995). The rise of the modern addict. *American Journal of Public Health, 85*(8), 1157–1162.

JOSHI, N. P., & SCOTT, M. (1988). Drug use, depression, and adolescents. *Pediatric Clinics of North America, 35*(6), 1349–1364.

JOYCE, C. (1989). The woman alcoholic. *American Journal of Nursing, 89,* 1314–1316.

JUDD, L. L., & HUEY, L. Y. (1984). Lithium antagonizes ethanol intoxication in alcoholics. *American Journal of Psychiatry, 141,* 1517–1521.

JUERGENS, S. M. (1993). Benzodiazepines and addiction. *Psychiatric Clinics of North America, 16,* 75–86.

JUERGENS, S. M., & MORSE, R. M. (1988). Alprazolam dependence in seven patients. *American Journal of Psychiatry, 145,* 625–627.

JULIEN, R. M. (1992). *A primer of drug action* (6th ed.). New York: Freeman.

JUST SAY BUPRENORPHINE. (1990). *The Economist, 313*(7626), 95.

KACSO, G., & TEREZHALMY, G. T. (1994). Acetylsalicylic acid and acetaminophen. *Dental Clinics of North America, 38,* 633–644.

KAHN, P. (1996). Gene hunters close in on elusive prey. *Science, 271,* 1352–1354.

KAISER, D. (1996). Not by chemicals alone: A hard look at "psychiatric medicine." *Psychiatric Times, XIII*(12), 41–44.

KALES, J. P., BARONE, M. A., BIXLER, E. O., MILJKOVIC, M. M., & KALES, J. D. (1995). Mental illness and substance use among sheltered homeless persons in lower-density population areas. *Psychiatric Services, 46,* 592–596.

KAMINER, W. (1992). *I'm dysfunctional, you're dysfunctional.* New York: Addison-Wesley.

KAMINER, Y. (1991). Adolescent substance abuse. In R. J. Frances & S. I. Miller (Eds.), *Clinical textbook of addictive disorders.* New York: Guilford Press.

KAMINER, Y. (1994). Adolescent substance abuse. In M. Galanter & H. D. Kleber (Eds.),*Textbook of substance abuse treatment.* Washington, DC: American Psychiatric Press.

KAMINER, Y., & FRANCES, R. J. (1991). Inpatient treatment of adolescents with psychiatric and substance abuse disorders. *Hospital and Community Psychiatry,* 42,894–896.

KAMINSKI, A. (1992). *Mind-altering drugs.* Madison: Wisconsin Clearinghouse, Board of Regents, University of Wisconsin System.

KANDALL, S. R., GAINES, J., HABEL, L., DAVIDSON, G., & JESSOP, D. (1993). The relationship of maternal substance abuse to subsequent sudden infant death syndrome in offspring. *Journal of Pediatrics, 123,* 120–126.

KANDEL, D. B., & DAVIES, M. (1996). High school students who use crack and other drugs. *Archives of General Psychiatry, 53,* 71–80.

KANDEL, D. B., & RAVEIS, V. H. (1989). Cessation of illicit drug use in young adulthood. *Archives of General Psychiatry, 46,* 109–116.

KANDEL, D. B., YAMAGUCHI, K., & CHEN, K. (1992). Stages of progression in drug involvement from adolescence to adulthood: Further evidence for the gateway theory. *Journal of Studies on Alcohol, 53*(5), 447–458.

KANOF, P. D., ARONSON, M. J., & NESS, R. (1993). Organic mood syndrome associated with detoxification from methadone maintenance. *American Journal of Psychiatry, 150,* 423–428.

KANWISCHER, R. W., & HUNDLEY, J. (1990). Screening for substance abuse in hospitalized psychiatric patients. *Hospital & Community Psychiatry, 41,* 795–797.

KAPLAN, H. I., & SADOCK, B. J. (1990). *Pocket handbook of clinical psychiatry.* Baltimore: Williams & Wilkins.

KAPLAN, H. I., SADOCK, B. J., & GREBB, J. A. (1994). *Synopsis of psychiatry* (7th ed.). Baltimore: Williams & Wilkins.

KARCH, S. B. (1996). *The pathology of drug abuse* (2nd ed.). New York: CRC Press.

KARHUNEN, P. J., ERKINJUNTTI, T., & LAIPPALA, P. (1994). Moderate alcohol consumption and loss of cerebellar Purkinje cells. *British Medical Journal, 308,* 1663–1667.

KARLEN, A. (1995). *Man and microbes.* New York: Putnam.

KASHKIN, K. B. (1992). Anabolic steroids. In J. H. Lowinson, P. Ruiz, R. B. Millman, & J. G. Langrod (Eds.), *Substance abuse: A comprehensive textbook* (2nd ed.). New York: Williams & Wilkins.

KASHKIN, K. B., & KLEBER, H. D. (1989). Hooked on hormones? An anabolic steroid addiction hypothesis. *Journal of the American Medical Association, 262,* 3166–3173.

KASSIRER, J. P. (1997). Federal foolishness and marijuana. *New England Journal of Medicine, 336,* 366–367.

KATZ, S. J., & LIU, A. E. (1991). *The codependency conspiracy.* New York: Warner Books.

KAUFFMAN, E., DORE, M. M., & NELSON-ZLUPKO, L. (1995). The role of women's therapy groups in the treatment of chemical dependence. *American Journal of Orthopsychiatry, 65,* 355–363.

KAUFMAN, E., & MCNAUL, J. P. (1992). Recent developments in understanding and treating drug abuse and dependence. *Hospital and Community Psychiatry, 43,* 223–236.

KAUFMAN, G. (1989). *The psychology of shame.* New York: Springer.

KAY, S. R., KALATHARA, M., & MEINZER, A. E. (1989). Diagnostic and behavioral characteristics of psychiatric patients who abuse substances. *Hospital and Community Psychiatry, 40,* 1062–1065.

KELLER, D. S. (1996). Exploration in the service of relapse prevention: A psychoanalytic contribution to substance abuse treatment. In F. Rotgers, D. S. Keller, & J. Morgenstern (Eds.), *Treating substance abuse.* New York: Guilford Press.

KELLY, J. A., MURPHY, D. A., SIKKEMA, K. J., & KALICYHMAN, S. C. (1993). Psychological interventions to prevent HIV infection are urgently needed. *American Psychologist, 48,* 1023–1034.

KELLY, V. A., & MYERS, J. E. (1996). Parental alcoholism and coping: A comparison of female children of alcoholics with female children of nonalcoholics. *Journal of Counseling & Development, 74,* 501–504.

KEMM, J. (1993). Alcohol and heart disease: The implications of the U-shaped curve. *British Medical Journal, 307,* 1373–1374.

KENDER, K. S., HEATH, A. C., NEALE, M. C., KESSLER, R. C., & EVES, J. (1992). A population based twin study of alcoholism in women. *Journal of the American Medical Association, 268,* 1877–1882.

KENFORD, S. L., FIORE, M. C., JORENBY, D. E., SMITH, S. S., WETTER, D., & BAKER, T. B. (1994). Predicting smoking cessation. *Journal of the American Medical Association, 271,* 589–594.

KERFOOT, B. P., SAKOULAS, G., & HYMAN, S. E. (1996). Cocaine. In L. Friedman, N. F. Fleming, D. H. Roberts, & S. E. Hyman (Eds.), *Source book of substance abuse and addiction.* New York: Williams & Wilkins.

KERMANI, E. J., & CASTANEDA, R. (1996). Psychoactive substance use in forensic psychiatry. *American Journal of Drug and Alcohol Abuse, 22,* 1–28.

KESSLER, D. A. (1995). Nicotine addiction in young people. *New England Journal of Medicine, 333,* 186–189.

KESSLER, R. C., CRUM, R. M., WARNER, L. A., NELSON, C. B., SCHULENBERG, J., & ANTHONY, J. C. (1997). Lifetime co-occurrence of *DSM-III-R* alcohol abuse and dependence with other psychiatric disorders in the National Comorbidity Survey. *Archives of General Psychiatry, 54,* 313–321.

KESSLER, R. C., McGONAGLE, K. A., ZHAO, S., NELSON, C. B., HUGHES, M., ESHLEMAN, S., HANS-ULRICH, W., & KENDLER, K. S. (1994). Lifetime and 12 month prevalence of *DSM-III-R* psychiatric disorders in the United States. *Archives of General Psychiatry, 51,* 8–19.

KING, G. R., & ELLINWOOD, E. H. (1992). Amphetamines and other stimulants. In J. H. Lowinson,,P. Ruiz, R. B. Millman, & J. G. Langrod (Eds.), *Substance abuse: A comprehensive textbook* (2nd ed.). New York: Williams & Wilkins.

KING, S. R. (1994). HIV: Virology and mechanisms of disease. *Annals of Emergency Medicine, 24,* 443–449.

KIRN, T. F. (1989). Studies of adolescents indicate just how complex the situation is for this age group. *Journal of the American Medical Association, 261,* 3362.

KIRSCH, M. M. (1986). *Designer drugs.* Minneapolis, MN: CompCare.

KISHLINE, A. (1996). A toast to moderation. *Psychology Today, 29*(1), 53–56.

KITCHENS, J. M. (1994). Does this patient have an alcohol problem? *Journal of the American Medical Association, 272,* 1782–1787.

KITRIDOU, R. C. (1993). The efficacy and safety of oxaproxzin versus aspirin: Pooled results of double-blind trials in rheumatoid arthritis. *Drug Therapy, 23*(Suppl.), 21–25.

KIVLAHAN, D. R., HEIMAN, J. R., WRIGHT, R. C., MUNDT, J. W., & SHUPE, J. A. (1991). Treatment cost and rehospitalization rate in schizophrenic outpatients with a history of substance abuse. *Hospital and Community Psychiatry, 42,* 609–614.

KLAG, M. J., & WHELTON, P. K. (1987). Risk of stroke in male cigarette smokers. *New England Journal of Medicine, 316,* 628.

KLAR, H. (1987). The setting for psychiatric treatment. In *American Psychiatric Association Annual Review* (Vol. 6). Washington, DC: American Psychiatric Association Press.

KLASS, P. (1989). Vital signs. *Discover, 10*(1), 12–14.

KLATSKY, A. L. (1990). Alcohol and coronary artery disease. *Alcohol Health & Research World, 14*(4), 289–300.

KLEBER, H. D. (1991). Tracking the cocaine epidemic. *Journal of the American Medical Association, 266,* 2272–2273.

KLEBER, H. D. (1994). Letter to the editor. *New England Journal of Medicine, 331,* 129.

KLEIN, J. M., & MILLER, S. I. (1986). Three approaches to the treatment of drug addiction. *Hospital and Community Psychiatry, 37,* 1083–1085.

KLINE, A. (1996). Pathways into drug user treatment: The influence of gender and racial/ethnic identity. *Substance Use & Misuse, 31,* 323–342.

KLINGER, R. L., & CABAJ, R. P. (1993). Characteristics of gay and lesbian relationships. In J. M. Oldham, M. B. Riba, & A. Tasman (Eds.), *Review of psychiatry* (Vol. 12). Washington, DC: American Psychiatric Association.

KLONOFF-COHEN, H. S., EDELSTEIN, S. L., LEFKOWITZ, E. S., SRINIVASEN, I. P., KAEGI, D., CHANG, J. C., & WILEY, K. J. (1995). The effect of passive smoking and tobacco exposure through breast milk on Sudden Infant Death Syndrome. *Journal of the American Medical Association, 173,* 795–798.

KNAPP, C. (1996). *Drinking: A love story.* New York: Dial Press.

KOCH, M., DEZI, A., FERRARIO, F., & CAPURSO, L. (1996). Prevention of Nonsteroidal antiinflammatory drug-induced gastrointestinal mucosal injury. *Archives of Internal Medicine, 156,* 2321–2331.

KOCUREK, K. (1996). Primary care of the HIV patient. *Medical Clinics of North America, 80,* 375–410.

KOFOED, L., KANIA, J., WALSH, T., & ATKINSON, R. M. (1986). Outpatient treatment of patients with substance abuse and coexisting psychiatric disorders. *American Journal of Psychiatry, 143,* 867–872.

KOFOED, L., & KEYS, A. (1988). Using group therapy to persuade dual-diagnosis patients to seek substance abuse treatment. *Hospital & Community Psychiatry, 39,* 1209 1211.

KOLODNER, G., & FRANCES, R. (1993). Recognizing dissociative disorders in patients with chemical dependency. *Hospital and Community Psychiatry, 44,* 1041–1044.

KOLODNY, R. C. (1985). The clinical management of sexual problems in substance abusers. In T. E. Bratter & G. G. Forrest (Eds.), *Alcoholism and substance abuse: Strategies for clinical intervention.* New York: Free Press.

KONSTAN, M. W., BYARD, P. J., HOPPEL, C. L., & DAVIS, P. B. (1995). Effect of high-dose ibuprofen in patients with cystic fibrosis. *New England Journal of Medicine, 332,* 848–854.

KONSTAN, M. W., HOPPEL, C. L., CHAI, B., & DAVIS, P. B. (1995). Ibuprofen in children with cystic fibrosis: Pharmacokinetics and adverse effects. *Journal of Pediatrics, 118,* 956–965.

KOTTLER, J. A. (1992). *Compassionate therapy.* New York: Jossey-Bass.

KOTULAK, R. (1992). Recent discoveries about cocaine may help unlock secrets of brain. *St. Paul Pioneer Press, 143*(345), 4C.

KOTZ, M., & COVINGTON, E. C. (1995). Alcoholism. In R. E. Rakel (Ed.), *Conn's current therapy.* Philadelphia: Saunders.

KOVASZNAY, B., BROMET, E., SCHWARTZ, J. E., RANGANATHAN, R., LAVELLE, J., & BRANDON, L. (1993). Substance abuse and onset of psychotic illness. *Hospital and Community Psychiatry, 44,* 567–571.

KOZLOWSKI, L. T., WILKINSON, A., SKINNER, W., KENT, W., FRANKLIN, T., & POPE, M. (1989). Comparing tobacco cigarette dependence with other drug dependencies. *Journal of the American Medical Association, 261,* 898–901.

KRANZLER, H. R., BURLESON, J. A., DEL BOCA, F. K., BABOR, T. F., KORNER, P., BROWN, J., & BOHN, T. F. (1994). Buspirone treatment of anxious alcoholics. *Archives of General Psychiatry, 51,* 720–731.

KRITZ, H., SCHMID, P., & SINZINGER, H. (1995). Passive smoking and cardiovascular risk. *Archives of Internal Medicine, 155,* 1942–1948.

KRUGER, T. E., & JERRELLS, T. R. (1992). Potential role of alcohol in human immunodeficiency virus infection. *Alcohol Health & Research World, 16*(1), 57–63.

KRUZICKI, J. (1987). Dispelling a myth: The facts about female alcoholics. *Corrections Today, 49,* 110–115.

KRYGER, M. H., STELJES, D., POULIOT, Z., JEUFELD, H., & ODYNSKI, T. (1991). Subjective versus objective evaluation of hypnotic efficacy: Experience with Zolpidem. *Sleep, 14*(5), 399–407.

KUNITZ, S. J., & LEVY J. E. (1974). Changing ideas of alcohol use among Navaho indians. *Quarterly Journal of Studies on Alcohol, 46,* 953–960.

KURTZ, E. (1979). *Not God: A history of Alcoholics Anonymous.* Center City, MN: Hazelden.

KURTZ, H. (1995). Everybody's got something to hide except me and my monkey. *Minneapolis Star-Tribune, XIV*(50), 12A.

KUSHNER, M. G., SHER, K. J., & BEITMAN, B. D. (1990). The relation between alcohol problems and the anxiety disorders. *American Journal of Psychiatry, 147,* 685–695.

KVIZ, F. J., CLARK, M. A., CRITTENDEN, K. S., WERNECKE, R. B., & FREELS, S. (1995). Age and smoking cessation behaviors. *Preventative Medicine, 24,* 297–307.

LACKRITZ, E. M., SATTEN, G. A., ABERLE-GRASSE, J., DODD, R. Y., RAIMONDI, V. P., JANSSEN, R. S., LEWIS, W. F., NOTARI, E. P., & PETERSEN, L. R. (1995). Estimated risk of transmission of the human immunodeficiency virus by screened blood in the United States. *New England Journal of Medicine, 333,* 1721–1725.

LACKS, P., & MORIN, C. M. (1992). Recent advances in the assessment and treatment of insomnia. *Journal of Consulting and Clinical Psychology, 60,* 586–594.

LACOMBE, P. S., VICENTE, J. A. G., PAGES, J. C., & MORSELLI, P. L. (1996). Causes and problems of nonresponse or poor response to drugs. *Drugs, 51,* 552–570.

LADER, M. (1987). Assessing the potential for buspirone dependence or abuse and effects of its withdrawal. *American Journal of Medicine, 82*(Suppl. 5A), 20–26.

LAEGREID, L., RAGNAR, O., NILS, C., HAGBERG, G., WAHLSTROM, J., & ABRAHAMSSON, L. (1990). Congenital malformations and maternal consumption of benzodiazepines: A case control study. *Developmental Medicine and Child Neurology, 32,* 432–442.

LAMAR, J. V., RILEY, M., & SMGHABADI, R. (1986). Crack: A cheap and deadly cocaine is spreading menace. *Time, 128,* 16–18.

LAND, W., PINSKY, D., & SALZMAN, C. (1991). Abuse and misuse of anticholinergic medications. *Hospital and Community Psychiatry, 42,* 580–581.

LANDRY, G. L., & PRIMOS, W. A. (1990). Anabolic steroid abuse. *Advances in Pediatrics, 7,* 185–205.

LANGE, R. A., CIGARROA, R. G., YANCY, C. W., WILLARD, J. E., POPMA, J. J., SILLS, M. N., MCBRIDE, W., KIM, A. S., & HILLIS, L. D. (1989). Cocaine induced coronary artery vasoconstriction. *New England Journal of Medicine, 321,* 1557–1562.

LANGE, W. R., WHITE, N., & ROBINSON, N. (1992). Medical complications of substance abuse. *Postgraduate Medicine, 92,* 205–214.

LANGONE, J. (1989). Hot to block a killer's path. *Time, 133*(5), 60–62.

LANGSTON, J. W., & PALFREMAN, J. (1995). *The case of the frozen addicts.* New York: Pantheon Books.

LARSON, K. K. (1982). Birthplace of "The Minnesota Model." *Alcoholism, 3*(2), 34–35.

LAURENCE, D. R., & BENNETT, P. N. (1992). *Clinical pharmacology* (7th ed.). New York: Churchill Livingstone.

LAWENTAL, E., MCLELLAN, A. T., GRISSOM, G. R., BRILL, P., & O'BRIEN, C. (1996). Coerced treatment for substance abuse problems detected through workplace urine surveillance: Is it effective? *Journal of Substance Abuse, 8,* 115–128.

LAWSON, C. (1994). Flirting with tragedy: Women who say yes to drugs. *Cosmopolitan, 217*(1), 138–141.

LAYNE, G. S. (1990). Schizophrenia and substance abuse. In D. F. O'Connell (Ed.), *Managing the dually diagnosed patient.* New York: Haworth Press.

LEDERBERG, M. S., & HOLLAND, J. C. (1989). Psycho-oncology. In H. I. Kaplan & B. J. Sadock (Eds.), *Comprehensive textbook of psychiatry* (Vol. V). Baltimore: Williams & Wilkins.

LEE, E. W., & D'ALONZO, G. E. (1993). Cigarette smoking, nicotine addiction, and its pharmacologic treatment. *Archives of Internal Medicine, 153,* 34–48.

LEEDS, J., & MORGENSTERN, J. (1996). Psychoanalytic theories of substance abuse. In F. Rotgers, D. S. Keller, & J. Morgenstern (Eds.), *Treating substance abuse.* New York: Guilford Press.

LEEPER, K. V., & TORRES, A. (1995). Community-acquired pneumonia in the intensive care unit. *Clinics in Chest Medicine, 16,* 155–171.

LEHMAN, A. F. (1996). Heterogeneity of person and place: Assessing co-occurring addictive and mental disorders. *American Journal of Orthopsychiatry, 66,* 32–41.

LEHMAN, A. F., MYERS, C. P., & CORTY, E. (1989) Assessment and classification of patients with psychiatric and substance abuse syndromes. *Hospital and Community Psychiatry, 40,* 1019–1025.

LEHMAN, L. B., PILICH, A., & ANDREWS, N. (1994). Neurological disorders resulting from alcoholism. *Alcohol Health & Research World, 17,* 305–309.

LEIGH, G. (1985) Psychosocial factors in the etiology of substance abuse. In T. E. Bratter & G. G. Forrest (Eds.), *Alcoholism and substance abuse: Strategies for clinical intervention.* New York: Free Press.

LELAND, J., KATEL, P., & HAGER, M. (1996). The fear of heroin is shooting up. *Newsweek, CXXVIII(9),* 55–56.

LENDER, M. E. (1981). The disease concept of alcoholism in the United States: Was Jellinek first? *Digest of Alcoholism Theory and Application, 1(1),* 25–31.

LEO, J. (1990). The it's-not-my-fault syndrome. *U.S. News & World Report, 109(12),* 16.

LEONARD, K. E., & ROBERTS, R. J. (1996). Alcohol in the early years of marriage. *Alcohol Health & Research World, 20,* 192–196.

LESHNER, A. I. (1996). Molecular mechanisms of cocaine addiction. *New England Journal of Medicine, 335(2),* 128–129.

LESSARD, S. (1989). Busting our mental blocks on drugs and crime. *Washington Monthly, 21(1),* 70.

LEVERS, L. L., & HAWES, A. R. (1990). Drugs and gender: A woman's recovery program. *Journal of Mental Health Counseling, 12,* 527–531.

LEVY, S. J., & RUTTER, E. (1992). *Children of drug abusers.* New York: Lexington Books.

LEWIS, D. C. (1996). *"First do no harm": A medical perspective on U.S. drug policy.* Seventh annual Norman E. Zinberg Memorial Lecture Award, symposium presented to the Department of Psychiatry at The Cambridge Hospital, Boston.

LEWIS, D. O. (1989). Adult antisocial behavior and criminality. In H. I. Kaplan & B. J. Sadock (Eds.), *Comprehensive textbook of psychiatry* (Vol. V). New York: Williams & Wilkins.

LEWIS, J. A., DANA, R. Q., & BLEVINS, G. A. (1988). *Substance abuse counseling.* Pacific Grove, CA: Brooks/Cole.

LEWIS, J. W. (1995). Buprenorphine—Medicinal chemistry. In A. Cowan & J. W. Lewis (Eds.), *Buprenorphine.* New York: Wiley Interscience.

LEWIS, R. (1989). Drug tolerance apparently works in Holland. *Minneapolis Star-Tribune, VIII(173),* 15A.

LEX, B. W. (1994). Alcohol and other drug abuse among women. *Alcohol Health & Research World, 18,* 212–219.

LIBERTO, J. G., OSLIN, D. W., & RUSKIN, P. E. (1992). Alcoholism in older persons: A review of the literature. *Hospital and Community Psychiatry, 43,* 975–984.

LICHTENSTEIN, E., & GLASGOW, R. E. (1992). Smoking cessation: What we have learned over the past decade. *Journal of Consulting and Clinical Psychology, 60,* 518–526.

LIEBER, C. S. (1995). Medical disorders of alcoholism. *New England Journal of Medicine, 333,* 1058–1065.

LIEBER, C. S. (1996). *Metabolic basis of alcoholic liver disease.* Paper presented at the 1996 annual Frank P. Furlano, M.D. memorial lecture, Gunderson-Lutheran Medical Center, La Crosse, WI.

LIEBERMAN, M. L. (1988). *The sexual pharmacy.* New York: New American Library.

LIEBSCHUTZ, J. M., MULVEY, K. P., & SAMET, J. H. (1997). Victimization among substance abusing women. *Archives of Internal Medicine, 157,* 1093–1097.

LIEVELD, P. E., & ARUNA, A. (1991). Diagnosis and management of the alcohol withdrawal syndrome. *U.S. Pharmacist, 16(1),* H1–H11.

LIMITS BY MANAGED CARE WORRY FEDERAL OFFICIALS. (1996). *Substance Abuse Letter, 3(11),* 1.

LING, W., WESSON, D. R., CHARUVASTRA, C., & KLETT, C. J. (1996). A controlled trial comparing buprenorphine and methadone maintenance in opioid dependence. *Archives of General Psychiatry, 53,* 401–407.

LINGEMAN, R. R. (1974). *Drugs from A to Z: A dictionary.* New York: McGraw-Hill.

LINNOILA, M., DEJONG, J., & VIRKKUNEN, M. (1989). Family history of alcoholism in violent offenders and impulsive fire setters. *Archives of General Psychiatry, 46,* 613–616.

LINSZEN, D. H., DINGEMANS, P. M., & LENIOR, M. E. (1994). Cannabis abuse and the course of recent-onset schizophrenic disorders. *Archives of General Psychiatry, 51,* 273–279.

LIPKIN, M. (1989). Psychiatry and medicine. In H. I. Kaplan & B. J. Sadock (Eds.), *Comprehensive textbook of psychiatry* (Vol. V). Baltimore: Williams & Wilkins.

LIPSCOMB, J. W. (1989). What pharmacists should know about home poisonings. *Drug Topics, 133(15),* 72–80.

LIT, E., WIVIOTT-TISHLER, W., WONG, S., & HYMAN, S. (1996). Stimulants: Amphetamines and caffeine. In L. Friedman, N. F. Fleming, D. H. Roberts, & S. H. Hyman (eds.), *Source book of substance abuse and addiction.* New York: Williams & Wilkins.

LITTLE, R. E., ANDERSON, K. W., ERVIN, C. H., WORTHINGTON-ROBERTS, B., & CLARREN, S. K. (1989). Maternal alcohol use during breast-feeding and infant mental and motor development at one year. *New England Journal of Medicine, 321,* 425–430.

LIU, S., SIEGEL, P. Z., BREWER, R. D., MOKDAD, A. H., SLEET, D. A., & SERDULA, M. (1997). Prevalence of alcohol-impaired driving. *Journal of the American Medical Association, 277,* 122–125.

LIVELY, K. (1996). The "date rape drug": Colleges worry about reports of use of Rohypnol, a sedative. *Chronicle of Higher Education, 42(42),* A29.

LØBERG, T. (1986). Neuropsychological findings in the early and middle phases of alcoholism. In I. Grant & K. M. Adams (Eds.), *Neuropsychological assessment of neuropsychiatric disorders.* New York: Oxford University Press.

LOEBL, S., SPRATTO, G. R., & WOODS, A. L. (1994). *The nurse's drug handbook* (7th ed.). New York: Delmar.

LOISELLE, J. M., BAKER, M. D., TEMPLETON, J. M., SCHWARTZ, G., & DROTT, H. (1993). Substance abuse in adolescent trauma. *Annals of Emergency Medicine, 22,* 1530 1534.

LOMBARD, J., LEVIN, I. H., & WEINER, W. J. (1989). Arsenic intoxication in a cocaine abuser. *New England Journal of Medicine, 320,* 869.

LOPEZ, W., & JESTE, D. V. (1997). Movement disorders and substance abuse. *Psychiatric Services, 48,* 634–636.

LOS ANGELES TIMES. (1996a). A very venerable vintage. *Minneapolis Star-Tribune, XV*(63), A16.

LOS ANGELES TIMES. (1996b). Tobacco smoke greatly increases SIDS risk, study finds. *Minneapolis Star-Tribune, X* (113), A1, A16.

LOSKIN, A., MAVIGLIA, S., & FRIEDMAN, L. S. (1996). Marijuana. In L. Friedman, N. F. Fleming, D. H. Roberts, & S. E. Hyman (Eds.), *Source book of substance abuse and addiction.* New York: Williams & Wilkins.

LOUIE, A. K. (1990). Panic attacks—when cocaine is the cause. *Medical Aspects of Human Sexuality, 24*(12), 44–46.

LOURWOOD, D. L., & RIEDLINGER, J. E. (1989). The use of drugs in the breast feeding mother. *Drug Topics, 133*(21), 77–85.

LOVETT, A. R. (1994, May 5). Wired in California. *Rolling Stone,* 39–40.

LUND, N., & PAPADAKOS, P. J. (1995). Barbiturates, neurloeptics, and propofol for sedation. *Critical Care Clinics, 11,* 875–885.

LYONS, J. S., & McGOVERN, M. P. (1989). Use of mental health services by dually diagnosed persons. *Hospital & Community Psychiatry, 40,* 1067–1069.

MAAS, E. F., ASHE, J., SPIEGEL, P., ZEE, D. S., & LEIGH, R. J. (1991). Acquired pendular nystagmus in toluene addiction. *Neurology, 41,* 282–286.

MACKENZIE, T. D., BARTECCHI, C. E., & SCHRIER, R. W. (1994a). The human costs of tobacco use (Part One). *New England Journal of Medicine, 330,* 907–912.

MACKENZIE, T. D., BARTECCHI, C. E., & SCHRIER, R. W. (1994b). The human costs of tobacco use (Part Two). *New England Journal of Medicine, 330,* 975–980.

MACKMAN, M. D. (1995). Managing the patient with anaphylaxis. *Emergency Medicine, 27*(2), 68–84.

MADDUX, J. F., DESMOND, D. P., & COSTELLO, R. (1987). Depression in opioid users varies with substance use status. *American Journal of Drug & Alcohol Abuse, 13*(4), 375–378.

MAGUIRE, J. (1990). *Care and feeding of the brain.* New York: Doubleday.

MAISTO, S. A., & CONNORS, G. J. (1988). Assessment of treatment outcome. In D. M. Donovan & G. A. Marlatt (Eds.), *Assessment of addictive disorders.* New York: Guilford Press.

MALES, M. (1992). Tobacco: Promotion and smoking. *Journal of the American Medical Association, 267,* 3282.

MANFREDI, R. L., KALES, A., VGONTZAS, A. N., BIXLER, E. O., ISAAC, M. A., & FALCONE, C. M. (1991). Buspirone: Sedative or stimulant effect? *American Journal of Psychiatry, 148,* 1213–1217.

MANN, C. C., & PLUMMER, M. L. (1991). *The aspirin wars.* New York: Knopf.

MANN, J. (1994). *Murder, magic and medicine.* New York: Oxford University Press.

MARANTO, G. (1985). Coke: The random killer. *Discover, 12*(3), 16–21.

MARGOLIN, A., KOSTEN, T., PETRAKIS, I., AVANTS, S. K., & KOSTEN, T. (1991). Bupropion reduces cocaine abuse in methadone-maintained patients. *Archives of General Psychiatry, 48,* 87.

MARIJUANA AND BREAST FEEDING. (1990). *Pediatrics for Parents, 11*(10), 1.

MARIJUANA INITIATIVE MAKES CALIFORNIA BALLOT. (1996). *Forensic Drug Abuse Advisor, 8*(6), 44–45.

MARKET UPDATE. (1993). *The Economist, 329*(7830), 68.

MARLATT, G. A. (1994). Harm reduction: A public health approach to addictive behavior. *Division on Addictions newsletter, 2*(1), 1, 3.

MARSANO, L. (1994). Alcohol and malnutrition. *Alcohol Health & Research World, 17,* 284–291.

MARSHALL, J. R. (1994). The diagnosis and treatment of social phobia and alcohol abuse. *Bulletin of the Menninger Clinic, 58,* A58–A66.

MARTENSEN, R. L. (1996). From Papal endorsement to southern vice. *Journal of the American Medical Association, 276,* 1615.

MARTIN, P. J., ENEVOLDSON, T. P., & HUMPHREY, P. R. D. (1997). Causes of ischaemic stroke in the young. *Postgraduate Medical Journal, 73,* 8–16.

MARVEL, B. (1995). AA's "higher power" challenged. *St. Paul Pioneer Press, 147*(44), 4A

MARZUK, M. M. (1996). Violence, crime and mental illness. *Archives of General Psychiatry, 53,* 481–486.

MARZUK, P. M., TARDIFF, K., LEON, A. C., HIRSCH, C. S., STAJIC, M., PORTERA, L., HARTWELL, N., & IQBAL, M. I. (1995). Fatal injuries after cocaine use as a leading cause of death among young adults in New York City. *New England Journal of Medicine, 332,* 1753–1757.

MARZUK, P. M., TARDIFF, K., LEON, A. C., STAJIC, M., MORGAN, E. B., & MANN, J. J. (1992). Prevalence of cocaine use among residents of New York City who committed suicide during a one-year period. *American Journal of Psychiatry, 149,* 371–375.

MASSACHUSETTS MEDICAL SOCIETY. (1994). *Morbidity and Mortality Weekly Report, 43*(SS-3).

MATHERS, D. C., & GHODSE, A. D. (1992). Cannabis and psychotic illness. *British Journal of Psychiatry, 161,* 648–653.

MATHEW, J., ADDAI, T., ASHWIN, A., MORROBEL, A., MA-HESHWARI, P., & FREELS, S. (1995). Clinical features, site of involvement, bacteriologic findings and outcome of infection endocarditis in intravenous drug users. *Archives of Internal Medicine, 155,* 1641–1649.

MATHEW, R. D., WILSON, W. H., BLAZER, D. G., & GEORGE, L. K. (1993). Psychiatric disorders in adult children of alcoholics: Data from the epidemiologic catchment area project. *American Journal of Psychiatry, 150,* 793–800.

MATHIAS, R. (1995). NIDA survey provides first national data on drug use during pregnancy. *NIDA Notes, 10*(1), 6–7.

MATSUDA, L. A., LOLAIT, S. J., BROWNSTEIN, M. J., YOUNG, A. C., & BONNER, T. I. (1990). Structure of a cannabinoid receptor and functional expression of the cloned cDNA. *Nature, 346,* 561–564.

MATTICK, R. P., & HALL, W. (1996). Are detoxification programs effective? *Lancet, 347,* 97–100.

MATTILA, M. A. K., & LARNI, H. M. (1980). Flunitrazepam: A review of its pharmacological properties and therapeutic use. *Drugs, 20,* 353–374.

MATTSON, S. N., & RILEY, E. P. (1995). Prenatal exposure to alcohol. *Alcohol Health & Research World, 19,* 273–278.

MATUSCHKA, P. R. (1985). The psychopharmacology of addiction. In T. E. Bratter & G. G. Forrest (Eds.), *Alcoholism and substance abuse: Strategies for clinical intervention.* New York: Free Press.

MAXMEN, J. S., & WARD, N. G. (1995). *Psychotropic drugs fast facts* (2nd ed.). New York: Norton.

MAY, G. G. (1988). *Addiction and grace.* New York: Harper & Row.

MAY, G. G. (1991). *The awakened heart.* New York: Harper & Row.

MAYES, L. C., GRANGER, R. H., FRANK, M. A., SCHOTTENFELD, R., & BORNSTEIN, M. H. (1993). Neurobehavioral profiles of neonates exposed to cocaine prenatally. *Pediatrics, 91,* 778–783.

MAYO CLINIC HEALTH LETTER. (1989). *America's drug crisis.* Rochester, MN: Mayo Foundation for Medical Education and Research.

MCCAFFERY, M., & FERRELL, B. R. (1994). Understanding opioids and addiction. *Nursing 94, 24*(8), 56–59.

MCCARTHY, J. J., & BORDERS, O. T. (1985). Limit setting on drug abuse in methadone maintenance patients. *American Journal of Psychiatry, 142,* 1419–1423.

MCCAUL, M. D., & FURST, J. (1994). Alcoholism treatment in the United States. *Alcohol Health & Research World, 18,* 253–260.

MCCRADY, B. S. (1993). Alcoholism. In D. H. Barlow (Ed.), *Clinical handbook of psychological disorders* (2nd ed.). New York: Guilford Press.

MCCRADY, B. S. (1994). Alcoholics Anonymous and behavior therapy: Can habits be treated as diseases? Can

diseases be treated as habits. *Journal of Consulting and Clinical Psychology, 62,* 1159–1166.

MCCRADY, B. S., & DELANEY, S. I. (1995). Self-help groups. In R. K. Hester & W. R. Miller (Eds.), *Handbook of alcoholism treatment approaches* (2nd ed.). New York: Allyn & Bacon.

MCCRADY, B. S., & EPSTEIN, E. E. (1995). Marital therapy in the treatment of alcoholism. In N. S. Jacobson & A. S. Gurman (Eds.), *Clinical handbook of couple therapy.* New York: Guilford Press.

MCCRADY, B. S., & IRVINE, S. (1989). Self-help groups. In R. K. Hester & W. R. Miller (Eds.), *Handbook of alcoholism treatment approaches.* New York: Pergamon Press.

MCCRADY, B. S., & LANGENBUCHER, J. W. (1996). Alcohol treatment and health care system reform. *Archives of General Psychiatry, 53,* 737–746.

MCCUSKER, J., STODDARD, A., FROST, R., & ZORN, M. (1996). Planned versus actual duration of drug abuse treatment. *Journal of Nervous and Mental Disease, 184,* 482–489.

MCCUTCHAN, J. A. (1990). Virology, immunology, and clinical course of HIV infection. *Journal of Clinical and Consulting Psychology, 58,* 5–12.

MCENROE, P. (1990). Hawaii is fighting losing battle against the popularity of drug "ice." *Minneapolis Star-Tribune, IX*(44), 1, 20A.

MCGINNIS, J. M., & FOEGE, W. H. (1993). Actual causes of death in the United States. *Journal of the American Medical Association, 270,* 2207–2212.

MCGUIRE, L. (1990). The power of non-narcotic pain relievers. *RN, 53*(4), 28–35.

MCGUIRE, P., & FAHY, T. (1991). Chronic paranoid psychosis after misuse of MDMA ("ecstacy"). *British Medical Journal, 302,* 697.

MCHUGH, M. J. (1987). The abuse of volatile substances. *Pediatric Clinics of North America, 34*(2), 333–340.

MCLELLAN, A. T., ARNDT, I. O., METZGER, D. S., WOODY, G. E., & O'BRIEN, C. P. (1993). The effects of psychosocial services in substance abuse treatment. *Journal of the American Medical Association, 269,* 1953–1959.

MCMICKEN, D. B. (1990). Alcohol withdrawal syndromes. *Emergency Medicine Clinics of North America, 8,* 805–819.

MCNAMARA, J. D. (1996). The war on drugs is lost. *National Review, XLVIII*(2), 42–44.

MCWILLIAMS, P. (1993). Ain't nobody's business. *Playboy, 40*(9), 49–52.

MDMA MAY NOT BE SO NEUROTOXIC AFTER ALL. (1996). *Forensic Drug Abuse Advisor, 8*(1), 5–6.

MEAD, R. (1993). Teen access to cigarettes in Green Bay, Wisconsin. *Wisconsin Medical Journal, 92,* 23–25.

MEDICAL BENEFITS OF MARIJUANA. (1991). *Health Facts, XVI*(147), 1, 4.

MEDICAL ECONOMICS COMPANY. (1989). Anabolic steroid abuse and primary care. *Patient Care, 23*(8), 12.

MEDICAL ECONOMICS COMPANY. (1995). *1995 Physician's Desk Reference* (49th ed.). Oradell, NJ: Author.

MEDICAL ECONOMICS COMPANY. (1997). *1997 Physician's Desk Reference* (51st ed.). Oradell, NJ: Author.

MEE-LEE, D. (1995). *Addiction treatment in a managed care environment.* Workshop presented by Institute for Behavioral Healthcare, Kansas City, KS.

MEER, J. (1986). Marijuana in the air: Delayed buzz bomb. *Psychology Today, 20,* 68.

MELZACK, R. (1990). The tragedy of needless pain. *Scientific American, 262*(2), 27–33.

MENDELSON, J. H., & MELLO, N. K. (1996). Management of cocaine abuse and dependence. *New England Journal of Medicine, 334,* 965–972.

MENDELSON, W. B., & RICH, C. L. (1993). Sedatives and suicide: The San Diego study. *Acta Psychiatrica Scandinavica, 88,* 337–341.

MENDOZA, R., & MILLER, B. L. (1992). Neuropsychiatric disorders associated with cocaine use. *Hospital and Community Psychiatry, 43,* 677–678.

MERLOTTI, L., ROEHRS, T., KOSHOREK, G., ZORICK, F., LAMPHERE, J., & ROTH, T. (1989). The dose effects of zolpidem on the sleep of healthy normals. *Journal of Clinical Psychopharmacology, 9*(1), 9–14.

MERTON, T. (1961). *New seeds of contemplation.* New York: New Directions.

MERTON, T. (1978). *No man is an island.* New York: New Directions.

METHADONE ALTERNATIVE NEARS APPROVAL. (1993). *Alcoholism & Drug Abuse Week, 5*(22), 4.

METHADONE CENTERS INEFFECTIVE IN TREATING HEROIN ADDICTS–GAO. (1989). *The Addiction Letter, 6*(5), 5.

"METH'S" REACH TO ADDICTS AND TREATMENT PROGRAMS IS GROWING (methamphetamine). (1995). *Alcoholism & Drug Abuse Week, 7*(31), 1–2.

MEYER, R. (1988). Intervention: Opportunity for healing. *Alcoholism & Addiction, 9*(1), 7.

MEYER, R. E. (1989a). Who can say no to illicit drug use. *Archives of General Psychiatry, 46,* 189–190.

MEYER, R. E. (1989b). What characterizes addiction? *Alcohol Health & Research World, 13*(4), 316–321.

MEYER, R. E. (1992). New pharmacotherapies for cocaine dependence . . . revisited. *Archives of General Psychiatry, 49,* 900–904.

MEYER, R. E. (1994). What for, alcohol research? *American Journal of Psychiatry, 151,* 165–168.

MEYER, R. E. (1995). Biology of psychoactive substance dependence disorders: Opiates, cocaine and ethanol. In A. F. Schatzberg & C. B. Nemeroff (Eds.), *Textbook of psychopharmacology.* Washington, DC: American Psychiatric Association.

MEYER, R. E. (1996). The disease called addiction: Emerging evidence is a 200 year debate. *Lancet, 347,* 162–166.

MEYERS, B. R. (1992). *Antimicrobial therapy guide.* Newtown, PA: Antimicrobial Prescribing.

MEZA, E., & KRANZLER, H. R. (1996). Closing the gap between alcoholism research and practice: The case for pharmacotherapy. *Psychiatric Services, 47,* 917–920.

MICHELSON, J. B., CARROLL, D., McLANE, N. J., & ROBIN, H. S. (1988). Drug abuse and ocular disease. In J. B. Michelson & R. A. Nozik (Eds.), *Surgical treatment of ocular inflammatory disease.* New York: J. B. Lippincott Co.

MIDDLEMAN, A. B., & DuRANT, R. H. (1996). Anabolic steroid use and associated health risk behaviors. *Sports Medicine, 21,* 251–255.

MIKKELSEN, E. (1985). Substance abuse in adolescents and children. In R. Michels, J. O. Cavenar, H. K. H. Brodie, A. M. Cooper, S. B. Guze, S. B. Judd, G. Klerman, & A. J. Solnit (Eds.), *Psychiatry.* New York: Basic Books.

MILBERGER, S., BIEDERMAN, J., FARAONE, S. V., CHEN, L., & JONES, J. (1996). Is maternal smoking during pregnancy a risk factor for attention deficit hyperactivity disorder in children? *American Journal of Psychiatry, 153,* 1138–1142.

MILBY, J. B., HOHMANN, A. A., GENTILE, M., HUGGINS, N., SIMS, M. K., McLELLAN, T., WOODY, G., & HAAS, N. (1994). Methadone maintenance outcome as a function of detoxification phobia. *American Journal of Psychiatry, 151,* 1031–1037.

MILHORN, H. T. (1991). Diagnosis and management of phenocyclidine intoxication. *American Family Physician, 43,* 1293–1302.

MILHORN, H. T. (1992). Pharmacologic management of acute abstinence syndromes. *American Family Physician, 45,* 231–239.

MILLER, A. (1988). *The enabler.* Claremont, CA: Hunter House.

MILLER, B. A., & DOWNS, W. R. (1995). Violent victimization among women with alcohol problems. In M. Galanter (Ed.), *Recent developments in alcoholism* (Vol. 12). New York: Plenum Press.

MILLER, F. T., & TANENBAUM, J. H. (1989). Drug abuse in schizophrenia. *Hospital and Community Psychiatry, 40,* 847–849.

MILLER, L. J. (1994). Psychiatric medication during pregnancy: Understanding and minimizing risks. *Psychiatric Annals, 24*(2), 69–75.

MILLER, N. S. (1994). Psychiatric comorbidity: Occurrance and treatment. *Alcohol Health & Research World, 18,* 261–264.

MILLER, N. S., & GOLD, M. S. (1991a). Organic solvent and aerosol abuse. *American Family Physician, 44,* 183–190.

MILLER, N. S., & GOLD, M. S. (1991b). Abuse, addiction, tolerance, and dependence to benzodiazepines in medical and nonmedical populations. *American Journal of Drug and Alcohol Abuse, 17*(1), 27–37.

MILLER, N. S., & GOLD, M. S. (1991c). Dual diagnosis: Psychiatric syndromes in alcoholism and drug addiction. *American Family Physician, 43,* 2071–2076.

MILLER, N. S., & GOLD, M. S. (1993). A hypothesis for a common neurochemical basis for alcohol and drug disorders. *Psychiatric Clinics of North America, 16,* 105–117.

MILLER, P. M., & FOY, D. W. (1981). Substance abuse. In S. M. Turner, K. S. Calhoun, & H. E. Adams (Eds.), *Handbook of clinical behavior therapy.* New York: Wiley.

MILLER, S. I., FRANCES, R. J., & HOLMES, D. J. (1988). Use of psychotropic drugs in alcoholism treatment: A summary. *Hospital & Community Psychiatry, 39,* 1251–1252.

MILLER, S. I., FRANCES, R. J., & HOLMES, D. J. (1989). Psychotropic medications In R. K. Hester & W. R. Miller (Eds.), *Handbook of alcoholism treatment approaches.* New York: Pergamon Press.

MILLER, W. R. (1976). Alcoholism scales and objective measures. *Psychological Bulletin, 83,* 649–674.

MILLER, W. R. (1992). Client/treatment matching in addictive behaviors. *Behavior Therapist, 15*(1), 7–8.

MILLER, W. R. (1995). Increasing motivation for change. In R. K. Hester & W. R. Miller (Eds.), *Handbook of alcoholism treatment approaches* (2nd ed.). New York: Allyn & Bacon.

MILLER, W. R., & CERVANTES, E. A. (1997). Gender and patterns of alcohol problems: Pretreatment responses of women and men to the comprehensive drinker profile. *Journal of Clinical Psychology, 53,* 263–277.

MILLER, W. R., GENEFIELD, G., & TONIGAN, J. S. (1993). Enhancing motivation for change in problem drinking: A controlled comparison of two therapist styles. *Journal of Consulting and Clinical Psychology, 61,* 455–462.

MILLER, W. R., & HESTER, R. K. (1980). Treating the problem drinker: Modern approaches. In W. R. Miller (Ed.), *The addictive behaviors.* New York: Pergamon Press.

MILLER, W. R., & HESTER, R. K. (1986). Inpatient alcoholism treatment. *American Psychologist, 41*(7), 794–806.

MILLER, W. R., & HESTER, R. K. (1995). Treating alcohol problems: Toward an informed eclectism. In R. K. Hester & W. R. Miller (Eds.), *Handbook of alcoholism treatment approaches* (2nd ed.). New York: Allyn & Bacon.

MILLER, W. R., & KURTZ, E. (1994). Models of alcoholism used in treatment: Contrasting AA and other perspectives with which it is often confused. *Journal of Studies on Alcohol, 55,* 159–166.

MILLER, W. R., & McCRADY, B. S. (1993). The importance of research on Alcoholics Anonymous. In B. S. McCrady & W. R. Miller (Eds.), *Research on Alcoholics Anonymous.* New Brunswick, NJ: Rutgers Center of Alcohol Studies.

MILLER, W. R., & ROLLNICK, S. (1991). *Motivational interviewing.* New York: Guilford Press.

MILLER, W. R., WESTERBERG, V. S., & WALDRON, H. B. (1995). Evaluating alcohol problems in adults and adolescents. In R. K. Hester & W. R. Miller (Eds.), *Handbook of alcoholism treatment approaches* (2nd ed.). New York: Allyn & Bacon.

MILLMAN, R. B., & BEEDER, A. B. (1994). Cannabis. In M. Galanter & H. D. Kleber (Eds.), *Textbook of substance abuse treatment.* Washington, DC: American Psychiatric Press.

MILLON, T. (1981). *Disorders of personality.* New York: Wiley.

MILLS, K. C. (1995). Serotonin syndrome. *American Family Physician, 52,* 1475–1482.

MILZMAN, D. P., & SODERSTROM, C. A. (1994). Substance use disorders in trauma patients. *Critical Care Clinics, 10,* 595–612.

MINKOFF, K. (1989). An integrated treatment model for dual diagnosis of psychosis and addiction. *Hospital and Community Psychiatry, 40,* 1031–1036.

MIRIN, S. M., WEISS, R. D., & GREENFIELD, S. F. (1991). Psychoactive substance use disorders. In A. J. Galenberg, E. L. Bassuk, & S. C. Schoonover (Eds.), *The practitioner's guide to psychoactive drugs* (3rd ed.). New York: Plenum Medical Book.

MITCHELL, J. R. (1988). Acetaminophen toxicity. *New England Journal of Medicine, 319,* 1601–1602.

MITRA, S. C., GANESH, V., & APUZZIO, J. J. (1994). Effect of maternal cocaine abuse on renal arterial flow and urine output in the fetus. *American Journal of Obstetrics and Gynecology, 171,* 1556–1560.

MIXED SIGNALS ON POSSIBLE UPSURGE IN HEROIN USE. (1991). *Alcoholism & Drug Abuse Week, 3*(24), 4–5.

MOLITERNO, D. J., WILLARD, J. E., LANGE, R. A., NEGUS, B. H., BOEHRER, J. D., GLAMANN, B., LANDAU, C., ROSSEN, J. D., WINNIFORD, M. D., & HOLLIS, L. D. (1994). Coronary-artery vasoconstriction induced by cocaine, cigarette smoking, or both. *New England Journal of Medicine, 330,* 454–459.

MONCHER, M. S., HOLDEN, G. W., & TRIMBLE, J. E. (1990). Substance abuse among native American youth. *Journal of Consulting and Clinical Psychology, 58,* 408–415.

MONFORTE, R., ESTRUCH, R., VALLS-SOLE, J., NICOLAS, J., VILLALTA, J., & URBANO-MARQUEZ, A. (1995). Autonomic and peripheral neuropathies in patients with chronic alcoholism. *Archives of Neurology, 51,* 45–51.

MONROE, J. (1994). Designer drugs: CAT & LSD. *Current Health, 20*(1), 13–16.

MONROE, J. (1995). Inhalants: Dangerous highs. *Current Health, 22*(1), 16–20.

MONTEITH, S. K. (1997). Aids: The untold story. *Medical Sentinel, 2*(3), 97–100.

MOORE, J. (1993). AIDS: Striking the happy media. *Nature, 363,* 391–392.

MOORE, M. H. (1991). Drugs, the criminal law, and the administration of justice. *Milbank Quarterly, 69*(4), 529–560.

MOORE, R. A. (1995). Analysis. In A. Cowan & J. W. Lewis (Eds.), *Buprenorphine.* New York: Wiley Interscience.

MOOS, R. H., KING, M. J., & PATTERSON, M. A. (1996). Outcomes of residential treatment of substance abuse in hospital and community-based programs. *Psychiatric Services, 47,* 68–74.

MOOS, R. H., & MOOS, B. S. (1995). Stay in residential facilities and mental health care as predictors of readmission for patients with substance use disorders. *Psychiatric Services, 46,* 66–72.

MORABIA, A., BERNSTEIN, M., HERITIER, S., & KHATCHATRIAN, N. (1996). Relation of breast cancer with passive and active exposure to tobacco. *American Journal of Epidemiology, 143,* 918–928.

MOREY, L. C. (1996). Patient placement criteria. *Alcohol Health & Research World, 20,* 36–44.

MORGENROTH, L. (1989). High-risk pain pills. *The Atlantic, 264*(6), 36–42.

MORRISON, M. A. (1990). Addiction in adolescents. *Western Journal of Medicine, 152,* 543–547.

MORRISON, S. F., ROGERS, P. D., & THOMAS, M. H. (1995). Alcohol and adolescents. *Pediatric Clinics of North America, 42,* 371–389.

MORSE, R. M., & FLAVIN, D. K. (1992). The definition of alcoholism. *Journal of the American Medical Association, 268,* 1012–1014.

MORTENSEN, M. E., & RENNEBOHM, R. M. (1989). Clinical pharmacology and use of nonsteroidal anti-inflammatory drugs. *Pediatric Clinics of North America, 36,* 1113–1139.

MORTON, H. G. (1987). Occurrence and treatment of solvent abuse in children and adolescents. *Pharmacological Therapy, 33,* 449–469.

MORTON, W. A., & SANTOS, A. (1989). New indications for benzodiazepines in the treatment of major psychiatric disorders. *Hospital Formulary, 24,* 274–278.

MOTT, S. H., PACKER, R. J., & SOLDIN, S. J. (1994). Neurologic manifestations of cocaine exposure in childhood. *Pediatrics, 93,* 557–560.

MOYER, T. P., & ELLEFSON, P. J. (1987). Marijuana testing—How good is it? *Mayo Clinic Procedures, 62,* 413–417.

MOYLAN, D. W. (1990). Court intervention. *Adolescent Counselor, 2*(5), 23–27.

MUELLER, T. I., LAVORI, P. W., KELLER, M. B., SWARTZ, A., WARSHAW, M., HASIN, D., CORYELL, W., ENDICOTT, J., RICE, J., & AKISKALL, H. (1994). Prognostic effect of the variable course of alcoholism on the 10 year course of depression. *American Journal of Psychiatry, 151,* 701–706.

MUESER, K. T., BELLACK, A. S., & BLANCHARD, J. J. (1992). Comorbidity of schizophrenia and substance abuse: Implications for treatment. *Journal of Counseling and Clinical Psychology, 60,* 845–856.

MUESER, K. T., YARNOLD, P. R., & BELLACK, A. S. (1992). Diagnostic and demographic correlates of substance abuse in schizophrenia and major affective disorder. *Acta Psychiatrica Scandinavica 85,* 48–55.

MURPHY, D. F. (1993). NSAIDs and postoperative pain. *British Medical Journal, 306,*1493.

MURPHY, G. E., WETZEL, R. D., ROBINS, E., & McEVOY, L. (1992). Multiple risk factors predict suicide in alcoholism. *Archives of General Psychiatry, 49,* 459–463.

MURPHY, S. L., & KHANTZIAN, E. J. (1995). Addiction as a self-medication disorder: Application of ego psychology to the treatment of substance abuse. In A. M. Washton (Ed.), *Psychotherapy and substance abuse.* New York: Guilford Press.

MURPHY, S. M., OWEN, R., & TYRER, P. (1989). Comparative assessment of efficacy and withdrawal symptoms after 6 and 12 weeks' treatment with diazepam or buspirone. *British Journal of Psychiatry, 154,* 529–534.

MURRAY, M. J., DERUYTER, M. L., & HARRISON, B. A. (1995). Opioids and benzodiazepines. *Critical Care Clinics, 11,* 849–873.

MUSCAT, J. E., STELLMAN, S. D., & WYNDER, E. L. (1995). Analgesic use and colonrectal cancer. *Preventive Medicine, 24,* 110–112.

MUSTO, D. F. (1991). Opium, cocaine and marijuana in American history. *Scientific American, 265*(1), 40–47.

MUSTO, D. F. (1996). Alcohol in American history. *Scientific American, 274*(4), 78–83.

MYERS, M. G., & BROWN, S. A. (1994). Smoking and health in substance-abusing adolescents: A two year follow-up. *Pediatrics, 93,* 561–566.

NACE, E. P. (1987). *The treatment of alcoholism.* New York: Brunner/Mazel.

NACE, E. P., & ISBELL, P. G. (1991). Alcohol. In R. J. Frances & S. I. Miller (Eds.), *Clinical textbook of addictive disorders.* New York: Guilford Press.

NADELMANN, E. (1997). Save money, cut crime, get real. *Playboy, 44*(1), 129, 193–194.

NADELMANN, E., & WENNER, J. S. (1994, May 5). Towards a sane national drug policy. *Rolling Stone,* 24–26.

NADELMANN, E. A. (1989). Drug prohibition in the United States: Costs, consequences,and alternatives. *Science, 245,* 939–946.

NADELMANN, E. A., KLEIMAN, M. A. R., & EARLS, F. J. (1990). Should some illegal drugs be legalized? *Issues in Science and Technology, VI*(4), 43–49.

NAHAS, G. G. (1986). Cannabis: Toxicological properties and epidemiological aspects. *Medical Journal of Australia, 145,* 82–87.

NAJM, W. (1997). Viral hepatitis: How to manage type C and D infections. *Geriatrics, 52*(5), 28–37.

NARCOTICS ANONYMOUS. (1982). Van Nuys, CA: Narcotics Anonymous World Service Office.

NASH, J. M., & PARK, A. (1997). Addicted. *Time, 149*(18), 68–76.

NATHAN, P. E. (1980). Etiology and process in the addictive behaviors. In W. R. Miller (Ed.), *Addictive behaviors.* New York: Pergamon Press.

NATHAN, P. E. (1988). The addictive personality *is* the behavior of the addict. *Journal of Consulting and Clinical Psychology, 56,* 183–188.

NATHAN, P. E. (1991). Substance use disorders in the *DSM-IV. Journal of Abnormal Psychology, 100,* 356–361.

NATIONAL ACADEMY OF SCIENCES. (1990). *Treating drug problems* (Vol. 1). Washington, DC: National Academy Press.

NATIONAL COMMISSION ON MARIHUANA AND DRUG ABUSE. (1972). *Marihuana: A signal of misunderstanding.* Washington, DC: U.S. Government Printing Office.

NATIONAL COMMISSION ON MARIHUANA AND DRUG ABUSE. (1973). *Drug use in America: Problem in perspective.* Washington, DC: U.S. Government Printing Office.

NATIONAL FOUNDATION FOR BRAIN RESEARCH. (1992). *The cost of disorders of the brain.*Washington, DC: Author.

NATIONAL INSTITUTE ON ALCOHOL ABUSE AND ALCOHOLISM. (1989). *Relapse and craving. Alcohol Alert (# 6).* Washington, DC: U.S. Department of Health and Human Services.

NATIONAL INSTITUTE ON DRUG ABUSE. (1991). *National household survey on drug abuse: Population estimates 1990.* Rockville, MD: U.S. Government Printing Office.

NATIONAL INSTITUTE ON DRUG ABUSE. (1994). *Monitoring the future study, 1975–1994.*Rockville, MD: U.S. Government Printing Office.

NEGUS, S. S., & WOODS, J. H. (1995). Reinforcing effects, discriminative stimulus effects, and physical dependence liability of buprenorphine. In A. Cowan & J. W. Lewis (Eds.), *Buprenorphine.* New York: Wiley Interscience.

NELIPOVICH, M., & BUSS, E. (1991). Investigating alcohol abuse among persons who are blind. *Journal of Visual Impairment & Blindness, 85,* 343–345.

NELSON, H. D., NEVITT, M. C., SCOTT, J. C., STONE, K. L., & CUMMINGS, S. R. (1994). Smoking,alcohol, and neuromuscular and physical function in older women. *Journal of the American Medical Association, 272,* 1825–1831.

NESSE, R. M., & WILLIAMS, G. C. (1994). *Why we get sick.* New York: Random House.

NESTLER, E. J., FITZGERALD, L. W., & SELF, D. W. (1995). Neurobiology. In J. M. Oldham & M. B. Riba (Eds.), *Review of psychiatry* (Vol. 14). Washington, DC: American Psychiatric Press.

NEWCOMB, M. D. (1996). Adolescence: Pathologizing a normal process. *Counseling Psychologist, 24,* 482–490.

NEWCOMB, M. D., & BENTLER, P. M. (1989). Substance use and abuse among children and teenagers. *American Psychologist, 44,* 242–248.

NEW DRUG "ICE" GRIPS HAWAII, THREATENS MAINLAND. (1989). *Minneapolis Star-Tribune, VIII*(150), 12a.

NEWELL, T., & COSGROVE, J. (1988). *Recovery of neuropsychological functions during reduction of PCP use.* Paper presented at the 1988 annual meeting of the American Psychological Association, Atlanta, GA.

NEWLAND, D. (1989). Alcohol and drug addiction—a disease or a crime? *Supervision, 50*(6), 16–19.

NEW LAW NETS MOSTLY MARIJUANA USERS. (1996). *Forensic Drug Abuse Advisor, 8*(3), 29.

NEWTON, R. E., MARUNYCZ, J. D., ALDERDICE, M. C., & NAPOLIELLO, M. J. (1986). Review of the side effects of buspirone. *American Journal of Medicine, 80*(Suppl. 3B).

NEY, J. A., DOOLEY, S. L., KEITH, L. G., CHASNOFF, I. J., & SOCOL, M. L. (1990). The prevalence of substance abuse in patients with suspected preterm labor. *American Journal of Obstetrics and Gynecology, 162,* 1562–1568.

NIAURA, R. S., ROHSENOW, D. J., BINKOFF, J. A., MONTI, P. M., PEDRAZA, M., & ABRAMS, D. B. (1988). Relevance of cue reactivity to understanding alcohol and smoking relapse. *Journal of Abnormal Psychology, 97*(2), 133–153.

NICASTRO, N. (1989). Visual disturbances associated with over-the-counter ibuprofen in three patients. *Annuals of Ophthalmology, 21,* 447–450.

NIGHTCAP DANGERS. (1989). *Science Digest, 2*(5), 90.

NISHINO, S., MIGNOT, E., & DEMENT, W. C. (1995). Sedative-hypnotics. In A. F. Schatzberg & C. B. Nemeroff (Eds.), *Textbook of psychopharmacology.* Washington, DC: American Psychiatric Association Press.

NIXON, S. J. (1994). Cognitive deficits in alcoholic women. *Alcohol Health & Research World, 18,* 228–231.

NOBLE, E. P., BLUM, K., RITCHIE, T., MONTGOMERY, A., & SHERIDAN, P. F. (1991). Allelic association of the D_2 dopamine receptor gene with receptor-binding characteristics in alcoholism. *Archives of General Psychiatry, 48,* 648–654.

NORRIS, D. (1994). War's "wonder" drugs. *America's Civil War, 7*(2), 50–57.

NORTH, C. S. (1996). Alcoholism in women. *Postgraduate Medicine, 100,* 221–224, 230–232.

NORTON, R. L., BURTON, B. T., & McGIRR, J. (1996). Blood lead of intravenous drug users. *Journal of Toxicology: Clinical Toxicology, 34*(4), 425–431.

NOT ENOUGH DATA ON HOW LONG MARIJUANA USERS TEST POSITIVE. (1995). *Forensic Drug Abuse Advisor, 7*(9), 66–68.

NOVELLO, A. C., & SHOSKY, J. (1992). From the Surgeon General, U.S. Public Health Service. *Journal of the American Medical Association, 268,* 961.

NOWAK, M. A., & MCMICHAEL, A. J. (1995). How HIV defeats the immune system. *Scientific American, 273*(2), 58–65.

NOWINSKI, J. (1996). Facilitating 12-Step recovery from substance abuse and addiction. In F. Rotgers D. S. Keller & J. Morgenstern (Eds.), *Treating substance abuse.* New York: Guilford Press.

NUNES, J. V., & PARSON, E. B. (1995). Patterns of psychoactive substance use among adolescents. *American Family Physician, 52,* 1693–1697.

NUTT, D. J. (1996). Addiction: Brain mechanisms and their treatment implications. *Lancet, 347,* 31–36.

O'BRIEN, C. P. (1996). Recent developments in the pharmacotherapy of substance abuse. *Journal of Consulting and Clinical Psychology, 64,* 677–686.

O'BRIEN, C. P., & MCLELLAN, A. T. (1996). Myths about the treatment of addiction. *Lancet, 347,* 237–240.

O'BRIEN, C. P., & MCLELLAN, A. T. (1997). Addiction medicine. *Journal of the American Medical Association, 277,* 1840–1841.

O'BRIEN, P. E., & GABORIT, M. (1992). Codependency: A disorder separate from chemical dependency. *Journal of Clinical Psychology, 48*(1), 129–136.

OCHS, L. (1992). EEG treatment of addictions. *Biofeedback, 20*(1), 8–16.

O'CONNOR, P. G., CHANG, G., & SHI, J. (1992). Medical complications of cocaine use. In T. R. Kosten & H. D. Kleber (Eds.), *Clinician's guide to cocaine addiction.* New York: Guilford Press.

O'CONNOR, P. G., SAMET, J. H., & STEIN, M. D. (1994). Management of hospitalized intravenous drug users: Role of the internist. *American Journal of Medicine, 96,* 551–558.

O'DONNELL, M. (1986). The executive ailment: "Curable only by death." *International Management, 41*(7), 64.

O'DONOVAN, M. C., & MCGUFFIN, P. (1993). Short acting benzodiazepines. *British Medical Journal, 306,* 182–183.

OETTING, E. R., & BEAUVAIS, F. (1990). Adolescent drug use: Findings of national and local surveys. *Journal of Consulting and Clinical Psychology, 58,* 385–394.

O'FARRELL, T. J. (1995). Marital and family therapy. In R. K. Hester & W. R. Miller (Eds.), *Handbook of alcoholism treatment approaches* (2nd ed.). New York: Allyn & Bacon.

OFFICE OF NATIONAL DRUG CONTROL POLICY. (1995). *Pulse check.* Washington, DC: U.S. Government Printing Office.

OFFICE OF NATIONAL DRUG CONTROL POLICY. (1996). *The national drug control strategy: 1996.* Washington, DC: U.S. Government Printing Office.

OGBORNE, A. C. (1993). Assessing the effectiveness of Alcoholics Anonymous in the community: Meeting the challenges. In B. S. McCrady & W. R. Miller (Eds.), *Research on Alcoholics Anonymous.* New Brunswick, NJ: Rutgers Center of Alcohol Studies.

OGBORNE, A. C., & GLASER, F. B. (1985). Evaluating Alcoholics Anonymous. In T. E. Bratter & G. G. Forrest (Eds.), *Alcoholism and substance abuse: Strategies for clinical intervention.* New York: Free Press.

OLDS, D. L., HENDERSON, C. R., & TATELBAUM, R. (1994). Intellectual impairment in children of women who smoke cigarettes during pregnancy. *Pediatrics, 93,* 221–227.

OLIWENSTEIN, L. (1988). The perils of pot. *Discover, 9*(6), 18.

OLIWENSTEIN, L. (1990). The kaposi's connection. *Discover, 11*(8), 28.

OLSON, J. (1992). *Clinical pharmacology made ridiculously simple.* Miami, FL: MedMaster.

O'MALLEY, S., ADAMSE, M., HEATON, R. K., & GAWIN, F. G. (1992). Neuropsychological impairment in chronic cocaine abusers. *American Journal of Drug and Alcohol Abuse, 18*(2), 131–144.

ONDCP GIVES RUNDOWN ON TREATMENT APPROACHES. (1990). *Alcoholism & Drug Abuse Week, 2*(26), 3–5.

ONDCP SAYS AMERICANS SPENT $41 BILLION ON DRUGS IN 1990. (1991). *Alcoholism & Drug Abuse Week, 3*(24), 3.

OSHER, F. C., & DRAKE, R. E. (1996). Reversing a history of unmet needs: Approaches to care for persons with co-occurring addictive and mental disorders. *American Journal of Orthopsychiatry, 66,* 4–11.

OSHER, F. C., DRAKE, R. E., NOORDSY, D. L., TEAGUE, G. B., HURLBUT, S. C., BIESANZ, J. C., & BEAUDETT, M. S. (1994). Correlates and outcomes of alcohol use disorder among rural outpatients with schizophrenia. *Journal of Clinical Psychiatry, 55,* 109–113.

OSHER, F. C., & KOFOED, L. L. (1989). Treating patients with psychiatric and psychoactive substance abuse disorders. *Hospital and Community Psychiatry, 40,* 1025–1030.

OTHER AAFS HIGHLIGHTS. (1995). *Forensic Drug Abuse Advisor, 7*(3), 18.

OTTO, R. K., LANG, A. R., MEGARGEE, E. I., & ROSENBLATT, A. I. (1989). Ability of alcoholics to escape detection by the MMPI. *Critical Items, 4*(2), 2, 7–8.

OUIMETTE, P. C., FINNEY, J. W., & MOOS, R. H. (1997). Twelve-step and cognitive-behavioral treatment for substance abuse: A comparison of treatment effectiveness. *Journal of Consulting and Clinical Psychology, 65,* 230–240.

OWEN, R. R., FISCHER, E. P., BOOTH, B. M., & CUFFEL, B. J. (1996). Medication noncompliance and substance abuse among patients with schizophrenia. *Psychiatric Services, 47,* 853–858.

OWINGS-WEST, M., & PRINZ, R. J. (1987). Parental alcoholism and child psychopathology. *Psychological Bulletin, 102*(2), 204–281.

PACKE, G. E., GARTON, M. J., & JENNINGS, K. (1990). Acute myocardial infarction caused by intravenous amphetamine abuse. *British Heart Journal, 64,* 23–24.

PALELLA, F. J., DELANEY, K. M., MOORMAN, A. C., LOVELESS, M. O., FUHRER, J., SATTEN, G. A., ASCHMAN, D. J., & HOLMBERG, S. D. (1998). Declining morbidity and mortality among patients with advanced human immunodeficiency virus infection. *New England Journal of Medicine, 338,* 853–860.

PAPE, P. A. (1988). EAP's and chemically dependent women. *Alcoholism & Addiction, 8*(6), 43–44.

PAPPAS, N. (1990). Dangerous liaisons: When food and drugs don't mix. *In Health, 4*(4), 22–24.

PAPPAS, N. (1995). Secondhand smoke: Is it a hazard? *Consumer Reports, 60*(1), 27–33.

PARIS, P. M. (1996). Treating the patient in pain. *Emergency Medicine, 28*(9), 66–76, 78–79, 83–86, 90.

PARKER, G. B., BARRETT, E. A., & HICKIE, I. B. (1992). From nurture to network: Examining links between perceptions of parenting received in childhood and social bonds in adulthood. *American Journal of Psychiatry, 149,* 877–885.

PARKER, R. N. (1993). The effects of context on alcohol and violence. *Alcohol Health & Research World, 17*(2), 117–122.

PARRAS, F., PATIER, J. L., & EZPELETA, C. (1988). Lead contaminated heroin as a source of inorganic lead intoxication. *The Staff, 316,* 755.

PARRY, A. (1992). Taking heroin maintenance seriously: The politics of tolerance. *Lancet, 339,* 350–351.

PARSIAN, A., & CLONINGER, C. R. (1991). Genetics of high-risk populations. *Addiction & Recovery, 11*(6), 9–11.

PARSIAN, A., TODD, R. D., DEVOR, E. J., O'MALLEY, K. L., SUAREZ, B. K., REICH, T., & CLONINGER, C. R. (1991). Alcoholism and alleles of the human D_2 dopanine receptor locus: Studies of association and linkage. *Archives of General Psychiatry, 48,* 655–663.

PARSONS, O. A., & NIXON, S. J. (1993). Neurobehavioral sequelae of alcoholism. *Behavioral Neurology, 11,* 205–218.

PATLAK, M. (1989). The fickle virus. *Discover, 10*(2), 24–25.

PATON, A. (1996). The detection of alcohol misuse in accident and emergency departments grasping the opportunity. *Journal of Accident & Emergency Medicine, 13,* 306–308.

PATRONO, C. (1994). Aspirin as an antiplatelet drug. *New England Journal of Medicine, 330,* 1287–1294.

PAUL, J. P., STALL, R., & BLOOMFIELD, K. A. (1991). Gay and alcoholic. *Alcoholic Health & Research World, 15,* 151–160.

PAULOS, J. A. (1994). Counting on dyscalculia. *Discover, 15*(3), 30, 34–36.

PAYAN, D. G., & KATZUNG, B. G. (1995). Nonsteroidal anti-inflammatory drugs: Nonopioid analgesics; drugs used in gout. In B. G. Katzung (Ed.), *Basic and clinical pharmacology.* Norwalk, CT: Appleton & Lange.

PEARLSON, G. D., JEFFERY, P. J., HARRIS, G. J., ROSS, C. A., FISCHMAN, M. W., & CAMARGO, E. E. (1993). Correlation of acute cocaine-induced changes in local cerebral blood flow with subjective effects. *American Journal of Psychiatry, 150,* 495–497.

PEARSON, M. A., HOYME, E., SEAVER, L. H., & RIMSZA, M. E. (1994). Toluene embryopathy: Delineation of the phenotype and comparison with Fetal Alcohol Syndrome. *Pediatrics, 93,* 211–215.

PECK, M. S. (1978). *The road less traveled.* New York: Simon & Schuster.

PECK, M. S. (1993). *Further along the road less traveled.* New York: Simon & Schuster.

PECK, M. S. (1997a). *The road less traveled and beyond.* New York: Simon & Schuster.

PECK, M. S. (1997b). *Denial of the soul.* New York: Harmony Books.

PEELE, S. (1984). The cultural context of psychological approaches to alcoholism. *American Psychologist, 39,* 1337–1351.

PEELE, S. (1985). *The meaning of addiction.* Lexington, MA: DC Heath.

PEELE, S. (1988). On the diseasing of America. *Utne Reader, 30,* 67.

PEELE, S. (1989). *Diseasing of America.* Lexington, MA: DC Heath.

PEELE, S. (1991). What we now know about treating alcoholism and other addictions. *Harvard Mental Health Letter, 8*(6), 5–7.

PEELE, S. (1994). Hype overdose: Why does the press automatically accept reports of heroin overdoses, no matter how thin the evidence? *National Review, 46*(21), 59–61.

PEELE, S. (1996). Recovering from an all-of-nothing approach to alcohol. *Psychology Today, 29*(5), 35, 37, 39, 41, 43, 70.

PEELE, S., BRODSKY, A., & ARNOLD, M. (1991). *The truth about addiction and recovery.* New York: Simon & Schuster.

PEGUES, D. A., HUGHES, B. J., & WOERNIE, C. H. (1993). Elevated blood lead levels associated with illegally distilled alcohol. *Archives of Internal Medicine, 153,* 1501–1504.

PELUSO, E., & PELUSO, L. S. (1988). *Women and dugs.* Minneapolis: CompCare.

PELUSO, E., & PELUSO, L. S. (1989). Alcohol and the elderly. *Professional Counselor, 4*(2), 44–46.

PENICK, E. C., NICKEL, E. J., CANTRELL, P. F., POWELL, B. J., READ, M. R., & THOMAS, M. M. (1990). The emerging concept of dual diagnosis: An overview and implications. In D. F. O'Connell (Ed.), *Managing the dually diagnosed patient.* New York: Haworth Press.

PENISTON, E. G., & KULKOSKY, P. J. (1990). Alcoholic personality and Alpha-Theta brain wave training. *Medical Psychotherapy, 3,* 37–55.

PENTZ, M. A., DWYER, J. H., MACKINNON, D. P., FLAY, B. R., HANDEN, W. B., WANG, E. Y. I., & JOHNSON, A. (1989). A multicommunity trial for primary prevention of adolescent drug abuse. *Journal of the American Medical Association, 261*(2), 3259–3266.

PERNEGER, T. V., WHELTON, P. K., & KLAG, M. J. (1994). Risk of kidney failure associated with the use of acetaminophen, aspirin, and nonsteroidal anti-inflammatory drugs. *New England Journal of Medicine, 331,* 1675–1679.

PEROUTKA, S. J. (1989). "Ecstacy": A human neurotoxin? *Archives of General Psychiatry, 46,* 191.

PERRY, J. C., & COOPER, S. H. (1989). An empirical study of defense mechanisms. *Archives of General Psychiatry, 46,* 444–452.

PETERS, H., & THEORELL, C. J. (1991). Fetal and neonatal effects of maternal cocaine use. *Journal of Obstetric, Gynecologic, and Neonatal Nursing, 20*(2), 121–126.

PETERSON, A. M. (1997). Analgesics. *RN, 60*(4), 45–50.

PETO, R., LOPEZ, A. D., BOREHAM, J., THUN, M., & HEATH, C. (1992). Mortality from tobacco in developed countries: Indirect estimation from national vital statistics. *Lancet, 339,* 1268–1278.

PETTINE, K. A. (1991). Association of anabolic steroids and avascular necrosis of femoral heads. *American Journal of Sports Medicine, 19*(1), 96–98.

PEYSER, H. S. (1989). Alcohol and drug abuse: Under recognized and untreated. *Hospital and Community Psychiatry, 40*(3), 221.

PHELPS, D. (1996). Records suggest nicotine enhanced. *Minneapolis Star-Tribune, XV*(5), 1A, 22A.

PHILLIPS, A., SAVIGNY, D., & LAW, M. M. (1995). As Canadians butt out, the developing world lights up. *Canadian Medical Journal, 153,* 1111–1114.

PHILLIPS, A. N., WANNAMETHEE, M. W., THOMSON, A., & SMITH, G. D. (1996). Life expectancy in men who have never smoked and those who have smoked continuously: 15 year follow up of large cohort of middle aged British men. *British Medical Journal, 313,* 907–908.

PICKENS, R. W., SVIKIS, D. S., MCGUE, M., LYKKEN, D. T., HESTON, L. L., & CLAYTON, P. J. (1991). Heterogeneity in the inheritance of alcoholism: A study of male and female twins. *Archives of General Psychiatry, 48,* 19–28.

PIERCE, J. P., GILPIN, E., BURNS, D. M., WHALEN, E., ROSBROOK, B., SHOPLAND, D., & JOHNSON, M. (1991). Does tobacco advertising target young people to start smoking? *Journal of the American Medical Association, 266,* 3154–3158.

PIHL, R. O., & PETERSON, J. B. (1993). Alcohol, serotonin, and aggression. *Alcohol Health & Research World, 17,* 113–116.

PINKNEY, D. S. (1990). Substance abusers seen shifting to "kitchen lab" drugs. *American Medical News, 33*(16), 5–7.

PIRKLE, J., FLEGAL, K. M., BERNERT, J. T., BRODY, D. J., ETZEL, R. A., & MAURER, K. R. (1996). Exposure of the US population to environmental tobacco smoke. *Journal of the American Medical Association, 275,* 1233–1240.

PIROZZOLO, F. J., & BONNEFIL, V. (1995). Disorders appearing in the perinatal and neonatal period. In E. S. Batchelor & R. S. Dean (Eds.), *Pediatric neuropsychology.* New York: Allyn & Bacon.

PLASKY, P., MARCUS, L., & SALZMAN, C. (1988). Effects of psychotropic drugs on memory: Part 2. *Hospital & Community Psychiatry, 39,* 501–502.

PLESSINGER, M. A., & WOODS, J. R. (1993). Maternal, placental, and fetal pathophysiology of cocaine exposure during pregnancy. *Clinical Obstetrics and Gynecology, 36,* 267–278.

POEL, VAN DER, C., CUYPERS, H. T., & REESINK, H. W. (1994). Hepatitis C virus six years on. *Lancet, 344,* 1475–1479.

POLEN, M. R., SIDNEY, S., TEKAWA, I. S., SADLER, M., & FRIEDMAN, G. D. (1993). Health care use by frequent marijuana smokers who do not smoke tobacco. *Western Journal of Medicine, 158,* 596–601.

POLITICIANS DISCOVER THE DRUG WAR. (1996). *Forensic Drug Abuse Advisor, 8*(9), 70–72.

POLLES, A. G., & SMITH, P. O. (1995). Treatment of coexisting substance dependence and posttraumatic stress disorder. *Psychiatric Services, 46,* 729–730.

POMERLEAU, O. D., COLLINS, A. C., SHIFFMAN, S., & POMERLEAU, C. S. (1993). Why some people smoke and others do not: New perspectives. *Journal of Clinical and Consulting Psychology, 61,* 723–731.

POPE, H. G., & KATZ, D. L. (1987). Bodybuilder's psychosis. *Lancet, 334,* 863.

POPE, H. G., & KATZ, D. L. (1988). Affective and psychotic symptoms associated with anabolic steroid use. *American Journal of Psychiatry, 145,* 487–490.

POPE, H. G., & KATZ, D. L. (1990). Homicide and near-homicide by anabolic steroid users. *Journal of Clinical Psychiatry, 51*(1), 28–31.

POPE, H. G., & KATZ, D. L. (1991). What are the psychiatric risks of anabolic steroids? *Harvard Mental Health Letter, 7*(10), 8.

POPE, H. G., & KATZ, D. L. (1994). Psychiatric and medical effects of anabolic-androgenic steroid use. *Archives of General Psychiatry, 51,* 375–382.

POPE, H. G., KATZ, D. L., & CHAMPOUX, R. (1986). Anabolic-androgenic steroid use among 1,010 college men. *Physician and Sports Medicine, 17*(7), 75–81.

POPE, H. G., & YURGELUN-TODD, D. (1996). The residual cognitive effects of heavy marijuana use in college students. *Journal of the American Medical Association, 275,* 521–527.

POPE, K. S., & MORIN, S. F. (1990). AIDS and HIV infection update: New research, ethical responsibilities, evolving legal frameworks, and published sources. *Independent Practitioner, 10*(4), 43–53.

PORTERFIELD, L. M. (1991). Steroid abuse. *Advancing Clinical Care, 6*(2), 44.

POST, R. M., WEISS, S. R. B., PERT, A., & UHDE, T. W. (1987). Chronic cocaine administration: Sensitization and kindling effects. In S. Fisher, A. Rashkin, & E. H. Unlenhuth (Eds.), *Cocaine: Clinical and behavioral aspects.*. New York: Oxford University Press.

POT SHOT. (1992). *Psychology Today, 25*(3), 8.

POTTER, W. Z., RUDORFER, M. V., & GOODWIN, F. K. (1987). Biological findings in bipolar disorders. In *American Psychiatric Association Annual Review* (Vol. 6). Washington, DC: American Psychiatric Association Press.

POTTERTON, R. (1992). A criminal system of justice. *Playboy, 39*(9), 46–47.

POWELL, B. J., READ, M. R., PENICK, E. C., MILLER, N. S., & BINGHAM, S. F. (1987). Primary and secondary depression in alcoholic men: An important distinction. *Journal of Clinical Psychiatry, 48*, 98–101.

PRATT, C. T. (1990). Addiction treatment for health care professionals. *Addiction & Recovery, 10*(3), 17–19, 38–41.

PRICE, L. H., RICAURTE, G. A., KRYSTAL, J. H., & HENINGER, G. R. (1989). Neuroendocrine and mood responses to intravenous L-tryptophan in 3, 4-Methylenedioxymethamphetamine (MDMA) users. *Archives of General Psychiatry, 46*, 20–22.

PRICE, L. H., RICAURTE, G. A., KRYSTAL, J. H., & HENINGER, G. R. (1990). In reply. *Archives of General Psychiatry, 47*, 289.

PRISTACH, C. A., & SMITH, C. M. (1990). Medication compliance and substance abuse among schizophrenic patients. *Hospital and Community Psychiatry, 41*, 1345–1348.

PRISTACH, C. A., & SMITH, C. M. (1996). Self-reported effects of alcohol use on symptoms of schizophrenia. *Psychiatric Services, 47*, 421–423.

PROCHASKA, J. O., DiCLEMENTE, C. C., & NORCROSS, J. C. (1992). In search of how people change. *American Psychologist, 47*, 1102–1114.

PRUMMEL, M. F., & WIERSINGA, W. M. (1993). Smoking and the risk of Graves' disease. *Journal of the American Medical Association, 269*, 479–482.

PURSCH, J. A. (1987). Mental illness and addiction. *Alcoholism & Addiction, 7*(6), 42.

PUTNAM, F. W. (1989). *Diagnosis and treatment of multiple personality disorder.* New York: Guilford Press.

QUINN, T. C. (1995). The epidemiology of the acquired immunodeficiency syndrome in the 1990's. *Emergency Medicine Clinics of North America, 13*, 1–25.

RACINE, A., JOYCE, T., & ANDERSON, R. (1993). The association between prenatal care and birth weigh among women exposed to cocaine in New York City. *Journal of the American Medical Association, 270*, 1581–1586.

RADETSKY, P. (1990). Closing in on an AIDS vaccine. *Discover, 11*(9), 71–77.

RADO, T. (1988). The client with a dual diagnosis—a personal perspective. *Alcohol Quarterly, 1*(1), 5–7.

RAINS, V. S. (1990). Alcoholism in the elderly—the hidden addiction. *Medical Aspects of Human Sexuality, 24*(10), 40–42, 43.

RALL, T. W. (1990). Hypnotics and sedatives. In A. G. Gilman, T. W. Rall, A. S. Nies, & P. Taylor (Eds.), *The pharmacological basis of therapeutics* (8th ed.). New York: Pergamon Press.

RAND, L. (1995). A different road. *Chicago Tribune, 148*(53), Tempo Sect., 1, 7.

RANDALL, T. (1992). Medical news and perspectives. *Journal of the American Medical Association, 268*, 1505–1506.

RAPOPORT, R. J. (1993). The efficacy and safety of oxaproxzin versus aspirin: Pooled results of double-blind trials in osteoarthritis. *Drug Therapy, 23*(Suppl.), 3–8.

RAPPORT, D. J., & COVINGTON, E. D. (1989). Motor phenomena in benzodiazepine withdrawal. *Hospital and Community Psychiatry, 40*, 1277–1280.

RASKIN, V. D. (1994). Psychiatric aspects of substance use disorders in childbearing populations. *Psychiatric Clinics of North America, 16*, 157–165.

RASYMAS, A. (1992). Basic pharmacology and pharmacokinetics. *Clinics in Podiatric Medicine and Surgery, 9*, 211–221.

RAUT, C. P., STEPHEN, A., & KOSOPSKY, B. (1996). Intrauterine effects of substance abuse. In L. Friedman, N. F. Fleming, D. H. Roberts, & S. E. Hyman (Eds.), *Source book of substance abuse and addiction.* New York: Williams & Wilkins.

RAVEL, R. (1989). *Clinical laboratory medicine: Clinical application of laboratory data* (5th ed.). Chicago: Year Book Medical Publishers.

RAW DATA. (1990). *Playboy, 37*(1), 16.

RAW DATA. (1993). *Playboy, 40*(12), 22.

RAW DATA. (1995). *Playboy, 42*(1), 16.

RAY, O. S., & KSIR, C. (1993). *Drugs, society and human behavior* (6th ed.). St. Louis: Mosby.

REDMAN, G. L. (1990). Adolescents and anabolics. *American Fitness, 8*(3), 30–33.

REEVES, D., & WEDDING, D. (1994). *The clinical assessment of memory.* New York: Springer.

REGIER, D. A., FARMER, M. E., RAE, D. S., LOCKE, B. Z., KIETH, S. J., JUDD, L. L., & GOODWIN, F. K. (1990). Comorbidity of mental disorders with alcohol and other drug abuse. *Journal of the American Medical Association, 264*, 2511–2518.

REINSCH, J. M., SANDERS, S. A., MORTENSEN, E. L., & RUBIN, D. B. (1995). In utero exposure to phenobarbital and intelligence deficits in adult men. *Journal of the American Medical Association, 174*, 1518–1525.

REISER, M. F. (1984). *Mind, brain, body.* New York: Basic Books.

REISINE, T., & PASTERNAK, G. (1995). Opioid analgesics and antagonists. In J. G. Hardman & L. E. Limbird (Editors-in-chief). *The pharmacological basis of therapeutics* (9th ed.). New York: McGraw-Hill.

RENAUD, S., & DeLORGERIL, M. (1992). Wine, alcohol, and the French paradox for coronary heart disease. *Lancet, 339,* 1523–1526.

RESEARCHERS CLAIM HAIR TESTING UNRELIABLE FOR QUANTITATING DRUG USE; RACIAL BIAS ALSO QUESTIONED. (1996). *Forensic Drug Abuse Advisor, 8*(3), 17–19.

RESEARCH ON NITRITES SUGGESTS DRUG PLAYS ROLE IN AIDS EPIDEMIC. (1989). *AIDS Alert, 4*(9), 153–156.

RESTAK, R. (1984). *The brain.* New York: Bantam Books.

RESTAK, R. (1991). *The brain has a mind of its own.* New York: Harmony Books.

RESTAK, R. (1993). Brain by design. *The Sciences, 33*(5), 27–33.

RESTAK, R. (1994). *Receptors.* New York: Bantam Books.

RESTAK, R. (1995). *Brainscapes.* New York: Hyperion Press.

REULER, J. B., GIRARD, D. E., & COONEY, T. G. (1985). Wernicke's encephalopathy. *New England Journal of Medicine, 316,* 1035–1039.

REVKIN, A. C. (1989). Crack in the cradle. *Discover, 10*(9), 63–69.

RHODES, J. E., & JASON, L. A. (1990). A social stress model of substance abuse. *Journal of Consulting and Clinical Psychology, 58,* 395–401.

RICE, C., & DUNCAN, D. F. (1995). Alcohol use and reported physician visits in older adults. *Preventative Medicine, 24,* 229–234.

RICE, D. P. (1993). The economic cost of alcohol abuse and alcohol dependence: 1990. *Alcohol Health & Research World, 17*(1), 10–11.

RICHARDSON, G. A., & DAY, N. L. (1994). Detrimental effects of prenatal cocaine exposure: Illusion or reality? *Journal of the American Academy of Child and Adolescent Psychiatry, 33*(1), 28–34.

RICHARDSON, S. (1995). The race against AIDS. *Discover, 16*(5), 28–32.

RICKELS, K., SCHWEIZER, E., & LUCKI, I. (1987). Benzodiazepine side effects. In R. E. Hales & A. J. Frances (Eds.), *American Psychiatric Association Annual Review* (Vol. 6). Washington, DC: American Psychiatric Association Press.

RICKELS, K., SCHWEIZER, E., CASE, W. G., & GREENBLATT, D. J. (1990). Long-term therapeutic use of benzodiazepines: I. Effects of abrupt discontinuation. *Archives of General Psychiatry, 47,* 899–907.

RICKELS, K., SCHWEIZER, E., CSANALOSI, I., CASE, W. G., & CHUNG, H. (1988). Long-term treatment of anxiety and risk of withdrawal. *Archives of General Psychiatry, 45,* 444–450.

RICKELS, L. K., GIESECKE, M. A., & GELLER, A. (1987). Differential effects of the anxiolytic drugs, diazepam and buspirone on memory function. *British Journal of Clinical Pharmacology, 23,* 207–211.

RIDKER, P. M., CUSHMAN, M., STAMPFER, M. J., TRACY, R. P., & HENNEKENS, C. H. (1997). Inflammation, aspirin, and the risk of cardiovascular disease in apparently healthy men. *New England Journal of Medicine, 336,* 973–979.

RIES, R. K., & ELLINGSON, T. (1990). A pilot assessment at one month of 17 dual diagnosis patients. *Hospital and Community Psychiatry, 41,* 1230–1233.

RIGGS, J. E. (1996). The "protective" influence of cigarette smoking on Alzheimer's and Parkinson's Diseases. *Neurologic Clinics, 14,* 353–358.

RILEY, J. A. (1994). Dual diagnosis. *Nursing Clinics of North America, 29,* 29–34.

RIMM, E. B., CHAN, J., STAMPFER, M. J., COLDITZ, G. A., & WILLETT, W. C. (1995). Prospective study of cigarette smoking, alcohol use, and the risk of diabetes in men. *British Medical Journal, 310,* 555–559.

ROBBINS, A. S., MANSON, J. E., LEE, I., SATTERFIELD, S., & HENNEKENS, C. H. (1994). Cigarette smoking and stroke in a cohort of U.S. male physicians. *Annals of Internal Medicine, 120,* 458–462.

ROBERTS, D. H., & BUSH, B. (1996). Inpatient management issues and pain management. In L. Friedman, N. F. Fleming, D. H. Roberts, & S. E. Hyman (Eds.), *Source book of substance abuse and addiction.* New York: Williams & Wilkins.

ROBERTS, D. J. (1995). Drug abuse. In R. E. Rakel (Ed.), *Conn's current therapy.* Philadelphia: Saunders.

ROBERTS, J. R., & TAFURE, J. A. (1990). Benzodiazepines. In L. Haddad & J. F. Winchester (Eds.), *Clinical management of poisoning and drug overdose* (2nd ed.). Philadelphia: Saunders.

ROBERTS, M. (1986). MDMA: "Madness, not ecstasy." *Psychology Today, 20,* 14–16.

ROBERTS, S. V., & WATSON, T. (1994). Teens on tobacco. *U.S. News & World Report, 116*(15), 38, 43.

RODGERS, J. E. (1994). Addiction—A whole new view. *Psychology Today, 27*(5), 32–38, 72, 74, 76, 79.

RODMAN, M. J. (1993). OCT interactions. *RN, 56*(1), 54–60.

RODRIGUES, C. (1990). Drug market runs on a cycle of poverty and greed. *Minneapolis Star-Tribune, IX*(155), 21A.

ROEHLING, P., KOELBEL, N., & RUTGERS, C. (1994). *Codependence—pathologizing feminity?* Paper presented at the 1994 annual meeting of the American Psychological Association, Los Angeles.

ROEHRS, T., & ROTH, T. (1995). Alcohol-induced sleepiness and memory function. *Alcohol Health & Research World, 19*(2), 130–135.

ROFFMAN, R. A., & GEORGE, W. H. (1988). Cannabis abuse. In D. M. Donovan & G. A. Marlatt (Eds.),

Assessment of addictive behaviors. New York: Guilford Press.

ROGERS, C. R. (1961). *On becoming a person.* Boston: Houghton-Mifflin.

ROGERS, P. D., HARRIS, J., & JARMUSKEWICZ, J. (1987). Alcohol and adolescence. *Pediatric Clinics of North America, 34*(2), 289–303.

ROHSENOW, D. J., & BACHOROWSKI, J. (1984). Effects of alcohol and expectancies on verbal aggression in men and women. *Journal of Abnormal Psychology, 93,* 418–432.

ROHYPNOL AND DATE RAPE. (1997). *Forensic Drug Abuse Advisor, 9*(1), 1–2.

ROHYPNOL USE SPREADING THROUGHOUT SOUTHERN U.S. (1995). *Substance Abuse Letter, 2*(1), 1, 6.

ROINE, R., GENTRY, T., HERNANDEZ-MUNOZ, R., BARAONA, E., & LIEBER, C. S. (1990). Aspirin increases blood alcohol concentrations in humans after ingestion of alcohol. *Journal of the American Medical Association, 264,* 2406–2408.

ROLD, J. F. (1993). Mushroom madness. *Postgraduate Medicine, 78*(5), 217–218.

ROMAN, P. M., & BLUM, T. C. (1996). *American Journal of Health Promotion, 11*(2),136–149.

ROME, H. P. (1984). Psychobotanica revisited. *Psychiatric Annals, 14,* 711–712.

ROOTS, L. E., & AANES, D. L. (1992). A conceptual framework for understanding self help groups. *Hospital and Community Psychiatry, 43,* 379–381.

ROSE, K. J., (1988). *The body in time.* New York: Wiley.

ROSEN, M. I., & KOSTEN, T. R. (1991). Buprenorphine: Beyond methadone? *Hospital and Community Psychiatry, 42,* 347–349.

ROSENBAUM, J. F. (1990). Switching patients from alprazolam to clonazepam. *Hospital and Community Psychiatry, 41,* 1302.

ROSENBAUM, J. F., & GELENBERG, A. J. (1991). Anxiety. In A. J. Gelenberg, E. L. Bassuk, & S. C. Schoonover (Eds.), *The practitioner's guide to psychoactive drugs* (3rd ed.). New York: Plenum Press.

ROSENBERG, A. (1996). Brain damage caused by prenatal alcohol exposure. *Scientific American Medicine, 3*(4), 42–51.

ROSENBERG, N. (1989). Nervous systems effects of toluene and other organic solvents. *Western Journal of Medicine, 150,* 571–573.

ROSENBLUM, M. (1992). Ibuprofen provides longer lasting analgesia than fentanyl after laparoscopic surgery. *Journal of the American Medical Association, 267,* 219.

ROSENTHAL, E. (1992). Bad fix. *Discover, 13*(2), 82–84.

ROSS, A. (1991). Poland's dark harvest. *In Health, 5*(4), 66–70.

ROSSE, R. B., COLLINS, J. P., FAY-MCCARTHY, M., ALIM, T. N., WYATT, R. J., & DEUTSCH, S. I. (1994). Phenomenologic comparison of the idiopathic psychosis of schizophrenia and drug-induced cocaine and

phencyclidine psychosis: A retrospective study. *Clinical Neuropharmacology, 17,* 359–369.

ROTHENBERG, L. (1988). The ethics of intervention. *Alcoholism & Addiction, 9*(1), 22 24.

ROTHWELL, P. M., & GRANT, R. (1993). Cerebral venous sinus thrombosis induced by "ecstacy." *Journal of Neurology, Neurosurgery and Psychiatry, 56,* 1035.

ROUNSAVILLE, B. J., ANTON, S. F., CARROLL, K., BUDDE, D., PRUSOFF, B. A., & GAWIN, F. (1991). Psychiatric diagnoses of treatment-seeking cocaine abusers. *Archives of General Psychiatry, 48,* 43–51.

ROY, A. (1993). Risk factors for suicide among adult alcoholics. *Alcohol Health & Research World, 17,* 133–136.

ROYCE, R. A., SENA, A., CATES, W., & COHEN, M. S. (1997). Sexual transmission of HIV. *New England Journal of Medicine, 336,* 1072–1078.

ROYKO, M. (1990). Drug war's over: Guess who won. *Playboy, 37*(1), 46.

RUBIN, E., & DORIA, J. (1990). Alcoholic cardiomyopathy. *Alcohol Health & Research World, 14*(4), 277–284.

RUBIN, R. H. (1993). Acquired immunodeficiency syndrome. In E. Rubenstein & D. D. Federman (Eds.), *Scientific American medicine.* New York: Scientific American Press.

RUBINO, F. A. (1992). Neurologic complications of alcoholism. *Psychiatric Clinics of North America, 15,* 359–372.

RUBINSTEIN, L., CAMPBELL, F., & DALEY, D. (1990). Four perspectives on dual diagnosis: Overview of treatment issues. In D. F.O'Connell (Ed.), *Managing the dually diagnosed patient.* New York: Haworth Press.

RUBY, M. (1993). Should drugs be legalized? *U.S. News & World Report, 115*(24), 80.

RUSSELL, J. M., NEWMAN, S. C., & BLAND, R. C. (1994). Drug abuse and dependence. *Acta Psychiatrica Scandinavica, 376*(Suppl.), 54–62.

RUSTIN, T. (1988). Treating nicotine addiction. *Alcoholism & Addiction, 9*(2), 18–19.

RUSTIN, T. (1992, August). *Review of nicotine dependence and its treatment. Consultation to La Crosse addiction treatment programs: Lutheran Hospital and St. Francis Hospital.* Symposium conducted for staff, Lutheran Hospital, La Crosse, WI.

RYGLEWICZ, H., & PEPPER, B. (1996). *Lives at risk.* New York: Free Press.

SABBAG, R. (1994, May 5). The cartels would like a second chance. *Rolling Stone, 3537,* 43.

SACCO, R. L. (1995). Risk factors and outcomes for ischemic stroke. *Neurology, 45*(Suppl. 1), S10–S14.

SACKS, O. (1970). *The man who mistook his wife for a hat.* New York: Harper & Row.

SAGAN, C. (1995). *The demon-haunted world.* New York: Random House.

SAGAR, S. M. (1991). Toxic and metabolic disorders. In M. A. Samuels (Ed.), *Manual of neurology.* Boston: Little, Brown.

SAGAR, S. M., & MCGUIRE, D. (1991). Infectious diseases. In M. A. Samuels (Ed.), *Manual of neurology.* Boston: Little, Brown.

SAITZ, R., MAYO-SMITH, M. F., ROBERTS, M. S., REDMOND, H. A., BERNARD, D. R., & CALKINS, D. R. (1994). Individualized treatment for alcohol withdrawal. *Journal of the American Medical Association, 272,* 519–523.

SALLOWAY, S., SOUTHWICK, S., & SADOWSKY, M. (1990). Opiate withdrawal presenting as posttraumatic stress disorder. *Hospital & Community Psychiatry, 41,* 666–667.

SALZMAN, C. (1990). What are the uses and dangers of the controversial drug Halcion? *Harvard Medical School Mental Health Letter, 6*(9), 8.

SAMET, J. H., ROLLNICK, S., & BARNES, H. (1996). Beyond CAGE. *Archives of Internal Medicine, 156,* 2287–2293.

SANDERS, S. R. (1990). Under the influence. *Family Therapy Networker, 14*(1), 32–37.

SANDS, B. F., CREELMAN, W. L., CIRAULO, D. A., GREENBLATT, D. J., & SHADER, R. I. (1995). Benzodiazepines. In D. A. Ciraulo, R. I. Shader, D. J. Greenblatt, & W. Creelman (Eds.), *Drug interactions in psychiatry* (2nd ed.). Baltimore: Williams & Wilkins.

SANDS, B. F., KNAPP, C. M., & CIRAULO, D. A. (1993). Medical consequences of alcohol drug interactions. *Alcohol Health & Research World, 17,* 316–320.

SARID-SEGAL, O., CREELMAN, W. L., & SHADER, R. I. (1995). Lithium. In D. A. Ciraulo, R. I. Shader, D. J. Greenblatt, & W. Creelman (Eds.), *Drug interactions in psychiatry* (2nd ed.). Baltimore: Williams & Wilkins.

SATEL, S. L. (1992). "Craving for and fear of cocaine": A phenomenologic update on cocaine craving and paranoia. In T. R. Kosten & H. D. Kleber (Eds.), *Clinician's guide to cocaine addiction.* New York: Guilford Press.

SATEL, S. L., & EDELL, W. S. (1991). Cocaine-induced paranoia and psychosis proneness. *American Journal of Psychiatry, 148,* 1708–1711.

SATEL, S. L., KOSTEN, T. R., SCHUCKIT, M. A., & FISCHMAN, M. W. (1993). Should protracted withdrawal from drugs be included in *DSM-IV? American Journal of Psychiatry, 150,* 695–704.

SATEL, S. L., PRICE, L. H., PALUMBO, J. M., MCDOUGLE, C. J., KRYSTAL, J. H., GAWIN, F., CHARNEY, D. S., HENINGER, G. R., & KLEBER, H. D. (1991). Clinical phenomenology and neurobiology of cocaine abstinence: A prospective inpatient study. *American Journal of Psychiatry, 148,* 1712–1716.

SAUM, C. A., & INCIARDI, J. A. (1997). Rohypnol misuse in the United States. *Substance Use & Misuse, 32,* 723–731.

SAUNDERS, J. B., AASLAND, O. G., BABOR, T. F., DE LA FUENTE, J. R., & GRANT, M. (1993). Development of the alcohol use disorders identification test (AUDIT): WHO collaborative project on early detection of persons with harmful alcohol consumption II. *Addiction, 88,* 791–804.

SAVAGE, S. R. (1993). Opium: The gift and its shadow. *Addiction & Recovery, 13*(1), 38–39.

SAWICKI, T. (1995). Tel Aviv's miracle cure for addicts. *World Press Review, 42*(9), 37–39.

SBRIGLIO, R., & MILLMAN, R. B. (1987). Emergency treatment of acute cocaine reactions. In A. M. Washton & M. S. Gold (Eds.), *Cocaine: A clinician's handbook.* New York: Guilford Press.

SCAFIDI, F. A., FIELD, T. M., WHEEDEN, A., SCHANBERG, S., KUHN, C., SYMANSKI, R., ZIMMERMAN, E., & BANDSTRA, E. S. (1996). Cocaine-exposed preterm neonates show behavioral and hormonal differences. *Pediatrics, 97,* 851–856.

SCARF, M. (1980). *Unfinished business.* New York: Ballantine Books.

SCAROS, L. P., WESTRA, S., & BARONE, J. A. (1990). Illegal use of drugs: A current review. *U.S. Pharmacist, 15*(5), 17–39.

SCHAFER, J., & BROWN, S. A. (1991). Marijuana and cocaine effect expectancies and drug use patterns. *Journal of Consulting and Clinical Psychology, 59,* 558–565.

SCHAUBEN, J. L. (1990). Adulterants and substitutes. *Emergency Medicine Clinics of North America, 8,* 595–611.

SCHEER, R. (1994a). The drug war's a bust. *Playboy, 41*(2), 49.

SCHEER, R. (1994b). Fighting the wrong war. *Playboy, 41*(10), 49.

SCHEER, R. (1995). Cracked Obsession. *Playboy, 42*(4), 49.

SCHENKER, S., & SPEEG, K. V. (1990). The risk of alcohol intake in men and women. *New England Journal of Medicine, 322,* 127–129.

SCHIAVI, R. C., STIMMEL, B. B., MANDELI, J., & WHITE, D. (1995). Chronic alcoholism and male sexual function. *American Journal of Psychiatry, 152,* 1045–1051.

SCHLOSSER, E. (1994). Marijuana and the law. *The Atlantic Monthly, 274*(3), 84–86,89–90, 92–94.

SCHMOKE, K. (1996). The war on drugs is lost. *National Review, XLVIII*(2), 40–42.

SCHMOKE, K. (1997). Save money, cut crime, get real. *Playboy, 44*(1), 129, 190–191.

SCHNEIDERMAN, H. (1990). What's your diagnosis? *Consultant, 30*(7), 61–65.

SCHREIBER, G. B., BUSCH, M. P., KLEINMAN, S. H., & KORELITZ, J. J. (1996). The risk of transfusion-transmitted viral infections. *New England Journal of Medicine, 334,* 1685–1690.

SCHROF, J. M. (1992). Pumped up. *U.S. News & World Report, 112*(21), 54–63.

SCHUCKIT, M. A. (1986). Primary men alcoholics with histories of suicide attempts. *Journal of Studies on Alcohol, 47,* 78–81.

SCHUCKIT, M. A. (1987). Biological vulnerability to alcoholism. *Journal of Consulting and Clinical Psychology, 55*, 301–309.

SCHUCKIT, M. A. (1994). Low level of response to alcohol as a predictor of future alcoholism. *American Journal of Psychiatry, 151*, 184–189.

SCHUCKIT, M. A. (1995a). Alcohol related disorders. In H. I. Kaplan & B. J. Sadock (Eds.), *Comprehensive textbook of psychiatry* (6th ed.). Baltimore: Williams & Wilkins.

SCHUCKIT, M. A. (1995b). *Drug and alcohol abuse: A clinical guide to diagnosis and treatment* (4th ed.). New York: Plenum Press.

SCHUCKIT, M. A. (1996a). Alcohol, anxiety and depressive disorders. *Alcohol Health & Research World, 20*, 81–86.

SCHUCKIT, M. A. (1996b). Recent developments in the pharmacology of alcohol dependence. *Journal of Consulting and Clinical Psychology, 64*, 669–676.

SCHUCKIT, M. A., KLEIN, J., TWITCHELL, G., & SMITH, T. (1994). Personality test scores as predictors of alcoholism almost a decade later. *American Journal of Psychiatry, 151*, 1038–1042.

SCHUCKIT, M. A., & SMITH, T. L. (1996). An 8-year follow-up of 450 sons of alcoholic and control subjects. *Archives of General Psychiatry, 53*, 202–210.

SCHUCKIT, M. A., SMITH, T. L., ANTHENELLI, R., & IRWIN, M. (1993). Clinical course of alcoholism in 636 male inpatients. *American Journal of Psychiatry, 150*, 786–792.

SCHUCKIT, M. A., ZISOOK, S., & MORTOLA, J. (1985). Clinical implications of *DSM-III* diagnoses of alcohol abuse and alcohol dependence. *American Journal of Psychiatry, 142*, 1403–1408.

SCHUSTER, C. R. (1990). The National Institute on Drug Abuse in the decade of the brain. *Neuropsychopharmacology, 3*, 315–318.

SCHUTTE, K. K., MOOS, R. H., & BRENNAN, P. L. (1995). Depression and drinking behavior among women and men: A three-wave longitudinal study of older adults. *Journal of Consulting and Clinical Psychology, 63*, 810–822.

SCHWARTZ, R. H. (1987). Marijuana: An overview. *Pediatric Clinics of North America, 34*(2), 305–317.

SCHWARTZ, R. H. (1989). When to suspect inhalant abuse. *Patient Care, 23*(10), 39–50.

SCHWARTZ, R. H. (1994). Letter to the editor. *New England Journal of Medicine, 331*, 126–127.

SCHWARTZ, R. H. (1995). LSD. *Pediatric Clinics of North America, 42*, 403–413.

SCHWARTZ, R. H. (1996). Let's help young smokers quit. *Patient Care, 30*(8), 45–51.

SCHWEIZER, E., & RICKELS, K. (1994). New and emerging clinical uses of buspirone. *Journal of Clinical Psychiatry, 55*(5)(Suppl.), 46–54.

SCHWEIZER, E., RICKELS, K., CASE, W. G., & GREENBLATT, D. J. (1990). Long term therapeutic use of benzodiazepines: II. Effects of gradual taper. *Archives of General Psychiatry, 47*, 908–916.

SCHWERTZ, D. W. (1991). Basic principles of pharmacologic action. *Nursing Clinics of North America, 26*, 245–262.

SCOTT, M. J., & SCOTT, M. J. (1989). HIV infection associated with injections of anabolic steroids. *Journal of the American Medical Association, 262*(2), 207–208.

SEARIGHT, H. R., & McLAREN, L. (1997). Behavioral and psychiatric aspects of HIV infection. *American Family Physician, 55*, 1227–1237.

SECONDHAND CRACK SMOKE IS NOT AN ACCEPTABLE EXCUSE. (1995). *Forensic Drug Abuse Advisor, 7*(10), 75–76.

SEGAL, R., & SISSON, B. V. (1985). Medical complications associated with alcohol use and the assessment of risk of physical damage. In T. E. Bratter & G. G. Forrest (Eds.), *Alcoholism and substance abuse: Strategies for clinical intervention.* New York: Free Press.

SEIDMAN, S. N., & RIEDER, R. O. (1994). A review of sexual behavior in the United States. *American Journal of Psychiatry, 151*, 330–341.

SEILHAMER, R. A., JACOB, T., & DUNN, N. J. (1993). The impact of alcohol consumption on parent-child relationships in families of alcoholics. *Journal of Studies on Alcohol, 54*(2), 189–198.

SEIVEWRIGHT, N., & GREENWOOD, J. (1996). What is important in drug misuse treatment? *Lancet, 347*, 373–376.

SELLERS, E. M., CIRAULO, D. A., DUPONT, R. L., GRIFFITHS, R. R., KOSTEN, T. R., ROMACH, M. K., & WOODY, G. E. (1993). Alprazolam and benzodiazepine dependence. *Journal of Clinical Psychiatry, 54*(10)(Suppl.), 64–74.

SELWYN, P. A. (1993). Illicit drug use revisited: What a long, strange trip its been. *Annals of Internal Medicine, 119*, 1044–1046.

SELZER, M. (1971). The Michigan Alcoholism Screening Test: The quest for a new diagnostic instrument. *American Journal of Psychiatry, 127*, 1653–1658.

SENCHAK, M., LEONARD, K. E., GREENE, B. W., & CARROLL, A. (1995). Comparisons of adult children of alcoholic, divorced and control parents in four outcome domains. *Psychology of Addictive Behaviors, 9*(3), 147–156.

SERFATY, M., & MASTERTON, G. (1993). Fatal poisonings attributed to benzodiazepines in Britain during the 1980's. *British Journal of Psychiatry, 163*, 386–393.

SEX-FOR-DRUGS PUSHES US SYPHILIS RATES UP. (1990). *The Nation's Health, 20*(1), 17.

SEXSON, W. R. (1994). Cocaine: A neonatal perspective. *International Journal of the Addictions, 28*, 585–598.

SEYMOUR, J. (1997). Old diseases, new danger. *Nursing Times, 93*(14), 22–24.

SHADER, R. I. (1994). A perspective on contemporary psychiatry. In *Manual of psychiatric therapeutics* (2nd ed.). Boston: Little, Brown.

SHADER, R. I., & GREENBLATT, D. J. (1993). Use of benzodiazepines in anxiety disorders. *New England Journal of Medicine, 328,* 1398–1405.

SHADER, R. I., GREENBLATT, D. J., & CIRAULO, D. A. (1994). Treatment of physical dependence on barbiturates, benzodiazepines, and other sedative-hypnotics. In *Manual of psychiatric therapeutics* (2nd ed.). Boston: Little, Brown.

SHAFER, J. (1985). Designer drugs. *Science '85, 12*(3), 60–67.

SHAFFER, H. J., & ROBBINS, M. (1995). Psychotherapy for addictive behavior: A stage change approach to meaning making. In A. M. Washton (Ed.), *Psychotherapy and substance abuse.* New York: Guilford Press.

SHANER, A., KHALSA, E., ROBERTS, L., WILKINS, J., ANGLIN, D., & HSIECH, S. C. (1993). Unrecognized cocaine use among schizophrenic patients. *American Journal of Psychiatry, 150,* 758–762.

SHANNON, M. T., WILSON, B. A., & STANG, C. L. (1995). *Drugs and nursing implications* (8th ed.). Norwalk, CT: Appleton & Lange.

SHAPIRO, D. (1981). *Autonomy and rigid character.* New York: Basic Books.

SHARARA, A. I., HUNT, C. M., & HAMILTON, J. D. (1996). Hepatitis C. *Annual of Internal Medicine, 125,* 658–668.

SHEDLER, J., & BLOCK, J. (1990). Adolescent drug use and psychological health. *American Psychologist, 45,* 612–630.

SHENKMAN, R. (1991). *I love Paul Revere, whether he rode or not.* New York: Harper-Collins.

SHEPHERD, S. M., & JAGODA, A. S. (1990). PCP. In L. D. Haddad & J. F. Winchester (Eds.), *Clinical management of poisoning and drug overdose* (2nd ed.). Philadelphia: Saunders.

SHER, K. J. (1991). *Children of alcoholics.* Chicago: University of Chicago Press.

SHER, K. J., WALITZER, K. S., WOOD, P. K., & BRENT, E. E. (1991). Characteristics of children of alcoholics: Putative risk factors, substance use and abuse, and psychopathology. *Journal of Abnormal Psychology, 100,* 427–448.

SHERIDAN, E., PATTERSON, H. R., & GUSTAFSON, E. A. (1982). *Falconer's The drug, the nurse, the patient* (7th ed.). Philadelphia: Saunders.

SHERMAN, C. (1994). Kicking butts. *Psychology Today, 27*(5), 40–45.

SHERMAN, C. B. (1991). Health effects of cigarette smoking. *Clinics in Chest Medicine, 12,* 643–658.

SHERMAN, D. I. N., WARD, R. J., WARREN-PERRY, M., WILLIAMS, R., & PETERS, T. J. (1993). Association of restriction fragment length polymorphism in alcohol dehydrogenase 2 gene with alcohol induced liver damage. *British Medical Journal, 307,* 1388–1390.

SHIELDS, R. O. (1990). Amphetamines. In L. M. Haddad & J. F. Winchester (Eds.), *Clinical management of poisoning and drug overdose* (2nd ed.). Philadelphia: Saunders.

SHIFFMAN, L. B., FISCHER, L. B., ZETTLER-SEGAL, M., & BENOWITZ, N. L. (1990). Nicotine exposure among nondependent smokers. *Archives of General Psychiatry, 47,* 333–340.

SHIFFMAN, S. (1992). Relapse process and relapse prevention in addictive behaviors. *Behavior Therapist, 15*(1), 99–11.

SHIH, R. D., & HOLLANDER, J. E. (1996). Management of cocaine-associated chest pain. *Hospital Physician, 32*(11), 11–20, 45.

SHINTON, R., SAGAR, G., & BEEVERS, G. (1993). The relation of alcohol consumption to cardiovascular risk factors and stroke. The west Birmingham stroke project. *Journal of Neurology, Neurosurgery and Psychiatry, 56,* 458–462.

SHOUMATOFF, A. (1995). Trouble in the land of Muy Verde. *Outside, XX*(3), 56–63, 149–154.

SICHERMAN, A. (1992). Two fingers of Tagamet. *Minneapolis Star-Tribune, X*(342), 1T.

SIEBERT, C. (1996). Are we more than ever at the mercy of our genes? *Minneapolis Star-Tribune, XIV*(286), A13.

SIEGEL, B. S. (1986). *Love, medicine and miracles.* New York: Harper & Row.

SIEGEL, B. S. (1989). *Peace, love and healing.* New York: Harper & Row.

SIEGEL, L. (1989). Want to take the risks? It should be your choice. *Playboy, 36*(1), 59.

SIEGEL, R. K. (1982). Cocaine smoking disorders: Diagnosis and treatment. *Psychiatric Annals, 14,* 728–732.

SIEGEL, R. K. (1991). Crystal meth or speed or crank. *Lear's, 3*(1), 72–73.

SIEGEL, R. L. (1986). Jungle revelers: When beasts take drugs to race or relax, things get zooey. *Omni, 8*(6), 70–74, 100.

SIERLES, F. S. (1984). Correlates of malingering. *Behavioral Sciences and the Law, 2*(1), 113–118.

SIGVARDSSON, S., BOHMAN, M., & CLONINGER, R. (1996). Replication of the Stockholm adoption study. *Archives of General Psychiatry, 53,* 681–687.

SILAGY, C. A., McNEIL, J. J., DONNAN, G. A., TONKIN, A. M., WORSAM, B., & CAMPION, K. (1993). Adverse effects of low-dose aspirin in a healthy elderly population. *Clinical Pharmacology Therapeutics, 54,* 84–89.

SILVERMAN, M. M. (1989). Children of psychiatrically ill parents: A prevention perspective. *Hospital & Community Psychiatry, 40,* 1257–1265.

SILVERS, J. (1990). Wounded country. *Playboy, 37*(8), 76–77, 80, 147–150.

SIMMONS, A. L. (1991). A peculiar dialect in the land of 10,000 treatment centers. *Minneapolis Star-Tribune*, X(24), 23A.

SIMON, E. J. (1992). Opiates: Neurobiology. In J. H. Lowinson, P. Ruiz, R. B. Millman, & J. G. Langrod (Eds.), *Substance abuse: A comprehensive textbook* (2nd ed.). New York: Williams & Wilkins.

SIMONS, A. M., PHILLIPS, D. H., & COLEMAN, D. V. (1993). Damage to DNA in cervical epithelium related to smoking tobacco. *British Medical Journal*, 306, 1444–1448.

SIMPLE WAY TO BEAT URINE TESTS-JUST DRINK WATER. (1994). *Forensic Drug Abuse Advisor*, 6(3), 17–18.

SIMPSON, D. D., CRANDALL, R. L., SAVAGE, J., & PAVA-KRUEGER, E. (1981). Leisure of opiate addicts at posttreatment follow-up. *Journal of Counseling Psychology*, 28, 36–39.

SIMS, A. (1994). "Psyche"—Spirit as well as mind? *British Journal of Psychiatry*, 165, 441–446.

SINGH, R. A., MATTOO, S. K., MALHOTRA, A., & VARMA,, V. K. (1992). Cases of buprenorphine abuse in India. *Acta Psychiatrica Scandinavica*, 86, 46–48.

60 MINUTES. (1992). *Rx drugs* (XXV, 15). Livingston, NJ: Burrelle's Information Services.

60 MINUTES. (1993). *The CIA's Cocaine* (XXVI, 10). Livingston, NJ: Burrelle's Information Services.

60 MINUTES. (1994). *Halcion* (XXVI, 42). Livingston, NJ: Burrelle's Information Services.

60 MINUTES. (1995). *Cigarettes* (XXVIII, 9). Livingston, NJ: Burrelle's Information Services.

60 MINUTES. (1996a). *Pain killer* (XXVIX, 13). Livingston, NJ: Burrelle's Information Services.

60 MINUTES. (1996b). *How he won the war* (XXVIX, 13). Livingston, NJ.: Burrelle's Information Services.

60 MINUTES. (1997a). *North of the border* (XXIX, 31). Livingston, NJ: Burrelle's Information Services.

60 MINUTES. (1997b). *The tobacco tapes* (XXIX, 33). Livingston, NJ: Burrelle's Information Services.

SJOGREN, M. H. (1996). Serologic diagnosis of viral hepatitis. *Medical Clinics of North America*, 80, 929–956.

SKOG, O. J., & DUCKERT, F. (1993). The development of alcoholics' and heavy drinkers' consumption: A longitudinal study. *Journal of Studies on Alcohol*, 54, 178–188.

SLABY, A. E., LIEB, J., & TANCREDI, L. R. (1981). *Handbook of psychiatric emergencies* (2nd ed.). Garden City, NY: Medical Examination.

SLADE, J., BERO, L. A., HANAUER, P., BARNES, D. E., & GLANTZ, S. A. (1995). Nicotine and addiction. *Journal of the American Medical Association*, 274, 225–233.

SLEEPING PILLS AND ANTIANXIETY DRUGS. (1988). *The Harvard Medical School Mental Health Letter*, 5(6), 1–4.

SLOVUT, G. (1992). Sports medicine. *Minneapolis Star-Tribune*, X(353), 20C.

SMITH, B. D., & SALZMAN, C. (1991). Do benzodiazepines cause depression? *Hospital and Community Psychiatry*, 42, 1101–1102.

SMITH, D. (1997, May). *Prescription drug abuse*. Paper presented at the WisSAM Symposium: "Still Getting High: A 30 year perspective on drug abuse," Gundersen-Lutheran Medical Center, La Crosse, WI.

SMITH, G. T., GOLDMAN, M. S., GREENBAUM, P. E., & CHRISTIANSEN, B. A. (1995). Expectancy for social facilitation from drinking: The divergent paths of high-expectancy and low-expectancy adolescents. *Journal of Abnormal Psychology*, 104, 32–40.

SMITH, R. (1990). Psychopathology and substance abuse: A psychoanalytic perspective. In D. F. O'Connell (Ed.),*Managing the dually diagnosed patient*. New York: Haworth Press.

SMITH, S. G. T., TOUQUET, R., WRIGHT, S., & DAS GUPTA, N. (1996). Detection of alcohol misusing patients in accident and emergency departments: The Paddington alcohol test (PAT). *Journal of Accident & Emergency Medicine*, 13, 308–312.

SMITH, T. (1994). How dangerous is heroin? *British Medical Journal*, 307, 807.

SMITH, T. (1994). Psychological expectancy as mediator of vulnerability to alcoholism. In T. F. Babor, V. Hesselbrock, R. E. Meyer, & W. Shoemaker (Eds.), *Types of alcoholics*. New York: New York Academy of Sciences.

SMITHSONIAN. (1989). Letters to the editor. *Smithsonian*, 20(6), 18.

SMOLOWE, J. (1993). Choose your poison. *Time*, 142(4), 56–57.

SNYDER, S. H. (1977). Opiate receptors and internal opiates. *Scientific American*, 260(3), 44–56.

SNYDER, S. H. (1986). *Drugs and the brain*. New York: Scientific American Books.

SOLOMON, J., ROGERS, A., KATEL, P., & LACH, J. (1997). Turning a new leaf. *Newsweek*, CXXIX(13), 50.

SOUTH AMERICAN DRUG PRODUCTION INCREASES. (1997). *Forensic Drug Abuse Advisor*, 9(3), 18.

SPANGLER, J. G., & SALISBURY, P. L. (1995). Smokeless tobacco: Epidemiology, health effects and cessation strategies. *American Family Physician*, 52, 1421–1430.

SPARADEO, F. R., & GILL, D. (1989). Effects of prior alcohol use on head injury recovery. *Journal of Head Trauma Rehabilitation*, 4(1), 75–82.

SPIEGEL, R. (1996). *Psychopharmacology: An introduction* (3rd ed.). New York: Wiley.

SPINDLER, K. (1994). *The man in the ice*. New York: Harmony Books.

SPODE, H. (1994). The first step toward sobriety: The "boozing devil" in sixteenth century Germany. *Contemporary Drug Problems*, 21(3), 454–483.

SPOHR, H. L., WILLIAMS, J., & STEINHAUSEN, H. C. (1993). Prenatal alcohol exposure and long-term consequences. *Lancet*, 341, 907–910.

SPORER, K. A., & KHAYAM-BASHI, H. (1996). Acetaminophen and salicylate serum levels in patients with suicidal ingestion or altered mental states. *American Journal of Emergency Medicine, 14,* 443–446.

SPRINGBORN, W. (1987). Step one: The foundation of recovery. In *The twelve steps of Alcoholics Anonymous.* New York: Harper & Row.

SQUIRES, S. (1990). Popular painkiller ibuprofen is linked to kidney damage. *Minneapolis Star-Tribune, VIII*(315), 1E, 4E.

STEELE, T. E., & MORTON, W. A. (1986). Salicylate-induced delirium. *Psychosomatics, 27*(6), 455–456.

STEIN, J. A., NEWCOMB, M. D., & BENTLER, P. M. (1993). Differential effects of parent and grandparent drug use on behavior problems of male and female children. *Developmental Psychology, 29,* 31–43.

STEIN, S. M., & KOSTEN, T. R. (1992). Use of drug combinations in treatment of opioid withdrawal. *Journal of Clinical Psychopharmacology, 12*(3), 203–209.

STEIN, S. M., & KOSTEN, T. R. (1994). Reduction of opiate withdrawal-like symptoms by cocaine abuse during methadone and buprenorphine maintenance. *American Journal of Drug and Alcohol Abuse, 20*(4), 445–459.

STEINBERG, A. D. (1993). Should chloral hydrate be banned? *Pediatrics, 92,* 442–446.

STEINBERG, L. (1991). Adolescent transitions and alcohol and other drug use prevention. In *Preventing adolescent drug use: From theory to practice.* Rockville, MD: U.S. Department of Health and Human Services.

STEINBERG, N. (1994, May 5). The cartels would like a second chance. *Rolling Stone,* 33–34.

STEINBERG, W., & TENNER, S. (1994). Acute pancreatitis. *New England Journal of Medicine, 330,* 1198–1210.

STEINGLASS, P., BENNETT, L. A., WOLIN, S. J., & REISS, D. (1987). *The alcoholic family.* New York: Basic Books.

STERNBACH, G. L., & VARON, J. (1992). "Designer drugs." *Postgraduate Medicine, 91,* 169–176.

STEVENS, R. S., ROFFMAN, R. A., & SIMPSON, E. E. (1994). Treating adult marijuana dependence: A test of the relapse prevention model. *Journal of Consulting and Clinical Psychology, 62,* 92–99.

STEVENS, V. J., & HOLLIS, J. F. (1989). Preventing smoking relapse, using an individually tailored skills-training technique. *Journal of Consulting and Clinical Psychology, 57,* 420–424.

STEWART, W. F., KAWAS, C., CORRADA, M., & METTER, E. J. (1997). Risk of Alzheimer's disease and duration of NSAID use. *Neurology, 48,* 626–632.

STINCHFIELD, R. D., NIFOROPULOS, L., & FEDER, S. H. (1994). Follow-up contact bias in adolescent substance abuse treatment research. *Journal of Studies on Alcohol, 55*(3), 285–270.

STIX, G. (1994). Lollipop, lollipop. *Scientific American, 270*(5), 113.

STOCKWELL, T., & TOWN, C. (1989). Anxiety and stress management. In H. K. Hester & W. R. Miller (Eds.), *Handbook of alcoholism treatment approaches.* New York: Pergamon Press.

STOFFELMAYR, B. E., BENISHEK, L. A., HUMPHREYS, K., LEE, J. A., & MAVIS, B. E. (1989). Substance abuse prognosis with an additional psychiatric diagnosis: Understanding the relationship. *Journal of Psychoactive Drugs, 21*(2), 145–152.

STOLBERG, S. (1994). Aspirin isn't just for headaches. *Minneapolis Star-Tribune, XIII*(179), 4A.

STONE, J. (1991). Light elements. *Discover, 12*(1), 12–16.

STRAIN, E. C., STRITZER, M. L., LIEBSON, I. A., & BIGELOW, G. E. (1994). Comparison of buprenorphine and methadone in the treatment of opioid dependence. *American Journal of Psychiatry, 151,* 1025–1030.

STRANG, J., GRIFFITHS, P., POWIS, B., & GOSSOP, M. (1992). First use of heroin: Changes in route of administration over time. *British Medical Journal, 304,* 1222–1223.

STRANG, J., JOHNS, A., & CAAN, W. (1993). Cocaine in the UK—1991. *British Journal of Psychiatry, 162,* 1–13.

STREISSGUTH, A. P., AASE, J. M., CLARREN, S. K., RANDELS, S. P., LADUE, R. A., & SMITH, D. F. (1991). Fetal alcohol syndrome in adolescents and adults. *Journal of the American Medical Association, 265,* 1961–1967.

STRONG MEDICINE. (1995). *Harvard Health Letter, 20*(6), 4–6.

STUART, R. B. (1980). *Helping couples change.* New York: Guilford Press.

STUDY: COCAINE TREATMENT MORE EFFECTIVE THAN SUPPLY CONTROL. (1994). *Alcoholism & Drug Abuse Week, 6*(24), 4.

STUDY: DRUG TREATMENT MAKES CENTS. (1994). *Minneapolis Star-Tribune, XIII*(71), 8a.

SULLUM, J. (1995). Weights and half-measures. *Reason, 27*(4), 15.

SUPERNAW, R. B. (1991). Pharmacotherapeutic management of acute pain. *U.S. Pharmacist, 16*(2), H1–H14.

SUSSMAN, N. (1988). Diagnosis and drug treatment of anxiety in the elderly. *Geriatric Medicine Today, 7*(10), 1–8.

SUSSMAN, N. (1994). The uses of buspirone in psychiatry. *Journal of Clinical Psychiatry, 55*(5)(Suppl.), 3–19.

SUTER, P. M., SCHULTZ, Y., & JEQUIER, E. (1992). The effect of ethanol on fat storage in healthy subjects. *New England Journal of Medicine, 326,* 983–987.

SUTHERLAND, G., STAPLETON, J. A., RUSSELL, M. A. H., JARVIS, M. J., HAJEK, P., BELCHER, M., & FEYERABEND, C. (1992). Randomized controlled trial of nasal nicotine spray in smoking cessation. *Lancet, 340,* 324–329.

SVANUM, S., & MCADOO, W. G. (1989). Predicting rapid relapse following treatment for chemical dependence: A matched-subjects design. *Journal of Consulting and Clinical Psychology, 34,* 1027–1030.

SWADI, H. (1993). Alcohol abuse in adolescence: An update. *Archives of Disease in Childhood*, 68, 341–343.

SWAIM, R. C., OETTING, R. W., EDWARDS, R. W., & BEAUVAIS, F. (1989). Links from emotional distress to adolescent drug use: A path model. *Journal of Consulting and Clinical Psychology*, 57, 227–231.

SWAN, N. (1994). Research demonstrates long-term benefits of methadone treatment. *NIDA Notes*, 9(4), 1, 4–5.

SWAN, N. (1995a). 31% of New York murder victims had cocaine in their bodies. *NIDA Notes*, 10(2), 1, 4.

SWAN, N. (1995b). NIDA plays key role in studying links between AIDS and drug abuse. *NIDA Notes*, 10(3), 1, 4.

SWIFT, R. M., WHELIHAN, W., KUZNETSOV, O., BUONGIORNO, G., & HSUING, H. (1994). Naltrexone-induced alterations in human ethanol intoxication. *American Journal of Psychiatry*, 151, 1463–1467.

SZAREWSKI, A., JARVIS, M. J., SASIENI, P., ANDERSON, M., EDWARDS, R., STEELE, S. J., & BUILLEBAUD, J. C. (1996). Effect of smoking cessation on cervical lesion size. *Lancet*, 347, 941–943.

SZASZ, T. S. (1972). Bad habits are not diseases: A refutation of the claim that alcoholism is a disease. *Lancet*, 319, 83–84.

SZASZ, T. S. (1988). A plea for the cessation of the longest war of the twentieth century—the war on drugs. *Humanistic Psychologist*, 16(2), 314–322.

SZASZ, T. S. (1991). Diagnoses are not diseases. *Lancet*, 338, 1574–1576.

SZASZ, T. S. (1994). Mental illness is still a myth. *Transaction Social Science and Modern Society*, 31(4), 34–39.

SZASZ, T. S. (1996). The war on drugs is lost. *National Review*, XLVIII(2), 45–47.

SZASZ, T. S. (1997). Save money, cut crime, get real. *Playboy*, 44(1), 129, 190.

SZUSTER, R. R., SCHANBACHER, B. L., & McCANN, S. C. (1990). Characteristics of psychiatric emergency room patients with alcohol- or drug-induced disorders. *Hospital and Community Psychiatry*, 41, 1342–1345.

SZWABO, P. A. (1993). Substance abuse in older women. *Clinics in Geriatric Medicine*, 9, 197–208.

TABAKOFF, B., & HOFFMAN, P. L. (1992). Alcohol: Neurobiology. In J. H. Lowinson, P. Ruiz, R. B. Millman, & J. G. Langrod (Eds.), *Substance abuse: A comprehensive textbook* (2nd ed.). New York: Williams & Wilkins.

TABOR, B. L., SMITH-WALLACE, T., & YONEKURA, M. L. (1990). Parinatal outcome associated with PCP versus cocaine use. *American Journal of Drug and Alcohol Abuse*, 16, 337–349.

TAHA, A. S., DAHILL, S., STURROCK, R. D., LEE, F. D., & RUSSELL, R. I. (1994). Predicting NSAID related ulcers—assessment of clinical and pathological risk factors and importance of differences in NSAID. *Gut*, 35, 891–895.

TAKANISHI, R. (1993). The opportunities of adolescence-research, interventions, and policy. *American Psychologist*, 48, 85–87.

TAKE TIME TO SMELL THE FENTANYL. (1994). *Forensic Drug Abuse Advisor*, 6(5), 34–35.

TAKE 2 ASPIRINS AND COME BACK IN 76 YEARS. (1994). *U.S. News & World Report*, 117(12), 24.

TALLEY, N. J. (1993). The effects of NSAIDs on the gut. *Contemporary Internal Medicine*, 5(2), 14–28.

TANNER, S. (1995). Steroids: A breakfast of champions. *Orthopaedic Nursing*, 14(6), 26–30.

TARTER, R. E. (1988). Are there inherited behavioral traits that predispose to substance abuse? *Journal of Consulting and Clinical Psychology*, 56, 189–197.

TARTER, R. E., OTT, P. J., & MEZZICH, A. C. (1991). Psychometric assessment. In R. J. Frances & S. I. Miller (Eds.), *Clinical textbook of addictive disorders*. New York: Guilford Press.

TASHKIN, D. P. (1990). Pulmonary complications of smoked substance abuse. *Western Journal of Medicine*, 152, 525–531.

TASHKIN, D. P. (1993). Is frequent marijuana smoking harmful to health? *Western Journal of Medicine*, 158, 635–637.

TATE, C. (1989). In the 1800's, antismoking was a burning issue. *Smithsonian*, 20(4), 107–117.

TATE, J. C., STANTON, A. L., GREEN, S. B., SCHMITZ, J. M., LE, T., & MARSHALL, B. (1994). Experimental analysis of the role of expectancy in nicotine withdrawal. *Psychology of Addictive Behaviors*, 8, 169–178.

TAVRIS, C. (1990). One more guilt trip for women. *Minneapolis Star-Tribune*, VIII(341), 21A.

TAVRIS, C. (1992). *The mismeasure of woman*. New York: Simon & Schuster.

TAYLOR, D. (1993). Addicts' abuse of sleeping pills brings call for tough curbs. *Observer*, 10531, 6.

TAYLOR, M. A. (1993). *The neuropsychiatric guide to modern everyday psychiatry*. New York: Free Press.

TAYLOR, W. A., & GOLD, M. S. (1990). Pharmacologic approaches to the treatment of cocaine dependence. *Western Journal of Medicine*, 152, 573–578.

TERWILLIGER, E. G. (1995). Biology of HIV-1 and treatment strategies. *Emergency Medicine Clinics of North America*, 13, 27–42.

TEST, M. A., WALLISCH, L. S., ALLNESS, D. J., & RIPP, K. (1990). Substance use in young adults with schizophrenic disorders. *Schizophrenia Bulletin*, 15, 465–476.

THACKER, W., & TREMAINE, L. (1989). Systems issues in serving the mentally ill substance abuser: Virgina's experience. *Hospital and Community Psychiatry*, 40, 1046–1049.

THE AGONY OF "ECSTASY." (1994). *Medical Update*, 17(11), 5–6.

THE BACK LETTER. (1994). Steroid-abusing patients: Handle with care. *Archives of General Psychiatry*, 51, 83.

THE CHANGING FACE OF AIDS. (1991). *The Wellness Letter*, 7(8), 6.

THE DRUG INDEX. (1995). *Playboy*, 42(9), 47.

THE MEN WHO CREATED CRACK. (1991). *U.S. News & World Report*, 11(8), 44–53.

THERAPEUTIC COMMUNITY RESEARCH YIELDS INTERESTING RESULTS. (1989). *The Addiction Letter*, 5(1), 2.

THE SAUNA DEFENSE. (1995). *Forensic Drug Abuse Advisor*, 7(6), 42.

THE SMOKING EPIDEMIC. (1991). *Lancet*, 338, 1387.

THOMASON, H. H., & DILTS, S. L. (1991). Opioids. In R. J. Frances & S. I. Miller (Eds.), *Clinical textbook of addictive disorders*. New York: Guilford Press.

THOMSON, A. D. (1994). Alcoholic hepatitis. *Lancet*, 343, 810.

THORNTON, J. (1990). Pharm aid: 10 new medicines you should know about. *Men's Health*, 5(4), 73–78.

THUN, M. J., NAMBOODIRI, M. M., & HEATH, C. W. (1991). Aspirin use and reduced risk of fatal colon cancer. *New England Journal of Medicine*, 325, 1593–1596.

TOBIN, J. W. (1992). Is AA "treatment"? You bet. *Addiction & Recovery*, 12(3), 40.

TOLMETIN FOILS EMIT ASSAY. (1995). *Forensic Drug Abuse Advisor*, 7(3), 23.

TONEATTO, T., SOBELL, L. C., SOBELL, M. B., & LEO, G. I. (1991). Psychoactive substance use disorder (Alcohol). In M. Hersen & S. M. Turner (Eds.), *Adult psychopathology and diagnosis* (2nd ed.). New York: Wiley.

TONIGAN, J. S., & HILLER-STURMHOFEL, S. (1994). Alcoholics Anonymous: Who benefits? *Alcohol Health & Research World*, 18, 308–310.

TORRENS, M., SAN, L., & CAMI, J. (1993). Buprenorphine verses heroin dependence: Comparison of toxicologic and psychopathologic characteristics. *American Journal of Psychiatry*, 150, 822–824.

TRABERT, W., CASPARI, D., BERNHARD, P., & BIRO, G. (1992). Inappropriate vasopressin secretion in severe alcohol withdrawal. *Acta Psychiatrica Scandinavica*, 85, 376 379.

TRACHTENBERG, M. C., & BLUM, K. (1987). Alcohol and opioid peptides: Neuropharmacolical rationale for physical craving of alcohol. *American Journal of Drug and Alcohol Abuse*, 13(3), 365–372.

TRACHTENBERG, M. C., & BLUM, K. (1988). Improvement of cocaine-induced neuromodulator deficits by the neuronutrient Tropamine. *Journal of Psychoactive Drugs*, 20(3), 315–331.

TRAYNOR, M. P., BEGAY, M. E., & GLANTZ, S. A. (1993). New tobacco industry strategy to prevent local tobacco control. *Journal of the American Medical Association*, 270, 479–486.

TREADWAY, D. (1990). Codependency: Disease, metaphor, or fad? *Family Therapy Networker*, 14(1), 39–43.

TREATING WOMEN EFFECTIVELY DOESN'T MEAN SIMPLY TREATING WOMEN. (1994). *Alcoholism & Drug Abuse Week*, 6(17), 1–3.

TREATMENT OF DRUG ABUSE AND ADDICTION—PART I. (1995). *The Harvard Mental Health Letter*, 12(2), 1–4.

TREATMENT PROTOCOLS FOR MARIJUANA DEPENDENCE ARE STARTING TO EMERGE. (1995). *The Addiction Letter*, 11(8), 1–2.

TRESCH, D. D., & ARONOW, W. S. (1996). Smoking and coronary artery disease. *Clinics in Geriatric Medicine*, 12, 23–32.

TRIANGLE OF SELF-OBSESSION, THE. (1983). New York: Narcotics Anonymous World Service Office.

TRICHOPOULOS, D., MOLLO, F., TOMATIS, L., AGAPITOS, E., DELSEDIME, L., ZAVITSANOS, X., KALANDIDI, A., KATSOUYANNI, K., RIBOLI, E., & SARACCI, R. (1992). Active and passive smoking and pathological indicators of lung cancer risk in an autopsy study. *Journal of the American Medical Association*, 268, 1697–1701.

TRUOG, R. D., BERDE, C. B., MITCHELL, C., & GRIER, H. E. (1992). Barbiturates in the care of the terminally ill. *New England Journal of Medicine*, 327, 1678–1682.

TSAI, G., GASTFRIEND, D. R., & COYLE, J. T. (1995). The glutamatergic basis of human alcoholism. *American Journal of Psychiatry*, 152, 332–340.

TSUANG, J. W., & LOHR, J. B. (1994). Effects of alcohol on symptoms in alcoholic and nonalcoholic patients with schizophrenia. *Hospital and Community Psychiatry*, 45, 1229–1230.

TUCKER, J. A., & SOBELL, L. C. (1992). Influences on help-seeking for drinking problems and on natural recovery without treatment. *Behavior Therapist*, 15(1), 12–14.

TURBO, R. (1989). Drying out is just a start: Alcoholism. *Medical World News*, 30(3), 56–63.

TURKINGTON, C. (1994). Study of xanthines could lead to drug discoveries. *APA Monitor*, 25(2), 18.

TWEED, S. H., & RYFF, C. D. (1991). Profiles of wellness amidst distress. *Journal of Studies on Alcohol*, 52, 133–141.

TWELVE STEPS AND TWELVE TRADITIONS. (1981). New York: Alcoholics Anonymous World Services.

TWERSKI, A. J. (1983). Early intervention in alcoholism: Confrontational techniques. *Hospital & Community Psychiatry*, 34, 1027–1030.

TWERSKI, A. J. (1989). Diagnosing and treating dual disorders. *Alcoholism & Addiction*, 9(3), 37–40.

TYAS, S., & RUSH, B. (!993). The treatment of disabled persons with alcohol and drug problems: Results of a survey of addiction services. *Journal of Studies on Alcohol*, 54, 275–282.

TYLER, D. C. (1994). Pharmacology of pain management. *Pediatric Clinics of North America*, 41, 59–71.

TYRER, P. (1993). Withdrawal from hypnotic drugs. *British Medical Journal*, 306, 706–708.

UHDE, T. W., & TRANCER, M. E. (1995). Barbiturates. In H. I. Kaplan & B. J. Sadock (Eds.), *Comprehensive textbook of psychiatry* (6th ed.). Baltimore: Williams & Wilkins.

UHL, G. R., PERSICO, A. M., & SMITH, S. S. (1992). Current excitement with D$_2$ dopamine receptor gene alleles in substance abuse. *Archives of General Psychiatry, 49,* 157–160.

UNDERSTANDING ANONYMITY. (1981). New York: Alcoholics Anonymous World Services.

UNITED STATES PHARMACOPEIAL CONVENTION, INC. (1990). *Advice for the patient* (10th ed.). Rockville, MD: USPC Board of Trustees.

UNIVERSITY OF CALIFORNIA, BERKELEY. (1990a). Codependency. *The Wellness Letter, 7*(1), 7.

UNIVERSITY OF CALIFORNIA, BERKELEY. (1990b). Marijuana: What we know. *The Wellness Letter, 6*(6), 2–4.

UNIVERSITY OF CALIFORNIA, BERKELEY. (1990c). Women's magazines: Whose side are they on? *The Wellness Letter, 7*(3), 7.

UPDATE ON GLOBAL AIDS SITUATION. (1992, August 13). *CDC AIDS Weekly,* 2–4.

URBANO-MARQUEZ, A., ESTRUCH, R., FERNANDEZ-SOLA, J., NICHOLAS, J. M., PARE, C., & RUBIN, E. (1995). The greater risk of alcoholic cardiomyopathy and myopathy in women compared with men. *Journal of the American Medical Association, 274,* 149–154.

U.S. DEATHS FROM TOBACCO AND OTHER DRUGS CIRCA 1990. (1994). *NIDA Notes, 9*(3), 5.

UVA, J. L. (1991). Alcoholics Anonymous: Medical recovery through a higher power. *Journal of the American Medical Association, 266,* 3065–3068.

VAILLANT, G. E. (1983). *The natural history of alcoholism.* Cambridge, MA: Harvard University Press.

VAILLANT, G. E. (1990). We should retain the disease concept of alcoholism. *Harvard Medical School Mental Health Letter, 9*(6), 4–6.

VAILLANT, G. E. (1996). A long-term follow-up of male alcohol abuse. *Archives of General Psychiatry, 53,* 243–249.

VAILLANT, G. E., & HILLER-STURMHOFEL, S. (1996). The natural history of alcoholism. *Alcohol Health & Research World, 20,* 152–161.

VANDEPUTTE, C. (1989). Why bother to treat older adults? The answer is compelling. *Professional Counselor, 4*(2), 34–38.

VEREBEY, K., & TURNER, C. E. (1991). Laboratory testing. In R. J. Frances, & S. I. Miller (Eds.), *Clinical textbook of addictive disorders.* New York: Guilford Press.

VICTOR, M. (1993). Persistent altered mentation due to ethanol. *Neurologic Clinics, 11,* 639–661.

VOELKER, R. (1994). Medical marijuana: A trial of science and politics. *Journal of the American Medical Association, 271,* 1645–1648.

VOLKOW, N. D., HITZEMANN, R., WANG, G. J., FOWLER, J. S., BURR, G., PASCANI, K., DEWEY, S. L., & WOLF, A. P. (1992). Decreased brain metabolism in neurologically intact healthy alcoholics. *American Journal of Psychiatry, 149,* 1016–1022.

VOLPE, J. J. (1995). *Neurology of the newborn* (3rd ed.). Philadelphia: Saunders.

VOLPICELLI, J. R., ALTERMAN, A. I., HAYASHIDA, M., & O'BRIEN, C. P. (1992). Naltrexone in the treatment of alcohol dependence. *Archives of General Psychiatry, 49,* 876 880.

VOLPICELLI, J. R., CLAY, K. L., WATSON, N. T., & VOLPICELLI, L. A. (1994). Naltrexone and the treatment of alcohol dependence. *Alcohol Health & Research World, 18,* 272–278.

WADLER, G. I. (1994). Drug use update. *Medical Clinics of North America, 78,* 439–455.

WALKER, C. E., BONNER, B. L., & KAUFMAN, K. I. (1988). *The physically and sexually abused child.* New York: Pergamon Press.

WALKER, J. D. (1993). The tobacco epidemic: How far have we come? *Canadian Medical Association Journal, 148,* 145–147.

WALKER, S. (1996). *A dose of sanity.* New York: Wiley.

WALLACE, J. (1996). Theory of 12-step oriented treatment. In F. Rotgers, D. S. Keller, & J. Morgenstern (Eds.), *Treating substance abuse.* New York: Guilford Press.

WALLACE, J. M., OISHI, J. S., BARBERS, R. G., SIMMONS, M. S., & TASHKIN, D. P. (1994). Lymphocytic subpopulation profiles in bronchoalveolar lavage fluid and peripheral blood from tobacco and marijuana smokers. *Chest, 105,* 847–852.

WALLEN, M. C., & WEINER, H. D. (1989). Impediments to effective treatment of the dually diagnosed patient. *Journal of Psychoactive Drugs, 21,* 161–168.

WALSH, D. C., HINGSON, R. W., MERRIGAN, D. M., LEVENSON, S. M., CUPPLES, L. A., HERREN, T., COFFMAN, G. A., BECKER, C. A., BARKER, T. A., HAMILTON, S. A., McGUIRE, T. G., & KELLY, C. A. (1991). A randomized trial of treatment options for alcohol-abusing workers. *New England Journal of Medicine, 325,* 775–782.

WALTER, D. S., & INTURRISI, C. E. (1995). Absorption, distribution, metabolism, and excretion of buprenorphine in animals and humans. In A. Cowan & J. W. Lewis (Eds.), *Buprenorphine.* New York: Wiley Interscience.

WALTERS, G. D. (1994). The drug lifestyle: One pattern or several? *Psychology of Addictive Behaviors, 8,* 8–13.

WANNAMETHEE, S. G., SHAPER, A. G., WHINCUP, P. H., & WALKER, M. (1995). Smoking cessation and the risk of stroke in middle-aged men. *Journal of the American Medical Association, 274,* 155–160.

WAR BY OTHER MEANS. (1990). *The Economist, 314*(7641), 50.

WARNER, E. A. (1995). Is your patient using cocaine? *Postgraduate Medicine, 98,* 173–180.

WARNER, L. A., KESSLER, R. C., HUGHES, M., ANTHONY, J. C., & NELSON, C. B. (1995). Prevalence and correlates of drug use and dependence in the United States. *Archives of General Psychiatry, 51,* 219–229.

WASHINGTON POST. (1995). Netherlands says that tolerating soft drugs aids decline in addicts. *Minneapolis Star-Tribune*, XIV(234), A31.

WASHTON, A. M. (1990). Crack and other substance abuse in the suburbs. *Medical Aspects of Human Sexuality*, 24,(5), 54–58.

WASHTON, A. M. (1995). Clinical assessment of psychoactive substance use. In A. M. Washton (Ed.), *Psychotherapy and substance abuse*. New York: Guilford Press.

WASHTON, A. M., STONE, N. S., & HENDRICKSON, E. C. (1988). Cocaine abuse. In D. M. Donovan & G. A. Marlatt (Eds.), *Assessment of addictive behaviors*. New York: Guilford Press.

WASMAN, H. (1991). Tobacco marketing. *Journal of the American Medical Association*, 266, 3186–3186.

WATSON, C. G., HANCOCK, M., GEARHART, L. P., MENDEZ, C. M., MALOVRH, P., & RADEN, M. (1997). A comparative outcome study of frequent, moderate, occasional, and nonattenders of Alcoholics Anonymous. *Journal of Clinical Psychology*, 53, 209–214.

WATSON, C. G., HANCOCK, M., MALOVRH, P., GEARHART, L. P.,& RADEN, M. (1996). A 48 week natural history follow-up of alcoholics who do and do not engage in limited drinking after treatment. *Journal of Nervous and Mental Disease*, 184(10), 623–627.

WATSON, J. M. (1984). Solvent abuse and adolescents. *The Practitioner*, 228, 487–490.

WEATHERS, W. T., CRANE, M. M., SAUVAIN, K. J., & BLACKHURST, D. W. (1993). Cocaine use in women from a defined population: Prevalence at delivery and effects on growth in infants. *Pediatrics*, 91, 350–354.

WEBB, E., ASHTON, C. H., & KAMALI, F. (1996). Alcohol and drug use in UK university students. *Lancet*, 348, 922–925.

WEBB, S. T. (1989). Some developmental issues of adolescent children of alcoholics. *Adolescent Counselor*, 1(6), 47–48, 67.

WECHSLER, H., DAVENPORT, A., DOWDALL, G., MOEYKENS, B., & CASTILLO, S. (1994). Health and behavioral consequences of binge drinking in college. *Journal of the American Medical Association*, 272, 1672–1677.

WEDDINGTON, W. W. (1993). Cocaine. *Psychiatric Clinics of North America*, 16, 87–95.

WEGSCHEIDER-CRUSE, S. (1985). *Choice-making*. Pompano Beach, FL: Health Communications.

WEGSCHEIDER-CRUSE, S., & CRUSE, J. R. (1990). *Understanding co-dependency*. Pompano Beach, FL: Health Communications.

WEIL, A. (1986). *The natural mind*. Boston: Houghton-Mifflin.

WEINER, N. (1985). Norepinephrine, epinephrine, and the sympathomimetic amines. In A. G. Gilman, L. S. Goodman, T. W. Rall, & F. Murad (Eds.), *The pharmacological basis of therapeutics* (7th ed.). New York: Macmillan.

WEINRIEB, R. M., & O' BRIEN, C. P. (1993). Persistent cognitive deficits attributed to substance abuse. *Neurologic Clinics*, 11, 663–691.

WEISNER, C., & SCHMIDT, L. (1992). Gender disparities in treatment for alcohol problems. *Journal of the American Medical Association*, 268, 1872–1876.

WEISS, R. (1994). Of myths and mischief. *Discover*, 15(10), 36–42.

WEISS, R. D., GREENFIELD, S. H., & MIRIN, S. M. (1994). Intoxication and withdrawal syndromes. In S. E. Hyman & G. E. Tesar (Eds.), *Handbook of psychiatric emergencies* (3rd ed.). Boston: Little, Brown.

WEISS, R. D., & MIRIN, S. M. (1988). Intoxication and withdrawal syndromes. In S. E. Hyman (Ed.), *Handbook of psychiatric emergencies* (2nd ed.). Boston: Little, Brown.

WEISS, R. D., MIRIN, S. M., & FRANCES, R. J. (1992). The myth of the typical dual diagnosis patient. *Hospital and Community Psychiatry* 43, 107–108.

WEISS, R. D., MIRIN, S. M., GRIFFIN, M. L., & MICHAEL, J. L. (1988). Psychopathology in cocaine users: Changing trends. *Journal of Nervous and Mental Disease*, 176, 719–725.

WELLS-PARKER, E. (1994). Mandated treatment. *Alcohol Health & Research World*, 18, 302–306.

WENDER, P. H. (1995). *Attention-deficit hyperactivity disorder in adults*. New York: Oxford University Press.

WERNER, E. E. (1989). Children of the garden island. *Scientific American*, 260(4),106–111.

WERNER, M. J., WALKER, L. S., & GREENE, J. W. (1995). Relation of alcohol expectancies to changes in problem drinking among college students. *Archives of Pediatric and Adolescent Medicine*, 149, 733–739.

WESSON, D. R., & LING, W. (1996). Addiction medicine. *Journal of the American Medical Association*, 275, 1792–1793.

WESTERMEYER, J. (1987). The psychiatrist and solvent-inhalant abuse: Recognition,assessment and treatment. *American Journal of Psychiatry*, 144, 903–907.

WESTERMEYER, J. (1995). Cultural aspects of substance abuse and alcoholism. *Psychiatric Clinics of North America*, 18, 589–620.

WESTMAN, E. C. (1995). Does smokeless tobacco cause hypertension? *Southern Medical Journal*, 88, 716–720.

WETLI, C. V. (1987). Fatal reactions to cocaine. In A. M. Washton & M. S. Gold (Eds.), *Cocaine: A clinician's handbook*. New York: Guilford Press.

WETTER, D. W., FIORE, M. C., BAKER, T. B., & YOUNG, T. B. (1995). Tobacco withdrawal and nicotine replacement influence objective measures of sleep. *Journal of Consulting and Clinical Psychology*, 63, 658–667.

WETTER, D. W., YOUNG, T. B., BIDWELL, T. R., BADR, M. S., & PALTA, M. (1994). Smoking as a risk factor for sleep-disordered breathing. *Archives of Internal Medicine*, 154, 2219–2224.

WHATEVER HAPPENED TO ICE? (1994). *Brown University Digest of Addiction Theory and Application, 13*(3), 6–8.

WHEELER, K., & MALMQUIST, J. (1987). Treatment approaches in adolescent chemical dependency. *Pediatric Clinics of North America, 34*(2), 437–447.

WHITCOMB, D. C., & BLOCK, G. D. (1994). Association of acetaminophen hepatoxicity with fasting and ethanol use. *Journal of the American Medical Association, 272*, 1845–1850.

WHITE, P. T. (1989) Coca. *National Geographic, 175*(1), 3–47.

WHITE, R. J. (1993). Washington figuring out it has fought drug war on wrong fronts. *Minneapolis Star-Tribune, XI*(351), 23A.

WHITEHEAD, R., CHILLAG, S., & ELLIOTT, D. (1992). Anabolic steroid use among adolescents in a rural state. *Journal of Family Practice, 35*, 401–405.

WHITMAN, D., FRIEDMAN, D., & THOMAS, L. (1990). The return of skid row. *U.S. News & World Report, 108*(2), 27–30.

WHITWORTH, A. B., FISCHER, F., LESCH, O. M., NIM-MERRICHTER, A., OBERBAUER, H., PLATZ, T., POT-GIETER, A., WALTER, H., & FLEISCHHACKER, W. W. (1996). Comparison of acamprosate and placebo in long-term treatment of alcohol dependence. *Lancet, 347*, 1438–1442.

WHY CONFIRMATORY TESTING IS ALWAYS A NECESSITY. (1997). *Forensic Drug Abuse Advisor, 9*(4), 25.

WILBUR, R. (1986). A drug to fight cocaine. *Science '86, 7*(2), 42–46.

WILCOX, C. M., SHALEK, K. A., & COTSONIS, G. (1994). Striking prevalence of over-the counter nonsteroidal anti-inflammatory drug use in patients with upper gastrointestinal hemorrhage. *Archives of Internal Medicine, 154*, 42–46.

WILL, G. F. (1993). U.S. drug policy sets off slew of unintended consequences. *Minneapolis Star-Tribune, XII*(84), 21A.

WILLIAMS, B. R., & BAER, C. L. (1994). *Essentials of clinical pharmacology in nursing* (2nd ed.). Springhouse, PA: Springhouse.

WILLIAMS, E. (1989). Strategies for intervention. *Nursing Clinics of North America, 24*(1), 95–107.

WILLIAMSON, D. F., MADANS, J., ANDA, R., KLEINMAN, J. C., GIOVINO, G. A., & BYERS, T. (1991). Smoking cessation and severity of weight gain in a national cohort. *New England Journal of Medicine, 324*, 739–745.

WILLOUGHBY, A. (1984). *The alcohol troubled person: Known and unknown.* Chicago: Nelson-Hall.

WILLS, T. A., McNAMARA, G., VACCARO, D., & HIRKY, A. E. (1996). Escalated substance use: A longitudinal grouping analysis from early to middle adolescence. *Journal of Abnormal Psychology, 105*, 166–180.

WILSNACK, S. C. (1991). Barriers to treatment for alcoholic women. *Addiction & Recovery, 11*(4), 10–12.

WILSNACK, S. C., & WILSNACK, R. W. (1995). Drinking and problem drinking in U.S. women. In M. Galanter (Ed.), *Recent developments in alcoholism* (Vol. 12). New York: Plenum Press.

WILSNACK, S. C., WILSNACK, R. W., & HILLER-STURMHOFFEL, S. (1994). How women drink. *Alcohol Health & Research World, 18*, 173–181.

WILSON, F., & KUNSMAN, K. (1997). The saliva solution: New choices for alcohol testing. *Occupational Health & Safety, 66*(4), 40–43.

WILSON-TUCKER, S., & DASH, J. (1995). Legal—but lethal: Fighting the newest health threat to our kids. *Family Circle, 108*(14), 21–24.

WINCHESTER, J. F. (1990). Barbiturates, methaqualone and primidone. In L. M. Haddad & J. F. Winchester (Eds.), *Clinical management of poisoning and drug overdose* (2nd ed.). Philadelphia: Saunders.

WINDLE, M., WINDLE, R. C., SCHEIDT, D. M., & MILLER, G. B. (1995). Physical and sexual abuse and associated mental disorders among alcoholic inpatients. *American Journal of Psychiatry, 152*, 1322–1328.

WING, D. M. (1995). Transcending alcoholic denial. *Image, 27*, 121–126.

WISNEIWSKI, L. (1994). Use of household products as inhalants rising among young teens. *Minneapolis Star-Tribune, XIII*(9), 8EX.

WITKIN, G. (1995). A new drug gallops through the west. *U.S. News & World Report, 119*(19), 50–51.

WITKIN, G., & GRIFFIN, J. (1994). The new opium wars. *U.S. News & World Report, 117*(114), 39–44.

WOITITZ, J. G. (1983). *Adult children of alcoholics.* Pompano Beach, FL: Health Communications.

WOLF-REEVE, B. S. (1990). A guide to the assessment of psychiatric symptoms in the addictions treatment setting. In D. F. O'Connell (Ed.), *Managing the dually diagnosed patient.* New York: Haworth Press.

WOLIN, S. J., & WOLIN, S. (1993). *The resilient self.* New York: Villard Books.

WOLIN, S. J., & WOLIN, S. (1995). Resilience among youth growing up in substance abusing families. *Pediatric Clinics of North America, 42*, 415–429.

WOLKOWITZ, O. M. (1990). Long-lasting behavioral changes following prednisone withdrawal. *Journal of the American Medical Association, 261*, 1731.

WOLKOWITZ, O. M., RUBINOW, D., DORAN, A. R., BREIER, A., BERRETTINI, W. H., KLING, M. A.,& PICKAR, D. (1990). Prednisone effects on neurochemistry and behavior: Preliminary findings. *Archives of General Psychiatry, 47*, 963–968.

WOMEN WITH AIDS: THE GROWING THREAT. (1990). *Medical Aspects of Human Sexuality, 24*(10), 68–69.

WOODS, J. H., KATZ, J. L., & WINGER, G. (1988). Use and abuse of benzodiazepines. *Journal of the American Medical Association, 260*(23), 3476–3480.

WOODS, J. H., WINGER, G. D., & FRANCE, C. P. (1987). Reinforcing and discriminative stimulus effects of cocaine: Analysis of pharmacological mechanisms. In S. Fisher, A. Raskin, & E. H. Unlenhuth (Eds.), *Cocaine: Clinical and behavioral aspects.* New York: Oxford University Press.

WOODY, G. (1996). The challenge of dual diagnosis. *Alcohol Health & Research World, 20,* 76–79.

WOODY, G. E., & MACFADDEN, W. (1995). Cannabis related disorders. In H. I. Kaplan & B. J. Sadock (Eds.), *Comprehensive textbook of psychiatry* (6th ed.). Baltimore: Williams & Wilkins.

WOODY, G. E., MCLELLAN, A. T., & BEDRICK, J. (1995). Dual diagnosis. In J. M. Oldham & M. B. Riba (Eds.), *Review of psychiatry* (Vol. 14). Washington, DC: American Psychiatric Association Press.

WOOLF, A. D., & SHANNON, M. W. (1995). Clinical toxicology for the pediatrician. *Pediatric Clinics of North America, 42,* 317–333.

WORMSLEY, K. G. (1993). Safety profile of ranitidine. *Drugs, 46,* 976–985.

WRAY, S. R., & MURTHY, N. V. A. (1987). Review of the effects of cannabis on mental and physiological functions. *West Indian Medical Journal, 36*(4), 197–201.

YABLONSKY, L. (1967). *Synanon: The tunnel back.* Baltimore: Penguin Books.

YALOM, I. D. (1985). *The theory and practice of group psychotherapy* (3rd ed.). New York: Basic Books.

YESALIS, C. E., KENNEDY, N. J., KOPSTEIN, A. N., & BAHRKE, M. S. (1993). Anabolic-androgenic steroid use in the United States. *Journal of the American Medical Association, 270,* 1217–1221.

YIP, L., DART, R. C., & GABOW, P. A. (1994). Concepts and controversies in salicylate toxicity. *Emergency Medical Clinics of North America, 12,* 351–364.

YOST, D. A. (1996). Alcohol withdrawal syndrome. *American Family Physician, 54,* 657–664.

YOUNGSTROM, N. (1990a). Debate rages on: In- or outpatient? *APA Monitor, 21*(10), 19.

YOUNGSTROM, N. (1990b). The drugs used to treat drug abuse. *APA Monitor, 21*(10), 19.

YOUNGSTROM, N. (1991). Field, APA address drug abuse in society. *APA Monitor, 22*(1), 14.

YOUNGSTROM, N. (1992). Fetal alcohol syndrome carries severe deficits. *APA Monitor, 23*(4), 32.

YOUR HEROIN, SIR. (1991). *Lancet, 337,* 402.

ZAREK, D., HAWKINS, D., & ROGERS, P. D. (1987). Risk factors for adolescent substance abuse. *Pediatric Clinics of North America, 34*(2), 481–493.

ZERWEKH, J., & MICHAELS, B. (1989). Co-dependency. *Nursing Clinics of North America, 24*(1), 109–120.

ZIMBERG, S. (1978). Psychosocial treatment of elderly alcoholics. In S. Zimberg, J. Wallace, & S. B. Blume (Eds.), *Practical approaches to alcoholism psychotherapy.* New York: Plenum Press.

ZIMBERG, S. (1995). The elderly. In A. M. Washton (Ed.), *Psychotherapy and substance abuse.* New York: Guilford Press.

ZIMBERG, S. (1996). Treating alcoholism: An age-specific intervention that works for older patients. *Geriatrics, 51*(10), 45–49.

ZISOOK, S., HEATON, R., MORANVILLE, J., KUCK, J., JERNIGAN, T., & BRAFF, D. (1992). Past substance abuse and clinical course of schizophrenia. *American Journal of Psychiatry, 149,* 552–553.

ZITO, J. M. (1994). *Psychotherapeutic drug manual* (3rd ed.). New York: Wiley.

ZUBARAN, C., FERNANDES, J. G., & RODNIGHT, R. (1997). Wernicke-Korsakoff syndrome. *Postgraduate Medical Journal, 73,* 27–31.

ZUCKER, R. A., & GOMBERG, E. S. L. (1986). Etiology of alcoholism reconsidered: The case for a biopsychosocial process. *American Psychologist, 41,* 783–794.

ZUCKERMAN, B., & BRESNAHAN, K. (1991). Developmental and behavioral consequences of prenatal drug and alcohol exposure. *Pediatric Clinics of North America, 38,* 1387–1406.

ZUGER, A. (1994). Meningitis mystery. *Discover, 15*(3), 40–43.

ZUKIN, S. R., & ZUKIN, R. S. (1992). Phencyclidine. In J. H., Lowinson, P. Ruiz, R. B. Millman, & J. G. Langrod (Eds.), *Substance abuse: A comprehensive textbook* (2nd ed.). New York: Williams & Wilkins.

ZWEBEN, J. E. (1995). Integrating psychotherapy and 12-step approaches. In A. M. Washton (Ed.), *Psychotherapy and substance abuse.* New York: Guilford Press.

Index

TO THE OWNER OF THIS BOOK:

I hope that you have found *Concepts of Chemical Dependency*, Fourth Edition, useful. So that this book can be improved in a future edition, would you take the time to complete this sheet and return it? Thank you.

School and address: _____

Department: _____

Instructor's name: _____

1. What I like most about this book is: _____

_____

_____

2. What I like least about this book is: _____

_____

_____

3. My general reaction to this book is: _____

_____

4. The name of the course in which I used this book is: _____

_____

5. Were all of the chapters of the book assigned for you to read? _____

   If not, which ones weren't? _____

6. In the space below, or on a separate sheet of paper, please write specific suggestions for improving this book and anything else you'd care to share about your experience in using the book.

_____

_____

_____

_____

Optional:

Your name: _____ Date: _____

May Brooks/Cole quote you, either in promotion for *Concepts of Chemical Dependency,*
Fourth Edition, or in future publishing ventures?

Yes: _____ No: _____

Sincerely,

Harold Doweiko

NO POSTAGE
NECESSARY
IF MAILED
IN THE
UNITED STATES

BUSINESS REPLY MAIL
FIRST CLASS   PERMIT NO. 358   PACIFIC GROVE, CA

POSTAGE WILL BE PAID BY ADDRESSEE

ATT: *Harold Doweiko* _____

**Brooks/Cole Publishing Company
511 Forest Lodge Road
Pacific Grove, California 93950-5098**